MATERIALS AND DEVICES FOR BONE DISORDERS

MATERIALS AND DEVICES FOR BONE DISORDERS

Edited by

SUSMITA BOSE
Washington State University, Pullman, WA, United States

AMIT BANDYOPADHYAY
Washington State University, Pullman, WA, United States

ELSEVIER

AMSTERDAM • BOSTON • HEIDELBERG • LONDON
NEW YORK • OXFORD • PARIS • SAN DIEGO
SAN FRANCISCO • SINGAPORE • SYDNEY • TOKYO
Academic Press is an imprint of Elsevier

Academic Press is an imprint of Elsevier
125 London Wall, London EC2Y 5AS, United Kingdom
525 B Street, Suite 1800, San Diego, CA 92101-4495, United States
50 Hampshire Street, 5th Floor, Cambridge, MA 02139, United States
The Boulevard, Langford Lane, Kidlington, Oxford OX5 1GB, United Kingdom

Notices
Knowledge and best practice in this field are constantly changing. As new research and experience broaden our understanding, changes in research methods, professional practices, or medical treatment may become necessary.

Practitioners and researchers must always rely on their own experience and knowledge in evaluating and using any information, methods, compounds, or experiments described herein. In using such information or methods they should be mindful of their own safety and the safety of others, including parties for whom they have a professional responsibility.

To the fullest extent of the law, neither the Publisher nor the authors, contributors, or editors, assume any liability for any injury and/or damage to persons or property as a matter of products liability, negligence or otherwise, or from any use or operation of any methods, products, instructions, or ideas contained in the material herein.

British Library Cataloguing-in-Publication Data
A catalogue record for this book is available from the British Library

Library of Congress Cataloging-in-Publication Data
A catalog record for this book is available from the Library of Congress

ISBN: 978-0-12-802792-9

Publisher: Matthew Deans
Acquisition Editor: Laura Overend
Editorial Project Manager: Natasha Welford
Production Project Manager: Nicky Carter
Designer: Mark Rogers

Typeset by MPS Limited, Chennai, India

CONTENTS

LIST OF CONTRIBUTORS

P.B. Aswath
Texas A&M University, Dallas, TX, United States

P. Baker
University of Alabama at Birmingham, Birmingham, AL, United States

A. Bandyopadhyay
Washington State University, Pullman, WA, United States

D. Banerjee
Washington State University, Pullman, WA, United States

S. Bose
Washington State University, Pullman, WA, United States

S.A. Catledge
University of Alabama at Birmingham, Birmingham, AL, United States

J.J. Dedania
Center for Devices and Radiological Health, Silver Spring, MD, United States

J. Gallo
Palacky University, Olomouc, Czech Republic

E. Gibon
Stanford University, Stanford, CA, United States

S.V. Gohil
University of Connecticut Health Center, Farmington, CT, United States

S.B. Goodman
Stanford University, Stanford, CA, United States

R.E. Guldberg
Georgia Institute of Technology, Atlanta, GA, United States

A. Ilyas
Texas A&M University, Dallas, TX, United States

S.M. Iqbal
University of Texas at Arlington, Arlington, TX, United States

A. Kashi
Private Practice, Rochester, NY, United States; Biomedical Research and Services, Brooklyn, NY, United States

D.R. Katti
North Dakota State University, Fargo, ND, United States

K.S. Katti
North Dakota State University, Fargo, ND, United States

B.S. Klosterhoff
Georgia Institute of Technology, Atlanta, GA, United States

M. Kumar
Zimmer Biomet, Warsaw, IN, United States

L. Lu
Mayo Clinic College of Medicine, Rochester, MN, United States

S. Nagaraja
Center for Devices and Radiological Health, Silver Spring, MD, United States

L.S. Nair
University of Connecticut Health Center, Farmington, CT, United States; University of Connecticut, Storrs, CT, United States

T. Odatsu
Nagasaki University, Nagasaki, Japan

S.M. Ott
University of Washington Medical Center, Seattle, WA, United States

J. Rose
University of Connecticut, Storrs, CT, United States

M. Roy
Indian Institute of Technology (IIT), Kharagpur, India

S. Saha
SUNY Downstate Medical Center, Brooklyn, NY, United States

A. Sharma
North Dakota State University, Fargo, ND, United States

G.P. Siegal
University of Alabama at Birmingham, Birmingham, AL, United States

S. Suhail
University of Connecticut, Storrs, CT, United States

V. Thomas
University of Alabama at Birmingham, Birmingham, AL, United States

V.G. Varanasi
Texas A&M University, Dallas, TX, United States

T. Vella
Simsbury High School, Simsbury, CT, United States

M.F. Velten
University of Texas at Arlington, Arlington, TX, United States

Y.K. Vohra
University of Alabama at Birmingham, Birmingham, AL, United States

N.J. Willett
Georgia Institute of Technology, Atlanta, GA, United States; Emory University, Decatur, GA, United States; Atlanta Veteran's Affairs Medical Center, Decatur, GA, United States

M.J. Yaszemski
Mayo Clinic College of Medicine, Rochester, MN, United States

J. Zang
Mayo Clinic College of Medicine, Rochester, MN, United States; Peking University, Beijing, China

BIOGRAPHY

Susmita Bose is Herman and Brita Lindholm Endowed Chair Professor in the School of Mechanical and Materials Engineering (MME) at Washington State University (WSU). Prof. Bose received BS in Chemistry from University of Kalyani (WB, India) in 1990, MS from the Indian Institute of Technology (IIT) Kanpur, India, in 1992, and PhD in Physical Organic Chemistry from Rutgers University, NJ, in 1998. Prof. Bose's interdisciplinary research interest lies at the interface of chemistry, biology, bio-engineering, materials science and engineering, focusing on different biomaterials, 3D printing of ceramic and composite materials for various applications including drug delivery, bone tissue engineering, and surface modification of bone implants. Prof. Bose received the prestigious Presidential Early Career Award for Scientists and Engineers (PECASE, the highest honor given to a young scientist by the US President at the White House) from the US National Science Foundation. Prof. Bose was named a "Kavli fellow" by the US National Academy of the Sciences in 2006. In 2009, she received the prestigious Schwartzwalder-Professional Achievement in Ceramic Engineering Award (PACE) and Richard M. Fulrath Award in 2014 from the American Ceramic Society. Prof. Bose is an editorial board member for several international journals. Prof. Bose holds seven issued US patents and has published over 220 technical papers, including over 170 journal articles, six edited books, with over 8200 citations, "h" index 51. Prof. Bose has advised over 40 graduate students for their PhD and MS degrees. Prof. Bose is a fellow of the American Institute for Medical and Biological Engineering (AIMBE) and the American Ceramic Society (ACerS). In 2015, she was named as Life Science Innovation Northwest (LSINW), Women to Watch in Life Science Honoree, by the Washington Biotechnology and Biomedical Association (WBBA). Prof. Bose's group research on 3D printed bone tissue engineering scaffolds with controlled chemistry has been featured by the AP, BBC, NPR, CBS, MSNBC, ABC, and many other TV stations, radio stations, magazines, and news sites all over the world.

Amit Bandyopadhyay, Herman and Brita Lindholm Endowed Chair Professor in the School of MME at WSU, received his BS in Metallurgical Engineering from Jadavpur University in 1989 (Kolkata, India), MS in Metallurgy from the Indian Institute of Science in 1992 (Bangalore, India), and PhD in Materials Science and Engineering from the University of Texas at Arlington in 1995. He joined the Center for Ceramics Research at Rutgers University for his postdoctoral training in 1995. In 1997, he joined the MME at WSU as an Assistant Professor and was promoted to an associate level in 2001 and to the full professor level in 2006. Prof. Bandyopadhyay's research expertise lies with biomaterials, additive manufacturing of metallic and ceramic materials and their composites for various applications. Prof. Bandyopadhyay has published over 260 technical papers including over 180 journal papers, is an inventor of 15 issued US patents, and has edited nine books. His research papers have been cited over 8700 times by various research groups and his current "h" index is 51. Prof. Bandyopadhyay is a member of the editorial board for more than 10 different journals. Among others, Prof. Bandyopadhyay received the CAREER award from the US National Science Foundation and the Young Investigator Program (YIP) Award from the US Office of Naval Research. Prof. Bandyopadhyay is a fellow of the ACerS, American Society for Materials (ASM International), AIMBE, American Association for the Advancement of Science (AAAS), and National Academy of Inventors (NAI).

PREFACE

The area of biomaterials and devices for bone disorders truly addresses a multidisciplinary theme in which researchers from physical, biological, and engineering sciences need to work together with perspectives from clinicians. During the past three decades, interest in biomaterials has grown at a very rapid rate to solve a variety of clinical challenges. With the aging population, longer life expectancy, more sports-related injuries, and active lifestyles, the need for biomedical devices that can improve the quality of life is also increasing. Innovative, low-cost devices that can be used to mitigate short- and long-term healthcare problems are changing healthcare practices around the world.

Our work is primarily focused on bone disorders and related biomaterials. Though there are many general books available on biomaterials, we felt that there is an unmet need for a book that is primarily focused on biomaterials and devices for bone disorders with the perspectives of scientists, engineers, and physicians. Bone disorders are quite common in patients of all ages. It is not the type of diseases that cause death, but in most cases, trauma from bone disorders impact significantly on the quality of human life. For example, if a person becomes wheelchair-bound at an early age due to lack of treatment of a long bone fracture, or after the first revision surgery, the poor quality of life for the patient as well as lost wages become a significant societal challenge. Similarly, millions of patients with hip and knee implants around the world almost got a second life back due to those procedures. However, researchers are still working on increasing the life of those implants. The success of these procedures depends not only on the patients' age, lifestyle, etc., but also on the surgeons' expertise and the procedure. Our aims to develop this book were not just to discuss various issues with biomaterials for bone disorders, but to first understand current needs from clinicians, and then focus on biomaterials researchers with different solutions. The first few chapters are written by renowned clinicians to share their outlooks toward the current state of biomaterials, bone biology, and various solution options for bone disorders. The second sets of chapters are developed by scientists and engineers to offer their views of different biomaterials. Finally, the ethics and regulatory aspects, which are critical to the successful application of synthetic biomaterials and devices in human health, are addressed. Overall, we feel that this is a book that can be read by engineers, scientists as well as clinicians to appreciate the inherent multidisciplinary aspects, critical issues and find the niche to contribute towards the next generation of biomaterials and devices. Though our book is focused on bone disorders and various treatment options, it is important to note that a lifestyle including healthy food habits and regular exercise are still the best practices to maintain good bone health.

We would like to thank our current and past students, colleagues and collaborators for their contributions to making this project viable. Without their contributions, we would not have been able to complete this book. Finally, we would like to recognize our boys, Shohom and Aditya, for their compassionate understanding and cooperation without which we could not have completed this work. We sincerely hope that this book will inspire the next generation of researchers to innovate safer biomaterials and biomedical devices that can solve long-standing as well as upcoming clinical challenges to improve quality of life.

Susmita Bose and Amit Bandyopadhyay
Washington State University,
Pullman, WA, United States
October 2016

CHAPTER 1

Introduction to Biomaterials and Devices for Bone Disorders

S. Bose, D. Banerjee and A. Bandyopadhyay
Washington State University, Pullman, WA, United States

Contents

1.1 INTRODUCTION

Trauma, degeneration of bone and other severe bone-related diseases like bone cancer and osteoporosis often call for medical intervention and sometimes surgical procedures. Oftentimes such procedures include repair or reconstruction of skeletal parts including hip, knee, skull, elbow, vertebrae, or the mandible. The materials that are widely used today to repair or reconstruct bone disorders have performed acceptably over many years, and are generally called "biomaterials." Over the years, the field of biomaterials has witnessed a steady growth involving a variety of disciplines from materials science to applied sciences and engineering to medical and clinical sciences [1].

The uses of different synthetic materials for medical devices can be traced back to the Etruscans, who substituted a missing tooth with bridges developed from bones of oxen. Furthermore, gold wires were utilized to tie loose artificial teeth to neighboring ones in ancient Phoenicia. The first usage of dental amalgam was reported by the Chinese in 659 for the repair of decayed tooth [2]. An iron dental implant has been found in a corpse dated to AD 200 [3]. By the early 1990s, bone plates were commonly used for accelerated healing of bone fractures, and by the 1950s blood vessel replacements were undergoing clinical trials while total hip replacements and heart valves were in a developmental stage. Even in those early developmental years of biomedical devices, physicians were able to identify and list a preliminary set of materials and design issues that were key to implant failure. Some of the pivotal factors were recognized as mechanical failure, biocompatibility, corrosion resistance, and biofunctionality.

Apart from medical devices, biomaterials also find extensive applications in cell growth, investigational cell-silicon biochips, therapeutic and diagnostic gene arrays, regulation of cattle fertility, and in equipment for biomolecule processing. To reconcile the diverse applications of biomaterials into one field, the interaction of the modified natural or synthetic materials with the biological systems has been considered. For orthopedic and dental applications, biomaterials are often integrated into implants or devices. The main focus of this chapter is on the materials aspect of biomaterials. Nevertheless, it would soon be evident that biomaterials as a subject cannot be inspected without considering the biological response. In fact, the effect of the implanted device on the host tissue, and the biological response of the tissue on the device work in tandem toward the success of an implant. Thus biomaterials science is the study of the mechanical and biological properties of the materials and their interaction with the biological systems in vivo. The field of biomaterials can be categorized as metals, ceramics, polymers, and composites. These materials are being employed as machined parts, films, or coatings in a device. For example, titanium and its alloys, stainless steel (SS), cobalt chrome alloys have been used in total hip or knee replacements, SS for bone plate toward fracture repair, titanium alloys coupled with calcium phosphate (CaP), or alumina for dental implants. This chapter will specifically focus on various types of materials employed in the development of implants for orthopedic and dental applications. Table 1.1 illustrates different materials, their advantages, disadvantages, and applications in bone disorders. Table 1.2 summarizes biomaterials market, by application, specific to the skeletal system [4]. Fig. 1.1 shows different implants used for bone disorders.

Before illustrating the usage of the biomaterials specific to any application, it has to be noted that the field is also impacted by several ethical considerations, such as whether sacrifice of an animal is justified enough for the experiment, minimization of risk in human trials, and increasing the benefit-to-risk ratio in trials to name a few. And with so many unanswered questions, in the absence of sufficient data and adequate experimental results, getting approvals from government agencies for safe usage

Table 1.1 Different materials, their advantages, disadvantages and applications in bone disorders

Materials	Advantages	Disadvantages	Applications
Metals: Stainless steel 316 L, titanium and its alloys, cobalt–chromium and molybdenum alloy, tantalum, NiTi shape memory alloy	• Good ductility • High mechanical strength • Excellent fatigue resistance • Good corrosion resistance	• Bioinert • High modulus compared to bone • Poor biocompatibility	Load-bearing implants, plates, nails and screws, staples, plaques, wires, articulation prostheses, dental implants, skull plaques, and mesh for face reconstruction
Ceramics: Calcium phosphates, bioglass, aluminum oxides, zirconia, calcium aluminates, titanium oxides, etc.	• Good biocompatibility • Compositions can be tailored for bioactivity and bioresorption • Good corrosion resistance • High compressive strength • Density can be similar to bone	• Brittle • Low fatigue resistance • Aniostropic mechanical properties under different loading conditions • Inherent difficulty in manufacturing	Dental parts, coatings for load-bearing implants and dental implant applications, ceramic ball in hip implants, bone fillings, spinal fusion, bone cements, craniomaxillofacial, applications
Polymers: Poly lactic-*co*-glycolic acid (PLGA), polycaprolactone (PCL), poly-propylene fumarate (PPF), poly methyl methacrylate (PMMA), polyethylene (PE), polypropylene, polytetrafluroethylene	• Easy to produce • Low density • Rate of bioresorption can be tailored • Can be made in a variety of forms; from powders to films to bulk structures	• Low mechanical strength • Degradation products can be of concern	Sutures, cements, artificial tendons, teeth implants, spacer in intervertebral implants, liner in acetabular cups for hip replacements, carrier for drug delivery
Composites: Metals with ceramic coatings, polymer ceramic composites	• High biocompatibility • Good corrosion resistance	• Lack of consistency/ homogeneity	Knee implants, hip implants, artificial articulations
Natural materials: Collagen, human tissue, hyaluronic acid, grafts	• Available in human body • Biocompatible	• Possible rejection by host body	Increase or substitution of hard and soft tissues, tendons, and ligaments

Table 1.2 Biomaterials market, by application, specific to the skeletal system [4]

Orthopedic	Joint replacement	Knee replacement
		Hip replacement Shoulder replacement Others (ankle arthoplasty, elbow arthoplasty, wrist arthroplasty, and finger arthroplasty)
	Spine	Spinal fusion Pedicle-based rod systems • Interspinous spacers • Disc arthroplasty • Motion preservation/dynamic stabilization Minimally invasive fusion surgery
	Bioresorbable	Suture anchors Interference screws Meniscal repair tacks Mesh
	Orthobiologics	Stem cell therapy Synthetics Allograft Bone morphogenetic proteins (BMP) Growth factors Autograft
	Viscosupplementation	Abdominal and pelvic surgeries Knee osteoarthritis
Dental	Dental implants Dental bone grafts and substitutes Dental membranes Tissue regeneration materials	

of implants clinically is also difficult. Like most ethical situations, a search for an absolute answer can be difficult and sometimes perhaps impossible. Yet further research may be able to employ specific data for clinical research [5,6].

No foreign materials placed in a biological system conform to complete biocompatibility. Only autogenous materials that are directly manufactured by the same body do not elicit any host tissue response. The materials and host tissue interactions are directly interlinked with the surface of the implant material. Based on different interactions with the implant, biomaterials are categorized into bioinert, bioactive, and bioresorbable. Materials that interact minimally with the surrounding tissue and remain in isolation are termed bioinert. Specific examples include alumina ceramic, SS metal, and polyethylene (PE) polymer. Bioinert materials can form a fibrous tissue around the implant in vivo. Bioactive materials interact with the host tissue

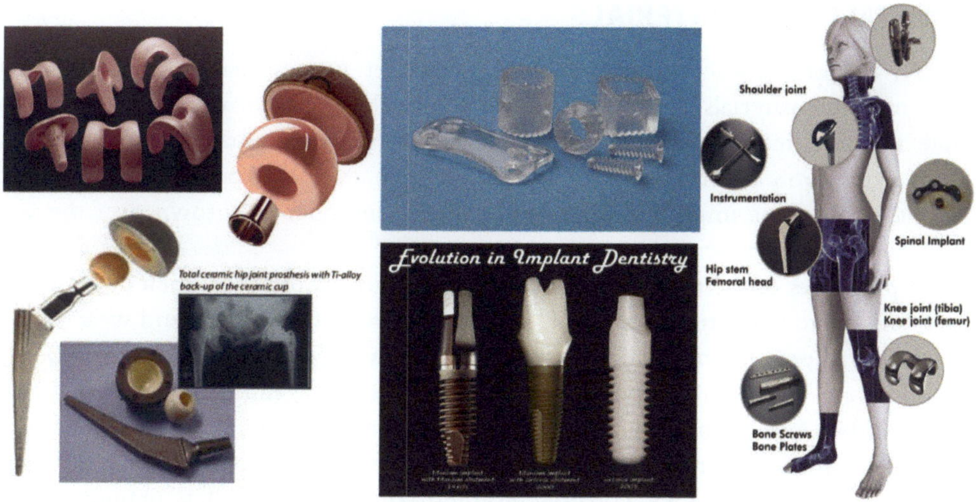

Figure 1.1 The variety of metallic, ceramic, and polymeric implants used for bone replacements. http://www.nemfi.com/uploads/5/4/5/4/54549909/orthopedicimplantandmedicaldevicefinishing.pdf.

surrounding them. A time-dependent kinetic modification and ion exchange reaction deposit bone-like apatite on the surface of these materials. This tissue integration into the implant improves the implant life. Specific examples include hydroxyapatite (HA) ceramic. Bioresorbable materials include materials which resorb gradually in vivo and are replaced by the host tissue. Bioresorbable materials do not produce any toxic byproducts on degradation. Specific examples include bioglass and tricalcium phosphate (TCP) ceramics.

As mentioned above, biomaterials can also be categorized into four major classes of materials namely metals, ceramics, polymers, and natural materials that are derived from plant and animals. Often two or more classes of biomaterials are incorporated together into composite materials to unfold a desired property for specific applications. Composites constitute a fifth class of biomaterials. Commendable technical and scientific progress in the field of biomaterials is evident from the distinct materials currently employed in medicine. Albeit till 1950s physicians rarely used commercially available biomaterials clinically, and there were meager government regulations; however, the earliest implants paved the way for further research. Continuous failure brought experts from a variety of fields together, and these collaborations identified primary factors required for the success of an implant. This interdisciplinary cooperation pointed out physical properties of materials along with their composition, density, and porosity as pivots for implant success. The need to develop new materials along with desired properties was also recognized. The following sections aim to discuss briefly fundamentals of biomaterials including some of their specific compositions, properties, processing issues, and principles governing their current usage.

1.2 METALLIC BIOMATERIALS

In 1991, the orthopedic and dental implant market was estimated at $2 billion in which metallic materials constituted about $1.4 billion. Approximately 3.6 million people in the United States undergo orthopedic surgery annually, where statistical analysis from 1988 reported that 4.6%, i.e., one in every 20 people in the United States has at least one implant [7]. It is believed that number has grown over the years due to our aging population.

The properties of the metallic implants are primarily governed by their composition, phases, and microstructures. Apart from mechanical properties, surface and wear properties are also important toward implant success in vivo. From the early days, metallic implants have been employed due to their availability as well as superior mechanical properties. An ideal metallic implant should have high strength, high fatigue resistance, and excellent corrosion resistance. The currently utilized and acceptable metallic materials for implant manufacturing are SS, cobalt–chromium–molybdenum alloy, titanium and its alloys, tantalum, gold, platinum, silver, and some of the noble metals. Among these, gold and silver do not possess adequate mechanical properties to be employed as structural implant materials. The most significant metallic materials have been grouped together under three subcategories of SSs, titanium alloys, and cobalt chromium alloys. These alloy systems are believed to have the optimal blend of mechanical properties and corrosion resistance, and are used in a large variety of devices.

Charnley reported the first successful implantation of a total hip replacement in the late 1950s. The replacement was a cemented prosthesis with a stem made of SS [8]. The most common SS used in biomedical applications is austenitic SS 316L (L stands for extra low carbon). The usage of SS in the field of biomaterials is restricted due to better mechanical and biological properties of titanium and cobalt chromium alloys. Currently manganese has been used to substitute the nickel in SS with a higher content of nitrogen. Such an approach minimizes concerns related to Ni^{+2} release in vivo. The higher content of nitrogen in the alloy stabilizes the austenitic phase at room temperature, enhancing the corrosion resistance and also ameliorates the yield stress of the implant. SS 316L is widely used as a temporary fixation device in trauma such as hip or knee nails or screws and bone plate fixations. Care needs to be taken in harnessing the impurity and carbon content in the alloy system, and also the melting and thermal treatment process to obtain the desired properties. The surface finish is acquired by removal of pits, marks, and contamination by mechanical and electropolishing processes. Final processing of the alloy is accomplished by removal of iron particles via surface passivation in nitric acid solution and artificial thickening of the chromium oxide layer. Due to poor bone bonding ability, SS 316L is an ideal material for fracture fixation devices that need to be removed after a few months without fracturing the bone.

Cobalt chromium alloy was developed by Elwood Haynes specially to meet resistance to oxidation, wear, and corrosive agents. The alloy gained importance after its first implantation as a heart valve in the 1960s which lasted for around 30 years and proved the high wear resistance of the alloy [9]. The cobalt chromium alloy exhibits a perfect blend of biocompatibility, higher mechanical strength, and corrosion resistance compared to 316L SS. This alloy manifests higher corrosion resistance even in chloride environments and has higher fatigue resistance compared to SS. Cobalt chromium alloys are manufactured both as cast and wrought variants. Cast cobalt chromium alloy cannot be contoured during processing because of its high work hardening rate. Hence, the cast variant of the alloy has been specifically used for implants with firm geometry-like hip stems. Furthermore, because of its high abrasion resistance, the alloy also finds its application extensively in articulating surfaces. The wrought alloys, containing around 35 wt.% of nickel, are often used in different orthopedic devices. Cobalt chromium alloys exhibit a very high elastic modulus, around 230 GPa, similar to SS that is 10 times higher than that of cortical bone. Due to the higher modulus compared to bone, the metal implant supports most of the load in vivo and causes stress shielding of the adjacent bone. The surrounding bone resorbs and a thick fibrous tissue growth is observed around the implant. This leads to the isolation of the implant material and also weakening of the surrounding bone that increases the chances of brittle fracture [10,11].

Titanium and its alloys are borrowed from the aerospace industry due to the unique blend of high corrosion resistance along with low elastic modulus of around 110 GPa. Brånemark, in 1964, first used titanium-based dental implants [12]. Titanium-based implants are able to tightly integrate with the host tissue, unlike SS and cobalt–chromium alloys. Due to the formation of an inherent TiO_2 bioactive layer at the Ti implant surface, titanium-based implants are viewed as bioactive metal implants that can enhance bone tissue integration. Commercially pure titanium (CpTi) and Ti6Al4V are the most commonly used titanium-based alloys for orthopedic or dental applications. In spite of an excellent blend of properties, harnessing processing parameters is very difficult. Ti is a difficult material to machine, and shows poor wear resistance. In most cases, Ti-based implants are either cast or forged to get the near net shape. Apart from CpTi and Ti6Al4V, many researchers have proposed other beta Ti-based alloys with lower modulus [13].

Shape memory effect refers to the self-recovery of a material's shape after plastic deformation. NiTi, a shape memory alloy, is currently used widely in a variety of applications including biomedical devices. In NiTi, in the martensitic state, NiTi exhibits an elastic modulus as low as 30 GPa and its recoverable elastic strain can be around 8% [14]. However, concerns related to release of nickel ions in the biological system posed a potential threat to cancer for these NiTi alloys [15]. This concern regarding Ni ion leaching restricted NiTi usage in the United States and Europe. However, NiTi-based implants have been successfully used in other parts of the world for over two decades, as well as cardiovascular devices around the world [16].

The metals discussed so far are not bioactive. Mostly, two pathways are adopted to ensure the bioactivity of the metallic implants. One includes the coating of the inert metal surface with bioactive ceramics like HAs and the other approach is to modify the surface of the implant chemically to ensure better adhesion of target proteins enhancing the healing process and accelerating tissue–material interactions. Several processing approaches have been explored to improve surface properties of biomaterials that remain in direct contact with the body fluid. Surface modification has been carried out in Ti alloys to improve the process of osteointegration via controlled oxidation [17,18]. Specific surface properties directly influencing the biological properties are identified as electrostatic charges [19], wettability [20], and roughness [21]. Hence to improve the bioactivity of the metallic implants, they are subjected to various surface modifications before implantation. Surface modification by modifying the surface roughness has been the most prevalent in cases of dental implants. Rough surfaces in cases of metallic dental implants have been achieved by passivation, shot peening, and shot blasting [22,23]. Some of the primary research was conducted on electrodeposition [24], ionic ray sputtering [25], plasma spraying [26], hot isostatic pressing [27], and laser ablation [28]. None of these coating methods bonds covalently with the substrate, creating a strong adherent layer and they are quite expensive for clinical uses. However, HA coating deposited by plasma spray method represents the most commonly used technique for clinical applications and also demonstrates enhanced osteogenesis compared to bare metallic substrates [29–31]. Oftentimes, incorporation of a variety of inorganic ions into the plasma spray HA coatings on metallic substrates also induces enhanced osteogenesis, angiogenesis, and antimicrobial property for secondary infection control [32–35]. Chemical treatments were also performed postfabrication to deposit CaP or apatite layer on the surface. Kokubo reported the etching of titanium alloy-based metals by NaOH followed by heat treatment to develop a thin titanate layer stimulating deposition of a bone-like apatite layer in a physiological medium [36]. Chemical etching using hydrogen peroxide and trace amount of tin chloride has also been reported [37]. Sol gel coating and biomimetic coating were further researched for the development of a strong interface between the CaP coating and the metallic substrate. Overall, metallic materials are widely used in treating bone disorders as implants or toward fracture fixation. Perhaps the most important issue in metallic implants today is its surface properties. Next-generation metallic implants with unique surface properties are being researched today to improve treatment options for various bone disorders.

1.3 CERAMIC BIOMATERIALS

The inorganic part of bone is a natural ceramic. In general, ceramics are ionic and/or covalently bonded materials that are inherently brittle, poor thermal and electrical conductors, and offer excellent corrosion resistance. Ceramics as biomaterials are typically used in articulating surfaces, bone cements, toward bone tissue engineering, drug delivery, and dental applications. Processing of a ceramic body starts from ceramic powders followed by shaping and then densifying at high temperature. Due to these multistep processing methods, manufacturing of ceramics is always challenging and sometimes riddled with low yield. Finally, inherent low fracture toughness of ceramics makes them unsuitable for any load-bearing applications unless the applied load is only compressive in nature. Ceramics are typically crystalline in nature; however the amorphous form is called glass. Glass-ceramics are those in which crystalline particles are embedded in an amorphous matrix.

One of the very first applications of ceramics in biomedical implants was high-density alumina in the femoral heads for total hip prostheses (THR) [38]. Good biocompatibility, high compressive strength, and excellent corrosion resistance surged the uses of ceramics in acetabular cups. A commercially available total hip alumina ball and socket with a metal stem has been used clinically. Christel et al. reported that alumina-based implants have a lifetime of 30 years with a 12,000 N load limit [39]. Alumina has been used as porous alumina spacers in cases of second revision surgery, coatings for hip stems, and in single and polycrystalline forms in dental implants. Albeit some dental implants have single crystal alumina, most often fine-grained polycrystalline alumina sintered around 1600°C are used [40]. The addition of trace amounts of magnesium oxide (less than 0.5 wt.%) abets the sintering and restricts grain growth during densification. Other clinical uses of alumina encompass maxillofacial implants, bone screws for knee prostheses, blades, and other dental implants. However, due to the high elastic modulus of alumina (380 GPa) compared to cortical bone, issues related to stress shielding can be of concern in people with rheumatoid arthritis and osteoporosis [40]. Although a ceramic—ceramic articulating surface offers the best possibility for load-bearing implants with the lowest metal ion release concern, the widespread applications of these ceramics will not happen due to fracture incidents in vivo, which is still a real concern and the major hurdle to overcome in the future.

Zirconia was introduced as a biomaterial especially for the femoral cups in 1985 to substitute alumina because of its apparent higher fracture toughness. Very low wear rates have been witnessed by the usage of zirconia against alumina in hip prostheses. The combination of alumina and zirconia as a ceramic-on-ceramic in the hip replacements was first introduced by Villermaux in 1998 [41]. It has also been used as the articulating ball in THR. Zirconia-based implants constitute 8% of the THR market in the United States and 25% of the total orthopedic surgery replacements in Europe. Zirconia offers a unique blend of very low elastic of modulus comparable to cortical bone and also excellent mechanical properties, i.e., strength and toughness. Zirconia has been proved to withstand a load limit of 250 kN which is significantly higher than that of alumina. The wear byproducts from zirconia degradation are nontoxic and do not elicit any adverse tissue response. However, care needs to be taken in regards to processing parameters for adequate quality control of the implants to ensure clinical success. Mostly the zirconia-based femoral heads contain 97% of zirconia oxide and 3% of yttrium oxide. Yttria-stabilized tetragonal polycrystalline zirconia has a fine grain size and hence improved mechanical properties. However, at lower temperature, tetragonal polycrystalline zirconia readily transforms to monoclinic phase. This transformation decreases the strength of zirconia. The wear rate of yttria-stabilized zirconia with ultrahigh-molecular-weight polyethylene (UHMWPE) is very low and hence the tribological debris has no untoward response to host tissue [42,43]. With regard to the concerns of metastable phases in zirconia, ongoing research tried to develop a degradation-free zirconia–alumina composite. Oxidized zirconium was introduced with the goal of achieving improved abrasion and wear resistance in knee implants and has shown great promise since then [44].

CaP-based ceramics have been extensively used for orthopedics and dentistry due to their inherent compositional similarity to bone. When the X-ray diffraction pattern for bone was demonstrated in 1926, it was seen that apatite constitutes a larger portion of the mineral phase [45]. However, the synthetic HA, a naturally occurring calcium apatite, was utilized for bone grafts in the 1970s. It was found to interact favorably with the human host tissue and yet remain stable under physiological conditions. Owing to the compositional similarities with natural bone [46], CaP ceramics integrate with host tissue without formation of a fibrous tissue layer. Reports have demonstrated CaP ceramics to be bioactive, biocompatible, and osteoconductive [47]. Osteoconductivity refers to the ability of bone growth in the surrounding regions of the implant. Natural bone is constituted of 67–70% CaP, 10% organic materials like collagen, 18–20% water, and trace amounts of inorganic ions like Na^{+}, Mg^{+2}, Cl^{-}, OH^{-}, and CO_3^{-2}. The incorporation of inorganic ions and drugs into CaP before implantation also plays an important role in both osteogenesis and angiogenesis as well as degradation of CaP ceramics [48–53]. The preliminary usage of CaP was restricted for low load-bearing applications in bone disorders, bone tissue engineering, and drug delivery, as well as coatings on metallic implants to enhance osseointegration [54].

Some of the CaP ceramics are biodegradable. Biodegradable ceramics can be used in bone tissue engineering in which body tissue can invade biodegradable scaffolds to repair bone disorders in vivo. The degradation kinetics and the phases of CaP are important issues for successful implementation of these materials. One approach to control the degradation kinetics in CaP ceramics is dopant addition. Small amounts of dopants can regulate degradation kinetics in CaP ceramics based on application needs. Reports have also shown that dopants can regulate the initial mechanical properties of scaffolds apart from degradation kinetics in vitro and in vivo [55–58]. A range of CaP ceramic compositions are used for various applications in orthopedics and dentistry, like TCP (Ca:P = 1.5:1), HA (Ca:P = 1.67:1), amorphous CaP, and others [59,60]. Some of these forms can also be successfully injected and used as a bone cement that can harden inside the damaged bone tissue.

The primary component of bone is the calcium-deficient crystalline apatite called HA ($Ca_{10}(PO_4)_6(OH)_2$). HA demonstrates superior bioactivity and gets integrated with bone tissue. Mechanical performance of devices made from HA varies remarkably due to the powder size, purity, and size distribution. It has been used for middle ear implants and alveolar ridge reconstruction in the dense sintered form and for filling bony defects in dental or orthopedic surgery in the porous form. It has also received widespread application as a coating material on metallic implants to enhance bone tissue integration. In general, HA-coated implants are preferred during revision surgery. Interestingly, HA-coated implants are more popular in Europe than in the United States.

TCP is another CaP phase that is bioresorbable and widely used in biomedical applications. β-TCP and α-TCP are two different phases of TCP in which α-TCP degrades faster than β-TCP. Due to their bioresorbable nature, these ceramics found applications in craniomaxillofacial and spinal fusion procedures. Nevertheless, synthetic TCP's in vivo performance is far worse than autografts. It is envisioned that doped TCP with improved biocompatibility and controlled resorbable rates may provide significant benefits in the development of future biodegradable bone grafts.

Hench et al. have shown the capacity of glass-based ceramics, bioglass, to bond with bone [61]. The time-dependent kinetic modification of the surface of bioglass-based ceramics on implantation in a biological system makes them bioactive and elicits favorable tissue responses, enhancing bone growth in the vicinity of the implants. The preliminary considerations for the bioactivity of these bioglass-based ceramics are less than 60 mol.% SiO_2, a high Ca/P ratio, and high contents of Na_2O and CaO. The most common bioglass composition is 45S5, which essentially refers to 45 wt.% of SiO_2 and CaO/P_2O_5 ratio of 5. The calcium to phosphorous ratio is very crucial in controlling the bioactivity of these materials. The additions of trace amounts of barium oxide to substitute silicon oxide, and calcium fluoride to substitute for calcium oxide, have shown no visible effects on the bioactivity of the materials. However, addition of 3 wt.% of aluminum to 45S5 composition of bioglass decreased bone bonding ability. Dissolution of bioglass and the ion release in the physiological system controls gene activation and apatite formation in the body. A key element in bioglass is silicon. The role of silicon in bone formation and bone calcification was demonstrated by Carlisle in 1970 in young bones [62]. The presence of silicon enhances osteogenesis and also incorporation of silicon has been shown to enhance bone formation compared to nondoped apatites [63]. Within 10 hours of implantation, the activation of osteogenic cascade occurs through protein and growth factor absorption. In the next 3–4 days, stem cells differentiate to osteoblasts and generate an extracellular matrix for new bone formation.

In spite of their excellent bone-regenerative properties, bioglass cannot be used in load-bearing applications due to low fracture toughness and poor mechanical properties. Bioglass finds success for low load-bearing applications such as in dental and craniomaxillofacial procedures. Ceravital and A-W glass-ceramics have just celebrated a decade of successful clinical usage for middle ear surgery and vertebral surgery, respectively. A-W was developed by Kokubo et al. in 1982 and contains oxyfluorapatite and wollastonite in a glassy matrix of magnesium calcium and silica oxide [64]. It bonds actively with living bone and inhibits fibrous tissue encapsulation and hence is used for artificial vertebral applications [65].

Apart from these compositions, several new bioceramic compositions are currently under development to promote bone tissue integration and angiogenesis, and are used in targeted drug or protein delivery [47,53,66]. Infusion of new manufacturing technologies such as additive manufacturing (AM) also added a new dimension to bioceramic materials toward patient-matched long bone defect repairs. However, the inherent brittle nature will be the most significant challenge that needs to be overcome to expand applications of bioceramics in bone disorders. The addition of a secondary material in ceramic scaffolds with controlled chemistry in presence of proteins and growth factors can further broaden their applications.

1.4 POLYMERIC BIOMATERIALS

Polymeric biomaterials form the largest class of biomaterials with a broad variety of applications. Polymers can be derived from natural or synthetic sources, and are classified into two categories according to their origin. The wide diversity of naturally occurring polymers includes collagen, heparin, and hyaluronic acid that are animal-derived, and natural rubber, sodium alginate, and cellulose that are plant-derived. These polymers find widespread uses in the field of biomaterials, however often they are obscured by the endless variety of synthetic polymers. Sometimes their uses are also limited by their availability and also eliciting immunogenic response in physiological systems. Synthetic polymers are an attractive candidate for biomaterials for their modifiable properties. They offer properties ranging from hydrophobic to water-soluble hydrophilic, and also from hydrolytically unstable (degrade in physiological conditions) to being stable through a patient's life time. Some of the polymers commonly used in the biomedical industry include silicone rubber, poly-vinyl chloride (PVC), poly-lactic-glycolic acid (PLGA), polycaprolactone (PCL), poly-ethylene (PE), and poly-methyl methacrylate (PMMA), nylons, just to name a few.

Impressed by the idea of dental cements, Charnley in 1960 first introduced self-polymerizing methyl methacrylate (MMA) into cemented orthopedic surgery [8]. PMMA is a transparent hydrophobic linear chain thermoplastic polymer and is amorphous at room temperature. PMMA has since been used in orthopedics, particularly in total hip replacements and spinal fractures, and also in the treatment of pathological fractures. Acrylic bone cements have also been widely used to anchor the implants to the host bone tissue in cases of cemented prostheses. It has also found usage in the internal fracture fixation plates to help allocate the forces evenly in the material bone interface, and inhibit premature plate failure. Very recently, PMMA has also been used in kyphoplasty and vertebroplasty for boosting the strength of weak vertebral column.

PMMA acts more or less like a grout in arthroplasty. It provides an excellent anchorage for the implants though it does not promote any biological fixation. Further complications arise with the possible release of residual monomer into the physiological system and cause problems with metabolism. PMMA is biologically compatible, however, the monomer, MMA, is considered an irritant and a potential carcinogen. MMA can cause a precipitous fall in blood pressure, which occasionally can be fatal.

PE is typically used in its higher density form, UHMWPE because the lower-density forms fail to endure higher sterilization temperatures and show poor wear resistance. It has been used widely as a liner for the acetabular cups in total hip replacements, as a spacer in intervertebral artificial disc replacements, and also in patellar and tibial inserts in total knee replacements. The quintessential blend of properties of high strength, processing ease, excellent toughness, low friction, wear and abrasion resistance, and biocompatibility makes PE an excellent candidate for orthopedic usage and resistance to lipid absorbance. Covalent crosslinking by radiation sterilization in an inert atmosphere enhances the strength and wear resistance of UHMWPE. However, wear debris due to the corrosive physiological conditions leads to undesirable effects. Gamma sterilization of the polymer increases the chances of wear from the polymer. The debris causes inflammatory responses at the surrounding bone and causes osteolysis, granulomatous lesions, and gradual bone resorption [67].

Silicones are synthetic polymers with a backbone of repeating silicon bonded to oxygen atoms. Alongside the backbone, silicones are also attached to a variety of organic groups, preferably methyl groups. Kipping named this category silicones with reference to their similarities to ketones [68]. With gradual development of silicones, the basic repeating unit was called siloxane and the most common silicone is polymethylsiloxae. Medical-grade silicone implants have been widely used in the replacement of diseased joints. Swanson in 1968 first introduced the usage of silicone implants in the replacement of hand joints [69]. Silicone implants have been reported to alleviate pain and amend ulnar drift in the fingers and enhance functional range of motion [70]. Their usability is enhanced by their stability in physiological conditions, lack of toxicity, and low surface tension. Introduction of tri or tetra functional siloxanes or substation of the methyl groups in siloxanes lead to diversified structures. At high temperature, these polymers crosslink to form elastomers without affecting their properties. However, implant mechanics and frequent fracture limit their usage in orthopedic surgeries. Dislocations, loosening of implant, and wear also pose as potential threats to the usage of these implants. A critical issue in regard to silicone implant success lies in the pertinent design mimicking the normal joint characteristics [71].

Various biodegradable polymers have been used to treat bone disorders including PCL, poly-glycolic acid (PGA), poly-dioxanone (PDS), poly-lactic acid (PLA), hyaluronic acid, chitosan, and PLGA. Introduced in the mid-1960s by Kulkarni, bioresorbable polymers found extensive uses in orthopedics, specifically in bone plates, pins, screws, and sutures for the replacement of bone, and repair of bone tissue, cartilage, and meniscus. For low load-bearing applications, bioresorbable polymers offer significant advantages over nonresorbable ones. It minimizes the effects of stress shielding and thus alleviates the need for a secondary surgery, and enables postoperative imaging. Although many macromolecules are bioresorbable, few offer the quintessential blend of properties required for the bone fixation process. PLA, PDS, and PGA are widely used in orthopedics. Mechanical properties of these polymers are enhanced by reinforcing them with oriented fibers of the same materials. These self-reinforcing mechanisms have been employed clinically since 1984 [72].

Bioresorbable polymers have been used for treating a variety of fractures like distal radius, femoral neck and head, tibial condyles, radial head, and malleolar fractures. It has currently been employed in bone fixation for reconstructive surgeries like osteotomics. Staples made from PLA have been used in foot surgery. Distal chevron osteotomy can be fixed by self-reinforced PDS, PLA, or PGA. PLA has been used in the fixation of shoulder dislocations and knee meniscus bucket handle lesions. Ulnar dislocations in the thumb can be fixed by using bioresorbable polymers as well. In recent times, bioresorbable polymers have also found applications in spinal surgery.

Bioresorbable polymers can be processed in a very similar manner as the thermoplastics. They can be melted, extruded, molded, and cast, however control of moisture is crucial in the processing of the polymers and controlling the molecular weight. Biodegradability occurs in the polymers by hydrolysis of the backbone chain and also by enzymatic activity. The degradation is influenced by the molecular weight of the polymer, crystallinity, porosity, and monomer concentration of the polymer as well as geometry and location of implantation. After implantation, water penetrates the bulk polymer and chemically hydrolyzes the bonds in the amorphous phase and thus gradually shortens the chain. The crystalline region of the polymer supports the implant until penetration of water disrupts the backbone. Further degradation occurs through the enzymatic activity in the physiological system. Implantation in the physiological system decreases the pH locally to a mildly acidic pH. Acidic pH autocatalyzes the rate of polymer degradation leaving more and more hydrophobic monomers and acidic groups which in turn accelerates the degradation process of these polymeric chains [73]. PLA and PGA degrade into acidic monomers of lactic acid and glycolic acid which are reused in the tricarboxylic pathway for oxygen production in the mitochondria.

Poly-ethylene glycol, chitosan, and hyaluronic acid are amongst the most researched hydrogels used for orthopedics. These hydrogels are capable of retaining a large amount of water in their structure. They have been used in ligaments, tendons, and cartilage repair applications. Biocompatible and highly hydrophilic hydrogel poly-hydroxyethylmethacrylate (PHEMA) is often augmented with PCL and reinforced by PGA and PET fibers for uses in ligament and tendon implants. This reinforced polymer has been researched as an alternative to metals and metal–polymer composites in intervertebral disc implants [74].

The usage of natural and synthetic polymers in the development of the three-dimensional scaffolds for ligaments and tendon applications opened a new horizon of research. Typically, synthetic polymers gained more attention from researchers due to tailorable properties of these polymers. PGA and PLA are most widely studied for ligament repair applications. A combination of PCL and hyaluronic acid has been proved successful in meniscus tissue engineering. The chemistry involved in the polymeric degradation and the mechanics of the polymers influence the performance of the implants to a huge extent. The presence of a variety of chemical groups on the side chains of these polymers allows chemical modification for tailorable properties. Immobilization of proteins and growth factors by biochemical or chemical interaction on the surface of these polymers can further enhance cell adhesion and bone regeneration, and further broadens their applications.

1.5 COMPOSITE BIOMATERIALS

As mentioned previously, bone, cartilage, and dentin are all natural composites. These natural composite materials have a hierarchical structure, in which porous, particulate, and fibrous structures are arranged into a complex geometry. The initial drive for the development of composites for orthopedics was concentrated in the advancements of materials for bioactive nondegradable materials. Developed by Bonfield, the first composite material was HAPEX, which was a reinforced PE matrix reinforced with HA. HA is a bioactive ceramic enhancing osteogenesis, whereas PE provides an enduring nondegradable inert polymer. HAPEX was commercialized soon after and witnessed successful middle ear implantation in more than 0.3 million patients [75]. Researches have shown that the incorporation of phosphorous in any polymers improves tissue adhesion and enhances osteogenesis. Essentially polymer composites constitute an inorganic phase and a polymer phase which are insoluble in each other [76]. The inorganic phase has higher elastic modulus and resistance to deformation than the polymeric phase. Hence, researches were involved in the adjustment of the mechanical properties between these phases to as close as bone, using other filling components as a composite.

Carbon fibers have also been utilized for reinforcing polymers and used successfully for spine surgery and other applications in orthopedics [77]. Acceptable results have also been witnessed by the usage of carbon—carbon implants for middle ear prostheses [78]. Nevertheless, the usage of these implants was limited by the release of carbon debris into the host tissue which elicits severe responses in the body and leads to collagenase synthesis in rare cases, and also cell apoptosis [79,80].

Composite reinforced with ceramic particles has been developed for both biodegradable and inert implantable materials for the last 30 years. Polymer matrix composites have been reinforced with ceramic particles for potential inert behavior in the physiological system, however from a chronological view, they were in usage at the same time when researches were in full swing for the development of bioactive materials. These implants constituted of polymer matrices of PE or polysulfone reinforced with glass or carbon fibers [81]. The reinforced biomaterials exhibited higher toughness and lower rigidity compared to metallic implants and thus showed mechanical properties closer to cortical bone [82]. These composites are nonresorbable and are stable in vivo in physiological conditions with no changes in stiffness over the implantation time. These composites are crosslinked and networked and do not involve problems associated with the release of toxic monomers into the body after implantation. The flexibility of these materials allows it to be molded into complex geometry, nevertheless, the lack of ductility often proves a problem while reshaping for uses in bone plates.

Carbon fiber-reinforced polyetherketone (PEEK) has improved mechanical properties, like low elastic modulus and high fatigue strength, and is significantly advantageous over the traditional implants used in orthopedic surgery. The radiolucent property of these materials also helps in artifact-free CT or MRI scan, and imaging for analyzing healing and repair. These carbon-reinforced PEEKs have been widely used for spinal interbody fusion implants. Further clinical examinations are required to ensure the usefulness of carbon-reinforced PEEK material in the fracture repair and in analyzing the progression of the bone infection through MRI images. Direct advantages of radiolucency of these materials in the fracture repair are still debated.

Further advancements in composite technology have resulted in the incorporation of undifferentiated bone marrow stromal cells into CaP suspension. Experimental results have shown improved osteogenesis and angiogenesis on implantation of the living cells along with the ceramic-reinforced polymer matrix. Thus it leads to research in a new era, which allows the development of composite with living cells [83].

1.6 ADDITIVE MANUFACTURING (AM) OF BIOMATERIALS

AM, the layer-by-layer manufacturing technique, allows fabrication of parts directly from a computer-aided design file without the usage of any part-specific tools. Conventional manufacturing limits implant design to a generalized form but fails to accommodate the individual needs of patients [84]. Such patient-matched devices may be needed for complex fractures, unique anatomical features, or patients with specific allergies to certain elements. AM has turned the dreams into reality for affordable complex custom implants which optimally cater to the individual needs of patients. Fig. 1.2 illustrates a CAD file and 3D printed jaw bone made from titanium alloy. Apart from patient-matched implants, controlled porosity scaffolds with similar mechanical and biological properties of bone can also be fabricated using AM for cranial and spinal implants [47]. Next-generation hip and knee implants that are lightweight and stiffness-matched can also be fabricated using AM by removing materials from noncritical areas, as shown in Fig. 1.3. With the advancements of the AM industry, a range of products can be custom-made depending on actual demands rather than the current practice of project-based manufacturing. Commonly, metallic implants are processed by solid-state and deposition-based AM processes like laser engineering net shaping (LENS), electron freeform fabrication (EFF), direct metal deposition (DMD), and laser-augmented manufacturing (LAM). Techniques used for AM of ceramics are based on extrusion (like fused deposition of ceramics), direct writing process (like ink-jet printing), photopolymerization (like stereolithography), and laser-aided sintering like solid laser sintering. Polymers can be additively manufactured by powder bed fusion, vat polymerization, binder jetting, and material extrusion. Often, these 3D printed scaffolds are used to act like multifunctional devices for enhanced osteogenesis, infection control, and blood vessel formation by the

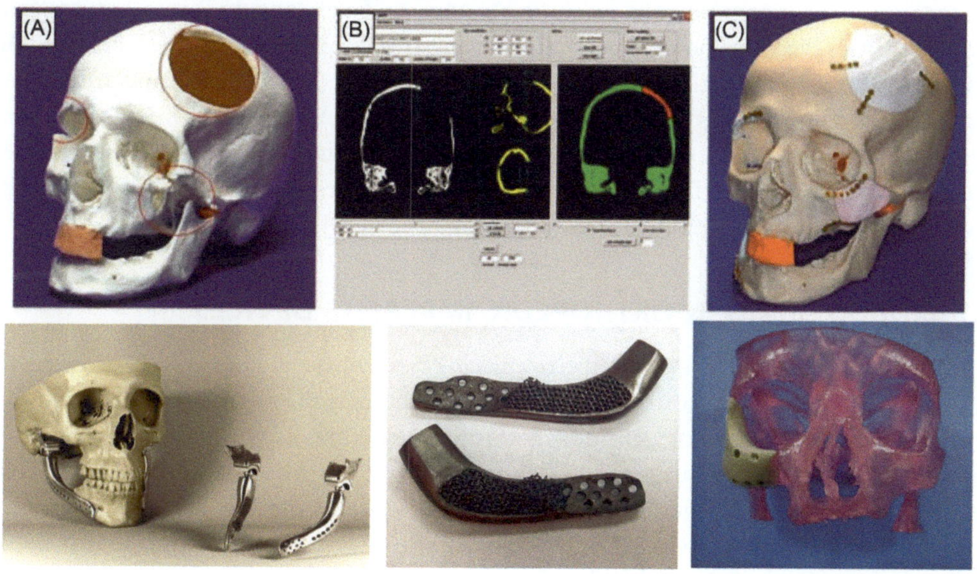

Figure 1.2 CAD file and 3D printed orthopedic implants of metals, ceramics, and polymers. *Picture credit: 3Dprint.com, www.dezeen.com, [97].*

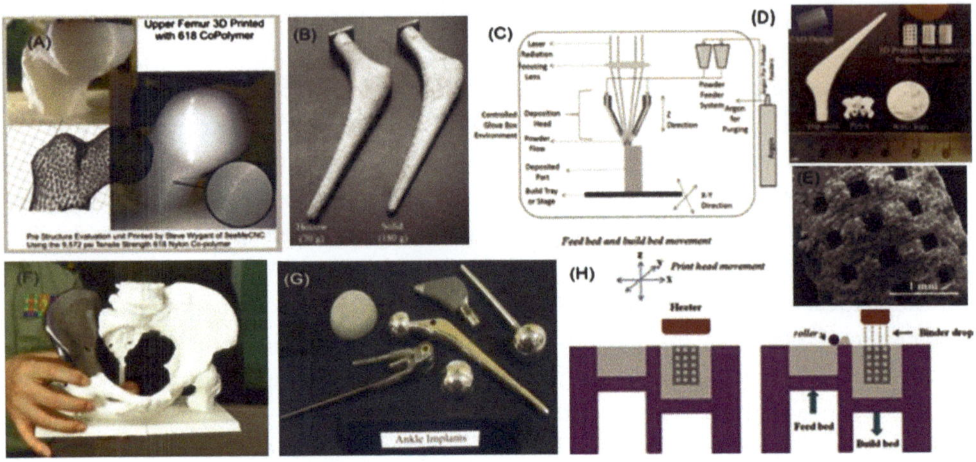

Figure 1.3 (A) Prestructure evaluation unit printed by Steve Wygant using 618 nylon copolymer (http://www.3ders.org/articles/20130218-3d-printing-bone-replacements-cartilage-replacements-medicaldevices-with-618-nylon.html), (B) LENS printed solid and hollow hip implant from commercially pure titanium (Bose and Bandyopadhyay, US Patent 9,327,056, 2016), (C) schematic representation of the LENS process [54, 98], (D, E) 3D printed porous ceramic scaffolds [87, 90, 91], (F) 3D printed metallic scaffolds for clinical use, (http://www.3ders.org/articles/20141215-researcher-earn-grant-to-create-better-3d-printed-bone-coating-material.html), Dec 15, 2014,(G) metallic ankle replacements (MediTeg, UTM), (H) schematic representation of ceramic powder-based inkjet 3D printer [90, 91].

incorporation of inorganic ions Si^{+4}, Sr^{+2}, Mg^{+2}, Zn^{+2}, and Li^{+} into the scaffolds [85–89]. Improved mechanical properties are also demonstrated in these ceramic 3D printed scaffolds due to the presence of these inorganic ions or by using microwave processing technique [87,89]. Specifically, AM, in the field of medical devices, is very dynamic and the progress of this field can be left to the author's view and imagination for phenomenal success. Table 1.3 illustrates briefly different AM processes along with their specific applications, advantages, and limitations [90].

1.7 BIOMATERIALS IN ORTHOPEDIC IMPLANTS DEVICES

An orthopedic device is fabricated to replace or repair an affected joint or damaged bone. Implantation of an orthopedic device encompasses the permanent or temporary restoration of the physiological and anatomical structure of the damaged bone. An implant is chosen by the surgeon according to the site of implantation, weight of the patient and the implant, age of the patient, and the size of the implant, along with the sensitivity of the patient to specific allergens. The usage of these implants for repair and replacement of a damaged or lost bone structure is referred to as internal fixation. Fig. 1.4 demonstrates the usage of a few orthopedic medical devices. External fixations are required to stabilize the bone and the soft tissue at a distance from the

Table 1.3 Additive manufacturing techniques, specific applications, advantages, and limitations [90]

Technique	Processed materials for bone tissue engineering	Advantages	Disadvantages
3D plotting/ direct ink writing	PCL, HA, bioactive glasses	Mild processing conditions, incorporation of drugs and biomolecules	Postprocessing required for few materials
Laser-assisted bioprinting	HA, zirconia, human osteoproginetor cell, HA/MG63 osteoblast-like cell	Ambient conditions, incorporation of drugs and biomolecules, quantitative control	Requirement of homogeneous ribbons
Selective laser sintering	PCL, nano HA, polymer ceramic composite, β-TCP	No requirement of postprocessing, support material not needed	Features in the part dependent on laser resolution
Stereolithography	β-TCP, polymer ceramic composites	Complex features can be made, incorporation of growth factors, proteins, cells possible	Limited to photopolymers
Fused deposition modeling	PCL, alumina, TCP, ceramic polymer composite	Support material not required	Restricted to few materials available in molten phase
Robocasting	HA/PCL composite, HA/ PLA composite, bioglass	Movement of 3D nozzle allows direct writing of liquid and then transformation to gel, control on thickness, support not required	Material restriction

damaged bone through surgical treatments. Orthopedic implants can be categorized into a few subcategories according to their usage and site of implantation.

1.7.1 Joint replacements

Joint replacements are implanted into the patient body with the aim of elimination or alleviating pain, replacing the affected joint and restoring normal functionalities for

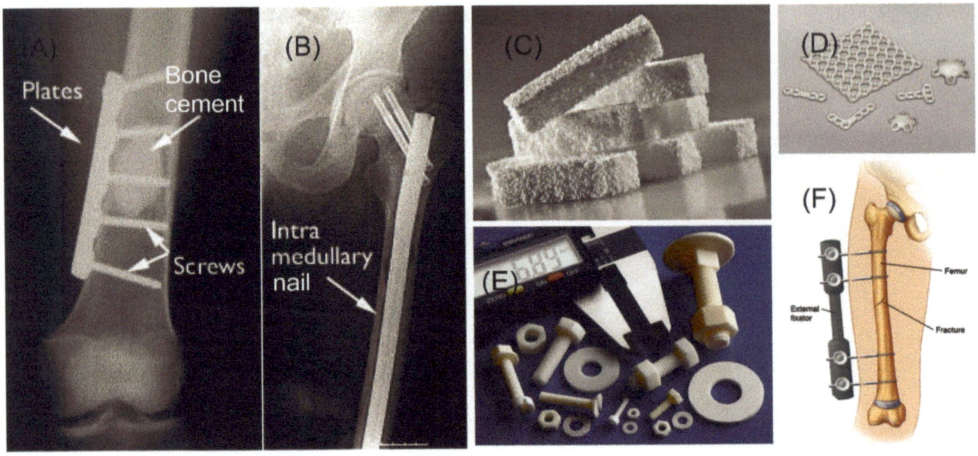

Figure 1.4 (A) Bone cement filling a large defect in the thigh bone. (B) Intramedullary nails and special screws used for stabilizing the thigh bone, picture credit: American Academy of Orthopedic Surgeons. (C) Hydroxyapatite used for large defect filling, picture credit: Ceraform – Teknimed ENTeknimed EN. (D) Various polymeric plates and screws used for implantation, picture credit: Evonik Industries. (E) Ceramic screws and washers, picture credit: Jset Company, Shanghai, China. (F) External metallic bone fixture, picture credit: https://www.fairview.org/HealthLibrary/Article/89347.

improved life quality. It is a surgical procedure in which the arthritic or damaged joint is removed and restored with a ceramic, metal, polymer, or composite part. These replacements are fabricated to recreate the activities of a normal healthy joint. Among the joint replacements, hip and knee replacements are the most widely used in orthopedics. Nevertheless, joint replacement can also be performed on the ankle, shoulder, wrist, or elbow. Through years of surgery, it is well known that femoral stem joint replacement has a limited lifespan after implantation due to aseptic loosening of implants caused by metal ion leaching, and wear particles induced osteolysis.

1.7.2 Implants used in osteosynthesis for stabilization and fracture repair

Bone is a living connective tissue and can heal by itself even when it is broken. Thus, in children, bone heals itself faster and in these cases or in mild fractures, splints and casts are used for support to allow the bone to heal. However, in most other fractures, internal fixations and open reduction are required for repair of the damaged bone. Orthopedic nails, pins, wires, and staples are used in these cases to support the fractured bone and help healing. These are available in a variety of shapes and sizes to fulfill the variety of fracture characteristics and strengthen the external and internal fracture fixations. Bone fixations have also been successfully used for the stabilization of multitraumatized patients and for correcting longitude discrepancies and deformities. Surgical techniques, application of biomaterials, and knowledge of biomechanical forces and patient diagnosis are a few of the rudimentary features used for bone fracture consolidation. These implants are sometimes removed once the bone is healed, depending on the clinical cases. Because of this, SS 316L is typically used in fracture management devices.

1.7.3 Spine implants

Developed in the 1950s by the eminent physician Paul Harrington, modern spine implants are used for the restoration of neuromuscular defects, specifically those associated with poliomyelitis. With a surge in spinal problems due to lethargic physical and postural habits and lifestyle, many sophisticated spinal implants have come into being to treat a variety of spine pathologies. Fig. 1.5 illustrates typical screws, hooks, plates, rods, and cages used as spine implants. To help treat spinal deformations in all dimensions, spinal implants are of two types: fusion implants which are used in tandem with bone grafts like rods, screws, and plates and nonfusion implants like artificial discs.

1.7.4 Nonconventional implants for bone tumor

Preservation of the affected parts remains the fundamental criterion for implant fabrication in cases of bone sarcoma. Most often, allografts are used in combination with the modular prosthesis. For children having bone sarcoma in their lower extremities

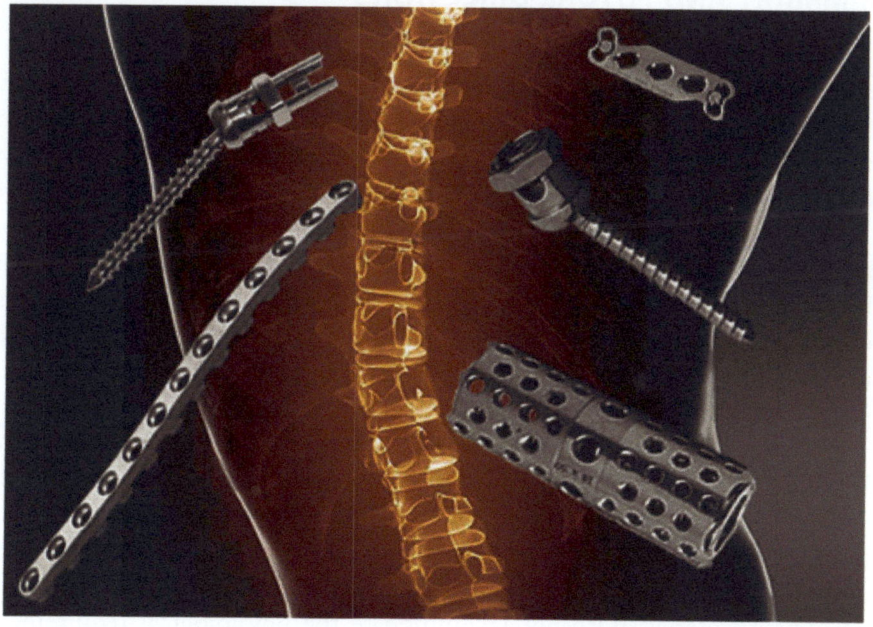

Figure 1.5 A variety of pins, hooks, cages, plates, and screws used for spinal implantation. *Picture credit: GPC. Medical Ltd.*

and developing length discrepancy, both noninvasive and invasive tumor modular prostheses can be used. This has been successful in many clinical cases; however, it requires a lot of research and experimental data for satisfactory day-to-day usage.

1.7.5 Multifunctional devices

Decision on the materials to be used for different medical devices is influenced by mechanical requirements as well as biological, structural, and chemical properties. Biomaterials developed for bone tissue engineering also play an important role in terms of drug delivery. Incorporation of a variety of biomolecules like drugs, growth factors, and inorganic ions into the scaffolds before implantation ensures transmittance to desired organs and release in a sustained manner [91−95]. Presence of inorganic ions those are found in physiological environment, e.g., Mg^{2+}, in metallic implants can also enhance bioactivity of metallic implants [96]. Magnetic nanoparticles can also be used as a carrier for drug molecules and directed to desired organs by control of the external magnetic particles. These particles also help in enhancing the imaging contrast and assist in MRI and CT scans [99]. These prove to be direct examples of multifunctional devices used for bone tissue engineering. Secondary infection poses as an insignificant threat to the success of joint replacements. Oftentimes, the scaffolds are utilized as multifunctional devices as carriers of infection control drugs.

1.8 SUMMARY AND FUTURE DIRECTIONS

Human bone has high regenerative capacity, especially in younger patients, and hence can heal the majority of fractures and defects without any major mediation. However, in the cases of large bone defects or complex fractures, surgical intervention may be required. For the past 100 years, different materials have been invented to treat various bone disorders and improve the quality of life. A key success story can be seen from over 1 million total hip and total knee implants that are being placed every year in the United States alone. However, compelling clinical needs for our aging population demand better treatment options in many cases that keeps the field of biomaterials very active and increasing. For example, even though SS 316L-based fracture management devices are widely used today, demand for infection-resistant nails or screws or plates keep the innovation going in this area. Similarly, clinical application of CaP-based bioceramic materials can be broaden by using a multimaterial-based device using beneficial properties of the components. In general, minimizing pain and faster healing are always a focus of biomaterials research for future treatment options.

For the last six decades, efforts behind advancements of biomaterials went from the industrial availability of materials to the ability to interact with the biological environment. These materials not only accommodate the physiological requirements but also advanced enough to elicit bioactive responses from the physiological systems to address a variety of issues like regenerative medicine, controlled delivery of therapeutic drugs, and biofouling. Moreover, most bone regeneration procedures are still limited by the requirement of angiogenesis, in addition to osteogenesis and proper load transfer between the host tissue and the implantable device, in the neo ECM which is crucial for healthy bone development. Albeit, most of the fabricated biomaterials are tested for their biological functionalities in vitro and in vivo; however, blood contact, appropriate waste removal, surgery details, inflammation, infection control, patient specific allergies, and lifestyle govern the final outcome of the implant behavior.

Thus, the significant conclusion appears to be that there is still a need for the development and introduction of biomaterials to mimic the physiological complexities at the micro and the macro level. Following the tissue engineering paradigm, development of materials with controlled biodegradation in vivo is still in demand. The synergistic interdisciplinary advancements in the fields of material science, applied sciences, biological sciences, and clinical sciences would perhaps make the tailoring of advanced materials to fit the need for biological complexities toward bone disorders in the coming days.

ACKNOWLEDGMENTS

The authors acknowledge financial support from National Institute of Arthritis and Musculoskeletal and Skin Diseases of the National Institutes of Health under Award Numbers R01 AR066361-01A1 and R01 AR067306-01A1. The content is solely the responsibility of the authors and does not necessarily represent the official views of the National Institutes of Health.

REFERENCES

[1] Bose S, Bandyopadhyay A. (2013). Introduction to biomaterials. Characterization of Biomaterials. Edited by Amit Bandyopadhyay and Susmita Bose, Elsevier. 1.
[2] Ring ME. Dentistry: an illustrated history, Harry N. Abrams, New York. Bobbio, A. (1970) The first endosseous alloplastic implant in the history of man, Bull Hist Dent 1992;20:1–6.
[3] Crubzy E, Murail P, Girard L, Bernadou JP. False teeth of the Roman world. Nature 1998;391 (6662):29.
[4] http://www.marketsandmarkets.com/Market-Reports/biomaterials-393.html.
[5] Saha S, Saha P. Bioethics and applied biomaterials. J Biomed Mater Res 1987;21(Suppl. A2):181–90.
[6] Schiedermayer DL, Shapiro RS. The artificial heart as a bridge to transplant: ethical and legal issues at the bedside. J Heart Transpl 1988;8(6):471–3.
[7] Moss AJ, Hamburger S, Moore Jr RM, Jeng LL, Howie LJ. Use of selected medical device implants in the United States, 1988. Adv Data 1991;191:1–24.
[8] Charnley J. Anchorage of the femoral head prosthesis to the shaft of the femur. J Bone Joint Surg 1960;42B(1):28–30.
[9] Tarzia V, Bottio T, Testolin L, Gerosa G. Extended (31 years) durability of a Starr-Edwards prosthesis in mitral position. Interact Cardiovasc Thorac Surg 2007;6(4):570–1.
[10] Huiskes R, Weinans H, Van Rietbergen B. The relationship between stress shielding and bone resorption around total hip stems and the effects of flexible materials. Clin Orthop Relat Res 1992;274:124–34.

[11] Bauer TW, Schils J. The pathology of total joint arthroplasty. Skeletal Radiol 1999;28(9):483−97.
[12] Brånemark PI, Breine U, Adell R, Hansson BO, Lindström J, Ohlsson Å. Intra-osseous anchorage of dental prostheses: I. Experimental studies. Scand J Plast Reconstr Surg 1969;3(2):81−100.
[13] Geetha M, Singh AK, Asokamani R, Gogia AK. Ti based biomaterials, the ultimate choice for orthopaedic implants—a review. Progress Mater Sci 2009;54(3):397−425.
[14] Krishna BV, Bose S, Bandyopadhyay A. Fabrication of porous NiTi shape memory alloy structures using laser engineered net shaping. J Biomed Mater Res B Appl Biomater 2009;89(2):481−90.
[15] Bernard SA, Balla VK, Davies NM, Bose S, Bandyopadhyay A. Bone cell—materials interactions and Ni ion release of anodized equiatomic NiTi alloy. Acta Biomater 2011;7(4):1902−12.
[16] Shabalovskaya SA. On the nature of the biocompatibility and on medical applications of NiTi shape memory and superelastic alloys. Biomed Mater Eng 1996;6(4):267−89.
[17] Das K, Bose S, Bandyopadhyay A. Surface modifications and cell—materials interactions with anodized Ti. Acta Biomater 2007;3(4):573−85.
[18] Das K, Bose S, Bandyopadhyay A. TiO_2 nanotubes on Ti: influence of nanoscale morphology on bone cell—materials interaction. J Biomed Mater Res A 2009;90(1):225−37.
[19] Shelton RM, Rasmussen AC, Davies JE. Protein adsorption at the interface between charged polymer substrata and migrating osteoblasts. Biomaterials 1988;9(1):24−9.
[20] Morra M, Cassinelli C. Bacterial adhesion to polymer surfaces: a critical review of surface thermodynamic approaches. Journal of Biomaterials Science, Polymer Edition 1998;9(1):55−74.
[21] Meyle J, Gültig K, Wolburg H, Von Recum AF. Fibroblast anchorage to microtextured surfaces. J Biomed Mater Res 1993;27(12):1553−7.
[22] Aparicio C, Gil FJ, Fonseca C, Barbosa M, Planell JA. Corrosion behaviour of commercially pure titanium shot blasted with different materials and sizes of shot particles for dental implant applications. Biomaterials 2003;24(2):263−73.
[23] Masmoudi M, Assoul M, Wery M, Abdelhedi R, El Halouani F, Monteil G. Friction and wear behaviour of cp Ti and Ti6Al4V following nitric acid passivation. Appl Surf Sci 2006;253 (4):2237−43.
[24] Lopez-Heredia MA, Sohier J, Gaillard C, Quillard S, Dorget M, Layrolle P. Rapid prototyped porous titanium coated with calcium phosphate as a scaffold for bone tissue engineering. Biomaterials 2008;29(17):2608−15.
[25] Ong JL, Lucas LC, Lacefield WR, Rigney ED. Structure, solubility and bond strength of thin calcium phosphate coatings produced by ion beam sputter deposition. Biomaterials 1992;13 (4):249−54.
[26] Xue W, Hosick HL, Bandyopadhyay A, Bose S, Ding C, Luk KDK, et al. Preparation and cell—materials interactions of plasma sprayed strontium-containing hydroxyapatite coating. Surf Coat Technol 2007;201(8):4685−93.
[27] Herø H, Wie H, Jørgensen RB, Ruyter I. Hydroxyapatite coatings on Ti produced by hot isostatic pressing. J Biomed Mater Res 1994;28(3):343−8.
[28] Cleries L, Martinez E, Fernandez-Pradas JM, Sardin G, Esteve J, Morenza JL. Mechanical properties of calcium phosphate coatings deposited by laser ablation. Biomaterials 2000;21(9):967−71.
[29] Roy M, Bandyopadhyay A, Bose S. Induction plasma sprayed nano hydroxyapatite coatings on titanium for orthopaedic and dental implants. Surface Coatings Technol 2011;205(8):2785−92.
[30] Capello WN, D'Antonio JA, Manley MT, Feinberg JR. Hydroxyapatite in Total Hip Arthroplasty: Clinical Results and Critical Issues. Clin Orthopaed Related Res 1998;355:200−11.
[31] Sun L, Berndt CC, Gross KA, Kucuk A. Material fundamentals and clinical performance of plasma-sprayed hydroxyapatite coatings: a review. J Biomed Mater Res 2001;58(5):570−92.
[32] Vahabzadeh S, Roy M, Bandyopadhyay A, Bose S. Phase stability and biological property evaluation of plasma sprayed hydroxyapatite coatings for orthopedic and dental applications. Acta Biomater 2015;17:47−55.
[33] Roy M, Bandyopadhyay A, Bose S. Induction plasma sprayed Sr and Mg doped nano hydroxyapatite coatings on Ti for bone implant. J Biomed Mater Res B Appl Biomater 2011;99(2):258−65.

[34] Fielding GA, Roy M, Bandyopadhyay A, Bose S. Antibacterial and biological characteristics of silver containing and strontium doped plasma sprayed hydroxyapatite coatings. Acta biomaterialia 2012;8(8):3144–52.

[35] Roy M, Fielding GA, Beyenal H, Bandyopadhyay A, Bose S. Mechanical, in vitro antimicrobial, and biological properties of plasma-sprayed silver-doped hydroxyapatite coating. ACS Appl Mater Interfaces 2012;4(3):1341–9.

[36] Kokubo T. Bioactive glass ceramics: properties and applications. Biomaterials 1991;12(2):155–63.

[37] Ohtsuki C, Iida H, Hayakawa S, Osaka A. Bioactivity of titanium treated with hydrogen peroxide solutions containing metal chlorides. J Biomed Mater Res 1997;35(1):39–47.

[38] Boutin P. Total arthroplasty of the hip by fritted aluminum prosthesis. Experimental study and 1st clinical applications. Revue de chirurgie orthopedique et reparatrice de l'appareil moteur 1972;58 (3):229.

[39] Christel P, Meunier A, Dorlot JM, Crolet JM, Witvoet J, Sedel L, et al. Biomechanical compatibility and design of ceramic implants for orthopedic surgery. Ann NY Acad Sci 1988;523(1):234–56.

[40] Hobkirk JA. In: McKinney RV, Lemons JE, editors. The dental implant. Clinical and biological response of oral tissues. Littleton, MA: PSG Publishing Company, Inc.; 1986. p. 205.

[41] Villermaux F, Cales B, Drouin JM. Zirconia-Alumina pairing for hip prosthesis applications: comparison to common head-cup systems on a hip joint simulator with different lubricants. Annual meeting-society for biomaterials in conjunction with the international biomaterials symposium 1998;21:215. Society for biomaterials.

[42] Clarke IC, Good V, Williams P, Schroeder D, Anissian L, Stark A, et al. Ultra-low wear rates for rigid-on-rigid bearings in total hip replacements. Proc Inst Mech Eng H 2000;214(4):331–47.

[43] Saikko V. Wear of polyethylene acetabular cups against zirconia femoral heads studied with a hip joint simulator. Wear 1994;176(2):207–12.

[44] Spector M, Ries MD, Bourne RB, Sauer WS, Long M, Hunter G. Wear performance of ultra-high molecular weight polyethylene on oxidized zirconium total knee femoral components. J Bone Joint Surg Am 2001;83(Suppl. 2):S80–6.

[45] De Jong WF. La substance minerale dans les os. Recueil des travaux chimiques des Pays-Bas 1926;45(6):445–8.

[46] Posner AS, Betts F. Synthetic amorphous calcium phosphate and its relation to bone mineral structure. Accoun Chem Res 1975;8(8):273–81.

[47] Meffert RM, Thomas JR, Hamilton KM, Brownstein CN. Hydroxylapatite as an alloplastic graft in the treatment of human periodontal osseous defects. J Periodontol 1985;56(2):63–73.

[48] Bose S, Fielding G, Tarafder S, Bandyopadhyay A. Understanding of dopant-induced osteogenesis and angiogenesis in calcium phosphate ceramics. Trends Biotechnol 2013;31(10):594–605.

[49] Vahabzadeh S, Hack VK, Bose S. Lithium-doped β-tricalcium phosphate: effects on physical, mechanical and in vitro osteoblast cell–material interactions. J Biomed Mater Res B Appl Biomater 2015;. Available from: http://dx.doi.org/10.1002/jbm.b.33485.

[50] Bandyopadhyay A, Bernard S, Xue W, Bose S. Calcium phosphate-based resorbable ceramics: influence of MgO, ZnO, and SiO_2 dopants. J Am Ceram Soc 2006;89(9):2675–88.

[51] Fielding G, Bose S. SiO_2 and ZnO dopants in three-dimensionally printed tricalcium phosphate bone tissue engineering scaffolds enhance osteogenesis and angiogenesis in vivo. Acta Biomater 2013;9(11):9137–48.

[52] Roy M, Fielding GA, Bandyopadhyay A, Bose S. Effects of zinc and strontium substitution in tricalcium phosphate on osteoclast differentiation and resorption. Biomater Sci 2013;1(1):74–82.

[53] Banerjee SS, Tarafder S, Davies NM, Bandyopadhyay A, Bose S. Understanding the influence of MgO and SrO binary doping on the mechanical and biological properties of β-TCP ceramics. Acta Biomater 2010;6(10):4167–74.

[54] Bandyopadhyay A, Shivaram A, Tarafder S, Sahasrabudhe H, Banerjee D, Bose S. In vivo response of laser processed porous titanium implants for load-bearing implants. Ann Biomed Eng 2016;1–12.

[55] Bose S, Tarafder S, Banerjee SS, Davies NM, Bandyopadhyay A. Understanding in vivo response and mechanical property variation in MgO, SrO and SiO_2 doped β-TCP. Bone 2011;48 (6):1282–90.

[56] Bandyopadhyay A, Petersen J, Fielding G, Banerjee S, Bose S. ZnO, SiO_2, and SrO doping in resorbable tricalcium phosphates: influence on strength degradation, mechanical properties, and in vitro bone–cell material interactions. J Biomed Mater Res B Appl Biomater 2012;100 (8):2203–12.

[57] Seeley Z, Bandyopadhyay A, Bose S. Influence of TiO_2 and Ag_2O addition on tricalcium phosphate ceramics. J Biomed Mater Res A 2007;82(1):113–21.

[58] Seeley Z, Bandyopadhyay A, Bose S. Tricalcium phosphate based resorbable ceramics: influence of NaF and CaO addition. Mater Sci Eng C 2008;28(1):11–17.

[59] Bose S, Saha SK. Synthesis and characterization of hydroxyapatite nanopowders by emulsion technique. Chem Mater 2003;15(23):4464–9.

[60] Banerjee A, Bandyopadhyay A, Bose S. Hydroxyapatite nanopowders: synthesis, densification and cell–materials interaction. Mater Sci Eng C 2007;27(4):729–35.

[61] Hench LL, Ethridge EC, Ethridge B. An interfacial approach. Biomaterials 1982;105–35.

[62] Carlisle EM. Silicon: a possible factor in bone calcification. Science 1970;167(3916):279–80.

[63] Patel N, Best SM, Bonfield W, Gibson IR, Hing KA, Damien E, et al. A comparative study on the in vivo behavior of hydroxyapatite and silicon substituted hydroxyapatite granules. J Mater Sci Mater Med 2002;13(12):1199–206.

[64] Kokubo T, Shigematsu M, Nagashima Y, Tashiro M, Nakamura T, Yamamuro T, Higashi S. Apatite-wollastonite containing glass—ceramic for prosthetic application. Bull Inst Chem Res, Kyoto Univ 1982;60:260–8.

[65] Reck R, Störkel S, Meyer A. Bioactive glass-ceramics in middle ear surgery an 8-year reviewa. Ann NY Acad Sci 1988;523(1):100–6.

[66] Wang C, Xue Y, Lin K, Lu J, Chang J, Sun J. The enhancement of bone regeneration by a combination of osteoconductivity and osteostimulation using β-CaSiO 3/β-Ca 3 (PO 4) 2 composite bioceramics. Acta Biomater 2012;8(1):350–60.

[67] Maloney WJ, Smith RL. Periprosthetic osteolysis in total hip arthroplasty: the role of particulate wear debris. J Bone Joint Surg Am 1995;77(9):1448–61.

[68] Kipping FS. Organic derivative of silicon. Preparation of alkylsilicon chlorides. Proc Chem Soc 1904;20:15.

[69] Swanson AB. Silicone rubber implants for replacement of arthritis or destroyed joints in the hand. Surg Clin North Am 1968;48(5):1113–27.

[70] Kirschenbaum D, Schneider LH, Adams DC, Cody RP. Arthroplasty of the metacarpophalangeal joints with use of silicone-rubber implants in patients who have rheumatoid arthritis. Long-term results. J Bone Joint Surg Am 1993;75(1):3–12.

[71] El-Gammal TA, Blair WF. Motion after metacarpophalangeal joint reconstruction in rheumatoid disease. J Hand Surg 1993;18(3):504–11.

[72] Törmälä P. Biodegradable self-reinforced composite materials; manufacturing structure and mechanical properties. Clin Mater 1992;10(1):29–34.

[73] Grizzi I, Garreau H, Li S, Vert M. Hydrolytic degradation of devices based on poly (DL-lactic acid) size-dependence. Biomaterials 1995;16(4):305–11.

[74] Taksali S, Grauer JN, Vaccaro AR. Material considerations for intervertebral disc replacement implants. Spine J 2004;4(6):S231–8.

[75] Bonfield W, Grynpas MD, Tully AE, Bowman J, Abram J. Hydroxyapatite reinforced polyethylene—a mechanically compatible implant material for bone replacement. Biomaterials 1981;2 (3):185–6.

[76] Gasser B. About composite materials and their use in bone surgery. Injury 2000;31:D48–53.

[77] Tullberg T. Failure of a carbon fiber implant: a case report. Spine 1998;23(16):1804–6.

[78] Adams D, Williams DF. The response of bone to carbon-carbon composites. Biomaterials 1984;5 (2):59–64.

[79] Brandwood A, Noble KR, Schindhelm K. Phagocytosis of carbon particles by macrophages in vitro. Biomaterials 1992;13(9):646–8.

[80] Olson EJ, Kang JD, Fu FH, Georgescu HI, Mason GC, Evans CH. The biochemical and histological effects of artificial ligament wear particles: in vitro and in vivo studies. Am J Sports Med 1988;16(6):558–70.
[81] Evans SL, Gregson PJ. Composite technology in load-bearing orthopaedic implants. Biomaterials 1998;19(15):1329–42.
[82] Lewandowska–Szumieł M, Komender J, Chłopek J. Interaction between carbon composites and bone after intrabone implantation. J Biomed Mater Res 1999;48(3):289–96.
[83] Trojani C, Boukhechba F, Scimeca JC, Vandenbos F, Michiels JF, Daculsi G, et al. Ectopic bone formation using an injectable biphasic calcium phosphate/Si-HPMC hydrogel composite loaded with undifferentiated bone marrow stromal cells. Biomaterials 2006;27(17):3256–64.
[84] Bandyopadhyay A, Vahabzadeh S, Shivaram A, Bose S. Three-dimensional printing of biomaterials and soft materials. MRS Bull 2015;40(12):1162–9.
[85] Fielding GA, Smoot W, Bose S. Effects of SiO_2, SrO, MgO, and ZnO dopants in tricalcium phosphates on osteoblastic Runx2 expression. J Biomed Mater Res A 2014;102(7):2417–26.
[86] Tarafder S, Dernell WS, Bandyopadhyay A, Bose S. SrO-and MgO-doped microwave sintered 3D printed tricalcium phosphate scaffolds: mechanical properties and in vivo osteogenesis in a rabbit model. J Biomed Mater Res B Appl Biomater 2015;103(3):679–90.
[87] Tarafder S, Balla VK, Davies NM, Bandyopadhyay A, Bose S. Microwave-sintered 3D printed tricalcium phosphate scaffolds for bone tissue engineering. J Tissue Eng Regenerat Med 2013;7 (8):631–41.
[88] Fielding GA, Bandyopadhyay A, Bose S. Effects of silica and zinc oxide doping on mechanical and biological properties of 3D printed tricalcium phosphate tissue engineering scaffolds. Dent Mater 2012;28(2):113–22.
[89] Tarafder S, Dernell WS, Bandyopadhyay A, Bose S. SrO-and MgO-doped microwave sintered 3D printed tricalcium phosphate scaffolds: Mechanical properties and in vivo osteogenesis in a rabbit model. Journal of Biomedical Materials Research Part B: Applied Biomaterials 2015;103 (3):679–90.
[90] Bose S, Vahabzadeh S, Bandyopadhyay A. Bone tissue engineering using 3D printing. Materials Today 2013;16(12):496–504.
[91] Bose S, Tarafder S. Calcium phosphate ceramic systems in growth factor and drug delivery for bone tissue engineering: a review. Acta biomaterialia 2012;8(4):1401–21.
[92] Tarafder S, Nansen K, Bose S. Lovastatin release from polycaprolactone coated β-tricalcium phosphate: Effects of pH, concentration and drug–polymer interactions. Materials Science and Engineering: C 2013;33(6):3121–8.
[93] Peter B, Pioletti DP, Laib S, Bujoli B, Pilet P, Janvier P, Gauthier O. Calcium phosphate drug delivery system: influence of local zoledronate release on bone implant osteointegration. Bone 2005;36 (1):52–60.
[94] Tarafder S, Bose S. Polycaprolactone-coated 3D printed tricalcium phosphate scaffolds for bone tissue engineering: in vitro alendronate release behavior and local delivery effect on in vivo osteogenesis. ACS Appl Mater Interfaces 2014;6(13):9955–65.
[95] Liu TY, Chen SY, Liu DM, Liou SC. On the study of BSA-loaded calcium-deficient hydroxyapatite nano-carriers for controlled drug delivery. J Control Release 2005;107(1):112–21.
[96] Roy M, Balla VK, Bandyopadhyay A, Bose S. MgO-doped tantalum coating on Ti: microstructural study and biocompatibility evaluation. ACS Appl Mater Interfaces 2012;4(2):577–80.
[97] Klammert U, Gbureck U, Vorndran E, Rödiger J, Meyer-Marcotty P, Kübler AC. 3D powder printed calcium phosphate implants for reconstruction of cranial and maxillofacial defects. J Cranio-Maxillofac Surg 2010;38(8):565–70.
[98] Bandyopadhyay A, Espana F, Balla VK, Bose S, Ohgami Y, Davies NM. Influence of porosity on mechanical properties and in vivo response of Ti6Al4V implants. Acta biomaterialia 2010;6 (4):1640–8.
[99] Sun C, Lee JS, Zhang M. Magnetic nanoparticles in MR imaging and drug delivery. Advanced drug delivery reviews 2008;60(11):1252–6.

CHAPTER 2

Bone Biology and Effects of Pharmaceutical Intervention on Bone Quality

S.M. Ott
University of Washington Medical Center, Seattle, WA, United States

Contents

2.1 BONE BIOLOGY

2.1.1 Bone functions

Bone tissue is a model of biological efficiency with multiple functions (Fig. 2.1). The skeleton as a structural material must be strong enough to support the body weight and

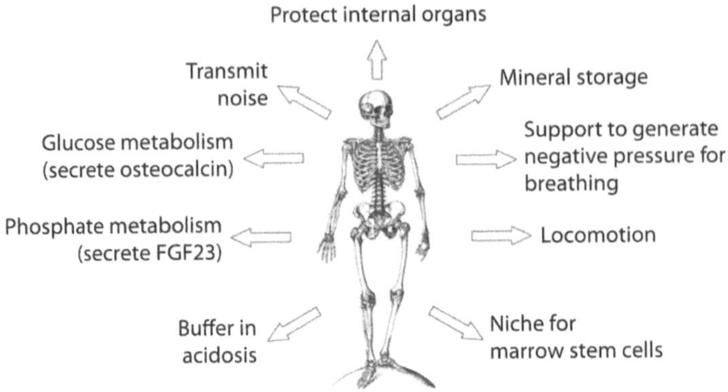

Figure 2.1 Functions of the skeleton.

light enough for efficient movement. Other functions depending on bone structure include protection of internal organs, especially the brain. The rib cage provides a firm structure to allow development of the negative pleural pressure that allows breathing. Specialized bone is found in the inner ear, where the function depends not on strength but on the ability to transmit sound. In addition to these structural functions, the bone acts as a reservoir for minerals and protein. Bone is an important buffer for acid loads. Bone cells secrete endocrine hormones which regulate mineral metabolism and influence energy metabolism. Bone cells form niches that protect the hematopoietic stem cells.

Bone as a material depends on the function [1,2]. Bones of the legs require strength; the stress to the third metacarpal of a thoroughbred racehorse during a gallop is on the order of 53 megapascals [3]. Bones in the ear are more like glass, able to transmit noise, and bones in the antlers of a deer are tough and flexible, made for fighting. Unlike other materials, the bone can adapt to external forces by changing shape and density. At repetitive loading equal to 100 miles of running fatigue damage will occur [4]. However, bone can repair itself by directing remodeling to the damaged site. In addition to directed remodeling, which repairs cracks and fatigue damage, there is apparently a random (Parfitt terms this stochastic) remodeling [5,6], which may act to continually renew bone. This will prevent accumulation of older, densely mineralized bone, which is more brittle [7].

Bones in the load-bearing skeleton must be strong (able to show stiffness under high loads) and tough (able to absorb energy without fracturing). As Currey stated, "Strength is usually measured in well-controlled situations, whereas toughness accords better with what goes on in the rough-and-tumble of real life" [8].

2.1.2 Composition

Bone is composed of water, organic matrix, and mineral. The percentage of mineral varies from about 50% to 90%, depending on the bone. Organic matrix accounts for 5–40% and the remainder is water (5–25%) [8,9].

The matrix, termed "osteoid," is predominantly protein, of which 90% is type I collagen [10]. Other proteins include fibronectin, osteonectin, thrombospondin, ameloblastin, osteocalcin, and matrix-gla-protein. These other proteins have various functions that act to stabilize the bone or regulate mineralization [11]. Some also signal the bone cells [12]. In addition, there are glycoproteins, such as sialoprotein, osteopontin, and matrix extracellular protein, and these also regulate mineralization as well as binding to the cells and signaling angiogenesis. Proteoglycans with attached sugar residues contribute to the complex bone matrix [13].

The mineral is mostly hydroxyapatite $Ca_{10}(PO_4)_6(OH)_2$, an insoluble salt of calcium and phosphorus. Small amounts of magnesium, sodium, and bicarbonate are also found in the crystal structure of the mineral [14].

2.1.3 Architecture

All bones have a solid outer layer (cortical bone) and many have an inner core which is honeycombed (called cancellous, spongy, or trabecular bone). The shafts of long bones may have only fatty bone marrow inside. The cortical bone is organized into Haversian systems, termed "osteons," consisting of concentric layers of bone and a central canal which supplies blood, which have a longitudinal orientation. Fig. 2.2 shows a cross section through cortical bone; the large black ovals are the central canals and the small black dots are the osteocyte lacunae. The darker color corresponds to lower mineralization density that is seen in the most recently formed osteons.

The trabecular bone is formed with interconnecting plate-like structures which tend to be oriented toward the stresses placed on the bone. Fig. 2.3 shows the proximal femur, with virtual biopsies in the different regions which have more bone and more strength in those regions that are subject to compressive forces, medium strength in those under tensile forces, and only a few trabecular structures in the "Ward's triangle" region that is not under any stress [15].

2.1.4 Bone cells

Two major families of cells control bone remodeling: the osteoclasts and the osteoblasts.

Fig. 2.4 shows the lineage of these cells. Osteoclasts originate from cells in the hematopoietic line, from precursors of macrophages. The precursors are found in the marrow and in the circulation. Osteoblasts are derived from mesenchymal stem cells in the marrow stroma that can alternatively differentiate into adipocytes or chondrocytes. Preosteoblasts differentiate into mature osteoblasts that secrete collagen and form bone. The osteoblasts either undergo apoptosis or further differentiate into lining cells or osteocytes. All of these steps are regulated by cytokines and hormones and the cells interact closely with each other [16,17] (Fig. 2.5).

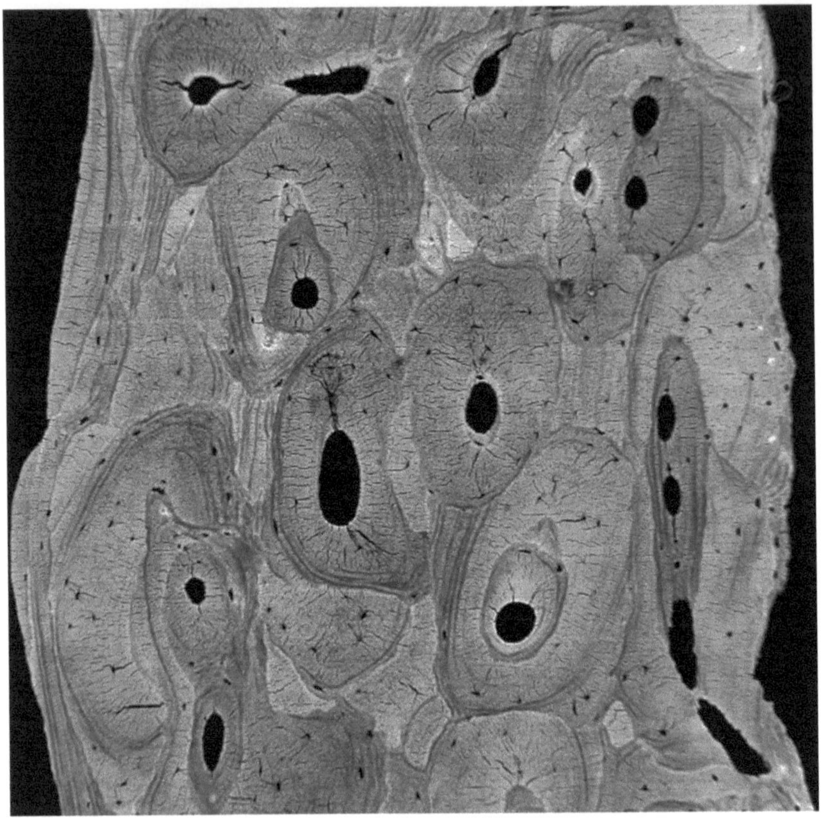

Figure 2.2 Cross section of cortical bone showing osteons with different mineralization densities.

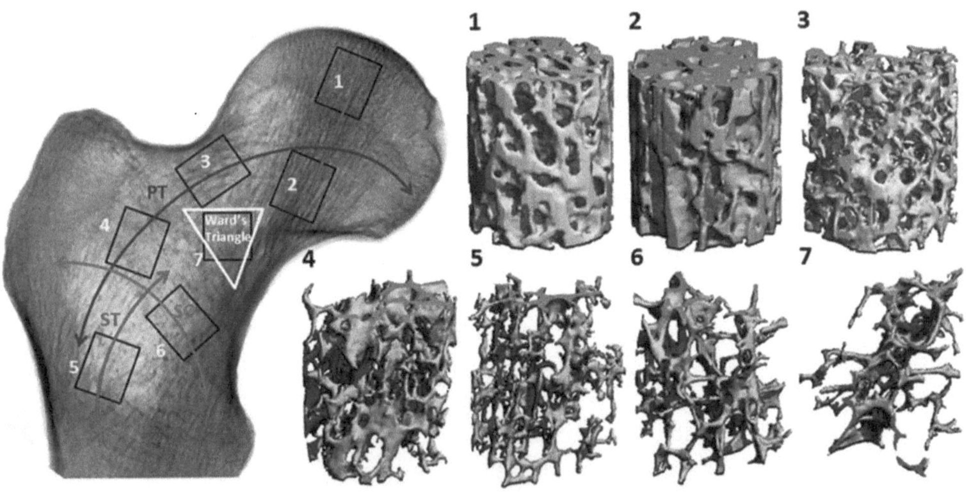

Figure 2.3 Trabecular structures within the proximal femur, showing denser bone where there are the compressive or tensile stresses [15]. Courtesy of Bone Bioengineering Laboratory, Columbia University.

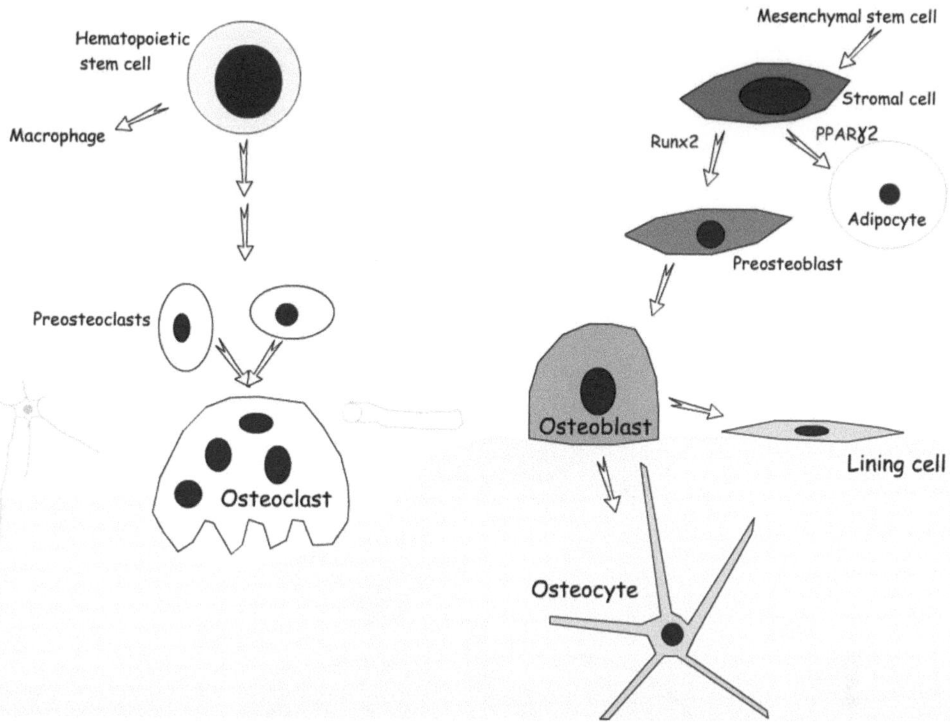

Figure 2.4 Bone cell origins and differentiation.

2.1.4.1 Osteoclasts

Osteoclast precursors circulate in the bloodstream. They have receptors for macrocyte colony-stimulating factor that is secreted by cells in the osteoblast line. The preosteoclasts express surface receptor activator of nuclear factor κ-B (RANK) [18]. When RANK-ligand (RANK-L) occupies these receptors the cells become active and merge with other preosteoclasts to form large, mature, multinucleated osteoclasts. The RANK-L is expressed on the surface of osteoblasts and osteocytes. Early studies found that osteoclasts were unable to resorb bone unless there was direct contact with cells in the osteoblast family. Recent studies have suggested that the osteocytes are the most important source of the RANK-L, and that the RANK-L is expressed as the osteocytes are undergoing apoptosis [19]. Since the osteocytes are able to sense damage or excess mechanical forces, this system allows resorption to be targeted to areas of need.

Many systemic hormones that eventually cause bone resorption do not act directly on osteoclasts but rather on osteoblast cells which then signal the osteoclasts via the RANK–RANK-L signaling.

The signaling pathway intracellularly is mediated by calcineurin; [20] thus, resorption is inhibited by medicines, such as FK506 and cyclosporin A, that used to prevent rejection in patients with organ transplantation.

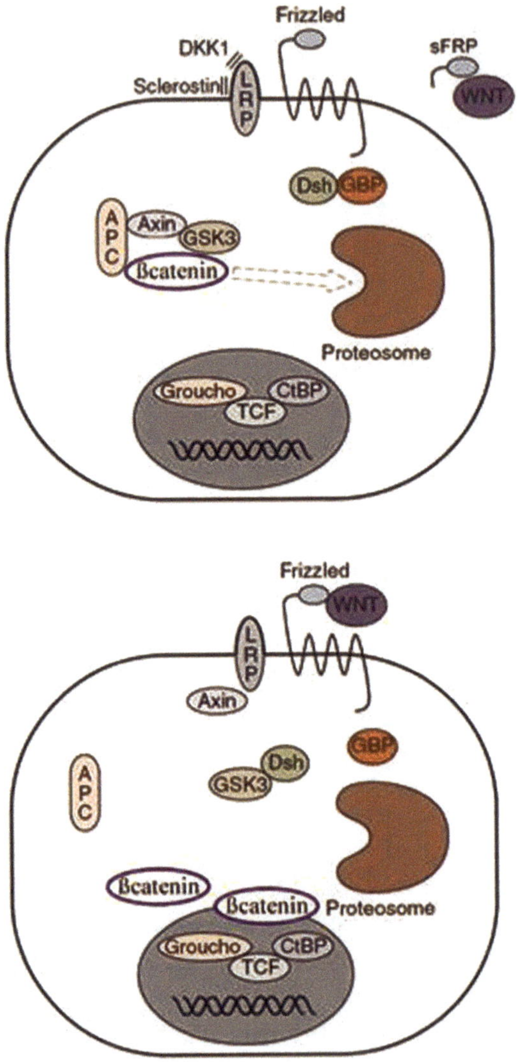

Figure 2.5 This is a simplified view of the canonical Wnt-signaling pathway. When inactive, a complex including Axin, GSK3, and APC phosphorylates ß-catenin so it is ubiquitinated and broken down by the proteosome. Frizzled is a seven-transmembrane domain receptor. LRP 5 and 6 are coreceptors necessary for signal transduction. When a Wnt ligand binds the Frizzled receptor, it phosphorylates and activates Disheveled (Dsh), which represses GSK3 which releases Axin from the ß-catenin. The Axin is then restrained by the intracellular part of LRP5, and so the ß-catenin accumulates and enters the nucleus and binds TCF transcription factors. Several extracellular proteins inhibit this process. Dickkopf (Dkk) ties up LRP5 by binding to it and another membrane protein called Kremen. Sclerostin also binds to the LRP5 protein (this is further discussed later in the chapter). These each prevent the LRP5 from restraining Axin. Secreted Frizzled-related protein (sFRP) acts as a decoy receptor and binds to Wnt, preventing signaling. In patients with high bone mass, the mutated LRP5 resists binding to Dkk. Therefore, the Wnt-signaling pathway is more active. In the patients with osteoporosis-pseudoglioma syndrome, the protein is nonfunctional, so the Wnt-signaling pathway is inhibited.

Other signaling pathways between the osteoblast and osteoclast include newly described immunoreceptor tyrosine-based activation motifs which are similar to systems found in immune cells and which modulate osteoclast fusion [21,22]. Recent interesting studies of spaceflight show that the osteoclastogenesis is enhanced with microgravity, and that this involves autophagy, the cellular process of recycling protein debris [23].

2.1.4.2 Osteoblast lineage

Stem cells near the vasculature within the bone marrow give rise to preosteoblasts [11,24], which can proliferate under the influence of local and systemic growth factors. Two transcription factors control the fate of the cells. RUNX2, the earliest marker of an osteoblast lineage cell, promotes maturation into osteoblasts, but PPAR-γ causes the stem cells to become adipocytes. The lipids in the environment partly determine which of these transcription factors is prominent.

2.1.4.2.1 The Wnt-signaling system

This signaling cascade was simultaneously discovered by one group of doctors studying a family with very high bone density and another studying children with a severe crippling bone disease. Both diseases were caused by a mutation in the receptor LRP-5 (lipoprotein receptor-related protein 5).

In 1997, clinicians from Creighton University reported a kindred with high bone mass [24,25]. The proband was an 18-year-old girl who had back pain after an automobile accident. Radiographs showed no fracture, dense but otherwise normal bones, and subsequent bone mineral density (BMD) was 5.6 standard deviations above average for age. Her mother had similarly dense bones. This led to an extended survey of this family whose members carried the "high bone mass" gene, which showed autosomal dominant inheritance. Using linkage analysis, they demonstrated that those with high bone mass had a single point mutation in the LRP5 gene [26]. Shortly afterwards, investigators reported an unrelated kindred with high bone mass which carried the identical mutation [27]. During this time a group from Belgium described a mutation in the SOST gene which caused severe bone thickening in patients with heterozygous inactivating mutations [28].

Meanwhile, another group discovered that a different mutation in the LRP5 gene caused the osteoporosis-pseudoglioma syndrome, a devastating autosomal recessive disorder manifested by multiple fractures [29]. Yet a different approach was being used in patients with multiple myeloma. Gene array analysis showed that the dickkopf gene was overexpressed in those with bone involvement.

These proteins are all part of the Wnt-signaling pathway [30,31]. The pathway had been described in *Drosophila* by embryologists, who named the genes after effects seen in the unfortunate fruitflies. Thus the ligand was "wingless" and the receptor "frizzled." The mouse analogue of wingless was "int" so the names were combined into "wnt." In the mouse, mutation of the dickkopf gene caused a thick head. LRP5 was called "arrow," and sclerostin was "wise." The current names are combinations of these original ones.

The Wnt-signaling pathway is involved in pleomorphic processes. These genes included ones that control cell differentiation (promotion of osteoblastic as opposed to adiopocytic phenotypes), inhibition of apoptosis (longer lifespan), and other proteins in the Wnt-signaling pathway (feedback). Of particular interest is the finding that Wnt3a upregulates osteoprotegerin (OPG), a secreted protein that inhibits bone resorption. Thus, the Wnt-signaling pathway not only increases osteoblastic cell differentiation and bone formation but also inhibits bone resorption by blocking the RANK–RANK-L interaction [32].

2.1.4.3 Preosteoblasts

The Wnt-signaling system is essential for differentiation of osteoblast cells. Other growth factors, such as transforming factor-beta (TGF-β), fibroblast growth factor, bone morphogenic proteins, platelet-derived growth factors, and colony-stimulating factors, can also increase proliferation of preosteoblasts. Bone morphogenic protein 7, which is made in the kidney, is necessary for the final differentiation of preosteoblasts into osteoblasts [32–35]. With deficiency, spindle-shaped preosteoblasts accumulate near the bone surface and have been misnamed "peritrabecular fibrosis" for years because early histologists thought that the inchoate preosteoblasts were fibroblasts.

The preosteoblasts have receptors for many of the hormones and cytokines that were classically felt to increase bone resorption (such as PTH, interleukins, and calcitriol). Preosteoblasts express RANK-L on their surface, which stimulates the preosteoclasts [36].

2.1.4.4 Reversal cells

Recent studies have shown that reversal cells express Runx2 and other gene markers that are in the osteoblast family [37,38]. These cells, which are especially located between the osteoclastic bone resorption surface and the osteoblast formation surface, may play an important role in coupling between the osteoclastic resorption and osteoblastic formation [39].

2.1.4.5 Mature osteoblasts

The mature osteoblasts secrete collagen and proteins into the bone matrix, including several growth factors. Osteocalcin and osteopontin are expressed in these mature cells, as well as OPG, a decoy receptor for RANK-L that will block osteoclast formation [16]. When a team of osteoblasts first starts forming matrix, the cells are cuboidal and plump and have many mitochondria. As they fill in the resorption cavity, they become flatter and less metabolically active [40]. Most eventually undergo apoptosis. Some of them stop making matrix and are left behind the other cells and surrounded by matrix and then differentiate into the osteocytes. When the resorption cavity is filled, the remaining cells differentiate into lining cells.

2.1.4.6 Lining cells

These cells are flat, pancake-like cells that form tight junctions with each other and essentially separate the bone from the rest of the body. The osteocytes remain in contact with the lining cells. The lining cells make alkaline phosphatase, which prevents pyrophosphate from entering the bone and dissolving the mineral. Patients with hypophosphatasia have mutations in the alkaline phosphatase and develop severe fatal osteomalacia [41].

The osteoblasts and the vascular sinusoids in the marrow function as a niche for the hematopoietic stem cells [42]. Recent studies using real-time imaging have shown that these cells home to the endosteal surface in irradiated mice, near preosteoblasts that are positive for N-cadherin. This special zone normally maintains the stem cells, but promotes their expansion in response to bone marrow damage [43].

2.1.4.7 Osteocytes

The osteocytes, once thought to be trapped in the bone mineral, are actually active within their lacunae and canaliculae [44,45]. They have multiple long cell processes that extend within the bone and form junctions with other osteocytes. The resulting network resembles a neuronal network, and the osteocytes are considered the brains of the bones (Fig. 2.6) [46].

A special cell process, like a cilia, can be found on these extensions, which is firmly attached to the mineral of the canalicular wall [47]. When mechanical loads are applied to the bone, the cilia can detect fluid movement [48], and thus the osteocytes can sense mechanical strains. They then stop secreting sclerostin, which releases inhibition of the osteoblasts. The osteocytes also secrete stimulatory factors into the marrow, including prostaglandins, nitric oxide, and IGF. The bone is also a hormone "gland" because the osteocytes secrete FGF23 that goes to the kidney and causes phosphate excretion [19]. Where there is microdamage, the osteocytes undergo apoptosis, and as they lay dying they express RANK-L to signal osteoclasts to come and start the repair process [49,50].

2.1.5 Bone remodeling

Healthy bone is a dynamic tissue, continually resorbing bone and replacing it with new bone in a sequence which is "highly coordinated in time and space" [37].

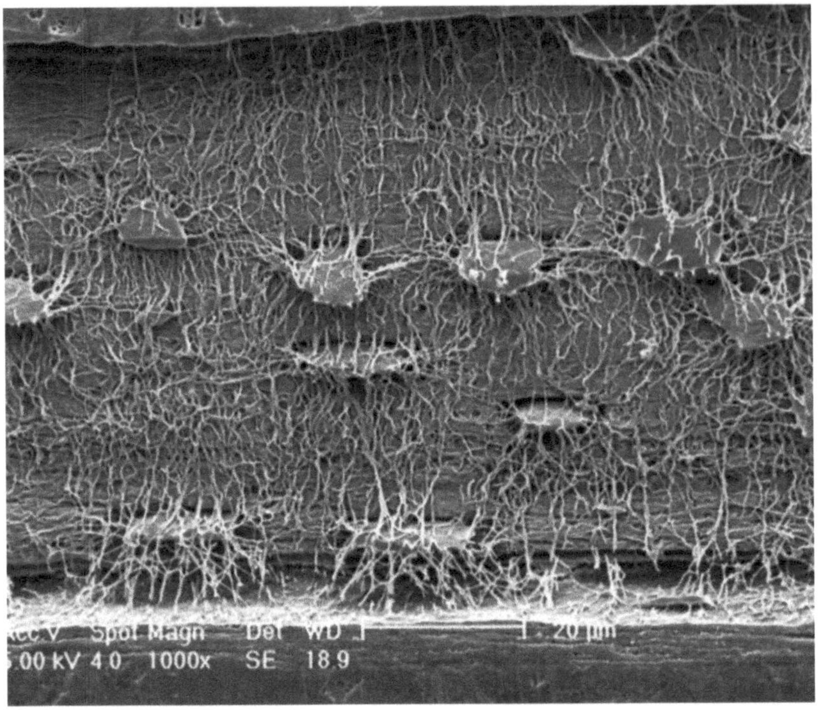

Figure 2.6 Osteocytes [46].

2.1.5.1 The basic multicellular unit

Harold Frost first noted that because tetracycline was fluorescent in bone, it could be used to label bone to measure the rates of bone formation [51]. Frost observed that the bone remodeling nearly always followed the same sequence and was performed by a team of osteoclasts and osteoblasts, which he termed the "basic multicellular unit (BMU)" (Fig. 2.7).

2.1.5.2 Sequence of bone remodeling

A BMU is not a permanent structure. It forms in response to a signal, performs its function, and disbands, leaving residual lining cells and osteocytes. Each BMU undergoes its functions in the same sequence: origination and organization of the BMU, activation of osteoclasts, resorption of old bone, recruitment of osteoblasts, formation of new bone matrix, and mineralization (see Fig. 2.8) [5,52]. Although bone formation follows bone resorption, the osteoblast maturation may be initiated before and during resorption. On the cancellous surfaces, a BMU does not only dissolve a pit on the surface, but it also spreads across the surface leaving behind an area filled with new bone [53]. In the cortex the osteoclasts form a cutting edge and bore a cylinder through the solid bone. Then osteoblasts follow, filling in the tunnel and leaving behind a small vascular channel.

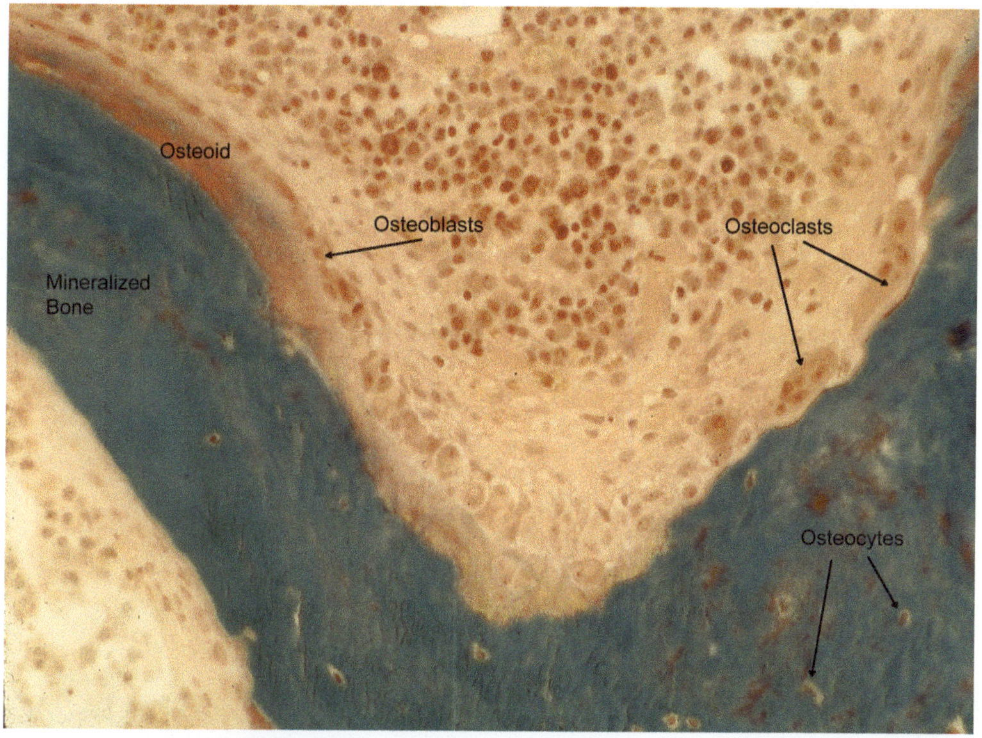

Figure 2.7 A basic multicellular unit.

The lifespan of a BMU is not well defined. Cortical BMUs can wander for months, usually in a straight line. Parfitt [54] estimates the duration as 2–8 months. This is harder to measure in cancellous bone because the two-dimensional sections do not capture the entire serpentine course of the BMU. More research is needed to understand the lifespan of a BMU and what controls its journey.

2.1.5.2.1 Origination

Some BMUs originate when the bone has been damaged (targeted remodeling) [6]; others may originate at random surfaces on the bone (stochastic remodeling) [5]. The osteocytes can initiate a BMU in response to microdamage or mechanical loading.

Osteocytes chronically inhibit lining cells by secreting sclerostin, and during origination of a BMU they stop secreting the sclerostin [55]. Also, osteocytes secrete paracrine factors when subjected to mechanical stimuli, e.g., IGF I expression increases 6 hours after mechanical loading [56]. Following more severe fatigue loading, osteocytes undergo apoptosis [50,57,58]. The apoptotic cells express RANK-L, which signals osteoclasts to resorb the bone.

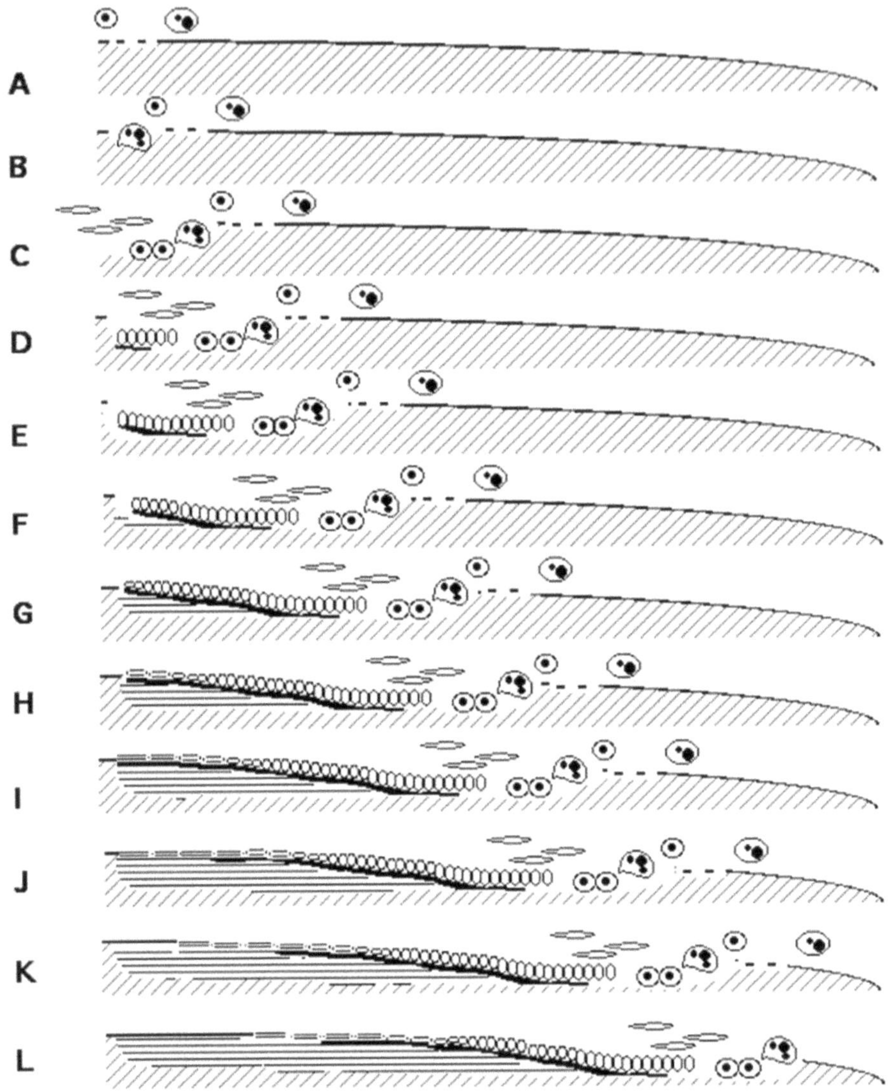

Figure 2.8 The remodeling sequence. (A) Origination, formation of multinucleated osteoclasts. (B) Osteoclasts resorb bone. (C) Reversal phase, preosteoblasts are multiplying. (D, E) Osteoblasts line cavity and start to make osteoid. (F—K) Bone formation, matrix formed and mineralized. (K, L) The remodeling cavity is filled at the original location, but the BMU continues to spread along the surface.

Mori and Burr [59] demonstrated an association between fatigue damage and intracortical remodeling. They anesthetized mature dogs and applied a cyclic load to the radius, which did not cause the animals to limp but did cause microscopic cracks. Eight days later an identical load was applied to the opposite radius and the animals were sacrificed. Histologic sections showed an equal number of cracks on each side. However, at the site with the earlier load, there was a significant increase in resorption cavities that were adjacent to the cracks. The temporal design of the study demonstrated that the resorption occurred after the fatigue damage.

Local and circulating hormones, cytokines, inflammatory factors, and growth factors certainly influence the early stages of the BMUs but it is not known which, if any, actually initiate resorption at a specific site. The hormones may increase the lifespan of the BMU, or the activity of cells, which will cause higher turnover but not necessarily an increased number of BMUs.

2.1.5.2.2 Activation

Activation is frequently confused with origination of a BMU [5]. A BMU originates at one point and then spreads. As it spreads the adjacent bone surface becomes activated. At the "cutting edge" the osteoclasts are recruited and preosteoblasts start proliferation and maturation. The lining cells change shape and form a canopy which is fused with endothelial cells, allowing access to bone collagen. The vasculature plays a necessary role in bone formation [60]. Osteocytes express RANK-L, which attracts more circulating preosteoclasts.

2.1.5.2.3 Resorption

Preosteoclasts fuse and form mature osteoclasts which resorb bone. At a given spot on the bone surface, resorption is rapid for the first 10 days, and continues for about a month. The osteoclasts eventually undergo apoptosis; the lifespan and activity of the osteoclasts determine the depth of the resorption cavity.

The apoptosis may be promoted by TGFß and estrogen [61]. The cells undergoing apoptosis have been located at the junction between the resorbing surface and the reversal surface, which suggests that the process might also be involved in signaling new osteoblasts.

Once activated, the osteoclast becomes polarized and undergoes cytoskeletal changes that allow it to attach to bone [62]. Small GTP-ases are necessary for these changes. The side of the osteoclast near the bone surface forms a "ruffled border" that will attach to integrins that were imbedded within mineralized bone matrix. The osteoclast seals off a circular surface of bone, creating a space between the bone and the ruffled border which is separated from the bone marrow, as shown in Fig. 2.9.

The integrins convey signals from the bone matrix to the osteoclast interior [63]. The osteoclast then pumps hydrogen ions into the resorbing space by a hydrogen ATP-ase (the same pump is used by renal tubular cells to secrete acid into the urine). These ions are generated from water and carbon dioxide by carbonic anhydrase, and the bicarbonate is secreted into the bone marrow. Chloride flows through a chloride channel to maintain electrical neutrality. The acid environment will then dissolve the

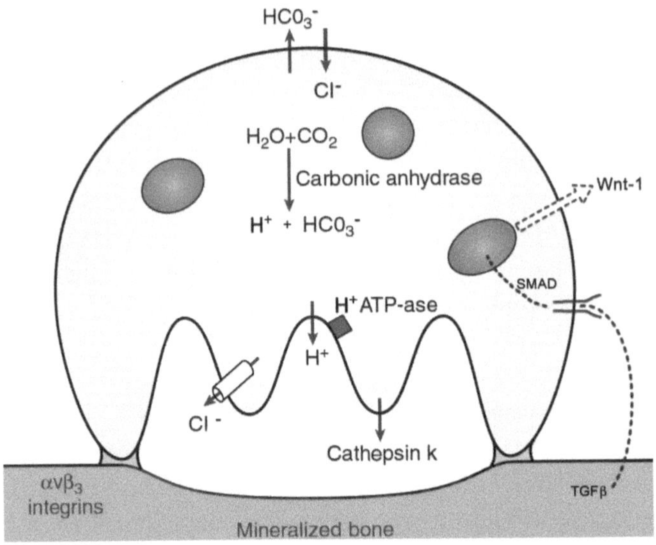

Figure 2.9 Osteoclast resorbing bone. The integrins allow attachment to the bone mineral and also signal the cell to form a ruffled border, creating a space into which the cell secretes cathepsin K. Hydrogen in pumped and chloride passively exits through a channel. Hydrogen is formed from water and carbon dioxide by carbonic anhydrase; this generates a bicarbonate ion that is secreted into the marrow. The acid environment activates TGFß which was deposited in the matrix; this can then bind to receptors on the osteoclast and signal the transcription of Wnt-1, which is secreted and can activate the signaling pathway on osteoblasts.

mineral from the bone. Also, the osteoclast secreted cathepsin K into the resorbing space; this degrades the collagen. The osteoclasts can also engulf debris through endocytosis, similar to macrophages, that are closely related cells.

The acid milieu of the resorbing space can activate the latent TGFß. The bone-derived TGFß can then activate receptors on the osteoclast surface, which signal via SMAD pathways and result in secretion of Wnt-1. The osteoblast precursors have Wnt receptors and will differentiate by Wnt signaling [64]. The osteoclasts also secrete several other factors that participate in osteoblast maturation, including sphingosine-1 phosphate, platelet-derived growth factor, interleukin-6, and annexin-II [65].

2.1.5.2.4 Reversal

Following osteoclast apoptosis, the bone surface is covered with cells that recently have been shown to have osteoblast markers. These cells function to clear out debris left by the osteoclasts and to prepare the surface for bone formation. They secrete collagenases and can also endocytose collagen fragments. During this phase a cement line is deposited, marking the end of the resorption and the beginning of the newly formed bone. The cement line can be seen histologically and the composition has been debated. These lines contain different protein concentrations than the lamellar bone, and they play a role in inhibiting crack propagation.

The reversal cells may be involved in the coupling between bone resorption and bone formation. A defect in this phase can result in bone loss [37,66,67].

2.1.5.2.5 Formation

During bone resorption, the preosteoblasts that were derived from the stromal stem cells have proliferated, and after the reversal phase a team of osteoblasts line the cavity along the cement lines. The osteoblasts form an osteoid matrix, and after about 14 days the matrix starts to mineralize. The osteoblasts continue to form osteoid until the cavity is filled, although in old age the cavities do not completely fill and each remodeling cycle results in loss of bone. The time to fill in the cavity at any given place on the surface is 124–168 days in normal individuals [68].

The apposition rate of matrix and of mineral is most rapid initially, as determined by measurements of osteoid seams that are very close to the cement lines. The initial rate is 1.2 μm/day, which gradually decreases to zero as the cavity is filled. The delay between osteoid formation and mineralization is 15 days initially, with an increase to 27 days, then a gradual decrease [68]. These rates were determined using reconstructive techniques. The average osteoid maturation time, which is the mean time interval between the onset of matrix deposition and the onset of mineralization, is 17–20 days [69].

At the bottom of the cavity, the new osteoblasts are plump and vigorous, they have tall nuclei, and they make a thick layer of osteoid. The cells then gradually flatten and finally become quiescent lining cells. Some of the osteoblasts differentiate into osteocytes and remain in the matrix. Adjacent osteoblasts appear to be the same age; plump and flat cells are not intermixed. This suggests that there are no replacement osteoblasts that join a team that is already filling the resorption space. Autoradiographic studies showing osteoblastic cells in teams of the same age confirm these observations [70]. As the BMU progresses, new osteoblasts are added only at the edge of the formation site.

The density of the osteoblasts at the formation site may vary. When the cells are more crowded they are taller and narrower, and they collectively can make more osteoid than when there are fewer cells. Parfitt et al. [71] have shown that osteoporotic patients have a normal rate of osteoid production per cell, but overall the wall thickness is decreased and the amount of newly formed bone is inadequate to fill the resorbed cavity. They suggest that when there are not enough osteoblasts, they must flatten out sooner to cover the bone.

The osteoblasts form collagen. This protein is formed from two collagen alpha-1 chains and one alpha-2 chain (derived from a different gene). The terminal ends are cleaved and can be used as serum markers for bone formation (P1NP, procollagen type 1 N-terminal propeptide). The tropocollagen molecules then precisely arrange into a fibril, as shown in Fig. 2.10. Pyridinoline or pyrrole rings form to covalently link the collagen into fibrils [72]. During bone resorption, the collagen is broken down by cathepsin K which cleaves the chains into fragments, but the crosslinks are stable and can be measured. They correlate with the rate of bone resorption.

The collagen fibrils then become fibers which are arranged in overlapping layers, giving the osteoid matrix a lamellar structure. When bone formation is abnormally high then the collagen is arranged in a more haphazard structure (woven bone) which is not as strong.

Collagen chains can also become glycosylated, which occurs in diabetes, and this can also weaken the structure [73].

Other proteins and growth factors are secreted into the osteoid along with the collagen [11,13].

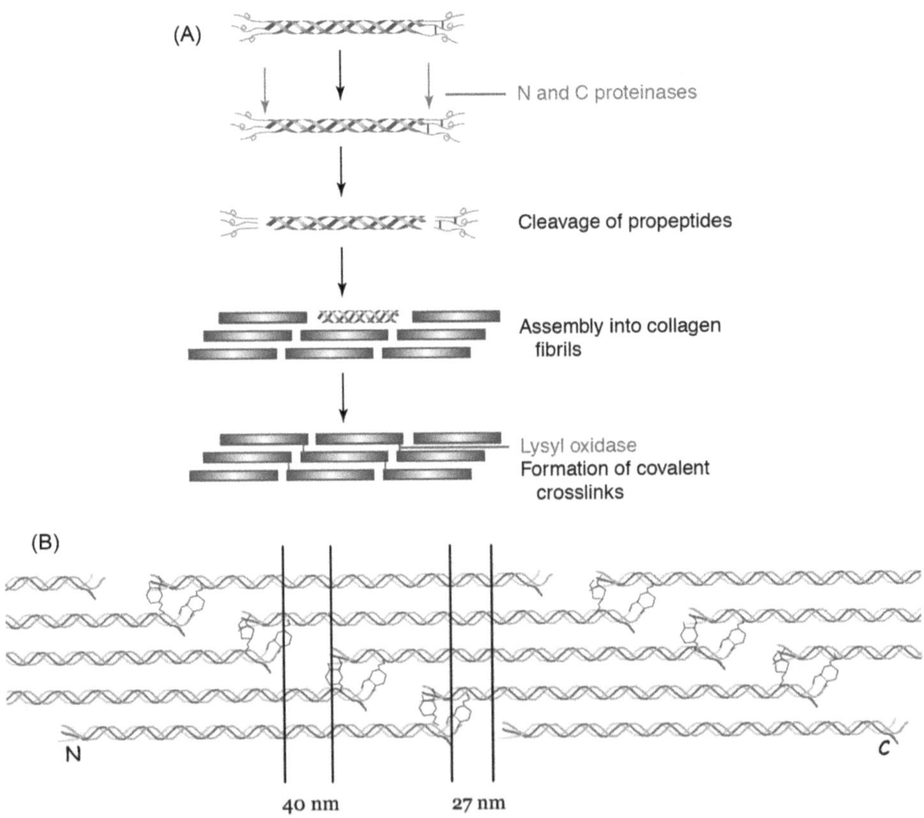

Figure 2.10 (A) Type I collagen comprises 90% of the protein in the bone matrix. The chains arrange in precise formations with overlap of 27 nm and space between ends of 40 nm. (B) Crosslinking is found at both N- and C-terminal ends.

2.1.5.2.6 Mineralization

In most situations (except osteomalacia), the average rate of osteoid formation and the rate of appearance of mineralization are the same and are measured by tetracycline labels. The labels are fluorescent. Tetracycline has the property of depositing where there is an active mineralization front. To measure the rate of bone formation, a patient is given tetracycline for 2 days and a repeat dose about 10 days later. Each dose deposits in a linear band along the interface between osteoid and mineralized osteoid. The distance between the labels is the volume of bone that was formed during the interval between labels. The length of labels throughout a biopsy sample reflects the surface that is forming bone (Fig. 2.11). This surface is termed the mineralizing surface and is normally about 6% of the cancellous bone surface.

The osteoid does not immediately mineralize, but "matures" for about 2 weeks and then mineral deposits between the collagen fibrils [74]. This mineralization of the osteoid matrix is a complexly controlled process [75]. The osteoblasts form small vesicles and secrete them into the matrix. These form the nidus of mineralization, which first occurs in the gaps between the tropocollagen molecules. The noncollagenous proteins influence the pattern of mineralization [11]. The calcium–phosphate product within the vasculature and extracellular fluids favors mineralization, which is prevented by circulating inhibitors, including pyrophosphate, matrix gal protein,

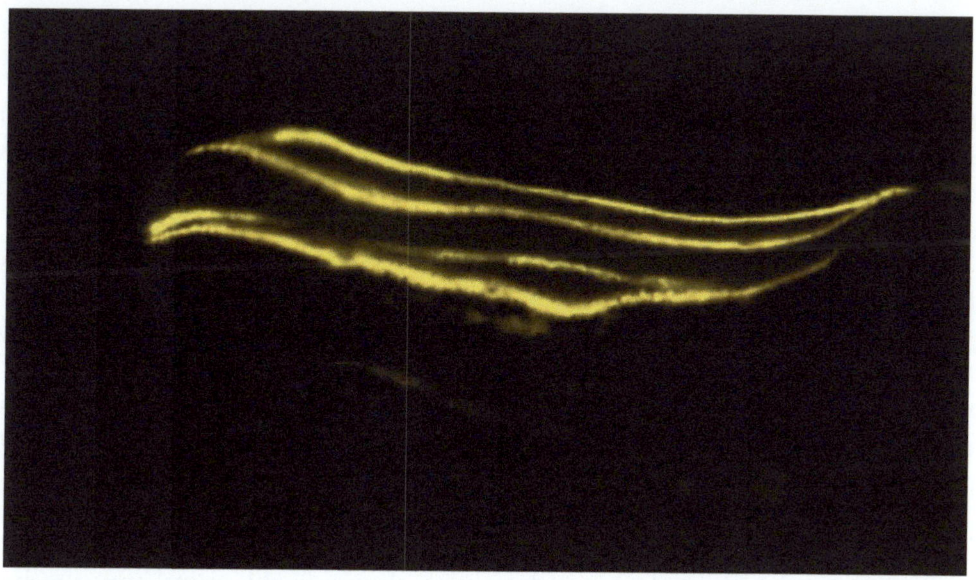

Figure 2.11 Tetracycline labels. This shows a bone surface undergoing formation. The patient was given four doses of tetracycline at 2, 12, 27, and 37 days before the biopsy.

osteonectin, fetuin A, and hydrogen sulfide. Therefore, the inhibitors must be removed within the bone to allow mineralization. One of the main inhibitors is pyrophosphate, which is cleaved by the alkaline phosphate secreted by osteoblasts and lining cells. Note that bisphosphonates are analogues of pyrophosphate that resist cleavage and can cause osteomalacia [76]. Patients with hypophosphatasia develop osteomalacia because they have low levels of alkaline phosphate [41].

The role of osteocalcin in mineralization remains uncertain but this protein contains carboxylated glutamic acid residues (gla) which bind to calcium. Vitamin K is necessary for this binding [77].

Crystal size and structure are also altered by concentrations of magnesium, sodium, and other minerals [78].

2.1.5.2.7 Reestablishing osteocyte network

Some of the osteoblasts further differentiate into osteocytes. As mineral is deposited, these cells become surrounded by mineralized matrix. Within their lacunae they remain active cells and extend cell processes through the bone to connect with neighboring osteocytes, and also the network extends to the bone surface and the lining cells [79].

The more mature osteocytes that are deeper in the matrix then start to secrete sclerostin which inhibits further bone formation [80].

2.1.5.2.8 Quiescence

Between remodeling cycles there is not much metabolic activity at the bone surfaces. The lining cells continue to make alkaline phosphatase to prevent pyrophosphate from entering the mineralized bone and dissolving the mineral. The osteocytes are active within the cannicular network, and are able to release mineral from the surrounding bone.

The mineralization within the newly formed osteoid continues to increase gradually for a prolonged time [81]. The length of time is uncertain but patients with osteoporosis who are treated with medicines that block bone formation increase density for at least 3 years before the density reaches a plateau. Older bone has more densely packed crystals, and microradiographic studies have shown that newly formed bone may be 25% less dense than older bone [82]. Backscattered electron micrographs demonstrate differences in the mineralization of osteoid (Fig. 2.12).

As individuals age, the interstitial bone (bone between newly remodeled osteons) becomes older and more densely mineralized [83,84]. The increased mineralization seen with more densely packed crystals or with change in the crystal structure itself may have several consequences. Schaffler et al. [85] reported observations of microcracks, which increased exponentially with aging. The overwhelming majority of microcracks (87%) were observed within the interstitial bone. Another consequence

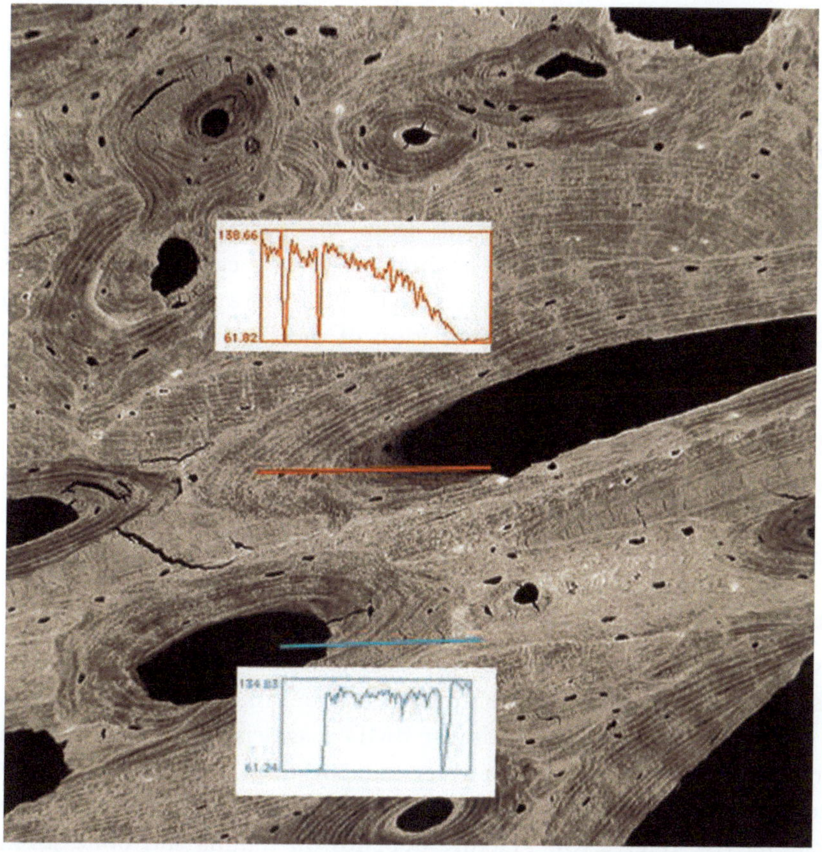

Figure 2.12 Backscattered electron micrograph of bone, showing different densities. The black regions are bone marrow. Line A is though an osteon that is still forming; the newest bone with darkest color is least mineralized, as shown in the corresponding graph above the line. Note the drop in mineralization when the line crosses over an osteocyte. As bone becomes older (further from the marrow) the density increases. Line B crosses a mature osteon and there is an abrupt edge at the Haversian canal, and the right side of line B shows the high bone density of the oldest interstitial bone.

of aging mineral is that it has less water and the minerals are less able to exchange with extracellular fluid [7].

2.1.6 Fracture repair

2.1.6.1 Stress fractures

Stress fractures are incomplete cracks caused by repetitive microdamage to the bone. Classic examples are "march fractures" seen in military recruits during basic training [86], or in athletes training for marathons. These fractures heal by forming woven bone which then undergoes bone remodeling, the osteoclasts resorb the damaged bone and osteoblasts form new bone [87]. If the process of remodeling cannot keep up with the damage then the stress fractures can eventually consolidate and cause a complete fracture.

2.1.6.2 Complete fractures

Fracture repair is a complex process [88]. Initially the gap between bone fragments is filled with blood clot. Fibroblastic cells from the periosteum will proliferate and secrete collagen in a rapid haphazard manner to form a callus which can bridge the gap and stabilize the bone. Chondrocytes then will form a layer of cartilage similar to the growth plate, and there is a recapitulation of the endochondrial bone formation. The chondrocytes line up, hypertrophy, undergo apoptosis, and marrow fills the spaces that were occupied by chondroblasts. The cartilage becomes calcified. Then osteoclasts will resorb calcified cartilage and osteoblasts form normal lamellar bone, eventually restoring the bone to its former shape and size. Signaling by the NOTCH pathway is necessary for repair of the fractures; this signaling is also important in maintaining the stem cell niche [89].

2.1.7 Aspects of bone strength

BMD, as measured by dual-energy X-ray absorptiometry (DEXA) is the most commonly used clinical test to assess bone strength and the risk of fracture. Studies involving millions of subjects have shown that lower BMD is associated with higher fracture risk [90]. For example, in elderly women every standard deviation decrease in the BMD is associated with 2.6 times the risk of a hip fracture. However, BMD does not explain all of the fracture risk (Fig. 2.13). Fracture depends on trauma and bone strength. The degree of trauma is a recognized factor, but too often bone strength is considered to be the BMD. But BMD is an imperfect predictor of fracture. For example, with normal aging, the fracture rate increases more rapidly than the rate of bone loss. A white woman with no clinical risks and body mass index of 23 with BMD T-score of −2.5 would have a hip fracture incidence of 2.2%/decade at age 60, but the risk would be 6.8% at age 80 (using the FRAX calculator at: https://www.shef.ac.uk/FRAX).

The bone density fails to predict bone failure in other clinical situations as well [91]. For example, patients with osteopetrosis have extremely high bone density, however, they also suffer from increased fracture rate because the bone quality is poor. Patients with diabetes also have more fractures than predicted by bone density.

Bone quality could be defined as the accumulation of aspects of bone that contribute to bone strength but are not measured by bone density [92,93]. Bone density is determined by the volume and the mineralization density of the bone, which are determined by growth, modeling, and remodeling. The rate of remodeling has two components, the rate of formation and the rate of resorption. If these are equal, then the term "turnover" is appropriate and would be measured by either one. Usually,

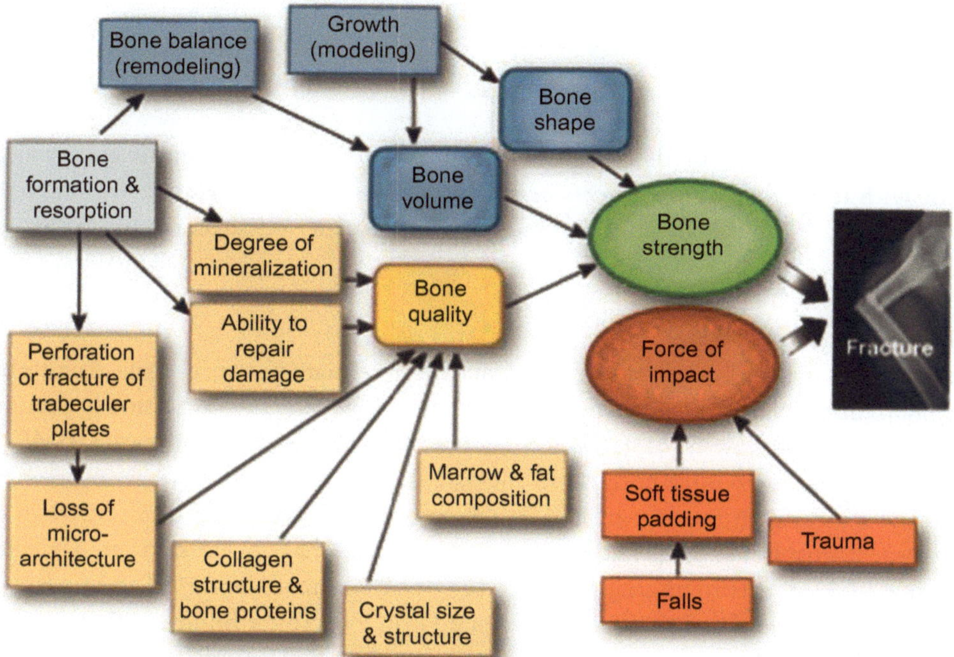

Figure 2.13 Factors that influence the risk of fracture. Bone mineral density is determined by both the bone volume and the degree of mineralization.

due to the complex intracellular communication, bone formation is coupled to resorption and these rates are similar. However, "turnover" is ambiguous when the formation and resorption are not coupled. For example, with myeloma the bone resorption is high but formation is low. In the year postweaning, women have high formation and low resorption.

2.1.7.1 Bone shape

The shape of the bone is determined by hormonal, nutritional, mechanical, and hereditary factors during growth. The diameter of the long bones continues to expand throughout life, although slowly after the maximum height is achieved. This compensates for the decreased bone mass and the deterioration of the material properties of bone with aging. Long bones are essentially like cylinders, and with the same amount of material, the resistance to bending is proportional to the fourth power of the distance from the center [2,92].

2.1.7.2 Bone volume

At the microscopic level bone shape continues to change to accommodate mechanical forces through bone modeling [94]. Bone formation can be more active on the side of a trabecular that experiences greater stress, and resorption more active on trabecular that have fewer stresses. This results in the changes seen in the proximal femur as shown in Fig. 2.3, where the bone volume in the "Ward's triangle" is lost more rapidly than in other locations [15].

Bone remodeling, as described above, removes packets of bone and replaces them with new bone. This process can result in loss of bone volume if the amount replaced is less than the amount formed (which is usually what happens with natural aging) [95].

2.1.7.3 Mineralization density

The BMD that is measured by DEXA cannot differentiate between bone volume and mineralization density. Thus there is low bone remodeling, the bone slowly accumulates mineral and loses water, which increases the density, causing the BMD to increase [96]. Many people confuse an increase in BMD with an increase in bone volume and interpret an increase in BMD as bone growth when it really is only hardening the existing bone. Mineralization density is measured by backscattered electron imaging [97] or microradiology (Fig. 2.12). The optimal degree of mineralization density depends on the function of the bone [7,98,99]. Some bones, such as those in the ear, have very high mineralization density in order to transmit noise, but they are brittle. Low mineralization density results in less stiffness which could lead to fracture, but high density results in less toughness that leads to fracture in different situations.

2.1.7.4 Microarchitecture

Other material properties of bone are also determined by the rate of bone formation and resorption. The microarchitecture, or the amount of connectivity of the trabecular plates, is directly determined by bone resorption rate and the likelihood of perforation [100]. Bone with the same overall volume that has more connectivity will be stronger. These properties are measured by high-resolution imaging such as microcomputed tomography [95,101]. These techniques can tell the dimensions of the trabeculae, whether they are connected, and the thickness of the cortex, all of which contribute to bone strength.

2.1.7.5 Collagen structure

Collagen structure, orientation, and crosslinking are important for bone strength. This may be independent of bone turnover. Several hereditary diseases, such as osteogenesis imperfecta, result in abnormal collagen structure. Diabetes and aging result in glycation end products within bone, which increases crosslinking but reduces strength [102]. The fibrils can be examined by electron microscopy. The crosslinking is measured with biochemistry or with Fourier transform infrared (FTIR) imaging, which can also measure other bone proteins that may play a role in bone strength [103].

D-periodicity is measured by scanning collagen fibrils at high resolution with atomic force microscopy. Normally collagen fibrils line up in precise repetitive patterns, forming stripes, and D-periodicity is the width of the stripe.

Imaging can evaluate collagen fiber arrangement with scanning electron microscopy, or with atomic force microscopy. Nuclear magnetic resonance spectroscopy measures the water that is bound to collagen molecules. The bound water decreases with aging and is strongly related to bone toughness [104].

2.1.7.6 Ability to repair damage

The number of microcracks and the accumulation of microdamage can also contribute to bone strength, and this is related to the bone turnover [102]. Bones with low turnover rates have more microcracks and the mineralization density is more homogeneous [7,105,106]. This can lead to increased propagation of a crack and eventually fracture [57]. These can be measured by special staining techniques, such as fuchsin red staining [107].

2.1.7.7 Crystal characteristics

The crystal structure is a material property that can change the bone strength [78]. Bones with larger crystals are more brittle. This is measured by Raman spectroscopy [103].

2.1.7.8 Bone marrow

Bone as an organ also contains marrow and fat. The contribution of fat to the mechanical strength of bone has not been studied very extensively. In some patients with severe osteoporosis, the fat cells themselves must be bearing a significant amount of the mechanical loading.

2.1.7.9 Overall bone strength

Biomechanical testing can be performed on a bone or a sample of bone, and the results normalized for bone density. The testing can be done with variously applied forces (bending, torsion, compression) and under different conditions (changing frequency and amplitude). The stiffness of bone is related to the amount of deformation caused by a force, and the toughness reflects the force required to complete failure of the bone. None of these tests are noninvasive and thus are done only in animal studies or on bone biopsies [2].

Nanoindentation measures the hardness of the bone (the force required to make a small indentation with a diamond point) [108].

2.2 PHARMACEUTICAL INTERVENTION

The main focus of this section is on the pharmaceutical medications that have been approved for osteoporosis, and how they affect bone quality. In addition, some toxins or agents which are used for other conditions that have effects on the bone will be briefly discussed. Other bone diseases, such as osteomalacia, osteosclerosis, or fibrous dysplasia, have complex pathophysiology and different treatments which are beyond the scope of this chapter.

But first it is important to understand how osteoporosis develops. Many of the medicines used to treat osteoporosis prevent the bone deterioration that occurs with aging or disease, without necessarily improving the bone strength.

2.2.1 Bone loss with aging or disease

Young healthy cancellous bone forms a well-connected lattice, with plate-shaped trabeculae. Remodeling does not necessarily change this overall structure, but when resorption exceeds formation, the bone loss leads to thinning of the trabecular plates and/or to perforations (Fig. 2.14) [95,109]. For the same amount of bone loss, the mechanical strength of the bone is impaired to a greater extent if the plate perforation causes structural loss.

Plates can perforate if the resorption depth of one BMU is deeper than the thickness of the plate, or if two BMUs on opposite sides of the plate resorb bone at the same time (Fig. 2.15). In any case, once the bone has perforated, further bone loss will be amplified because there is no more scaffolding to support a team of osteoblasts.

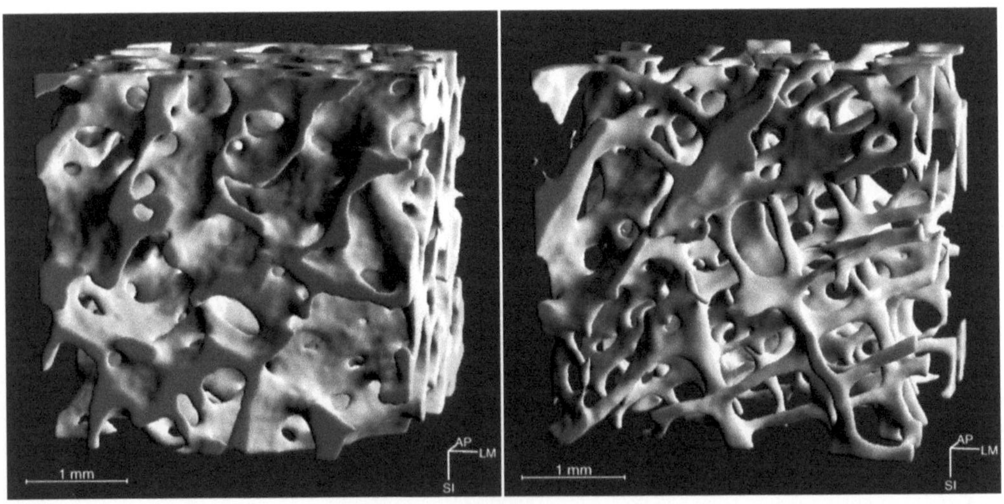

Figure 2.14 Microcomputed tomography of bone from young person (left) and older person (right) [109].

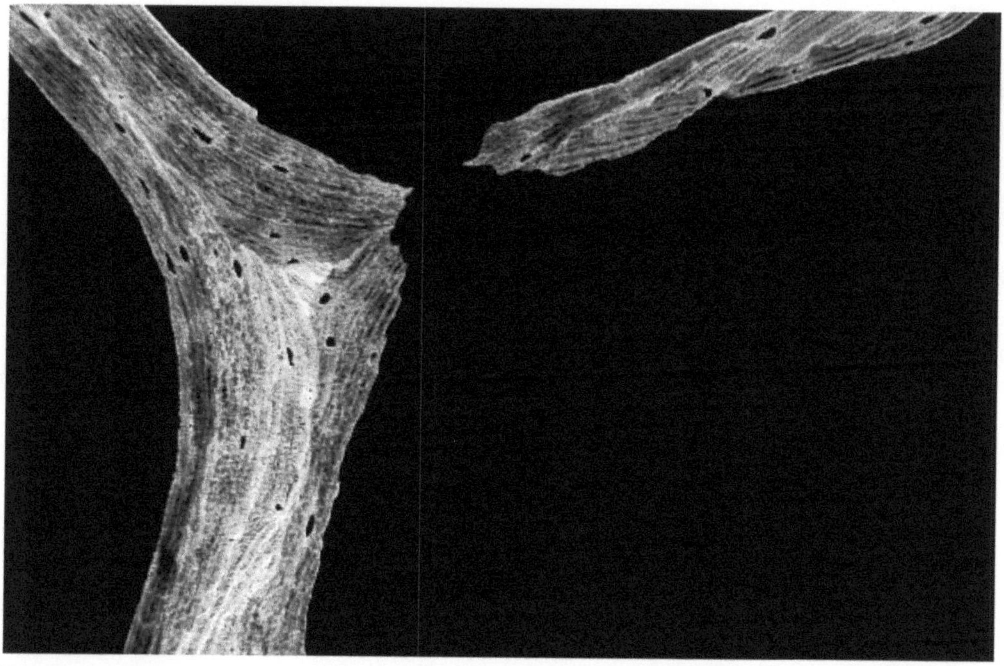

Figure 2.15 Trabecular perforation caused by resorption from both sides.

Instead of a cement line, there is empty marrow space. By this process, the plate-shaped trabecular bone is converted into a rod-shaped structure with loss of surface available for formation [7].

Once the plates have become rods, they may become disconnected. This has been demonstrated by scanning electron micrographs [110] and by examination of thick, superficially stained bone sections [111]. The isolated trabecular rods have no mechanical stimuli and are severed from the osteocyte network, and they are rapidly resorbed [112].

Thus there can be a vicious cycle of bone loss: as there is less and less bone to bear the body weight, the remaining bone is more likely to sustain damage, which increases bone resorption and further bone loss occurs. If the osteoblast response is not normally vigorous, then the bone loss proceeds even more quickly.

2.2.2 Actions of systemic hormones and local cytokines

2.2.2.1 Estrogen

New studies have not tarnished the important role of estrogen in maintaining bone health. Even in males, estrogens are important regulators of bone resorption, and testosterone is converted into estrogen by aromatases. Several mechanisms are involved: (1) estrogen increases osteoclast apoptosis; (2) by suppressing interleukins and proinflammatory cytokine expression in bone marrow cells, estrogen decreases the number of osteoclasts; (3) by inhibiting the production of RANK-ligand, estrogen reduces the number and activity of osteoclasts; and (4) by increasing stromal cell/osteoblast cell expression of TGFß, estrogen inhibits osteoclast activity. Estrogen also has some positive effects on bone formation by acting as a mitogen to cells early in the osteoblast line, reducing apoptosis of osteoblasts, and increasing expression of TGFβ, bone morphogenetic proteins, and IGF-I [113].

There may be anabolic as well as antiresorptive effects of very high-dose estrogen. In one study from 1999 (which is unlikely to be repeated), high doses of estrogen (100 mg every 6 months) were implanted into postmenopausal women for at least 14 years, and bone biopsies showed evidence of increased wall thickness [114]. These women also had high bone density, and the cortical width was substantially higher than in a group of untreated women (2.29 ± 0.78 mm vs 1.36 ± 0.60 mm) [115]. Studies of conventional doses of estrogen showed no anabolic effects, but suggested lower resorption [116].

Women who go through natural menopause lose bone rapidly, and imaging techniques can detect perforations of trabecular walls [101] and loss of cortical thickness. These changes are reversible with estrogen replacement.

2.2.2.2 Glucocorticosteroids

The steroid hormones synthesized in the adrenal cortex have powerful systemic actions on all systems. Prednisone, the synthetic analogue, is widely used to treat immune diseases, organ transplantation, and asthma. These hormones cause devastating loss of bone mineral and increase in fracture rates [117,118]. In the past it was thought that they increased bone resorption rates. Now it has been shown that the major physiologic action of these steroids is to inhibit bone formation [119]. A study of healthy men found that prednisolone decreased bone density up to 7.5% within 6 months. The osteocalcin decreased dramatically but there was no change in markers of bone resorption [119]. This effect is so strong that decreased markers of bone formation can be detected in healthy volunteer subjects after 1 week of oral prednisone. Contrary to popular opinion, the direct effect of glucocorticoids on osteoclasts is actually an inhibition of resorption [21,120].

Fractures occur even in patients with normal bone density (Fig. 2.16), which indicates that glucocorticosteroids have negative effects on the quality of bone in addition to causing loss of bone mass. This could be due to the fact that the drugs increase apoptosis of osteocytes [121]. Without the actions of osteocytes to direct bone remodeling, the bone loses strength.

The low bone formation and poorly functioning bone cells also slow healing of fractures. Prednisone also decreases gastrointestinal absorption of calcium, reducing mineral availability to the bone.

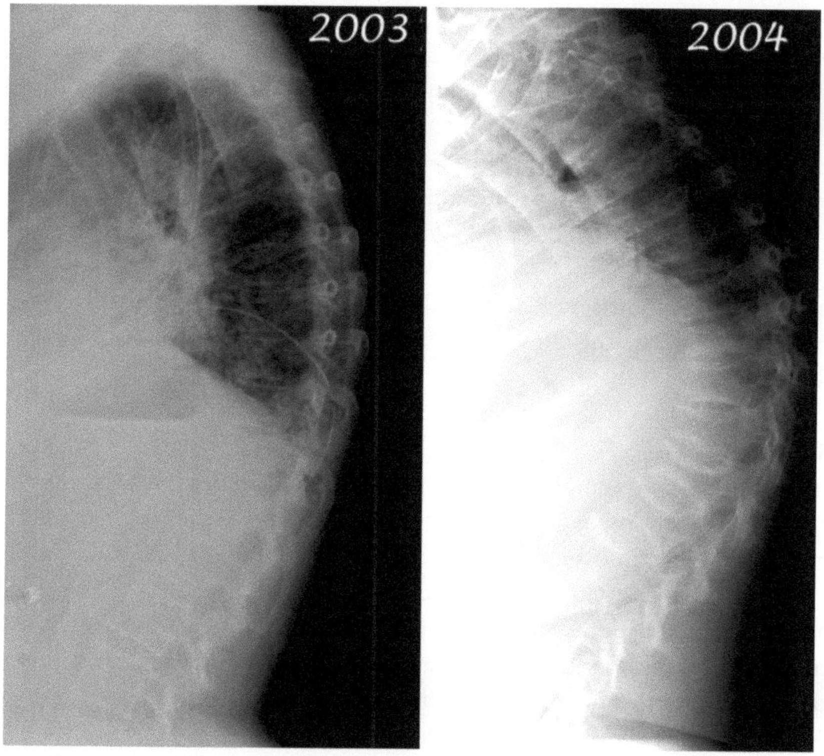

Figure 2.16 Effect of prednisone treatment in a patient who had a transplant. In 2003 the bone density was normal. A year later she had multiple vertebral compression fractures.

2.2.2.3 Thyroid

Thyroid hormone increases the metabolic rates of both the osteoclasts and the osteoblasts [122]. As a result there is a higher rate of bone resorption, and the resorption cavities fill more rapidly. The depth of resorption is normal, but the osteoblasts do not completely fill the cavity. There is also increased origination of BMUs with a higher percentage of surface forming or resorbing bone. Since each BMU results in a loss of bone, and there are increased surfaces engaged in bone remodeling, there will be loss of bone volume. This high turnover also results in bone that has lower mineralization density. The bone density by DEXA decreases, and the fracture risk is increased [123].

2.2.2.4 Parathyroid

Parathyroid hormone has complex effects on bone cells, which depend on the clinical circumstances as well as the level of hormone [124,125]. In primary hyperparathyroidism caused by an adenoma the continuous hypersecretion of PTH strongly increases bone resorption, but the effect is not directly on the osteoclasts. The osteoblasts and osteocytes express RANK-L when exposed to PTH. The increased resorption could increase subsequent osteoblast formation by a coupling mechanism, but the PTH could also directly increase activity of these cells. Through unknown mechanisms PTH increases trabecular bone volume by increasing the trabecular width, but at the same time causes increased cortical porosity and resorption at the endocortical surface. In secondary hyperparathyroidism from chronic kidney disease, the PTH levels become very high. In some cases, the bone samples show no distinction between cortical and trabecular bone. Patients with hyperparathyroidism have an increased fracture risk.

When PTH is administered as a daily subcutaneous injection, causing a cyclic spike in the PTH levels, the effect is different [126]. This pharmacological effect is discussed below.

2.2.2.5 Calcitonin

Calcitonin is a hormone secreted by the thyroid gland in response to hypercalcemia. Osteoclasts have receptors for calcitonin; when activated the cells shrink from the bone surface and stop resorbing bone, thereby reducing serum calcium. This drug does not have as strong antiresoprtive action as other medications.

In clinical trials of patients with osteoporosis or steroid osteoporosis, the vertebral fracture rate is decreased compared to placebo [127]. The hip fracture rates have not been shown to decrease. Calcitonin also has been used to block osteoclast resorption in Paget's disease, but currently the stronger medications are preferred.

2.2.2.6 1,25 $(OH)_2$-Cholecalciferol (1,25D)

This active form of vitamin D is a systemic secosteroid that has a final hydroxylation step in the renal tubules in a reaction that is regulated by calcium, PTH, FGF23, and several other factors. The osteoblast secretion of osteocalcin and FGF23 are increased by 1,25D, but there is no increase in the bone formation rates in patients treated with this drug [128]. 1,25D also increases the formation of preosteoblasts, thereby increasing bone resorption. The major effects on bone are to supply adequate serum levels of calcium and phosphate for mineralization. Patients with low 1,25D levels develop osteomalacia, with increased unmineralized osteoid, and this is reversed with treatment. The effect is probably not directly on the cells, because the osteomalacia can also be reversed with infusions of calcium.

In patients with secondary hyperparathyroidism, the net effect of 1,25D is to reduce bone formation and resorption, because this hormone lowers serum PTH levels.

2.2.2.7 Insulin and insulin-like growth factor

The skeleton consumes a large amount of energy, especially during remodeling, so it is not surprising that hormones that regulate energy would also effect the bone [129].

Osteoblasts have insulin receptors. IGF-1 is synthesized in the liver in response to growth hormone, but it is also a local hormone that can be secreted by the osteocytes. The IGF-1 from osteocytes is necessary for bone mechanosensitivity [130]. IGF-1 is also a stimulator of osteoblast proliferation. Osteoblast precursors require autophagy for differentiation, and this is stimulated by IFG-1 [131].

2.2.2.8 Serotonin

A recent series of genetic studies has suggested a role for gut-derived serotonin in the control of bone formation [88,132]. Mice with knockout of the LRP5, as well as humans with inactivating mutation of LRP5, have increased serum serotonin levels and serious osteoporosis. Serotonin receptors were identified in the osteoblasts, and when activated they inhibited osteoblast activity.

2.2.2.9 Local cytokines

Many of the cytokines that are increased during inflammation also have skeletal effects, mostly to increase bone resorption.

Interleukin 6 is one of the more important factors derived from marrow cells, that can stimulate the osteoblasts to form RANK-L, thus leading to increased bone resorption. Estrogen inhibits the IL-6 production, and tocilzumab (an inhibitor used to treat rheumatoid arthritis) increases the bone formation and stabilizes the bone density [133,134].

Tumor necrosis factor (TNF) is another important cytokine that increases bone resorption via the RANK-L pathway. In addition, TNF is a regulator of DKK-1, an inhibitor of the Wnt-signaling pathway, blocking osteoblast function and causing further decreases in bone resorption because the osteoblasts do not secrete osteoprotegerin. Patients treated with TNF-inhibitors show increases in bone density [135,136]

2.2.3 Calcium supplementation

Calcium supplements are frequently prescribed for patients with metabolic bone disease. Many clinical trials have been done in patients with osteoporosis, with results that are still debated [137–139]. The most consistent findings are that fracture rates are decreased in those women who had inadequate calcium intake before the study. Calcium is necessary for mineralization. Calcium also indirectly reduces bone resorption by decreasing PTH levels. The osteoblasts have calcium-sensing receptors on the surface, but it is not clear if these modify the cellular actions or the bone strength.

2.2.4 Bone formation with osteoporosis medications

Fig. 2.17 shows the bone formation rates in normal individuals and in patients with osteoporosis with or without bisphosphonate therapy. The effect of treatment with osteoporosis drugs from clinical trials is also shown.

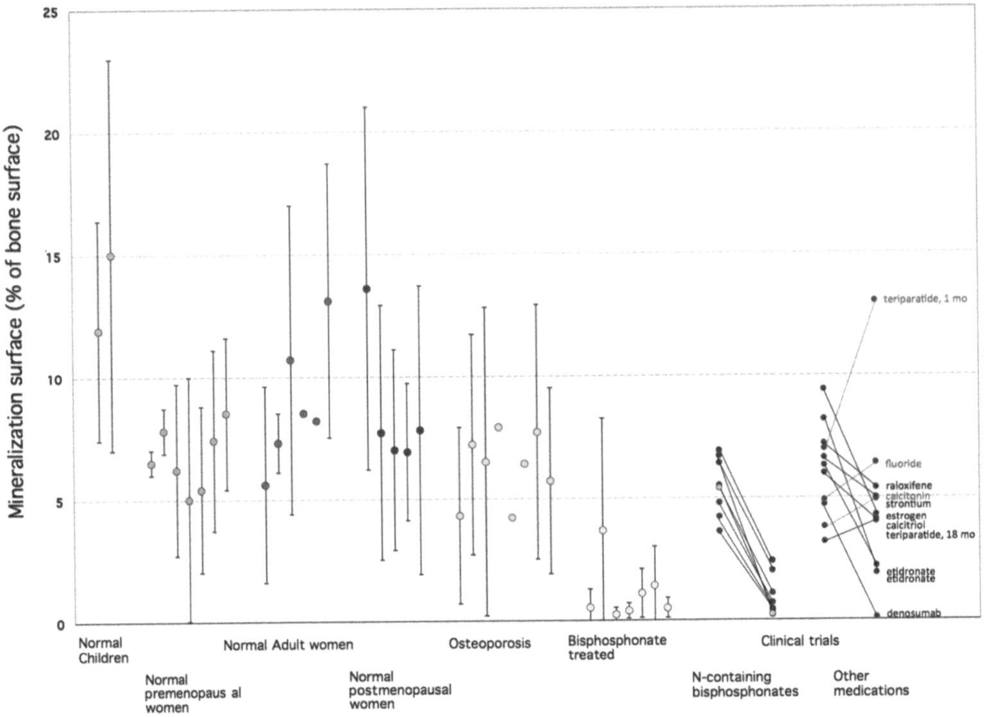

Figure 2.17 Bone formation from clinical bone biopsies of normal women, women with osteoporosis, and clinical trials of medications. Each dot is a separate study, and the error bars are one standard deviation.

2.2.5 Raloxifene

Raloxifene is a medication which activates the estrogen receptors on bone cells, and the effects on the skeleton are similar to those seen with estrogen. Clinical trials in patients with osteoporosis show decreased vertebral fracture rate, with modest increases in the bone density [140,141].

Histomorphology studies showed moderate decreases in the bone formation rate (Fig. 2.17) [142]. The bone resorption rate is not measured directly by this method, but a decrease is implied by the fact that formation decreased but bone mass increased. Also, the biochemical markers for bone resorption (urine NTX) decrease with raloxifene [140]. Raloxifene has been shown to reduce the sclerostin levels [143].

Raloxifene does not interfere with fracture healing. In a rat spinal arthrodesis model, raloxifene mildly suppressed bone remodeling but did not inhibit the ossification process, leading to a fusion mass comparable to that of sham animals. In the same model, bisphosphonates inhibited the endochondrial ossification and graft bone resorption [144]. Also, the fatigue life was not worsened with raloxifene [145].

Microradiography studies from bone biopsies in women with osteoporosis show an increase in the mineralization density after treatment with raloxifene. This is consistent with the decreased bone turnover in these patients [146].

Biomechanical studies in animal models show increased stiffness and toughness with raloxifene treatment [108].

With raloxifene nanoindentation studies show increased hardness in an ovine [108] and a canine [147] model. Infrared imaging in biopsies from humans showed no difference in the mineral crystallinity [103]. In sheep with osteoporosis caused by metabolic acidosis, FTIR imaging after raloxifene treatment showed decreased mineral/matrix ratio, increased crystallinity, and increased collagen maturity. The carbonate content was decreased compared to nontreated sheep [108,148].

Studies of the collagen fibrils measure the distance between bands (D-periodicity) [10]. In rats with CKD treated with vehicle the D-periodicity was slightly lower and with raloxifene it was slightly higher than normal. This is consistent with raloxifene treatment in a canine study [149]. In a canine model ex vivo raloxifene increased the matrix-bound water, which improves the bone toughness [149]. A new in vivo technique, ultrashort echotime magnetic resonance imaging was used to show that raloxifene-treated beagles had higher bound water [150]. Although it is not yet clear how this increases bone toughness, it is possible that raloxifene weakens the collagen hydroxyapatite bonding [104], which changes the collagen spacing and reduces formation of microcracks.

2.2.6 Bisphosphonates

Bisphosphonates are the most widely used medications to prevent or treat osteoporosis. They are analogues of pyrophosphate, which is an important endogenous inhibitor of ectopic mineralization. Alkaline phosphatase hydrolyzes the pyrophosphate and prevents it from entering bone mineral. Substitution of carbon for an oxygen molecule results in bisphosphonates, which cannot be hydrolyzed and therefore readily enter bone mineral, where they bind avidly [151,152].

All bisphosphonates have the phosphate—carbon—phosphate structure, with side chains bonded to the carbon. These side chains confer different properties which affect the ability to resorb bone with a very large range of potencies. Compared to etidronate, alendronate is 100-fold more potent and zoledronic acid 10,000-fold more potent. The compounds vary both in tightness of binding to hydroxyapatite and to binding to enzymes within the osteoclast [153].

The first bisphosphonates to be developed, etidronate and clodronate, are taken up by osteoclasts and metabolized into nonfunctional analogues of ATP that disrupt several cellular processes, leading to apoptosis of osteoclasts. Etidronate inhibits mineralization with a similar potency to pyrophosphate. As a result, it causes osteomalacia when used for longer than 6 months, and is no longer used in clinical practice. Nitrogen-containing bisphosphonates have a different mechanism of action. They bind to bone hydroxyapatite, and the closer they bind the longer they remain in the bone. Zoledronate binds with the highest affinity, followed by alendronate, ibandronate, risedronate, etidronate, and finally, clodronate. The bisphosphonates remain in the skeleton for many years. For example, the half-life of alendronate is more than 10 years [153].

Because the drugs are bound to the calcium, osteoclasts are the major cells that are exposed to these drugs. The bisphosphonates enter the cell by fluid-phase endocytosis. The intracellular nitrogen-containing bisphosphonates inhibit farnesyl pyrophosphate synthase, an enzyme in the mevalonate pathway that is necessary for osteoclast ruffled border formation. Zoledronate and risedonate fit more closely into the site (and, therefore, inhibit bone resorption at a lower dose) than do ibandronate, pamidronate, or alendronate. Because nitrogen-containing bisphosphonates are effective at doses several orders of magnitude below those required for etidronate, they do not inhibit mineralization to the extent that osteomalacia develops [153,154].

2.2.6.1 Short-term effects

In many large, randomized clinical trials, rates of osteoporotic fractures are reduced by about 50% in patients treated with bisphosphonates [155–158]. In all these studies there is a significant increase in the BMD, usually more improvement in the spine than in the hip or radius. These medications markedly decrease the bone resorption rate by direct inhibition of osteoclasts. It is likely that these medications prevent fractures because they prevent the microarchitectural deterioration that occurs with untreated osteoporosis. In bone biopsies from a clinical trial, micro-CT analysis showed stable bone structure in the risedronate-treated patients but deterioration in the placebo-treated patients [159].

Although they consistently increase the bone density, the change in bone volume, as measured from bone biopsies, is not significant in most studies [160]. The increased bone density is predominantly due to further mineralization of the bone matrix, as more water molecules are replaced by mineral [161].

The osteoblasts are not directly inhibited, and during the first 3–6 months the bone continues to fill resorption cavities that were present when drug initiated, thus modestly increasing the bone volume. However, when bone resorption ceases, the formation of new osteoblast teams will eventually stop, and in biopsies from bisphosphonate-treated patients the bone formation is about 90% lower than before therapy (see Fig. 2.17) [160]. The biochemical markers of bone resorption (C-telopeptide and N-telopeptide) decrease rapidly after initiation of bisphosphonates, but the markers of bone formation (bone alkaline phosphatase and P1NP) decrease gradually over 6 months and then reach a low level [162]. These findings suggest that the initial increase in bone volume would be greater if the initial volume of resorption cavities were high. This has been shown in patients with osteoporosis, in whom the improvement in bone density is greater with those who had either high bone turnover rates or increased loss of bone density prior to treatment [163,164].

Biochemical testing shows increased stiffness and increased force to fracture. A primate study showed improved strength as measured by three-point bending and compression to failure [165]. In sheep with osteoporosis caused by metabolic acidosis, zoledronic acid decreased the yield strain, increased mineralization on the bone surface, and did not alter the collagen crosslinking network or the crystallinity measured by FRIR [108]. In osteoporotic patients with pertrochanteric hip fractures treated with external fixation, a randomized trial of alendronate showed that after 3 months there was a twofold increase in extraction torque of the pins [166].

2.2.6.2 Long-term effects

With increased duration of bisphosphonate exposure, the bone formation seen by tetracycline-labeled bone biopsies remains suppressed. As many as 30% of osteoporotic patients have no measurable bone formation after 5 years of bisphosphonate therapy [167].

Decreased bone turnover leads to more mineralization. Backscattered electron microscopy and microradiography show increased mineralization density [168,169]. This may lead to more brittle bone.

The reduced turnover also results in accumulation of microcracks seen in bone biopsies from patients after 5 years of alendronate [170], although another did not find the increase was significant [167]. In beagles, microdamage accumulation after bisphosphonates was associated with increased stiffness but reduced toughness [105,171].

In osteoporotic patients, the risk of atypical femoral fractures (Fig. 2.18) increases with the duration of bisphosphonate use. The risk in patients treated for 1–2 years is 1.78/100,000/year and increases to 113.1/100,000/year after 8 years [172]. In some patients a focal thickening of the lateral cortical bone precedes the fracture. There may be a fracture line resembling a stress fracture. Patients often feel painful aching in the thigh, and the fractures occur spontaneously or with mild trauma. If bisphosphonates are continued, over half experience another fracture on the contralateral femur. Bone biopsies near the fracture site show a layer of debris which is not resorbed, surrounded by bone with poor bone formation. Patients of Asian heritage have a higher risk of developing these fractures. Also, patients with a more valgus femoral shaft angle are more prone to the atypical fractures.

Biomechanical studies of bone properties after alendronate treatment may explain these findings. In a rat model long-term pamidronate caused a decrease in ultimate load to failure of the femur [173]. Ribs from dogs who had been exposed to alendronate for 3 years showed that resistance of cortical bone tissue to failure under cyclic loading was

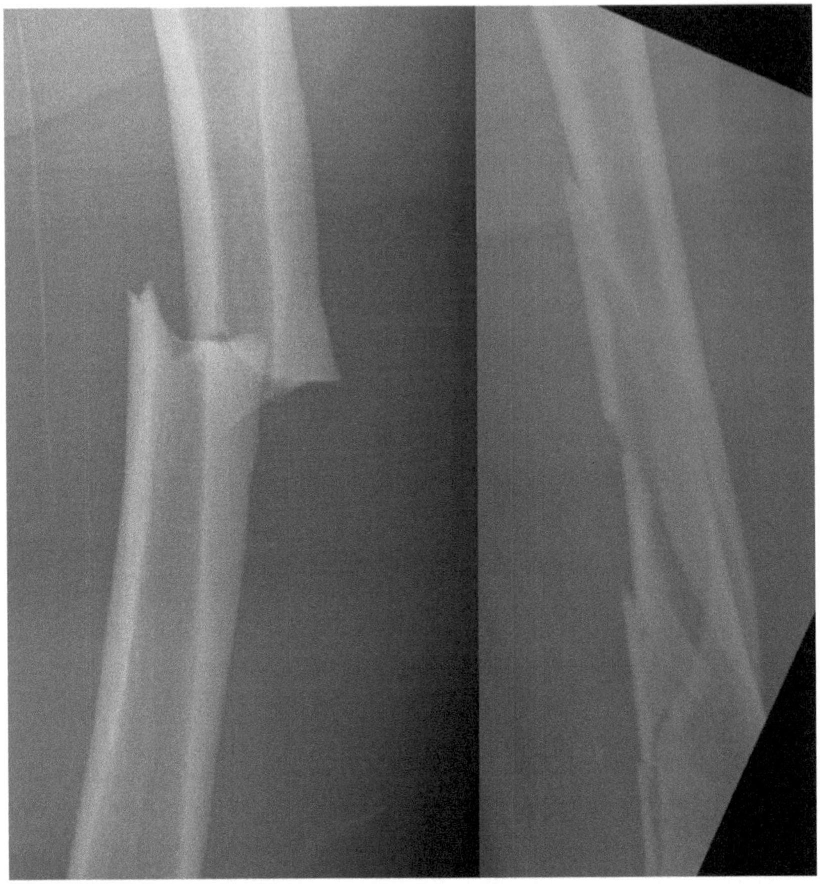

Figure 2.18 An atypical fracture with focal thickening at the fracture site, location in the femoral shaft, an initial sharp transverse break originating on the lateral cortex, and a medial spike. The right image is a typical fracture seen in a patient with osteoporosis, with thin cortices and comminuted pattern.

reduced compared to controls [174]. In another study of sheep, four-point bending fatigue testing showed that alendronate caused a significant loss in fatigue life. Zoledronic acid did not show this loss. This is possibly because the zoledronic acid does not penetrate as far into the bone due to its higher affinity for mineral [145,175].

2.2.6.3 Fracture healing

Nonunion of ordinary fractures was not noted in the clinical trials of bisphosphonates. Most studies report that fracture callus formation is larger but healing is not impaired [176,177]. However, for radial fractures a literature review suggested that there was an increased risk of nonunion [178]. One case-control study showed increased risk of nonunion in humerus fractures [179]. In controlled animal experiments the initial callus is actually even more abundant in experimental fractures comparing bisphosphonate treatment to estrogen or raloxifene. However, there is no remodeling of the woven bone of the callus into the lamellar bone that is seen with normal fracture healing [180]. In a rat arthrodesis model alendronate inhibited endochondrial ossification and graft bone resorption, but induced the growth of a larger, denser fusion mass compared to control rats by strongly suppressing osteoclastic activity [144]. Ibandronate inhibited direct fracture healing in a rat model [181]. Stress fracture healing of the rat ulna was delayed by risedronate [182]. In patients who had an atypical femur fracture, healing is delayed, surgical revisions are required in a third of patients [183].

2.2.7 Denosumab

Denosumab is a relatively new medication that blocks the formation of osteoclasts. It is an antibody against RANK-L. This results in more potent suppression of bone resorption than the bisphosphonates, and eventually in greater suppression of the bone formation. The fracture rate was significantly decreased compared to placebo-treated patients in a large 3-year study [184].

Clinical trials show increases in bone density that are greater during the first year of treatment but do not plateau after 8 years [185]. Bone biopsies show very low bone formation rates (see Fig. 2.17). In the clinical trials of denosumab in patients with osteoporosis, double labeling in trabecular bone was observed in 94% of placebo bones, and in only 19% of those treated with denosumab [186]. The mechanism for increasing BMD despite the absence of bone formation is unclear; some of the increase is caused by increased mineralization of the existing bone tissue. In a primate model, the drug does not inhibit the periosteal bone formation, so the cortical bone can increase in thickness [187].

QCT measurements show increased cortical thickness [188]. Biomechanical testing in a primate model showed improved strength as measured by three-point bending and by failure with compression [189].

Since the drug has not been on the market as long as the bisphosphonates there are less long-term data, but there are reports of atypical fractures of the femur [190–194]. The mechanism is probably similar to the suppression of bone formation seen with bisphosphonates.

This antibody is given as an injection which lasts 6 months; thereafter the osteoclasts appear to rebound and rapid resorption is seen, with reversal of the bone density to baseline levels. Several reports of multiple fractures during this interval have been reported [195,196].

2.2.8 Teriparatide

Teriparatide is a recombinant protein consisting of the first 34 amino acids of parathyroid hormone. This drug was developed after the serendipitous discovery in rats that

PTH administered continuously resulted in increased bone resorption and bone loss, whereas PTH administered by a daily injection had an anabolic effect, with increases in both resorption and formation, favoring the latter. In these rats the bone mass was markedly greater than in controls [197].

Teriparatide is the only anabolic medicine approved for treatment of osteoporosis [198]. The reason the daily injections are anabolic is still not known. In clinical trials the fracture rates are significantly decreased and the bone density increases. In this case, there is more bone volume as well. Bone biopsies show a marked increase in the bone formation rate with over 13% of the bone surface taking tetracycline labels a month after initiating the drug (see Fig. 2.17) [199]. However, this anabolic effect diminishes with time, and by 18 months the bone formation rate is similar to the baseline value [200]. The reason for the transient effect is also not understood.

Finite element analysis from QCT scans of patients treated with teriparatide showed increases in vertebral body strength [201,202] and hip strength [203].

Micro-CT analysis of bone biopsies shows increased improved trabecular microarchitecture, with a trend toward increased bone volume. Cortical bone showed increased thickness on 3D measurements but not 2D; porosity showed a trend toward increase on 2D but not on 3D [200]. In other studies the porosity is increased mainly near the endocortex, so the overall effect on bending strength of the long bones is not decreased [2,204]. In a study of sheep, four-point bending fatigue testing showed that teriparatide caused a significant improvement in fatigue life [145].

Backscattered electron microscopy shows the expected decrease in the mineralization density, as the newly formed bone is not as mineralized as the older bone [205].

Bone biopsies from patients in the randomized trial were analyzed with FTIR which found lower matrix mineralization, mineral crystallinity, and collagen crosslink ratio when compared with placebo. These findings indicate that the bone-forming effect of teriparatide results in bone with a molecular profile reminiscent of younger bone [206]. In another study, bone biopsies from patients who had received 2 years of teriparatide were analyzed by Raman and FTIR spectroscopy to determine mineral/matrix ratio, proteoglycan content, crystallinity, as well as collagen maturity within only the newly formed bone. Some of the patients were previously treated with alendronate. Comparing baseline to final biopsies from the treatment-naïve patients, there was a decrease in collagen maturity, a decrease in the crystal size, an increase in endosteal mineral content without a change in matrix, and no change in proteoglycan content. Pretreatment with alendronate did not affect most of these measurements, which indicate positive effects on the bone quality [207].

Because teriparatide has anabolic actions there is interest in ability to heal fractures more quickly [208–211]. This has been shown in some animal models. A trial in women with pelvic fractures showed faster healing with teriparatide [212]. However, a clinical study of humerus fractures in women with osteoporosis did not show evidence of more rapid healing with 1 month of teriparatide [213]. In distal radial fractures there was no overall benefit in a clinical trial using two doses, but posthoc analysis showed shorter healing with the 20 μg/day dose [214].

Teriparatide has not been used for long durations because the FDA mandated a limit of 2 years because animal studies showed an increase in osteosarcoma [215].

2.2.9 Strontium

Strontium ranelate is a compound that is approved for use in treating osteoporosis in some countries (but not in the United States). Its use is currently limited by the increased incidence of cardiovascular disease. Clinical trials have suggested a decreased fracture rate [216]. The mechanism of action is not known.

The bone density increases, but in this case much of the increase is due to the fact that strontium accumulates within the bone crystal. Since it is a heavier atom than calcium, it absorbs more of the radiation when using DEXA, and this is interpreted by the software as denser bone.

Bone biopsies before and after strontium treatment have shown mild decreases in the resorption rate, and decreases in the bone formation rates. Therefore, this is not an anabolic drug, but a mild antiresorptive drug [217]. Strontium does not change measurements of crystal characteristics or mineralization density [218,219].

Some studies have suggested that in patients with kidney disease, strontium can accumulate and contribute to osteomalacia [220–222].

2.2.10 Emerging therapies

2.2.10.1 Cathepsin K inhibitors

Cathepsin K is secreted by osteoclasts in order to break down collagen during bone resorption (see Fig. 2.9). Mutation in this protein results in a disease with high bone density called pycnodysostosis [223,224]. Despite the high bone mass these patients have poor bone quality and suffer from skeletal deformities and painful bone. Inhibitors of cathepsin K increase BMD because they block the bone resorption. The osteoclasts themselves are still present and may still be able to participate in cell signaling to the osteoblasts. These inhibitors are being studied as osteoporosis treatments [225] In a 5-year trial, odanacatib reduced fracture rates. Bone biopsies from treated patients show decreased resorption and formation [123]. However, these drugs cause an increased in morphia, a painful thickening of the skin [226]. Currently none are approved for use.

2.2.10.2 Romosozumab

Sclerosteosis is a rare, serious, autosomal recessive disease. Most of the patients are Afrikaans from South Africa [227]. They have thick bones with very high bone density, especially in the skull, with entrapment of cranial nerves leading to deafness and facial nerve palsy and increased intracranial pressure. Bones in the rest of the skeleton are also thick and dense, and frequently syndactyly is present. The bones are markedly different from those in another disease of high bone density called osteopetrosis, in which osteoclasts fail to form, the bone is all mineralized cartilage, which is fragile, brittle, and prone to "chalk-stick" fractures. The sclerosteosis patients do not fracture their bones, the bones have normal lamellar structure and good quality. Relatives of these patients who are heteozygous carriers also have increased bone density, although the thickness is not as great as in the homozygous patients. These relatives have no medical problems and they rarely have fractures [228]. Yet another bone disease with high bone mass is Van Buchem's disease; patients have abnormally thick skulls, square jaws, and may have abnormalities in fingers [229]. Patients with sclerosteosis were found to have homozygous mutations in the SOST gene [28], and those with Van Buchem's disease had mutations in an area on the same chromosome as SOST, which is upstream and is involved in regulation of the SOST gene transcription [230].

Sclerostin, the SOST gene product, is a circulating inhibitor of the Wnt-signaling pathway (see Fig. 2.5), which acts to inhibit LRP5 function. Sclerostin is expressed almost exclusively in mature osteocytes. Sclerostin plays an important role in skeletal adaptation to mechanical forces. An elegant study by Robling and colleagues established the importance of sclerostin as a mechanism to link biomechanical forces to bone formation. They studied mice and rats whose forelimbs were loaded by mild bending. The opposite limbs were used as controls. In the control limb, the osteocytes diffusely expressed sclerostin. This was seen by immunohistochemistry and also documented by in situ hydridization. In the loaded forearm, the osteocytes appeared normal on routine staining, but the sclerostin secretion was inhibited. Furthermore, the suppression of sclerostin secretion was very specifically located to the area of the bone that was most stressed. The mRNA for sclerostin was decreased in locations corresponding to the decreased immunohistochemistry, so the mechanical loading response of the SOST gene was partly at the transcriptional level. The animals were labeled with fluorochrome, and the bone formation rates 10 days later were increased in proportion to the decrease in the sclerostin, at precisely the same location as the mechanical stress.

Antibodies against sclerostin have been given to normal mice and rats, and their bone density increases. Bone biopsies in the animals show normal lamellar bone.

A larger study of 419 women with osteoporosis showed a 1-year increase in BMD of 11.3% that was greater than that seen in those randomly assigned to teriparatide or alendronate [231]. Markers of bone formation were increased and, importantly, markers of bone resorption were decreased. This is because the Wnt-signaling pathway results in both increased osteoblast activity and secretion of osteoprotegerin, which blocks RANK-L and inhibits osteoclasts. A phase 3 trial is underway. Sclerostin inhibition has potential for becoming a useful anabolic agent because it is targeted to the bone, and because there is a genetic model of partial suppression in which bones are strong but otherwise the people are healthy.

2.2.11 Other medications or substances that affect bone strength

Many medications are associated with increased fracture rates. They do not all affect the bone directly, and in many cases the underlying disease is responsible for both decreased bone density and increased fracture risk. Some drugs also increase the risk of falling by affecting neurologic or muscular systems, thereby increasing fracture risk without any effect on the bone. Several drugs reduce the estrogen levels and thereby cause bone loss as discussed above. Others do not have specific effects on the bone but cause fractures because they are generally toxic (such as cancer drugs), cause gastrointestinal side effects, weakness, or weight loss. But there are several medications listed below that directly affect various aspects of bone physiology.

2.2.11.1 Anticonvulsants

Patients with seizures have increased risk of fractures due to the seizures themselves. However, the anticonvulsants decrease bone strength and contribute to fracture [232]. Patients have lower bone density and higher bone resorption rates [233]. The mechanisms are not clearly defined. They can inhibit vitamin D metabolism, but this is not the only explanation because bone density decreases even when vitamin D levels are normal [234].

2.2.11.2 Selective serotonin reuptake inhibitors

Depression itself is associated with increased fracture rates and the causes are multifactorial. Observational studies suggest that the fracture rates are increased independently of the depression [235,236]. A potential mechanism is that the peripheral serotonin levels increase (i.e., the drugs are not as selective as their name implies). Recent studies have found serotonin receptors on osteoblasts, and serotonin directly inhibits the function of the osteoblast cells and therefore reduces the bone formation rates [237].

Selective serotonin reuptake inhibitors could also have central effects by stimulating the sympathetic nervous system. This inhibits bone formation.

2.2.11.3 Carbonic anhydrase inhibitors

Usually metabolic acidosis decreases bone density, decreases osteoblast activity, and increases bone resorption. Part of this is related to the skeleton's role of buffer in acidosis, and as bone is resorbed, bicarbonate is released. The acidosis that results from carbonic anhydrase inhibition is an exception. The osteoclasts are not able to effectively secrete hydrogen and therefore bone resorption is decreased. It is interesting that patients with a rare mutation in the gene for carbonic anhydrase have osteosclerosis with very dense bones [238,239].

2.2.11.4 *Thiazide diuretics*

Thiazide diuretics have also been associated with a reduction in hip fracture rates and a modest decrease in the rate of aging bone loss [240–242]. Bone biopsies show a mild decrease in the osteoclastic bone resorption rate [243]. In healthy older patients, bone density showed mild increases compared to losses seen with placebo [244]. These drugs directly increase the renal reabsorption of calcium, which can increase bone density by making calcium available and decreasing PTH [245]. But they also have a weak effect on carbonic anhydase and could reduce bone resorption by that mechanism as well. In one clinical trial the most long-lasting effect was a mild increase in the serum bicarbonate, suggesting a chronic effect to reduce metabolic acidosis [245].

2.2.11.5 *Rosiglitazone*

Treatment of diabetic patients with roziglitazone, a PPAR-γ agonist, increased the incidence of fractures in a large randomized clinical trial [246]. However, the bone density does not show serious loss; a recent meta-analysis shows only modest changes [247], while another meta-analysis showed increases risk of fracture [248]. Animal studies show that this drug increases the number of marrow adipocytes but decreases the number of preosteoblasts [249].

2.2.11.6 *Bortezomib*

On the other hand, bortezomib, a proteasome inhibitor used in the treatment of multiple myeloma, induces the mesenchymal stem cells to differentiate into the osteoblastic pathway, and this improves the bone mass in mice with osteoporosis [250].

2.2.11.7 *Lithium*

Lithium is used to treat manic-depressive illness. It acts intracellularly to inhibit GSK, one of the proteins involved in the Wnt-signaling pathway [36,251]. Therefore, more ß-catenin is available to enter the nucleus and increase signaling through the pathway. The result is greater bone formation and decreased bone resorption and in patients treated with lithium bone density is higher than in controls [252]. In animal models lithium accelerated bone regeneration [253].

2.2.11.8 *Elements toxic to the bone*

Aluminum deposition in the bone causes osteomalacia [254]. This is seen in dialysis patients who were exposed to aluminum in the dialysate, and in patient receiving parenteral nutrition that was contaminated with aluminum [255]. Bone biopsies show osteoid accumulation without bone resorption or formation, and aluminum deposition in the cement lines. Parathyroid hormone levels are also decreased and aluminum accumulates in the parathyroid glands, contributing to the low bone turnover. The mechanism of aluminum osteomalacia is not fully understood, because low PTH alone does not cause this.

Iron is stored in the reticuloendothelial cells in the bone marrow. Excessive iron loads will also deposit in bones, in the same locations as aluminum [256]. In dialysis patients, stains show that these are both on the interface between osteoid and mineralized bones, and within the cement lines. Rarely, osteomalacia is the result of excess iron accumulation. More often, patients with hemochomatosis or thalassemia have osteoporosis, and the bone improves with chelation [257]. Iron inhibits the osteoblast function [258], and also when estrogen is deficient iron increases osteoclast differentiation through production of reactive oxygen species [259].

Cadmium caused an epidemic of bone disease in a town in Japan, that was called "Itai-Itai disease" meaning "ouch-ouch" because the legs were painful due to multiple pseudofractures [260]. The cadmium came from a nearby industrial plant that contaminated the drinking water. Patients developed Fanconi's syndrome, a disease of the proximal renal tubules, resulting in acidosis and hypophosphatemia. This in turn caused the osteomalacia. More recently, even low levels of cadmium in blood have been associated with increased risk of fractures in elderly men [261].

Cobalt toxicity has been reported in patients who had undergone hip replacement [262]. As the metal surfaces of the replaced hip wear down, they release cadmium into the local bone and the circulation. This can result in failure of the prosthesis, or development of pseudotumors [263]. Cobalt is found within the mineralized bone [264]. This causes a decrease in osteogenic differentiation of stromal stem cells [265] and toxicity to the osteocytes [266] and osteoblasts [267].

2.2.11.9 Fluoride

This chapter ends with a discussion of fluoride, a drug that was once used to treat postmenopausal osteoporosis. It is a lesson that should not be forgotten, although many young physicians have never heard about it.

Scientists have realized that fluoride had effects to increase bone density for over 70 years. Small studies documented an increase in bone density with fluoride and it was commonly used as a treatment for osteoporosis.

Then, in 1990, an NIH-sponsored randomized placebo-controlled trial of fluoride in women with postmenopausal osteoporosis documented a dramatic improvement in the spine BMD, which steadily increased over 4 years, resulting in BMD that was 35% greater than baseline. The bone density at the hip increased by 12%, greater than with any drug used since then [268]. However, there were significantly more fractures in the fluoride group compared to the placebo group! Bone biopsies from patients treated with fluoride show abnormal osteoid accumulation and disorganized bone lamellar structure [269,270]. Mineralization density is increased [271]. Bone crystal size is larger than in untreated osteoporotic patients [272]. These important study results provide the most clear-cut evidence that bone density is not the same as bone strength.

2.3 SUMMARY

Many drugs, other exogenous substances, and endogenous hormones and cytokines can affect the quality of bone. Learning about these effects will allow design of better treatments for bone diseases.

REFERENCES

[1] Currey JD. The design of mineralised hard tissues for their mechanical functions. J Exp Biol 1999;202(Pt 23):3285–94.
[2] Turner CH. Biomechanics of bone: determinants of skeletal fragility and bone quality. Osteoporosis Int 2002;13:97–104.
[3] Rubin CT, Lanyon LE. Limb mechanics as a funtion of speed and gait. J Exp Biol 1982;101:187–211.
[4] Marcus R. Normal and abnormal bone remodeling in man. Ann Rev Med 1987;38:129–41.
[5] Parfitt AM. Targeted and nontargeted bone remodeling: relationship to basic multicellular unit origination and progression. Bone 2002;30:5–7.
[6] Burr D. Targeted and nontargeted remodeling. Bone 2002;30:2–4.
[7] Parfitt AM. Bone age, mineral density, and fatigue damage. Calcif Tissue Int 1993;53(Suppl 1): S82–5. discussion S5-6.
[8] Currey JD, Brear K, Zioupos P. The effects of ageing and changes in mineral content in degrading the toughness of human femora. J Biomech 1996;29:257–60.
[9] Boskey AL, Robey PG. The composition of bone. In: Rosen C, editor. Primer on the metabolic bone diseases and disorders of mineral metabolism. 8th ed Hoboken, NJ: Wiley; 2013. p. 49–58.
[10] Garnero P. The role of collagen organization on the properties of bone. Calcif Tissue Int 2015;97 (3):229–40.
[11] Gorski J. Biomineralization of bone: a fresh view of the roles of non- collagenous proteins. Front Biosci 2015;18:2598–621.
[12] Lu X, Fukumoto S, Yamada Y, Evans CA, Diekwisch TG, Luan X. Ameloblastin, an extracellular matrix protein, affects long bone growth and mineralization. J Bone Miner Res 2016;31 (6):1235–46.
[13] Wang X, Xu H, Huang Y, Gu S, Jiang JX. Coupling effect of water and proteoglycans on the in situ toughness of bone. J Bone Miner Res 2016;31(5):1026–9.
[14] Burnell JM, Baylink DJ, Chestnut CHd, Mathews MW, Teubner EJ. Bone matrix and mineral abnormalities in postmenopausal osteoporosis. Metabolism 1982;31(11):1113–20.
[15] Wang J, Zhou B, Guo XE. Trabecular microstructure differs greatly between trabecular groups in proximal femurs of postmenopausal women. Orth Res Soc Ann Meet 2013;0724.
[16] Crockett JC, Rogers MJ, Coxon FP, Hocking LJ, Helfrich MH. Bone remodelling at a glance. J Cell Sci 2011;124(Pt 7):991–8.
[17] Henriksen K, Neutzsky-Wulff AV, Bonewald LF, Karsdal MA. Local communication on and within bone controls bone remodeling. Bone 2009;44(6):1026–33.
[18] Kearns AE, Khosla S, Kostenuik PJ. Receptor activator of nuclear factor kappaB ligand and osteoprotegerin regulation of bone remodeling in health and disease. Endocr Rev 2008;29(2):155–92.
[19] Dallas SL, Prideaux M, Bonewald LF. The osteocyte: an endocrine cell . . . and more. Endocr Rev 2013;34(5):658–90.
[20] Kato. Promotion of osteoclast differentiation and activation in spite of impeded osteoblast-lineage differentiation under acidosis: effects of acidosis on bone metabolism. BioScience Trends 2013;7 (1):33–41.
[21] Novack DV, Teitelbaum SL. The osteoclast: friend or foe? Annu Rev Pathol 2008;3:457–84.
[22] Takayanagi H. Osteoimmunology: shared mechanisms and crosstalk between the immune and bone systems. Nat Rev Immunol 2007;7(4):292–304.

[23] Sambandam Y, Townsend MT, Pierce JJ, Lipman CM, Haque A, Bateman TA, et al. Microgravity control of autophagy modulates osteoclastogenesis. Bone 2014;61:125–31.
[24] Sacchetti B, Funari A, Michienzi S, Di Cesare S, Piersanti S, Saggio I, et al. Self-renewing osteoprogenitors in bone marrow sinusoids can organize a hematopoietic microenvironment. Cell 2007;131(2):324–36.
[25] Johnson ML, Gong G, Kimberling W, Recker SM, Kimmel DB, Recker RB. Linkage of a gene causing high bone mass to human chromosome 11 (11q12-13). Am J Hum Genet 1997;60 (6):1326–32.
[26] Little RD, Carulli JP, Del Mastro RG, Dupuis J, Osborne M, Folz C, et al. A mutation in the LDL receptor-related protein 5 gene results in the autosomal dominant high-bone-mass trait. Am J Hum Genet 2002;70:11–19.
[27] Boyden LM, Mao J, Belsky J, Mitzner L, Farhi A, Mitnick MA, et al. High bone density due to a mutation in LDL-receptor-related protein 5. N Eng J Med 2002;346:1513–21.
[28] Balemans W, Ebeling M, Patel N, Van Hul E, Olson P, Dioszegi M, et al. Increased bone density in sclerosteosis is due to the deficiency of a novel secreted protein (SOST). Hum Mol Genet 2001;10 (5):537–43.
[29] Gong Y, Slee RB, Fukai N, Rawadi G, Roman-Roman S, Reginato AM, et al. LDL receptor-related protein 5 (LRP5) affects bone accrual and eye development. Cell 2001;107:513–23.
[30] Johnson ML, Harnish K, Nusse R, Van Hul W. LRP5 and Wnt signaling: a union made for bone. J Bone Miner Res 2004;19(11):1749–57.
[31] Baron R, Kneissel M. WNT signaling in bone homeostasis and disease: from human mutations to treatments. Nat Med 2013;19(2):179–92.
[32] Glass II DA, Bialek P, Ahn JD, Starbuck M, Patel MS, Clevers H, et al. Canonical Wnt signaling in differentiated osteoblasts controls osteoclast differentiation. Dev Cell 2005;8(5):751–64.
[33] Gonzalez EA, Lund RJ, Martin KJ, McCartney JE, Tondravi MM, Sampath TK, et al. Treatment of a murine model of high-turnover renal osteodystrophy by exogenous BMP-7. Kidney Int 2002;61(4):1322–31.
[34] Li T, Surendran K, Zawaideh MA, Mathew S, Hruska KA. Bone morphogenetic protein 7: a novel treatment for chronic renal and bone disease. Curr Opin Nephrol Hypertens 2004;13(4):417–22.
[35] Gonzalez EA, Lund RJ, Martin KJ, McCartney JE, Tondravi MM, Sampath TK, et al. Treatment of a murine model of high-turnover renal osteodystrophy by exogenous BMP-7. Kidney Int 2002;61(4):1322–31.
[36] Khosla S, Westendorf JJ, Oursler MJ. Building bone to reverse osteoporosis and repair fractures. J Clin Invest 2008;118(2):421–8.
[37] Abdelgawad ME, Delaisse JM, Hinge M, Jensen PR, Alnaimi RW, Rolighed L, et al. Early reversal cells in adult human bone remodeling: osteoblastic nature, catabolic functions and interactions with osteoclasts. Histochem Cell Biol 2016;145(6):603–15.
[38] Jensen PR, Andersen TL, Hauge EM, Bollerslev J, Delaisse JM. A joined role of canopy and reversal cells in bone remodeling - Lessons from glucocorticoid-induced osteoporosis. Bone 2015;73:16–23.
[39] Delaisse JM. The reversal phase of the bone-remodeling cycle: cellular prerequisites for coupling resorption and formation. BoneKEy reports 2014;3:561.
[40] Parfitt M, Qiu S, Palnitkar S, Rao DS. Abnormal bone remodeling in patients with spontaneous painful vertebral fracture. J Bone Miner Res 2011;26(3):475–85.
[41] Whyte MP. Hypophosphatasia—aetiology, nosology, pathogenesis, diagnosis and treatment. Nat Rev Endocrinol 2016;12(4):233–46.
[42] Weber JM, Calvi LM. Notch signaling and the bone marrow hematopoietic stem cell niche. Bone 2010;46(2):281–5.
[43] Xie Y, Yin T, Wiegraebe W, He XC, Miller D, Stark D, et al. Detection of functional haematopoietic stem cell niche using real-time imaging. Nature 2009;457(7225):97–101.
[44] Atkins GJ, Findlay DM. Osteocyte regulation of bone mineral: a little give and take. Osteoporsis Int 2012;23(8):2067–79.

[45] Rochefort GY, Pallu S, Benhamou CL. Osteocyte: the unrecognized side of bone tissue. Osteoporsis Int 2010;21(9):1457–69.
[46] Manolagas SC, Parfitt AM. What old means to bone. Trends Endocrinol Metab 2010;21 (6):369–74.
[47] McNamara LM, Majeska RJ, Weinbaum S, Friedrich V, Schaffler MB. Attachment of osteocyte cell processes to the bone matrix. Anat Rec (Hoboken) 2009;292(3):355–63.
[48] Santos A, Bakker AD, Zandieh-Doulabi B, Semeins CM, Klein-Nulend J. Pulsating fluid flow modulates gene expression of proteins involved in Wnt signaling pathways in osteocytes. J Orthop Res 2009.
[49] Cabahug-Zuckerman P, Frikha-Benayed D, Majeska RJ, Tuthill A, Yakar S, Judex S, et al. Osteocyte apoptosis caused by hindlimb unloading is required to trigger osteocyte RANKL production and subsequent resorption of cortical and trabecular bone in mice femurs. J Bone Miner Res 2016;31(7):1356–65.
[50] Manolagas SC, Parfitt AM. For whom the bell tolls: distress signals from long-lived osteocytes and the pathogenesis of metabolic bone diseases. Bone 2013;54(2):272–8.
[51] Frost HM. Tetracycline-base histological analysis of bone remodeling. Calc Tiss Res 1969;3:211–37.
[52] Ott SM. Dynamics of bone remodeling. In: Martini L, editor. Encyclopedia of endocrine diseases. San Diego, CA: Academic Press, Elsevier; 2004. p. 386–91.
[53] Jayasinghe JAP, Jones SJ, Boyde A. Scanning electron microscopy of human lumbar vertebral trabecular bone surfaces. Virchows Archiv A Pathol Anat 1993;422:25–34.
[54] Parfitt AM. Osteonal and hemi-osteonal remodeling: the spatial and temporal framework for signal traffic in adult human bone. J Cellular Biochemistry 1994;55:273–86.
[55] Robling AG, Niziolek PJ, Baldridge LA, Condon KW, Allen MR, Alam I, et al. Mechanical stimulation of bone in vivo reduces osteocyte expression of sost/sclerostin. J Biol Chem 2008;283 (9):5866–75.
[56] Turner CH, Forwood MR. What role does the osteocyte network play in bone adaptation? Bone 1995;16:283–5.
[57] Verborgt O, Gibson GJ, Schaffler MB. Loss of osteocyte integrity in association with microdamage and bone remodeling after fatigue in vivo. J Bone Miner Res 2000;15:60–7.
[58] Noble BS, Reeve J. Osteocyte function, osteocyte death and bone fracture resistance. Mol Cell Endocrinol 2000;159:7–13.
[59] Mori S, Burr DB. Increased intracortical remodeling following fatigue damage. Bone 1993;14 (2):103–9.
[60] Towler D. <Towler bone repair angiogenic.pdf>. 2008.
[61] Janssens K, ten Dijke P, Janssens S, Van Hul W. Transforming growth factor-beta1 to the bone. Endocr Rev 2005;26(6):743–74.
[62] Teitelbaum SL. Osteoclasts: what do they do and how do they do it? Am J Pathol 2007;170 (2):427–35.
[63] Teitelbaum SL. Osteoclasts and integrins. Ann N Y Acad Sci 2006;1068:95–9.
[64] Weivoda MM, Ruan M, Pederson L, Hachfeld C, Davey RA, Zajac JD, et al. Osteoclast TGF-β receptor signaling induces wnt1 secretion and couples bone resorption to bone formation. J Bone Miner Res 2015;31(1):76–85.
[65] Pederson L, Ruan M, Westendorf JJ, Khosla S, Oursler MJ. Regulation of bone formation by osteoclasts involves Wnt/BMP signaling and the chemokine sphingosine-1-phosphate. Proc Natl Acad Sci U S A 2008;105(52):20764–9.
[66] Andersen TL, Abdelgawad ME, Kristensen HB, Hauge EM, Rolighed L, Bollerslev J, et al. Understanding coupling between bone resorption and formation: are reversal cells the missing link? Am J Pathol 2013;183(1):235–46.
[67] Andreasen CM, Ding M, Overgaard S, Bollen P, Andersen TL. A reversal phase arrest uncoupling the bone formation and resorption contributes to the bone loss in glucocorticoid treated ovariectomised aged sheep. Bone 2015;75:32–9.

[68] Eriksen EF, Gundersen HJG, Melsen F, Mosekilde L. Reconstruction of the formative site in iliac trabecular bone in 20 normal individuals employing a kinetic model for matrix and mineral apposition. Metab Bone Dis Rel Res 1984;5:243–52.
[69] Parfitt AM, Han ZH, Palnitkar S, Rao DS, Shih MS, Nelson D. Effects of ethnicity and age or menopause on osteoblast function, bone mineralization, and osteoid accumulation in iliac bone. J Bone Miner Res 1997;12(11):1864–73.
[70] Parfitt AM, Mundy GR, Roodman GD, Hughes DE, Boyce BF. A new model for the regulation of bone resorption with particular reference to the effects of bisphosphonates. J Bone Mineral Res 1996;11:150–9.
[71] Parfitt AM, Villanueva AR, Foldes J, Sudhaker Rao D. Relations between histologic indices of bone formation : implications for the pathogenesis of spinal osteoporosis. J Bone Mineral Res 1995;10:466–73.
[72] Hanson DA, Weis MA, Bollen AM, Maslan SL, Singer FREDR. A specific immunoassay for monitoring human bone resorption: quantitation of type I collagen cross-linked N-telopeptides in urine. J Bone Miner Res 1992;7(11):1251–8.
[73] Hammond MA, Gallant MA, Burr DB, Wallace JM. Nanoscale changes in collagen are reflected in physical and mechanical properties of bone at the microscale in diabetic rats. Bone 2014;60:26–32.
[74] Nudelman F, Lausch AJ, Sommerdijk NA, Sone ED. In vitro models of collagen biomineralization. J Struct Biol 2013;183(2):258–69.
[75] Atkins GJ, Rowe PS, Lim HP, Welldon KJ, Ormsby R, Wijenayaka AR, et al. Sclerostin is a locally acting regulator of late-osteoblast/preosteocyte differentiation and regulates mineralization through a MEPE-ASARM-dependent mechanism. J Bone Miner Res 2011;26(7):1425–36.
[76] Otero JE, Gottesman GS, McAlister WH, Mumm S, Madson KL, Kiffer-Moreira T, et al. Severe skeletal toxicity from protracted etidronate therapy for generalized arterial calcification of infancy. J Bone Miner Res 2013;28(2):419–30.
[77] Lombardi G, Perego S, Luzi L, Banfi G. A four-season molecule: osteocalcin. Updates in its physiological roles. Endocrine 2014.
[78] Burnell JM, Teubner EJ, Miller AG. Normal maturational changes in bone matrix, mineral, and crystal size in the rat. Calcif Tissue Int 1980;31(1):13–19.
[79] Kazama JJ, Fukagawa M. In and out of the bone: can the osteocyte escape skeletal jail and yet regulate mineralization? Kidney Int 2014;85(1):11–12.
[80] Poole KE, van Bezooijen RL, Loveridge N, Hamersma H, Papapoulos SE, Lowik CW, et al. Sclerostin is a delayed secreted product of osteocytes that inhibits bone formation. FASEB J 2005.
[81] Bala Y, Farlay D, Delmas PD, Meunier PJ, Boivin G. Time sequence of secondary mineralization and microhardness in cortical and cancellous bone from ewes. Bone 2010;46(4):1204–12.
[82] Jowsey J. Age changes in human bone. Clin Orthop Rel Res 1960;17:210–17.
[83] Boyde A, Elliott JC, Jones SJ. Stereology and histogram analysis of backscattered electron images: age changes in bone. Bone 1993;14(3):205–10.
[84] Reid SA, Boyde A. Changes in the mineral density distribution in human bone with age: image analysis using backscattered electrons in the SEM. J Bone Mineral Res 1987;2:13–22.
[85] Schaffler MB, Choi K, Micgrom C. Aging and matrix microdamage accumulation in human compact bone. Bone 1995;17:521–5.
[86] Cosman F, Ruffing J, Zion M, Uhorchak J, Ralston S, Tendy S, et al. Determinants of stress fracture risk in United States Military Academy cadets. Bone 2013;55(2):359–66.
[87] Uthgenannt BA, Kramer MH, Hwu JA, Wopenka B, Silva MJ. Skeletal self-repair: stress fracture healing by rapid formation and densification of woven bone. J Bone Miner Res 2007;22(10):1548–56.
[88] Gerstenfeld LC, Wronski TJ, Hollinger JO, Einhorn TA. Application of histomorphometric methods to the study of bone repair. J Bone Miner Res 2005;20(10):1715–22.
[89] Wang C, Inzana JA, Mirando AJ, Ren Y, Liu Z, Shen J, et al. NOTCH signaling in skeletal progenitors is critical for fracture repair. J Clin Invest 2016;126(4):1471–81.
[90] Cummings SR, Bates D, Black DM. Clinical use of bone densitometry: scientific review. JAMA 2002;288(15):1889–97.

[91] Ott SM. When bone mass fails to predict bone failure. Calcif Tissue Int 1993;53(Suppl 1):S7−13.
[92] Davison KS, Siminoski K, Adachi JD, Hanley DA, Goltzman D, Hodsman AB, et al. Bone strength: the whole is greater than the sum of its parts. Semin Arthritis Rheum 2006;36 (1):22−31.
[93] Ott SM. Bone strength: more than just bone density. Kidney Int 2016;89(1):16−19.
[94] Jee W. Cancellous bone minimodeling-based formation: a Frost, Takahashi Legacy. J Musculoskelet Neuronal Interact 2007;7:232−9.
[95] Muller R. Bone microarchitecture assessment: current and future trends. Osteoporsis Int 2003;14 (Suppl. 5):S89−95. discussion S-9.
[96] Boivin G, Farlay D, Bala Y, Doublier A, Meunier PJ, Delmas PD. Influence of remodeling on the mineralization of bone tissue. Osteoporsis Int 2009;20(6):1023−6.
[97] Bloebaum RD, Skedros JG, Vajda EG, Bachus KN, Constantz BR. Determining mineral content variations in bone using backscattered electron imaging. Bone 1997;20(5):485−90.
[98] Currey JD. Effects of differences in mineralization on the mechanical properties of bone. Philos Trans R Soc Lond B Biol Sci 1984;304:509−18.
[99] Vajda EG, Bloebaum RD. Age-related hypermineralization in the female proximal human femur. Anat Rec 1999;255(2):202−11.
[100] Mosekilde L, Ebbesen EN, Tornvig L, Thomsen JS. Trabecular bone structure and strength—remodelling and repair. J Musculoskelet Neuronal Interact 2000;1(1):25−30.
[101] Wehrli FW, Ladinsky GA, Jones C, Benito M, Magland J, Vasilic B, et al. In vivo magnetic resonance detects rapid remodeling changes in the topology of the trabecular bone network following menopause and protective effect of estradiol. J Bone Miner Res 2008;23(5):730−40.
[102] Tang SY, Vashishth D. Non-enzymatic glycation alters microdamage formation in human cancellous bone. Bone 2010;46(1):148−54.
[103] Faibish D, Ott SM, Boskey AL. Mineral changes in osteoporosis: a review. Clin Orthop Relat Res 2006;443:28−38.
[104] Luo Q, Leng H, Wang X, Zhou Y, Rong Q. The role of water and mineral-collagen interfacial bonding on microdamage progression in bone. J Orthop Res 2014;32(2):217−23.
[105] Mashiba T, Turner CH, Hirano T, Forwood MR, Johnston CC, Burr DB. Effects of suppressed bone turnover by bisphosphonates on microdamage accumulation and biomechanical properties in clinically relevant skeletal sites in beagles. Bone 2001;28:524−31.
[106] Schaffler MB. Role of bone turnover in microdamage. Osteoporsis Int 2003;14(Suppl. 5):S73−7. discussion S7-80.
[107] Napoli N, Novack D, Armamento-Villareal R. Bisphosphonate-associated femoral fracture: implications for management in patients with malignancies. Osteoporsis Int 2009.
[108] Burket JC, Brooks DJ, MacLeay JM, Baker SP, Boskey AL, van der Meulen MC. Variations in nanomechanical properties and tissue composition within trabeculae from an ovine model of osteoporosis and treatment. Bone 2013;52(1):326−36.
[109] Muller R, Van Campenhout H, Van Damme B, Van Der Perre G, Dequeker J, Hildebrand T, et al. Morphometric analysis of human bone biopsies: a quantitative structural comparison of histological sections and micro-computed tomography. Bone 1998;23:59−66.
[110] Dempster DW. The contribution of trabecular architecture to cancellous bone quality. J Bone Miner Res 2000;15(1):20−3.
[111] Aaron JE, Shore PA, Shore RC, Beneton M, Kanis JA. Trabecular architecture in women and men of similar bone mass with and without vertebral fracture: II. Three-dimensional histology. Bone 2000;27(2):277−82.
[112] Mosekilde L. Vertebral structure and strength in vivo and in vitro. Calcif Tissue Int 1993;53: S121−6.
[113] Modder UI, Roforth MM, Hoey K, McCready LK, Peterson JM, Monroe DG, et al. Effects of estrogen on osteoprogenitor cells and cytokines/bone-regulatory factors in postmenopausal women. Bone 2011;49(2):202−7.

[114] Vedi S, Purdie DW, Ballard P, Bord S, Cooper A, Compston J. Bone remodeling and structure in postmenopausal women treated with long-term, high-dose estrogen therapy. Osteoporsis Int 1999;10:52–8.

[115] Vedi S, Bell KL, Loveridge N, Garrahan N, Purdie DW, Compston JE. The effects of hormone replacement therapy on cortical bone in postmenopausal women. Bone 2003;33(3):330–4.

[116] Vedi S, Compston JE. The effects of long-term hormone replacement therapy on bone remodeling in postmenopausal women. Bone 1996;19:535–9.

[117] Van Staa TP, Abenhaim L, Cooper C, Zhang B, Leufkens HG. The use of a large pharmacoepidemiological database to study exposure to oral corticosteroids and risk of fractures: validation of study population and results. Pharmacoepidemiol Drug Saf 2000;9(5):359–66.

[118] Frenkel B. Glucocorticoid-induced osteoporosis. Adv Exp Med Biol 2015;872:179–214.

[119] Pearce G, Tabensky DA, Delmas PD, Baker HW, Seeman E. Corticosteroid-induced bone loss in men. J Clin Endocrinol Metab 1998;83:801–6.

[120] Teitelbaum SL. Glucocorticoids and the osteoclast. Clin Exp Rheumatol 2015;33(4 Suppl. 92): S37–9.

[121] Weinstein RS, Nicholas RW, Manolagas SC. Apoptosis of osteocytes in glucocorticoid-induced osteonecrosis of the hip. J Clin Endocrinol Metab 2000;85(8):2907–12.

[122] Eriksen EF, Mosekilde L, Melsen F. Trabecular bone remodeling and bone balance in hyperthyroidism. Bone 1985;9:421–8.

[123] Chavassieux P, Seeman E, Delmas PD. Insights into material and structural basis of bone fragility from diseases associated with fractures: how determinants of the biomechanical properties of bone are compromised by disease. Endocr Rev 2007;28(2):151–64.

[124] Bilezikian JP, Brandi ML, Eastell R, Silverberg SJ, Udelsman R, Marcocci C, et al. Guidelines for the management of asymptomatic primary hyperparathyroidism: summary statement from the Fourth International Workshop. J Clin Endocrinol Metab 2014;99(10):3561–9.

[125] Silverberg SJ, Clarke BL, Peacock M, Bandeira F, Boutroy S, Cusano NE, et al. Current issues in the presentation of asymptomatic primary hyperparathyroidism: proceedings of the Fourth International Workshop. J Clin Endocrinol Metab 2014;99(10):3580–94.

[126] Misof BM, Roschger P, Cosman F, Kurland ES, Tesch W, Messmer P, et al. Effects of intermittent parathyroid hormone administration on bone mineralization density in iliac crest biopsies from patients with osteoporosis: a paired study before and after treatment. J Clin Endocrinol Metab 2003;88:1150–6.

[127] Cranney A, Welch V, Adachi JD, Homik J, Shea B, Suarez-Almazor ME, et al. Calcitonin for the treatment and prevention of corticosteroid-induced osteoporosis. Cochrane Database Syst Rev 2000; CD001983.

[128] Ott SM, Chesnut CH. Calcitriol treatment is not effective in postmenopausal osteoporosis. Ann Intern Med 1989;110:267–74.

[129] Riddle RC, Clemens TL. Insulin, osteoblasts, and energy metabolism: why bone counts calories. J Clin Invest 2014;124(4):1465–7.

[130] Lau KH, Baylink DJ, Zhou XD, Rodriguez D, Bonewald LF, Li Z, et al. Osteocyte-derived insulin-like growth factor I is essential for determining bone mechanosensitivity. Am J Physiol Endocrinol Metab 2013;305(2):E271–81.

[131] Xi G, Rosen CJ, Clemmons DR. IGF-I and IGFBP-2 stimulate AMPK activation and autophagy which are required for osteoblast differentiation. Endocrinology 2015; en20151690.

[132] Yadav VK, Ryu JH, Suda N, Tanaka KF, Gingrich JA, Schutz G, et al. Lrp5 controls bone formation by inhibiting serotonin synthesis in the duodenum. Cell 2008;135(5):825–37.

[133] Briot K, Rouanet S, Schaeverbeke T, Etchepare F, Gaudin P, Perdriger A, et al. The effect of tocilizumab on bone mineral density, serum levels of Dickkopf-1 and bone remodeling markers in patients with rheumatoid arthritis. Joint, Bone, Spine 2015;82(2):109–15.

[134] Suzuki M, Yoshida H, Hashizume M, Tanaka K, Matsumoto Y. Blockade of interleukin-6 receptor enhances the anti-arthritic effect of glucocorticoids without decreasing bone mineral density in mice with collagen-induced arthritis. Clin Exp Immunol 2015;182(2):154–61.

[135] Kang KY, Ju JH, Park SH, Kim HY. The paradoxical effects of TNF inhibitors on bone mineral density and radiographic progression in patients with ankylosing spondylitis. Rheumatology (Oxford) 2013;52(4):718–26.
[136] Mauro M, Radovic V, Armstrong D. Improvement of lumbar bone mass after infliximab therapy in Crohn's disease patients. Can J Gastroenterol 2007;21(10):637–42.
[137] Weaver CM, Alexander DD, Boushey CJ, Dawson-Hughes B, Lappe JM, LeBoff MS, et al. Calcium plus vitamin D supplementation and risk of fractures: an updated meta-analysis from the National Osteoporosis Foundation. Osteoporsis Int 2016;27(1):367–76.
[138] Hirsch C. Review: calcium supplementation and risk for fracture in persons >50 years of age. Ann Intern Med 2016;164(2):JC4.
[139] Reid IR, Bristow SM, Bolland MJ. Cardiovascular complications of calcium supplements. J Cell Biochem 2015;116(4):494–501.
[140] Ettinger B, Black DM, Mitlak BH. Reduction of vertebral fracture risk in postmenopausal women with osteoporosis treated with raloxifene. JAMA 1999;282:637–45.
[141] Barrett-Connor E, Mosca L, Collins P, Geiger MJ, Grady D, Kornitzer M, et al. Effects of raloxifene on cardiovascular events and breast cancer in postmenopausal women. N Eng J Med 2006;355(2):125–37.
[142] Ott SM, Oleksik A, Lu Y, Harper K, Lips P. Bone histomorphometric and biochemical marker results of a 2-year placebo-controlled trial of raloxifene in postmenopausal women. J Bone Miner Res 2002;17:341–8.
[143] Chung YE, Lee SH, Lee SY, Kim SY, Kim HH, Mirza FS, et al. Long-term treatment with raloxifene, but not bisphosphonates, reduces circulating sclerostin levels in postmenopausal women. Osteoporsis Int 2011.
[144] Takahata M, Ito M, Abe Y, Abumi K, Minami A. The effect of anti-resorptive therapies on bone graft healing in an ovariectomized rat spinal arthrodesis model. Bone 2008;43(6):1057–66.
[145] Brock GR, Chen JT, Ingraffea AR, MacLeay J, Pluhar GE, Boskey AL, et al. The Effect of Osteoporosis Treatments on Fatigue Properties of Cortical Bone Tissue. Bone Reports 2015;2:8–13.
[146] Boivin G, Lips P, Ott SM, Harper KD, Sarkar S, Pinette KV, et al. Contribution of raloxifene and calcium and vitamin D3 supplementation to the increase of the degree of mineralization of bone in postmenopausal women. J Clin Endocrinol Metab 2003;88(9):4199–205.
[147] Aref M, Gallant MA, Organ JM, Wallace JM, Newman CL, Burr DB, et al. In vivo reference point indentation reveals positive effects of raloxifene on mechanical properties following 6 months of treatment in skeletally mature beagle dogs. Bone 2013;56(2):449–53.
[148] Calton EF, Macleay J, Boskey AL. Fourier transform infrared imaging analysis of cancellous bone in alendronate- and raloxifene-treated osteopenic sheep. Cells Tissues Organs 2011;194(2-4):302–6.
[149] Gallant MA, Brown DM, Hammond M, Wallace JM, Du J, Deymier-Black AC, et al. Bone cell-independent benefits of raloxifene on the skeleton: a novel mechanism for improving bone material properties. Bone 2014;61:191–200.
[150] Allen MR, Territo PR, Lin C, Persohn S, Jiang L, Riley AA, et al. In vivo UTE-MRI reveals positive effects of raloxifene on skeletal-bound water in skeletally mature beagle dogs. J Bone Miner Res 2015;30(8):1441–4.
[151] Russell RG. Bisphosphonates: from bench to bedside. Ann N Y Acad Sci 2006;1068:367–401.
[152] Russell RG. Bisphosphonates: the first 40 years. Bone 2011;49(1):2–19.
[153] Rogers MJ, Crockett JC, Coxon FP, Monkkonen J. Biochemical and molecular mechanisms of action of bisphosphonates. Bone 2011;49(1):34–41.
[154] Russell RG, Watts NB, Ebetino FH, Rogers MJ. Mechanisms of action of bisphosphonates: similarities and differences and their potential influence on clinical efficacy. Osteoporsis Int 2008;19 (6):733–59.
[155] Bilezikian JP. Efficacy of bisphosphonates in reducing fracture risk in postmenopausal osteoporosis. Am J Med 2009;122(Suppl. 2):S14–21.

[156] Black DM, Cummings SR, Karpf DB, Cauley JA, Thompson DE, Nevitt MC, et al. Randomised trial of effect of alendronate on risk of fracture in women with existing vertebral fractures. Fracture Intervention Trial Research Group. Lancet 1996;348(9041):1535–41.

[157] Black DM, Delmas PD, Eastell R, Reid IR, Boonen S, Cauley JA, et al. Once-yearly zoledronic acid for treatment of postmenopausal osteoporosis. N Eng J Med 2007;356(18):1809–22.

[158] McClung MR, Geusens P, Miller PD, Zippel H, Bensen WG, Roux C, et al. Effect of risedronate on the risk of hip fracture in elderly women. Hip Intervention Program Study Group. N Eng J Med 2001;344:333–40.

[159] Borah B, Dufresne TE, Chmielewski PA, Johnson TD, Chines A, Manhart MD. Risedronate preserves bone architecture in postmenopausal women with osteoporosis as measured by three-dimensional microcomputed tomography. Bone 2004;34(4):736–46.

[160] Chavassieux PM, Arlot ME, Reda C, Wei L, Yates AJ, Meunier PJ. Histomorphometric assessment of the long-term effects of alendronate on bone quality and remodeling in patients with osteoporosis. J Clin Invest 1997;100(6):1475–80.

[161] Boivin GY, Chavassieux PM, Santora AC, Yates J, Meunier PJ. Alendronate increases bone strength by increasing the mean degree of mineralization of bone tissue in osteoporotic women. Bone 2000;27:687–94.

[162] Eastell R, Barton I, Hannon RA, Chines A, Garnero P, Delmas P. Relationship of early changes in bone resorption to the reduction in fracture risk with risedronate*. J Bone Mineral Res 2003;18:1051–6.

[163] Eastell R, Boonen S, Cosman F, Reid IR, Palermo L, Cummings SR, et al. Relationship between pretreatment rate of bone loss and bone density response to once-yearly ZOL: HORIZON-PFT extension study. J Bone Miner Res 2015;30(3):570–4.

[164] Bauer DC, Garnero P, Hochberg MC, Santora A, Delmas P, Ewing SK, et al. Pretreatment levels of bone turnover and the antifracture efficacy of alendronate: the fracture intervention trial. J Bone Miner Res 2006;21(2):292–9.

[165] Balena R, Toolan BC, Shea M, Markatos A, Myers ER, Lee SC, et al. The effects of 2-year treatment with the aminobisphosphonate alendronate on bone metabolism, bone histomorphometry, and bone strength in ovariectomized nonhuman primates. J Clin Invest 1993;92(6):2577–86.

[166] Moroni A, Faldini C, Hoang-Kim A, Pegreffi F, Giannini S. Alendronate improves screw fixation in osteoporotic bone. J Bone Joint Surg Am 2007;89(1):96–101.

[167] Chapurlat RD, Arlot M, Burt-Pichat B, Chavassieux P, Roux JP, Portero-Muzy N, et al. Microcrack frequency and bone remodeling in postmenopausal osteoporotic women on long-term bisphosphonates: a bone biopsy study. J Bone Miner Res 2007;22(10):1502–9.

[168] Meunier PJ, Boivin G. Bone mineral density reflects bone mass but also the degree of mineralization of bone: therapeutic implications. Bone 1997;21:373–7.

[169] Boivin G, Meunier PJ. Changes in bone remodeling rate influence the degree of mineralization of bone. Connect Tissue Res 2002;43:535–7.

[170] Stepan JJ, Burr DB, Pavo I, Sipos A, Michalska D, Li J, et al. Low bone mineral density is associated with bone microdamage accumulation in postmenopausal women with osteoporosis. Bone 2007;41(3):378–85.

[171] Allen MR, Iwata K, Phipps R, Burr DB. Alterations in canine vertebral bone turnover, microdamage accumulation, and biomechanical properties following 1-year treatment with clinical treatment doses of risedronate or alendronate. Bone 2006;39(4):872–9.

[172] Dell RM, Adams AL, Greene DF, Funahashi TT, Silverman SL, Eisemon EO, et al. Incidence of atypical nontraumatic diaphyseal fractures of the femur. J Bone Miner Res 2012;27(12):2544–50.

[173] Yang KH, Won JH, Yoon HK, Ryu JH, Choo KS, Kim JS. High concentrations of pamidronate in bone weaken the mechanical properties of intact femora in a rat model. Yonsei Med J 2007;48 (4):653–8.

[174] Bajaj D, Geissler JR, Allen MR, Burr DB, Fritton JC. The resistance of cortical bone tissue to failure under cyclic loading is reduced with alendronate. Bone 2014;64:57–64.

[175] Roelofs AJ, Stewart CA, Sun S, Blazewska KM, Kashemirov BA, McKenna CE, et al. Influence of bone affinity on the skeletal distribution of fluorescently labeled bisphosphonates in vivo. J Bone Miner Res 2012;27(4):835−47.

[176] Kates SL, Ackert-Bicknell CL. How do bisphosphonates affect fracture healing? Injury 2016;47: S65−8.

[177] Xue D, Li F, Chen G, Yan SG, Pan Z. Do bisphosphonates affect bone healing? A meta-analysis of randomized controlled trials. J Orthop Surg 2014;9. 45-.

[178] Molvik H, Khan W. Bisphosphonates and their influence on fracture healing: a systematic review. Osteoporsis Int 2015.

[179] Solomon DH, Hochberg MC, Mogun H, Schneeweiss S. The relation between bisphosphonate use and non-union of fractures of the humerus in older adults. Osteoporsis Int 2009;20 (6):895−901.

[180] Cao Y, Mori S, Mashiba T, Westmore MS, Ma L, Sato M, et al. Raloxifene, estrogen, and alendronate affect the processes of fracture repair differently in ovariectomized rats. J Bone Miner Res 2002;17:2237−46.

[181] Savaridas T, Wallace RJ, Salter DM, Simpson AH. Do bisphosphonates inhibit direct fracture healing?: a laboratory investigation using an animal model. Bone Joint J 2013;95-b(9):1263−8.

[182] Kidd LJ, Cowling NR, Wu AC, Kelly WL, Forwood MR. Bisphosphonate treatment delays stress fracture remodeling in the rat ulna. J Orthop Res 2011.

[183] Teo BJX, Koh JSB, Goh SK, Png MA, Chua DTC, Howe TS. Post-operative outcomes of atypical femoral subtrochanteric fracture in patients on bisphosphonate therapy. Bone Joint J 2014; 96-B:658−64.

[184] Cummings SR, San Martin J, McClung MR, Siris ES, Eastell R, Reid IR, et al. Denosumab for prevention of fractures in postmenopausal women with osteoporosis. N Eng J Med 2009;361 (8):756−65.

[185] Papapoulos S, Lippuner K, Roux C, Lin CJ, Kendler DL, Lewiecki EM, et al. The effect of 8 or 5 years of denosumab treatment in postmenopausal women with osteoporosis: results from the FREEDOM Extension study. Osteoporsis Int 2015;26(12):2773−83.

[186] Reid I, Miller P, Brown J, Kendler D, Fahrleitner-Pammer A, Valter I, et al. Effects of denosumab on bone histomorphometry: the freedom and stand studies. J Bone Miner Res 2010.

[187] Ominsky MS, Libanati C, Niu Q-T, Boyce RW, Kostenuik PJ, Wagman RB, et al. Sustained modeling-based bone formation during adulthood in cynomolgus monkeys may contribute to continuous BMD gains with denosumab. J Bone Miner Res 2015;30(7):1280−9.

[188] Genant HK, Engelke K, Hanley DA, Brown JP, Omizo M, Bone HG, et al. Denosumab improves density and strength parameters as measured by QCT of the radius in postmenopausal women with low bone mineral density. Bone 2010;47(1):131−9.

[189] Ominsky MS, Stouch B, Schroeder J, Pyrah I, Stolina M, Smith SY, et al. Denosumab, a fully human RANKL antibody, reduced bone turnover markers and increased trabecular and cortical bone mass, density, and strength in ovariectomized cynomolgus monkeys. Bone 2011;49 (2):162−73.

[190] Selga J, Nunez JH, Minguell J, Lalanza M, Garrido M. Simultaneous bilateral atypical femoral fracture in a patient receiving denosumab: case report and literature review. Osteoporsis Int 2016;27(2):827−32.

[191] Edwards BJ, Sun M, West DP, Guindani M, Lin YH, Lu H, et al. Incidence of atypical femur fractures in cancer patients: the MD Anderson cancer center experience. J Bone Miner Res 2016.

[192] Thompson RN, Armstrong CL, Heyburn G. Bilateral atypical femoral fractures in a patient prescribed denosumab - A case report. Bone 2014;61:44−7.

[193] Paparodis R, Buehring B, Pelley EM, Binkley N. A case of an unusual subtrochanteric fracture in a patient receiving denosumab. Ende Pract 2013;19(3):e64−8.

[194] Singer FR. Metabolic bone disease: atypical femoral fractures. J Biomech 2011;44(2):244−7.

[195] Popp AW, Zysset PK, Lippuner K. Rebound-associated vertebral fractures after discontinuation of denosumab-from clinic and biomechanics. Osteoporsis Int 2016;27(5):1917−21.

[196] Aubry-Rozier B, Gonzalez-Rodriguez E, Stoll D, Lamy O. Severe spontaneous vertebral fractures after denosumab discontinuation: three case reports. Osteoporsis Int 2016;27(5):1923–5.
[197] Tam CS, Heersche JN, Murray TM, Parsons JA. Parathyroid hormone stimulates the bone apposition rate independently of its resorptive action: differential effects of intermittent and continuous administration. Endocrinology 1982;110(2):506–12.
[198] Neer RM, Arnaud CD, Zanchetta JR, Prince R, Gaich GA, Reginster JY, et al. Effect of parathyroid hormone (1-34) on fractures and bone mineral density in postmenopausal women with osteoporosis. N Eng J Med 2001;344:1434–41.
[199] Hodsman AB, Kisiel M, Adachi JD, Fraher LJ, Watson PH. Histomorphometric evidence for increased bone turnover without change in cortical thickness or porosity after 2 years of cyclical hPTH(1-34) therapy in women with severe osteoporosis. Bone 2000;27(2):311–18.
[200] Jiang Y, Zhao J, Mitlak B, Wang O, Genant H, Eriksen EF. Recombinant human parathyroid hormone (1-34) [teriparatide] improves both cortical and cancellous bone structure. J Bone Miner Res 2003;18:1932–41.
[201] Graeff C, Chevalier Y, Charlebois M, Varga P, Pahr D, Nickelsen TN, et al. Improvements in vertebral body strength under teriparatide treatment assessed in vivo by finite element analysis: results from the EUROFORS study. J Bone Miner Res 2009;24(10):1672–80.
[202] Keaveny TM, Donley DW, Hoffmann PF, Mitlak BH, Glass EV, San Martin JA. Effects of teriparatide and alendronate on vertebral strength as assessed by finite element modeling of QCT scans in women with osteoporosis. J Bone Miner Res 2007;22(1):149–57.
[203] Keaveny TM, Hoffmann PF, Singh M, Palermo L, Bilezikian JP, Greenspan SL, et al. Femoral bone strength and its relation to cortical and trabecular changes after treatment with PTH, alendronate, and their combination as assessed by finite element analysis of quantitative CT scans. J Bone Miner Res 2008;23(12):1974–82.
[204] Burr DB, Hirano T, Turner CH, Hotchkiss C, Brommage R, Hock JM. Intermittently administered human parathyroid hormone(1-34) treatment increases intracortical bone turnover and porosity without reducing bone strength in the humerus of ovariectomized cynomolgus monkeys. J Bone Miner Res 2001;16:157–65.
[205] Roschger P, Paschalis EP, Fratzl P, Klaushofer K. Bone mineralization density distribution in health and disease. Bone 2008;42(3):456–66.
[206] Paschalis EP, Glass EV, Donley DW, Eriksen EF. Bone mineral and collagen quality in iliac crest biopsies of patients given teriparatide: new results from the fracture prevention trial. J Clin Endocrinol Metab 2005;90(8):4644–9.
[207] Hofstetter B, Gamsjaeger S, Varga F, Dobnig H, Stepan JJ, Petto H, et al. Bone quality of the newest bone formed after two years of teriparatide therapy in patients who were previously treatment-naive or on long-term alendronate therapy. Osteoporsis Int. 2014.
[208] Pietrogrande L, Raimondo E. Teriparatide in the treatment of non-unions: scientific and clinical evidences. Injury 2013;44(Suppl. 1):S54–7.
[209] Barnes GL, Kakar S, Vora S, Morgan EF, Gerstenfeld LC, Einhorn TA. Stimulation of fracture-healing with systemic intermittent parathyroid hormone treatment. J Bone Joint Surg Am 2008;90 (Suppl. 1):120–7.
[210] Mancilla EE, Brodsky JL, Mehta S, Pignolo RJ, Levine MA. Teriparatide as a systemic treatment for lower extremity nonunion fractures: a case series. Endocrine Practice 2015;21(2):136–42.
[211] Zhang D, Potty AG, Vyas PA, Lane J. The role of recombinant PTH in human fracture healing: a systematic review. J Orthop Trauma 2014;28:57–62.
[212] Peichl P, Holzer LA, Maier R, Holzer G. Parathyroid hormone 1-84 accelerates fracture-healing in pubic bones of elderly osteoporotic women. J Bone Joint Surg Am 2011;93(17):1583–7.
[213] Johansson T. PTH 1-34 (teriparatide) may not improve healing in proximal humerus fractures. A randomized, controlled study of 40 patients. Acta Orthop 2016;87(1):79–82.
[214] Aspenberg P, Genant HK, Johansson T, Nino AJ, See K, Krohn K, et al. Teriparatide for acceleration of fracture repair in humans: a prospective, randomized, double-blind study of 102 postmenopausal women with distal radial fractures. J Bone Miner Res 2010;25(2):404–14.

[215] Vahle JL, Zuehlke U, Schmidt A, Westmore M, Chen P, Sato M. Lack of bone neoplasms and persistence of bone efficacy in cynomolgus macaques after long-term treatment with teriparatide [rhPTH(1-34)]. J Bone Miner Res 2008;23(12):2033–9.

[216] Reginster JY, Kaufman JM, Goemaere S, Devogelaer JP, Benhamou CL, Felsenberg D, et al. Maintenance of antifracture efficacy over 10 years with strontium ranelate in postmenopausal osteoporosis. Osteoporsis Int 2012;23(3):1115–22.

[217] Chavassieux P, Meunier PJ, Roux JP, Portero-Muzy N, Pierre M, Chapurlat R. Bone histomorphometry of transiliac paired bone biopsies after 6 or 12 months of treatment with oral strontium ranelate in 387 osteoporotic women. Randomized comparison to alendronate. J Bone Miner Res 2013.

[218] Boivin G, Meunier PJ. The mineralization of bone tissue: a forgotten dimension in osteoporosis research. Osteoporsis Int 2003;14(Suppl. 3):S19–24.

[219] Doublier A, Farlay D, Khebbab MT, Jaurand X, Meunier PJ, Boivin G. Distribution of strontium and mineralization in iliac bone biopsies from osteoporotic women treated long-term with strontium ranelate. Eur J Endocrinol 2011;165(3):469–76.

[220] Cohen-Solal M. Strontium overload and toxicity: impact on renal osteodystrophy. Nephrol Dialysis Transpl 2002;17(Suppl. 2):30–4.

[221] Oste L, Bervoets AR, Behets GJ, Dams G, Marijnissen RL, Geryl H, et al. Time-evolution and reversibility of strontium-induced osteomalacia in chronic renal failure rats. Kidney Int 2005;67 (3):920–30.

[222] D'Haese PC, Schrooten I, Goodman WG, Cabrera WE, Lamberts LV, Elseviers MM, et al. Increased bone strontium levels in hemodialysis patients with osteomalacia. Kidney Int 2000;57 (3):1107–14.

[223] Bor N, Rubin G, Rozen N. Fracture management in pycnodysostosis: 27 years of follow-up. J Pediatr Orthop B 2011;20(2):97–101.

[224] Alves Pereira D, Berini Aytes L, Gay Escoda C. Pycnodysostosis. A report of 3 clinical cases. Med Oral Patol Oral Cir Bucal 2008;13(10):E633–5.

[225] Appelman-Dijkstra NM, Papapoulos SE. From disease to treatment: from rare skeletal disorders to treatments for osteoporosis. Endocrine 2016;52(3):414–26.

[226] Bromme D, Panwar P, Turan S. Cathepsin K osteoporosis trials, pycnodysostosis and mouse deficiency models: commonalities and differences. Exp Opin Drug Discov 2016;11(5):457–72.

[227] Hamersma H, Gardner J, Beighton P. The natural history of sclerosteosis. Clin Genet 2003;63 (3):192–7.

[228] Gardner JC, van Bezooijen RL, Mervis B, Hamdy NA, Lowik CW, Hamersma H, et al. Bone mineral density in sclerosteosis; affected individuals and gene carriers. J Clin Endocrinol Metab 2005;90(12):6392–5.

[229] Wergedal JE, Veskovic K, Hellan M, Nyght C, Balemans W, Libanati C, et al. Patients with Van Buchem disease, an osteosclerotic genetic disease, have elevated bone formation markers, higher bone density, and greater derived polar moment of inertia than normal. J Clin Endocrinol Metab 2003;88(12):5778–83.

[230] Loots GG, Kneissel M, Keller H, Baptist M, Chang J, Collette NM, et al. Genomic deletion of a long-range bone enhancer misregulates sclerostin in Van Buchem disease. Genome Res 2005;15 (7):928–35.

[231] McClung MR, Grauer A, Boonen S, Bolognese MA, Brown JP, Diez-Perez A, et al. Romosozumab in postmenopausal women with low bone mineral density. N Eng J Med 2014;370(5):412–20.

[232] Ensrud KE, Walczak TS, Blackwell TL, Ensrud ER, Barrett-Connor E, Orwoll ES. Antiepileptic drug use and rates of hip bone loss in older men: a prospective study. Neurology 2008;71 (10):723–30.

[233] Kulak CA, Borba VZ, Silvado CE, Paola L, Seibel MJ, Bilezikian JP, et al. Bone density and bone turnover markers in patients with epilepsy on chronic antiepileptic drug therapy. Arq Bras Endocrinol Metabol 2007;51(3):466–71.

[234] Schelleman H, Pollard JR, Newcomb C, Markowitz CE, Bilker WB, Leonard MB, et al. Exposure to CYP3A4-inducing and CYP3A4-non-inducing antiepileptic agents and the risk of fractures. Pharmacoepidemiol Drug Saf 2011;20(6):619–25.
[235] Rabenda V, Nicolet D, Beaudart C, Bruyere O, Reginster JY. Relationship between use of antidepressants and risk of fractures: a meta-analysis. Osteoporsis Int 2013;24(1):121–37.
[236] Wu Q, Bencaz AF, Hentz JG, Crowell MD. Selective serotonin reuptake inhibitor treatment and risk of fractures: a meta-analysis of cohort and case-control studies. Osteoporsis Int 2012;23 (1):365–75.
[237] Kode A, Mosialou I, Silva BC, Rached MT, Zhou B, Wang J, et al. FOXO1 orchestrates the bone-suppressing function of gut-derived serotonin. J Clin Invest 2012;122(10):3490–503.
[238] Alhuzaim ON, Almohareb OM, Sherbeeni SM. Carbonic anhydrase II deficiency in a saudi woman. Clin Med Insights Case Rep 2015;8:7–10.
[239] Sly WS, Whyte MP, Sundaram V, Tashian RE, Hewett-Emmett D, Guibaud P, et al. Carbonic anhydrase II deficiency in 12 families with the autosomal recessive syndrome of osteopetrosis with renal tubular acidosis and cerebral calcification. N Eng J Med 1985;313(3):139–45.
[240] Jones G, Nguyen T, Sambrook PN, Eisman JA. Thiazide diuretics and fractures: can meta-analysis help?. J Bone Miner Res 1995;10(1):106–11.
[241] Rejnmark L, Vestergaard P, Mosekilde L. Reduced fracture risk in users of thiazide diuretics. Calcif Tissue Int 2005;76(3):167–75.
[242] Wiens M, Etminan M, Gill SS, Takkouche B. Effects of antihypertensive drug treatments on fracture outcomes: a meta-analysis of observational studies. J Intern Med 2006;260(4):350–62.
[243] Steiniche T. Bone histomorphometry in the pathophysiological evaluation of primary and secondary osteoporosis and various treatment modalities. APMIS 1995;51:1–44.
[244] LaCroix AZ, Ott SM, Ichikawa L, Scholes D, Barlow WE. Low-dose hydrochlorothiazide and preservation of bone mineral density in older adults. A randomized, double-blind, placebo-controlled trial. Ann Intern Med 2000;133(7):516–26.
[245] Ott SM, Lacroix AZ, Scholes D, Ichikawa LE, Wu K. Effects of three years of low-dose thiazides on mineral metabolism in healthy elderly persons. Osteoporsis Int 2008;19(9):1315–22.
[246] Kahn SE, Zinman B, Lachin JM, Haffner SM, Herman WH, Holman RR, et al. Rosiglitazone-associated fractures in type 2 diabetes: an analysis from A Diabetes Outcome Progression Trial (ADOPT). Diabetes Care 2008;31(5):845–51.
[247] Billington EO, Grey A, Bolland MJ. The effect of thiazolidinediones on bone mineral density and bone turnover: systematic review and meta-analysis. Diabetologia 2015;58(10):2238–46.
[248] Zhu ZN, Jiang YF, Ding T. Risk of fracture with thiazolidinediones: an updated meta-analysis of randomized clinical trials. Bone 2014;68:115–23.
[249] Kawai M, Rosen CJ. PPARgamma: a circadian transcription factor in adipogenesis and osteogenesis. Nat Rev Endocrinol 2010;6(11):629–36.
[250] Mukherjee S, Raje N, Schoonmaker JA, Liu JC, Hideshima T, Wein MN, et al. Pharmacologic targeting of a stem/progenitor population in vivo is associated with enhanced bone regeneration in mice. J Clin Invest 2008;118(2):491–504.
[251] Li J, Khavandgar Z, Lin SH, Murshed M. Lithium chloride attenuates BMP-2 signaling and inhibits osteogenic differentiation through a novel WNT/GSK3- independent mechanism. Bone 2011;48(2):321–31.
[252] Zamani A, Omrani GR, Nasab MM. Lithium's effect on bone mineral density. Bone 2009;44 (2):331–4.
[253] Arioka M, Takahashi-Yanaga F, Sasaki M, Yoshihara T, Morimoto S, Hirata M, et al. Acceleration of bone regeneration by local application of lithium: wnt signal-mediated osteoblastogenesis and Wnt signal-independent suppression of osteoclastogenesis. Biochem Pharmacol 2014;90 (4):397–405.
[254] Ott SM, Maloney NA, Coburn JW, Alfrey AC, Sherrard DJ. The prevalence of bone aluminum deposition in renal osteodystrophy and its relation to the response to calcitriol therapy. N Eng J Med 1982;307:709–13.

[255] Ott SM, Maloney NA, Klein GL, Alfrey AC, Ament ME, Coburn JW, et al. Aluminum is associated with low bone formation in patients receiving chronic parenteral nutrition. Ann Intern Med 1983;98:910–14.

[256] D'Haese PC, Couttenye MM, Lamberts LV, Elseviers MM, Goodman WG, Schrooten I, et al. Aluminum, iron, lead, cadmium, copper, zinc, chromium, magnesium, strontium, and calcium content in bone of end-stage renal failure patients. Clin Chem 1999;45(9):1548–56.

[257] Casale M, Citarella S, Filosa A, De Michele E, Palmieri F, Ragozzino A, et al. Endocrine function and bone disease during long-term chelation therapy with deferasirox in patients with beta-thalassemia major. Am J Hematol 2014;89(12):1102–6.

[258] Doyard M, Chappard D, Leroyer P, Roth MP, Loreal O, Guggenbuhl P. Decreased bone formation explains osteoporosis in a genetic mouse model of hemochromatosiss. PLoS One 2016;11(2): e0148292.

[259] Xiao W, Beibei F, Guangsi S, Yu J, Wen Z, Xi H, et al. Iron overload increases osteoclastogenesis and aggravates the effects of ovariectomy on bone mass. J Endocrinol 2015;226(3):121–34.

[260] Baba H, Tsuneyama K, Kumada T, Aoshima K, Imura J. Histopathological analysis for osteomalacia and tubulopathy in itai-itai disease. J Toxicol Sci 2013;39:91–6.

[261] Wallin M, Barregard L, Sallsten G, Lundh T, Karlsson MK, Lorentzon M, et al. Low-level cadmium exposure is associated with decreased bone mineral density and increased risk of incident fractures in elderly men: the MrOS Sweden study. J Bone Miner Res 2016;31(4):732–41.

[262] Allen LA, Ambardekar AV, Devaraj KM, Maleszewski JJ, Wolfel EE. Clinical problem-solving. Missing elements of the history. N Eng J Med 2014;370(6):559–66.

[263] van der Veen HC, Reininga IH, Zijlstra WP, Boomsma MF, Bulstra SK, van Raay JJ. Pseudotumour incidence, cobalt levels and clinical outcome after large head metal-on-metal and conventional metal-on-polyethylene total hip arthroplasty: mid-term results of a randomised controlled trial. Bone Joint J 2015;97-b(11):1481–7.

[264] Hahn M, Busse B, Procop M, Zustin J, Amling M, Katzer A. Cobalt deposition in mineralized bone tissue after metal-on-metal hip resurfacing: quantitative mu-X-ray-fluorescence analysis of implant material incorporation in periprosthetic tissue. J Biomed Mater Res B Appl Biomater 2016. Available from: http://dx.doi.org/10.1002/jbm.b.33667.

[265] Rakow A, Schoon J, Dienelt A, John T, Textor M, Duda G, et al. Influence of particulate and dissociated metal-on-metal hip endoprosthesis wear on mesenchymal stromal cells in vivo and in vitro. Biomaterials 2016;98:31–40.

[266] Kanaji A, Orhue V, Caicedo MS, Virdi AS, Sumner DR, Hallab NJ, et al. Cytotoxic effects of cobalt and nickel ions on osteocytes in vitro. J Orthop Surg 2014;9:91.

[267] Shah KM, Wilkinson JM, Gartland A. Cobalt and chromium exposure affects osteoblast function and impairs the mineralization of prosthesis surfaces in vitro. J Orthop Res 2015;33(11):1663–70.

[268] Riggs BL, Hodgson SF, O'Fallon WM, Chao EY, Wahner HW, Muhs JM, et al. Effect of fluoride treatment on the fracture rate in postmenopausal women with osteoporosis. N Eng J Med 1990;322(12):802–9.

[269] Balena R, Kleerekoper M, Foldes JA, Shih MS, Rao DS, Schober HC, et al. Effects of different regimens of sodium fluoride treatment for osteoporosis on the structure, remodeling and mineralization of bone. Osteoporsis Int 1998;8:428–35.

[270] Lundy MW, Stauffer M, Wergedal JE, Baylink DJ, Featherstone JD, Hodgson SF, et al. Histomorphometric analysis of iliac crest bone biopsies in placebo-treated versus fluoride-treated subjects. Osteoporsis Int 1995;5(2):115–29.

[271] Roschger P, Fratzl P, Klaushofer K, Rodan G. Mineralization of cancellous bone after alendronate and sodium fluoride treatment: a quantitative backscattered electron imaging study on minipig ribs. Bone 1997;20(5):393–7.

[272] Fratzl P, Roschger P, Eschberger J, Abendroth B, Klaushofer K. Abnormal bone mineralization after fluoride treatment in osteoporosis: a small-angle x-ray-scattering study. J Bone Miner Res 1994;9(10):1541–9.

CHAPTER 3

Bone Disorders

J. Zang[1,2], L. Lu[1] and M.J. Yaszemski[1]
[1]Mayo Clinic College of Medicine, Rochester, MN, United States
[2]Peking University, Beijing, China

Contents

3.1 INTRODUCTION

Bone is the most well-differentiated organ that originates from mesenchymal tissue. It is alive and dynamic. In terms of function, bone is primarily a structural, load-bearing organ. It provides protection to vital organs and bears loads that the body experiences, both from external forces and those that occur from muscle contraction. Bone provides the anchor point for that muscle contraction through its specialized tendon insertion sites (entheses). Bone's ligament insertion sites, which have the same structure as its tendon insertion sites (and are also classified as entheses), are essential to the function of joints. The articular cartilage that covers the ends of long bones, and which constitutes the bearing surfaces of joints, allows locomotion by the lower extremities and the positioning of the hands in space by the upper extremities. Bone also acts as a metabolic organ in its role as the storage depot of calcium and phosphate. It is the largest reservoir of calcium in the body, and the constant remodeling of bone mobilizes its calcium as one component of the process that tightly mediates calcium homeostasis. Bone remodeling also serves a structural purpose. The remodeling process positions the available mineralized bone tissue in an optimum distribution to bear the loads experienced by the skeleton. The spaces between bony struts and plates that make up trabecular bone (also called spongy or cancellous bone) contain the bone marrow, which produces and stores cells with multiple hematologic and regenerative body functions [1].

Bone disorders are very common. They occur at a rate of about 124/1000 persons in the United States [2]. They are among the most common causes of severe long-term pain and physical disabilities. The most common bone disease is osteoporosis, and the most common consequence of this disease is fracture. There are 1.5 million osteoporotic fractures in the United States annually. It is estimated that 40% of all women over 50 years of age will suffer from an osteoporotic fracture. Back pain is the second leading cause for visits to the doctor's office in the United States, outnumbered only by upper-respiratory infections. Joint diseases account for half of all chronic conditions in persons aged 65 and above [3]. Bone disease impacts not only the affected individuals and their families, but it also impacts society at large. From an individual's perspective, bone disorders can result in limitations on their activities of daily living and mobility, and in decreased quality of life. From society's perspective, bone disorders inflict a direct economic burden on both the affected families and society. Bone disorders also result in an indirect economic loss due to reduced participation in the labor force [2]. During the period 2009–2011, the average annual direct and indirect (lost work) costs in the United States attributable to persons with a musculoskeletal disease were $213 billion [4]. Fractures in the United States that result from osteoporosis lead annually to more than half a million hospitalizations, over 800,000 emergency room encounters, more than 2,600,000 physician office visits, and the placement of nearly 180,000 individuals into nursing homes. This burden will continue to rise as the frequency of bone disease increases in the future with the anticipated growth of the elderly population [5]. Although back pain is something that people often suffer in silence, its costs are large based on lost income and the consumption of health and social resources.

Due to the substantial burdens that result from bone disorders and the high prevalence of those disorders, more attention needs to be directed toward prevention and the development of more effective treatment modalities. There has been a global campaign, named "The Bone and Joint Decade," with the goals of raising awareness of the growing burden of bone disorders on society, promoting cost-effective prevention and treatment, and improving prevention and treatment by research [3]. The Decade is a global campaign, not a new organization. It provides opportunities and builds up a framework for cooperation. No one single organization is able to accomplish the desired benefits for the patients. The Decade is a multidisciplinary initiative involving those who participate in musculoskeletal care including communities, patients, healthcare providers, and researchers. There are now over 650 national and international organizations that represent such groups and have joined this campaign. The number of involved groups keeps rising, as the goal of the Decade is to include all such relevant organizations all over the world. In the spirit of the US Bone and Joint Decade, this chapter introduces several common bone disorders; osteoporosis, degenerative disc disease (DDD), osteoarthritis (OA), fractures, Paget's disease, and bone cancer. It will contain a brief description of current clinical practices to treat these bone disorders, critical issues surrounding them, and future directions in both clinical care and research.

3.2 METABOLIC DISEASES

Osteoporosis and Paget's disease are among the most common metabolic diseases in the United States. Osteoporosis is characterized by a systemic decrease in bone mass and strength. Paget's disease of bone (PDB) is characterized by localized areas of excessive bone resorption as well as increased bone formation, resulting in new bone which is less organized from a structural perspective and is weaker than normal bone.

3.2.1 Osteoporosis

Osteoporosis is the most common metabolic disease in the United States (Fig. 3.1) [6]. Patients with osteoporosis are at some level of increased risk for suffering an insufficiency (fragility) fracture. A fall or even slight stresses like bending over or coughing

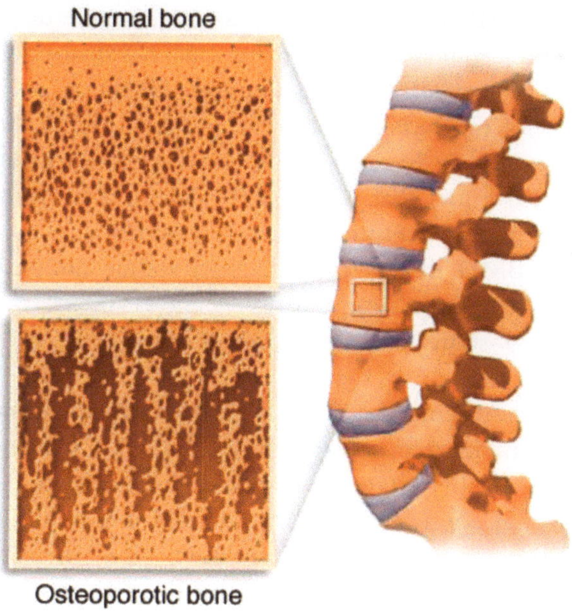

Figure 3.1 Normal bone has the appearance of a honeycomb matrix (top). Osteoporotic bone (bottom) is porous. In osteoporosis, the bone microstructure is normal; there is, however, less total bone mass. *From: Mayo Clinic.*

can cause such fractures. They can occur in multiple locations that include the hip, wrist and spine. In 2010, the US Department of Health and Human Services reported that osteoporosis affected more than 9 million women who were older than 50 years [7]. It has also been reported that more than 1.5 million people have osteoporosis-related fractures in the United States every year [8].

There are three types of osteoporosis, including primary, secondary, and idiopathic [9]. Primary osteoporosis occurs as a natural consequence of aging. It is subdivided into senile and postmenopausal varieties. Senile osteoporosis is due to the gradual loss of bone mass, and it affects both men and women. The postmenopausal type of osteoporosis occurs in women. Women's bone is sensitive to the estrogen withdrawal that is a component of menopause. Estrogen plays an important role in bone remodeling via its inhibition of bone resorption. Women undergo a rapid loss of their bone mass after menopause.

Secondary osteoporosis occurs in patients with chronic diseases that result in loss of bone mass. These conditions include nutritional deficiencies, anorexia, alcoholism, and chronic liver disease. Several categories of drugs, such as gonadotropin-releasing hormone agonists and steroids, have effects on bone formation and thus contribute to the loss of bone mass.

Idiopathic osteoporosis is a subtype that occurs primarily in young adults or children in whom there is no identifiable endocrine abnormality or risk factor.

Bone mineral density (BMD) evaluation is essential for the diagnosis of osteoporosis. Currently, the golden standard of measuring BMD is dual-energy X-ray absorptiometry (DEXA) scans. The DEXA scan evaluates BMD at any site; however, the bone mineral content of the lumbar spine, the proximal femur, and the distal radius are the three sites that are usually evaluated in current clinical practice. A DEXA scan report consists of several values that include a T score, a Z score, and a measurement of BMD in grams per square centimeter. The T score is a comparison of the BMD results to the average BMD in a gender-matched young adult cohort. T scores are reported as standard deviations from the expected BMD of that gender-matched young adult cohort. A T score that is less than or equal to −2.5 defines osteoporosis [10] (Table 3.1).

A Fracture Risk Assessment Tool (FRAX) was proposed by the WHO to predict the fracture risk in patients with osteoporosis. The FRAX takes the T score into account as well as several other osteoporosis risk factors, including age, gender, height, weight, smoking, alcohol consumption, corticosteroid use, family history of fractures, personal history of fractures, other health conditions (e.g., rheumatoid arthritis), and ethnicity. These factors enable FRAX to calculate the 10-year risk of a major osteoporotic fracture of the spine, shoulder, hip, or wrist. FRAX is available at the Foundation for Osteoporosis Research and Education website: https://riskcalculator.fore.org/.

Table 3.1 Diagnostic criteria for osteoporosis

T score	Diagnosis
0 to −0.99	Normal
−1 to −2.499	Osteopenia
≤−2.5	Osteoporosis
≤−2.5 accompanied by fracture or history of fracture	Severe osteoporosis

Source: World Health Organization Scientific Group. WHO Technical Report Series 921. Prevention and Management of Osteoporosis. Geneva, Switzerland: World Health Organization; 2003.

The initiation of treatment for both men and postmenopausal women with osteoporosis is commonly based on the following criteria: (1) T scores ≤− 2.5 at the lumbar spine, femoral neck, or total hip region; (2) T scores between − 1.0 and − 2.5 plus a FRAX score showing that the person is at risk for a major osteoporotic fracture of at least 20% or a hip fracture of at least 3% within 10 years; or (3) a personal history of an insufficiency vertebral or hip fracture (a fracture that occurs under "minimal energy trauma" circumstances that would ordinarily not be expected to result in fracture). An example of a vertebral insufficiency fracture would be a fracture that occurs as a result of coughing or sneezing. Insufficiency fractures are also called "fragility fractures" [11]. The National Osteoporosis Foundation suggests that treatment can be given to postmenopausal women aged over 50 years meeting any one of the above three criteria [12]. The treatment options for patients with osteoporosis include both nonpharmacologic and pharmacologic treatments.

The nonpharmacologic methods encompass the use of oral calcium and vitamin D supplementation, improving lighting, and fall prevention (removing loose rugs, as well as adding grab bars in bathtubs, toilets, and stairways can all contribute to fall prevention) [13]. The recommended minimum daily calcium dose for all women with osteoporosis is 1200 mg [6]. Most postmenopausal women have inadequate daily dietary calcium intake, and supplementation is needed for adequate bone mineral metabolism. Vitamin D is essential for calcium absorption. The National Osteoporosis Foundation suggests 800−1000 IU of vitamin D daily for persons 50 years and older [14].

Bisphosphonates represent the first-line strategy for combating osteoporosis, and they are the most commonly used drugs in its treatment. These agents bind to hydroxyapatite and block the enzyme farnesyl pyrophosphate synthase in bone tissue. They inhibit, via this mechanism, bone resorption mediated by osteoclasts. Bisphosphonates can both increase BMD and reduce the incidence of hip and nonvertebral fractures. To date, there are four bisphosphonate drugs approved by the FDA for the treatment of osteoporosis, including alendronate, risedronate, ibandronate, and zoledronic acid. Alendronate, risedronate, and ibandronate can be given by both daily and intermittent (weekly or monthly) dosage forms. Zoledronic acid is given by an annual intravenous infusion.

There are additional pharmacologic methods that can be used in patients with osteoporosis. Salmon calcitonin is, like the bisphosphonates, an antiresorptive therapy for osteoporosis. It increases BMD by inhibiting the activity of osteoclasts, and it decreases the risk of vertebral fractures. Raloxifene, a selective estrogen receptor modulator, is approved for the treatment of postmenopausal osteoporosis. It acts as an estrogen agonist on both bone and fat tissue, and as an estrogen antagonist on breast and uterine tissue. Teriparatide is recombinant human parathyroid hormone. It demonstrates anabolic effects on bone tissue by stimulating the activity of osteoblasts. Teriparatide is currently the only anabolic agent available for the treatment of osteoporosis. Denosumab, an antiresorptive agent, is a human monoclonal antibody against the receptor activator of nuclear factor-kappa ligand (RANKL), an osteoclast differentiating factor. Denosumab inhibits osteoclast formation via this mechanism, and thus decreases bone resorption.

3.2.2 Paget's disease

PDB is the second most common metabolic bone disease in the United States. The etiology of Paget's continues to be controversial. Some studies suggest that it is caused by a slow virus infection. The suspected viruses include paramyxovirus, respiratory syncytial virus, canine distemper virus, and the measles virus. However, there are studies that do not support the viral infection hypothesis [15,16].

Genetic factors also contribute to the development of Paget's, and 15–40% patients with Paget's have a positive family history for it. There are three gene mutations that are identified in Paget's disease and related syndromes, such as familial expansile osteolysis and idiopathic hyperphosphatasia. These mutations affect the receptor activator of nuclear factor kappa b (RANK), osteoprotegerin, and sequestosome 1. RANK is expressed on the surface of osteoclasts and is a critical regulator of the formation and function of osteoclasts. Osteoprotegerin is a decoy receptor for RANK. Sequestosome 1 is a protein involved in mediating NFκB signaling [17].

The incidence of Paget's disease varies remarkably with geographic location. It occurs commonly in the populations of the United States, England, Australia, New Zealand, Canada, France, and South Africa. It is rare throughout Asia and Scandinavia. The most recent estimated incidence in the United States is 1–2% [18,19]. Paget's disease rarely happens in people less than 55 years old, and the prevalence increases with age. One study from the United States showed that Paget's more commonly affects male patients [20]. A typical feature of the disease is its clustering in families, demonstrating that genetic factors play a role in its development.

Paget's can involve a single bone (monostotic) or multiple bones (polyostotic). In polyostotic Paget's, the axial skeleton is usually involved, and the most affected sites in polyostotic patients include the pelvis (70%), femur (55%), lumbar spine (53%), skull (42%), and tibia (32%) [21].

The most common symptom is bone pain, resulting from microfractures and periosteal tension produced by the enlarging bone. Pain occurs in 40–45% of Paget's patients. Bone deformities are the second most common finding; they occur in 12–36% of patients. The femur and tibia are the most common locations for pagetoid bone deformities. The usual deformity is bowing, which is characteristically apex anterolateral in the femur and apex anterior in the tibia.

As most patients with Paget's are asymptomatic, evaluation is recommended for individuals over 50 years of age who present with an unexplained elevation of serum alkaline phosphatase, with or without bone deformities.

Paget's features increase bone metabolic activity, in which bone formation and resorption are not coordinated as they normally are in the process of bone remodeling. Serum alkaline phosphatase, a bone formation marker, is useful for both diagnosis and monitoring of patients with the disease. Serum alkaline phosphatase has a sensitivity of 78% and a specificity of almost 100% for the diagnosis of Paget's. However, it may be normal in up to 20% of patients with monostotic disease [22].

The radiographic features of Paget's disease vary with its disease stages, including osteolytic, osteosclerotic, and mixed lesions (Fig. 3.2). In the earlier stages of Paget's, the lesions are osteolytic due to the increased activity of osteoclasts. These appearances can commonly be identified in the skull and the lesions are known as "osteoporosis circumscripta." This radiologic appearance may also be seen in the long bones. The lesions usually originate from the metaphysis pointing toward the diaphysis. At the junction of the lesion with normal bone, the osteolytic lesion shows the shape of a flame or inverted "V." The average rate of the lesion extending into the normal bone is about 1 cm per year [23]. Later, the compensatory osteoblastic response starts, resulting in the development of osteosclerotic lesions in the previous osteolytic areas.

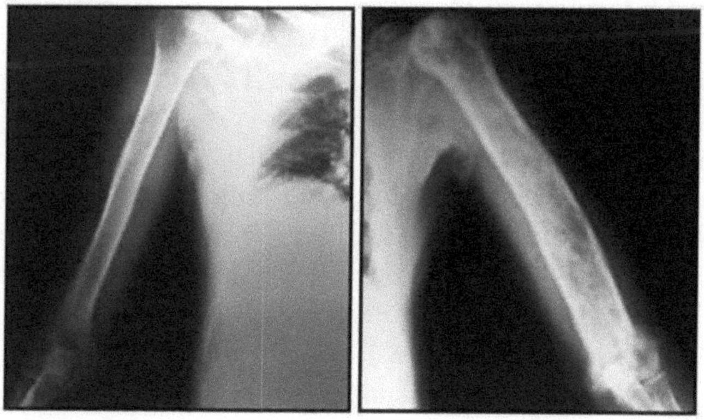

Figure 3.2 On the right, an X-ray of an upper arm bone (humerus) shows the abnormal growth associated with Paget's disease. The same person's other, normal humerus is shown in the X-ray on the left. *From: Mayo Clinic.*

The advancing front of osteolysis is trailed by patchy sclerosis superimposed on the earlier osteolytic process. The characteristic features of the late stage include coarsening of the trabeculae, blurring of the cortical–medullary junction, narrowing of the medullary cavity, and thickening or enlargement of the bone.

A CT scan can detect subtle fractures, spinal stenosis, and secondary neoplasms. An MRI scan may be helpful in evaluating spinal involvement by Paget's [24]. A bone scan will show increased uptake in skeletal areas of active Paget's due to the high rate of bone formation and blood flow in those areas. It is a sensitive method to detect the absence or quiescence of the disease. It can be positive even before the lytic changes are seen on plain radiography. It is also helpful to determine the extent of the involvement of the skeleton [25].

The histological appearances can be divided into three phases: the hot phase, the intermediate phase, and the cold phase. The hot phase is characterized by bone resorption. An increased number of osteoclasts are present and they are commonly larger than normal, having up to 100 nuclei in a single cross section rather than the 3–10 found in normal osteoclasts. The marrow is replaced by a vascular fibrous tissue. The histologic features of this phase are similar to those of secondary hyperparathyroidism. The characteristic intranuclear and cytoplasmic components can be observed via electron microscopy. The intranuclear components are tight bundles of microfilaments, and the cytoplasm shows randomly distributed filaments.

The appearance of the intermediate phase results from the compensatory osteoblastic response. The osteoblasts develop irregular, thick seams of osteoid, which are mineralized at twice the normal rate. The functional trabecular arrangement is obviously altered, and marrow fibrosis with increased vascularity is present. Woven bone (i.e., newly formed bone that has not yet been remodeled) is prominent, especially beneath the periosteum. In the cold phase, the active remodeling is less prominent. However, evidence of prior chaotic remodeling is obvious. Many intersecting cement lines form a "mosaic" pattern throughout the coarsely thickened trabeculae. The woven bone deposited in the intermediate phase has been remodeled into lamellar bone. These changes obliterate the distinction between the medullary bone and highly porous cortex.

The complications resulting from Paget's disease are classified as skeletal (bone pain, osteoarthrosis, deformities, fractures, and hypercalcemia), cardiovascular (high output heart failure, vascular calcifications, and valvular stenosis), neurological (deafness, increased intracranial pressure, and cranial nerve dysfunction), metabolic (hyperuricemia, hypercalciuria, hypercalcemia, and nephrolithiasis), and neoplastic (osteosarcoma (OS) and giant cell tumors) [25].

The pharmacological treatment methods target the osteoclasts and are responsible for slowing down the process of the disease, rather than acting as definitive therapy [26].

To date, there is no consensus regarding the indications for drug treatment. Based on a review of the literature, we propose that the indications can be grouped as follows: (1) bone pain; (2) hypercalcemia; (3) neurologic deficits associated with vertebral disease; (4) high-output congestive heart failure; (5) preparation for orthopedic surgery; and (6) prevention of complications, including hearing loss and skeletal deformity [24].

Calcitonin is used in the treatment of Paget's disease, and it acts by binding to the calcitonin receptors located on the osteoclasts. Due its short duration of action, partial response, and acquired resistance, it is used only in those with intolerance to bisphosphonates [27].

Currently, bisphosphonates are the most commonly used drugs for treating the disease. They act by inhibiting the activity of osteoclastic bone resorption. Generally, there are two types of bisphosphonates: nitrogenous (alendronate, risedronate, pamidronate, and zoledronic acid) and nonnitrogenous (etidronate, clodronate, and tiludronate). Nitrogenous bisphosphonates have higher efficiency and lower side effects. Therefore, the use of nitrogenous bisphosphonates is recommended for the treatment of Paget's disease, and zoledronic acid is the most potent bisphosphonate for use with this disease [25].

Surgical treatment can be considered in selected patients. For patients who have pathologic fractures, surgery can help achieve bone healing in a better position. Joint replacements of the hips and knees are used for patients with severe OA. For patients with bone deformities, osteotomies may play a role in helping to reduce the deformity and produce better function of the joints.

The level of serum alkaline phosphatase is used to monitor the treatment effect. It can be evaluated every 3 months after the initiation of the treatment and can be extended to every 6–12 months after a nadir has been reached. Remission is defined as a return of the level of alkaline phosphatase to normal, and partial remission as a decrease in levels greater than 75% of the distance to normal after 3–6 months of treatment. Treatment should be restarted when alkaline phosphatase levels begin to rise again (when treatment involves normalization), or when there is a 25% increase compared to posttreatment levels [28]. If a patient has a well-defined osteolytic lesion on plain X-ray images, it can be assessed annually to assure that the disease is well-controlled. It is not essential to perform regular scheduled bone scans for follow-up.

3.3 DEGENERATIVE DISC DISEASE

DDD is a pathologic process that may cause acute or chronic low back pain. It is not actually a disease, but rather a medical condition in which the spinal discs "degenerate," or lose their ability to perform their mechanical function in the spine. It is one of the most common causes for spine pain (neck pain and low back pain), which is the second leading cause for visits to the doctor's office. Up to 84% of adults have low back pain at some time in their lives [29]. Low back pain occurs in individuals of all ages, and it happens more commonly in individuals between 55 and 64 years of age [30]. Low back pain is also costly. In 1998, the expenditures for low back pain in the United States were estimated at 90 billion dollars and the amount is rising every year [31].

The intervertebral disc is made of nearly 80% water. As it degenerates, it slowly loses water, leading to a decrease in its viscoelastic properties. There are a series of spinal changes that can occur due to the process of disc degeneration. The most common diseases resulting from disc degeneration are herniated disc and spinal stenosis (Fig. 3.3). The nucleus pulposus may herniate through a tear in the disc wall (the annulus) and compress a nerve or more than one nerve. It causes pain in two ways. First, the nucleus pulposus that has ruptured into the spinal canal directly compresses the nerve roots. Second, the nucleus pulposus causes a chemical irritation of the nerve roots. The combination of the two can cause pain, weakness, and numbness in the area where the compromised nerve supplies sensation and movement. The herniated nucleus pulposus may also compress the spinal cord or cauda equina in addition to its ability to compress the nerve roots, especially in a congenitally narrow spinal canal. The degeneration of a disc causes the ligaments and facet joints to enlarge (hypertrophy) as they try to compensate and spread the load over a larger area. This overgrowth of facet joint bone, capsular ligaments, and yellow ligament causes the spinal canal to narrow, which can compress the spinal cord, cauda equina, and spinal nerves, causing pain and loss of function.

Several factors are involved in the genesis of disc degeneration. Age and genetic factors can affect the process of disc degeneration. Nutritional and mechanical factors

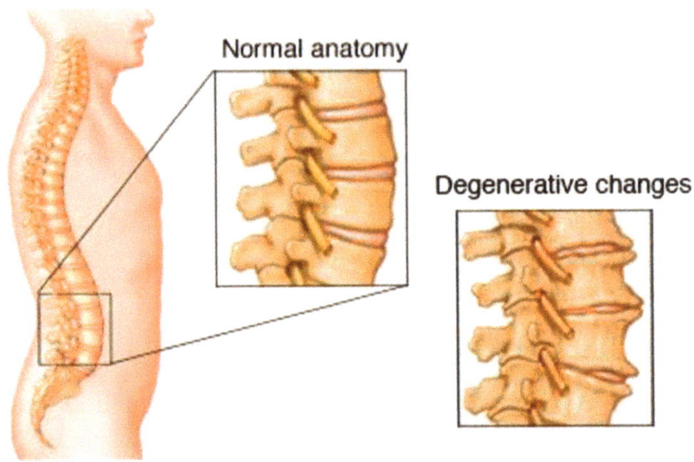

Figure 3.3 As the spine degenerates, it undergoes changes that include osteophytes (bone spurs), disc herniations, hypertrophied facet joint capsules, and thickened yellow ligaments. These normally occurring degenerative changes that accompany aging reduce the amount of space available for the spinal cord, cauda equina, and nerve roots. *From: Mayo Clinic.*

are also able to accelerate the process primarily. Moreover, other factors such as toxic and metabolic influences play a role in accelerating the degenerative process [32].

The symptoms and signs come from the compression of affected nerve roots, spinal cord, cauda equina, and vary with the compression sites. As for lumbosacral disc degeneration, patients often have low back pain, sometimes radiating to one or both legs. Some will be subjected to numbness in certain areas of one or both legs, or muscle weakness in certain muscles near the affected nerves. Bladder, bowel, and/or sexual function can be compromised due to cauda equina compression. Cervical disc degeneration causes neck pain and/or pain traveling into the arms. Numbness and weakness can also be observed in the distributions of the affected nerves. Spastic paresis of the lower limbs or quadriparesis can occur if the cervical spinal cord is compressed.

Plain X-ray images cannot reveal disc degeneration directly, and is done to exclude other medical conditions, such as fracture, tumor, or infection. It can show indirect findings of disc degeneration in the form of loss of intervertebral disc height and end-plate osteophytes. The oblique views of the plain X-ray imaging series are commonly used to assess narrowing of the neuroforaminal spaces.

CT has proven to be helpful in the diagnosis of disc degenerative disease. In disc herniation, it can show the displacement of the disc margin into the spinal canal or the neural foramen. It can demonstrate the displacement of the thecal sac and calcification within the disc herniation. In spinal stenosis, the CT scan shows the osteophytes around the vertebral body, the diminished diameters of the spinal canal, and the hypertrophy of the facet joints. It can also show the relationship between the osteophytes and the vital neural structures: spinal cord, cauda equina, and nerve roots.

MRI is the best tool to show the herniated nucleus pulposus. The herniations appear as focal protrusions of disc material beyond the extent of the annulus fibrosus. MRI can show the relationship between the herniated disc and the affected nerve root or the thecal sac. In spinal stenosis, MRI shows the osteophytes around the vertebral body, with dark signal on the T2 weighted images. It also can demonstrate the relationship between the osteophytes and the thecal sac. Moreover, it is used in the evaluation of cervical spinal stenosis by assessment of the cerebrospinal fluid distribution in the area of stenosis.

The initial treatment for patients with low back pain includes self-care advice, nonnarcotic medication, activity modifications and physical treatments, and noninvasive physical modalities. Acetaminophen and nonsteroidal antiinflammatory medications are considered to be the first-line pharmacologic options for low back pain. Other drugs used for low back pain include opioids, antidepressants, and antiepileptic medications [33]. The activity modifications and physical treatments include spinal manipulation, traction, acupuncture, and massage. The physical modalities involve low-level laser therapy, ultrasound, transcutaneous electrical nerve stimulation, and percutaneous electrical nerve stimulation [34,35]. For patients with neck pain, medications and physical treatments can be performed initially. Modalities such as trigger point injections, cervical medial branch blocks, and percutaneous radiofrequency neurotomy can also be performed if patients do not respond well to the methods described above.

Surgery is reserved for patients with severe or progressive motor weakness, myelopathic signs, or cauda equina syndrome. It is also an alternative option for patients with a significantly compromised quality of life and no response to the nonoperative treatments described above.

For patients with nonspecific low back pain, which is related to degenerative changes in the intervertebral discs or facet joints, spinal fusion is the most common surgical procedure. The aim is to restrict spinal movement and remove the degenerative disc and facet joints (the speculated pain generators) in order to alleviate symptoms. A bone graft is inserted into the space from which the affected disc is removed. Spinal fusion changes the normal mechanics of the spine and is related to long-term degenerative alterations in adjacent spine segments. Artificial disc replacement is a newer option as an alternative to fusion. It may theoretically reduce the long-term degenerative changes in adjacent vertebral segments by preserving the normal range of motion (ROM) and spine mechanics of the treated functional spinal unit (a disc and its two associated vertebral bodies). However, current studies show that the effect of this procedure is similar to spinal fusion. Disc replacement is approved by the FDA for patients with good health, ≤ 60 years old, with disease limited to one disc between L3 and S1 and no associated deformity, spondylolisthesis, facet arthritic changes, or neurologic deficit [36].

In patients who have a lumbar disc herniation with radiculopathy, discectomy may be performed to relieve symptoms by removing part of, or the whole, disc. The discectomy techniques include traditional open microdiscectomy and minimally invasive techniques. The traditional microdiscectomy involves visualizing the spine through an operating microscope or a loupe-headlight combination, followed by a hemilaminotomy and removal of the disc fragment compressing the compromised nerves. Minimally invasive techniques use microscopic microdiscectomy via transmuscular tube retraction [37]. Compared with microdiscectomy, minimally invasive techniques have the advantages of less trauma and quicker recovery from surgery; the disadvantages include less visualization and a smaller working space [36].

In patients with cervical radiculopathy, there are two surgical approaches: anterior cervical discectomy and fusion, and posterior laminoforaminotomy. Anterior cervical discectomy and fusion is the most commonly used decompressive procedure in the cervical spine. It can remove both lateral and midline disc herniations and osteophytes. A posterior surgical approach is used more often for patients with a far lateral disc herniation.

For patients with cervical myelopathy, there are two surgical procedures. Anterior surgeries include cervical discectomy with or without corpectomy, combined with a strut graft reconstruction using bone or synthetic materials, and plate fixation. Posterior surgeries include laminectomy and laminoplasty (decompression and reconstruction of the laminae) [38].

3.4 OSTEOARTHRITIS

OA is the most common adult joint disease, appearing as a progressive disorder of joints that results from gradual loss of cartilage, and from the development of bony spurs and synovial cysts at the ends of the joints (Fig. 3.4). It affects all the upper and lower extremity joints as well as the spinal and pelvic joints. Nearly 90% of Americans will have some features of OA in their weight-bearing joints by age 40. Clinical OA involves up to 30 million Americans, including one-third of seniors aged 65 or older and about 14% of all adults 25 years of age and older [39]. Disease progression may eventually reach a level at which joint replacement surgery is a reasonable option to restore lost function and alleviate pain. In 2009, the expenditure for hip and knee joint replacement surgery reached approximately $42 billion in the United States.

Cartilage is the predominant target of the harmful influences that cause OA and the biologic structure in which OA occurs. There are both endogenous and exogenous risk factors for OA. The endogenous factors include age, obesity, sex, heredity, ethnic origin (more common in persons of European lineage), and postmenopausal alterations. There are also some exogenous factors that contribute to the development

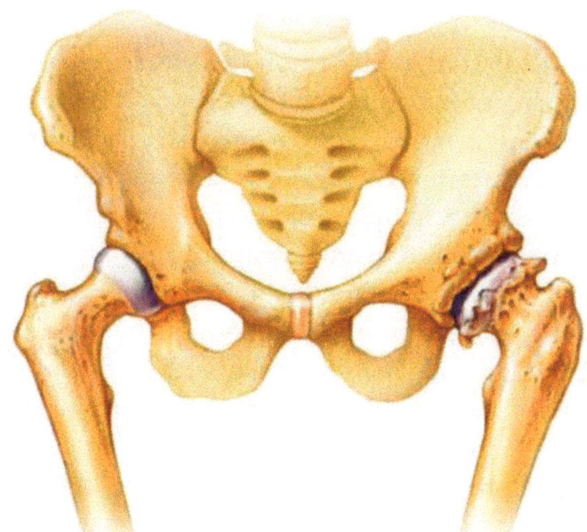

Figure 3.4 The hip joint shown on the left side of the image is normal, but the hip joint shown on the right side of the image shows deterioration of cartilage and the formation of bone spurs due to osteoarthritis. *From: Mayo Clinic.*

of OA, including repetitive microtrauma, macrotrauma, prior joint surgery, and lifestyle factors (alcohol, tobacco) [40].

OA is classified as primary and/or secondary OA. Primary OA results from heredity, without obvious local or systemic causes. It commonly affects people aged 50 years and above. Secondary OA results from certain diseases, such as congenital malformations of joints, trauma, malposition (varus/valgus angulation), metabolic diseases, endocrine disorders, and osteonecrosis.

OA patients usually have pain on movement, often occurring at the beginning of movement (start-up pain). The pain is often described as a dull ache and is relieved by rest. As OA progresses, the pain becomes more persistent and may occur at rest and during the night. These patients are also subjected to functional deficits that include stiffness, decreased ROM, and impairment in everyday activities. Additional symptoms include crepitus, joint-line tenderness and elevated sensitivity to cold and/or dampness. Blood tests may help exclude other causes of joint pain, such as any of the inflammatory arthritis. Synovial fluid examination can often determine the cause of a joint disorder such as gout or an infection.

Plain X-ray images are used for primary diagnosis and to evaluate the progression of OA. The typical plain X-ray signs of OA include joint space narrowing, subchondral sclerosis, osteophyte formation, subchondral cysts, and joint subluxation. Additional radiological studies may include an MRI, to image the hyaline cartilage and other joint soft tissues [40].

To date, OA is not a curable disease, and the goal of treatment is to moderate the patient's symptoms. The therapeutic modalities consist of nonsurgical modalities and surgical procedures.

Nonsurgical treatment options are based on the severity and distribution of symptoms as well as individual patient comorbidities. Modalities include physiotherapies, orthopedic aids, weight loss, pharmacological methods, and intraarticular corticosteroid injections. Physiotherapies for OA include exercise therapy, muscle stimulation, transverse friction (a massage technique), ultrasound application (to relieve pain and support endogenous healing processes), acupuncture, stretching, and walking. Exercises have been proven to be effective for alleviating pain and improving joint function [41]. Exercises may benefit from supervision by a physiotherapist until the patient and therapist are confident that the patient can perform the exercises correctly independently. Orthopedic aids are also used for the purpose of reducing pain and improving joint function. Orthopedic aids include cushioned heels (providing a shock-absorbing function) and wedges to elevate the inner or outer side of the shoe.

As for pharmacological treatment, the medications that are commonly used to treat OA can be classified as analgesics/antiinflammatory agents, glucocorticoids, and, occasionally, opioids. When signs of inflammation appear, intraarticular glucocorticoid injections can decrease a joint effusion and reduce the patient's pain significantly. Current guidelines from the American Academy of Orthopedic Surgeons suggested that intraarticular corticosteroid injections for the treatment of OA should be performed in the short term [42]. Septic arthritis is a serious potential complication of intraarticular steroid injection, and this procedure must be performed selectively and with the appropriate sterile technique.

Surgery is an option for patients when all the nonoperative methods have not provided appropriate relief of the patient's pain, and not allowed the patient to perform her/his required activities of daily living with a tolerable level of pain. Surgical procedures include joint-preserving treatment and joint replacement. There are multiple joint-preserving treatment methods that include lavage, cartilage shaving, debridement, microfracture, bone-stimulating modalities, joint surface restoration, and corrective osteotomy near the joint.

Most of the intraarticular procedures are performed via arthroscopy due to its advantages of minimal surgical trauma and low infection rate. Arthroscopic lavage is used to remove the inflammatory mediators and detritus [43]. Cartilage shaving is performed to remove frayed and fragmented cartilage and to smooth the edges of the remaining cartilage [44]. Debridement is used to treat meniscal damage, remove free-floating bodies within the joint, and reduction of the number of symptomatic osteophytes [45].

Bone-stimulating techniques refer to opening the subchondral cartilage and planting pluripotential stem cells into the joint surface, where they are then thought to form fiber bundles under the influence of mechanical and biological forces. The specific modalities include drilling, microfracturing, and abrasion arthroplasty [40].

Joint surface restoration techniques include autologous chondrocyte transplantation and autologous osteochondrocyte transplantation. In these techniques, cartilage and bone or cartilage alone are taken from a part of the joint that is not affected, and then transplanted into the cartilage defect [46].

Corrective osteotomy near the knee joint can be applied in the frontal, sagittal, or transverse plane, in either the distal portion of the femur or the proximal portion of the tibia. The aim is to redirect the weight-bearing axis toward the portion of the joint that still has functional cartilage and provides appropriate lower-extremity balance for standing and walking [40].

Joint replacement surgery has been proven, over the past five decades, to reduce pain and improve function. This type of surgery has long-term beneficial effects. In joint replacement surgery (arthroplasty), the surgeon removes the damaged joint surfaces and replaces them with plastic and metal parts. Postoperative joint motion exercises and muscle-strengthening exercises are important to improve the function of the new joint.

3.5 FRACTURE

A fracture is a complete or incomplete discontinuity of a bone that has been generated by a direct or indirect force. The predominant cause of fracture is musculoskeletal injury. More than 50 million Americans each year receive medical treatment for fractures. The estimated lifetime cost of these injuries is over $400 billion [47]. The WHO estimates that injuries account for 12% of all disability-adjusted life years lost, and that fractures are present in a significant number of these injuries [48]. In the United States, 5.6 million fractures happen each year, corresponding to a 2% incidence [49].

Bone fractures can be classified by a variety of methods, of which the following are examples. Based on the mechanism, fractures can be classified as either traumatic or pathologic. A traumatic fracture is when a degree of force acting on the bone exceeds the bone's ultimate stress. These injuries can be caused by falls or traffic accidents. A pathologic fracture is a bone fracture that results from a level of force that would not be sufficient to fracture a normal bone. In these instances, the fractured bone has been previously weakened by bone disorders such as osteoporosis, bone cancer, or osteogenesis imperfecta.

Another fracture classification component is the soft tissue involvement. Fractures can be classified as either closed or open. A closed fracture refers to fractures in which the overlying skin is intact. An open fracture, previously known as a "compound fracture," refers to a fracture in which the skin in the region of the fracture has been injured, and the fractured bone is either exposed or communicated directly with the outside environment via the skin laceration. In an open fracture situation, pathogenic bacteria from outside can enter the wound directly. For this reason, antibiotic drugs are used during the initial treatment of an open fracture.

Fractures may also be classified according to their pattern: a transverse fracture, an oblique fracture, a spiral fracture, a compression fracture, an avulsion fracture, or a comminuted fracture. A transverse fracture refers to a fracture line that is perpendicular to the long axis of the bone. An oblique fracture has a fracture line that is located between the long axis and the transverse axis of the bone. An impacted fracture refers to a fracture in which bone fragments have been driven into each other. A compression fracture is similar to an impaction fracture, but the term is applied to describe a fracture in which cancellous bone collapses and compresses upon itself. It usually describes fractures in vertebral bodies following trauma to the spine. An avulsion fracture refers to a fracture where a fragment of bone is separated from the main bone mass. This often occurs at the ligamentous or tendinous insertions into bone, and is sometimes caused by muscular contraction. A comminuted fracture is a fracture where the bone is broken into multiple fragments, and is often caused by high-energy trauma.

Fractures can also be divided into incomplete fractures and complete fractures. An incomplete fracture is one in which a bone has not completely lost its continuity;

some portion of the bone remains intact. The so-called "greenstick" fracture of children is one type of incomplete fracture. The extremely elastic periosteal tube may keep the bone ends together as a bending force on the bone generates a bone fracture. A complete fracture is a bone fracture in which a bone has lost its continuity completely. It is more common than an incomplete fracture. It can be subdivided by the shape of the fracture line as mentioned above.

The most common symptom of patients with bone fracture is pain. There are also some physical signs including deformity, swelling, tenderness, and crepitus of the affected sites that lead to X-ray examination of those sites. Concomitantly, it is essential to evaluate whether the nerves, vessels, and tendons near the fracture sites are affected, as well as if there is an injury to any joint adjacent to a fractured bone.

Plain X-ray images are the most important initial radiological studies for suspected bone fractures or dislocations. CT or MRI is used as needed depending on the initial X-rays and the specific patient's needs. One such situation occurs when a fracture is not visible on plain film but is strongly suspected clinically. CT and/or MRI are also used if more details are needed for further treatment planning and execution.

Although there are a variety of types of bone fractures, the main treatment principles are the same: reduction, immobilization, and rehabilitation. The aim of reduction is to restore the normal alignment of the affected bone. It can be achieved either by closed manipulation or by an open surgical procedure. Manipulative reduction is the standard initial treatment modality for reducing most fractures. When a satisfactory reduction cannot be accomplished, open reduction should be performed. Open reduction is also performed for other reasons, such as concomitant nerve or vessel damage that require repair.

The goals of fracture immobilization include the prevention of angulation or displacement of the fragments, the limitation of movement that may decrease the chance of union, and the alleviation of pain. The methods used for immobilization include casting with plaster or fiberglass, bracing, traction, external fixation, or internal fixation.

The rehabilitation that begins after reduction and immobilization is at least as important as those two initial principles of fracture treatment, as the end results of fracture treatment often depend heavily on the rehabilitation program. It should start as soon as the fracture receives appropriate treatment, and it includes both active and passive exercises.

For patients who have open fractures, there are additional measures that are needed, in addition to the three principles describes above, for comprehensive fracture treatment. The additional measures include cleaning the wound, removing all dead and devitalized tissue, closing the skin at the proper time and via the appropriate method, and delivering antibiotics to the area of the open fracture by either systemic means, local application at the time of surgery, or both.

The complications that may occur as a result of bone fractures can be classified as immediate, early, and late complications [50]. The immediate complications include soft tissue damage, nerve injury, and hemorrhage. The early postfracture complications include infection, neurovascular compromise, fat embolism, deep vein thrombosis, compartment syndrome, pressure ulcers, and pulmonary embolism. The late complications include delayed union, nonunion, malunion, posttraumatic OA, joint contractures, and osteonecrosis.

3.6 BONE CANCERS

Primary bone cancers are rare, accounting for less than 0.2% of all cancers. In 2014, an estimated 3020 people were diagnosed with primary bone cancers in the United States [51]. The most common forms of bone cancer include OS (35%), chondrosarcoma (30%), and Ewing's sarcoma (16%) [52]. Primary bone cancers usually affect adolescents and young adults. Patients with rapidly growing, destructive bone tumors present most frequently with pain. At first, the pain may be related to activity. However, it usually progresses to pain at rest, and often wakes the patient from sleep.

3.6.1 Osteosarcoma

OS is a sarcoma (malignant neoplasm of connective tissue) that produces osteoid (the initial tissue of newly formed bone that mineralizes to become mature bone). These tumors are generally locally aggressive and show a tendency toward early systemic metastases. The WHO (2013) classification of bone tumors classifies OS into eight subtypes: conventional, teleangiectatic, parosteal, periosteal, low-grade central, small cell, secondary, and high-grade surface OS. The conventional type is the most common, accounting for 90% of all OSs. OS has been further subdivided into osteoblastic, chondroblastic, and fibroblastic OS according to the predominant elements, with some differences of clinical outcome [53].

The etiology of OS is not yet clear. Although genetic studies have identified some chromosomal abnormalities, none of them is specific. Two genes—a hereditary mutation of retinoblastoma, and an autosomic recessive mutation of p53 in the Li–Fraumeni syndrome—localized in 13q14 and 17p13, respectively, are currently proposed to be involved in a stepwise accumulation of genomic defects [54,55].

Based on data from the Surveillance, Epidemiology, and End Results (SEER) program of the National Cancer Institute, there is an estimate of 4.4 new cases of OS per million people aged 0–24 years in the United States each year [56]. Most OSs occur in children and young adults between the ages of 10 and 30. However, OS can develop in people of any age. About 10% of all OSs develop in people over the age of 60 [57]. The patients with OS show a mild male predominance (60%) [58].

More than half of the OS primary sites are around the knee, and the three most common primary OS sites are the distal femur, the proximal tibia, and the proximal humerus [54,59]. The metaphyseal part of the long bones is affected most commonly.

About 10% of OSs occur in the axial skeleton, most commonly the pelvis [60,61]. An analysis from the SEER database showed a higher percentage of axial OS tumors in patients aged 60 and above (39.7%) when compared to patients less than 25 years of age (12.2%) or 25–59 years of age (35.3%) [62].

Pain and swelling are the most common symptoms. Many patients first present with pain, which initially may be intermittent and worse at night. It is uncommon for a pathologic fracture to be the presenting symptom for an OS, but it does occasionally occur. A painful mass is often seen at the affected site. There may also be overlying prominent veins and edema distal to an extremity tumor due to vascular compression from the mass [63].

The plain radiograph is the most useful method of localizing and reaching a presumptive diagnosis of OS. Typical appearances of conventional OS include medullary and cortical bone destruction, a wide zone of transition between zones of obvious lysis to zones of normal bone ("permeative" or "moth-eaten" appearance), aggressive periosteal reaction ("sunburst" type of tumor bone formation, Codman's triangle), soft-tissue mass, tumor matrix ossification/calcification. The appearance of tumor matrix ossification and/or calcification varies depending on the amount of tumor bone production, calcified matrix, and osteoid. The bone produced by tumor cells characteristically shows a "cloud-like" appearance and ill-defined margins.

The use of the CT scan is quite helpful in optimizing both the location of the biopsy tract and that of the harvested specimen from within the tumor. The biopsy tract must be positioned, to the greatest extent possible, so that it can be removed en bloc with the tumor at the time of surgery. The choice of specimen from within the tumor should optimally be from a part of the tumor that is at the growing edge of the tumor. The CT scan of chest, abdomen, and pelvis is a standard component of staging the extent of the tumor beyond its primary location. MRI is necessary for accurate local tumor assessment, particularly for determination of the intraosseous tumor extent and soft tissue involvement.

For conventional OS, the tumor cells vary from spindled to polyhedral with pleomorphic and hyperchromatic nuclei. Mitotic figures are present, and atypical mitotic figures may also be identified. Extracellular matrix produced by the tumor cells contains osseous, cartilaginous, or fibrous components in various proportions. The production of osteoid by the tumor cells somewhere within the tumor is necessary for a diagnosis of OS.

Histologic grading for OS is crucial in the oncologic staging of the tumor and for determining adjuvant treatment. There are several grading systems for OS. The four-tiered grading system popularized by the Mayo Clinic group is based on the original Broders grading of squamous cell carcinomas of the lip. In Broders' classification scheme, the tumor is graded from 1 to 4, based on the percentage of anaplasia in the tumor (from $\leq 25\%$ to 100%).

Complete surgical resection remains an essential treatment method for patients with OS [64]. It has been reported that there has not been any significant difference in local recurrence rates and survival between limb-salvage surgery and amputation in patients with high-grade, nonmetastatic OS [65,66]. However, the patients with limb-salvage surgery have better functional outcomes [67]. With the help of advanced imaging techniques and the use of preoperative (neoadjuvant) chemotherapy, nearly 80% of patients with extremity OSs are candidates for limb-savage surgery [68]. The local recurrence rate correlates with the surgical margins. The margins are defined as intralesional (within the tumor), marginal (within the reactive zone of the tumor), wide (through normal tissue beyond the reactive zone of the tumor), and radical (outside of the soft tissue and/or bony compartment of the tumor—"extracompartmental"). Either a wide margin or an extracompartmental margin is appropriate for the surgical treatment of OS [69,70].

For patients with pulmonary metastases, thoracotomy remains an essential and effective adjunct to multiagent chemotherapy. Surgical resection is preferred if all lung nodules can be resected and sufficient normal pulmonary tissue can be preserved to maintain adequate pulmonary function [54,69].

With the use of multiagent chemotherapy in the 1970s, the 5-year survival rate increased from about 20% to 65–70% [71]. The gold standard of chemotherapy includes high-dose methotrexate (HDMTX) with leucovorin rescue, doxorubicin (adriamycin), and cisplatin. Depending on the response to this triple-agent preoperative regimen (assessed by the percentage of tumor necrosis in the resected specimen, which usually occurs after the second or third cycle of chemotherapy), ifosfamide and/or etoposide may be added to the chemotherapy regimen. Combinations of these classic drugs serve to be the most effective method to reduce tumor growth and increase the survival rate of OS patients. Preoperative chemotherapy (neoadjuvant) is usually performed for about two or three cycles before surgery. Neoadjuvant chemotherapy provides an opportunity to allow time for planning limb-salvage surgery and reconstructive methods, and to study the histological effect of preoperative chemotherapy on the primary tumor when it is analyzed after resection. Patients with better responses to chemotherapy show a trend toward better survival outcome. After local treatment, postoperative adjuvant chemotherapy is administered for about 12–29 weeks, which could be modified based on the response to neoadjuvant chemotherapy [58,72].

OS is a radioresistant tumor. However, radiotherapy can be a treatment choice for local treatment in patients with "unresectable" tumors (those tumors for which resection is such a large and dangerous operation, or which gives the patient such large functional and/or cosmetic deficits that the patient and his/her physician team decide against surgery), following intralesional resection, or as palliation of symptomatic metastases [73–75]. Some chemotherapeutic agents (e.g., ifosfamide, cisplatin, HDMTX) show a sensitizing effect on the improvement of local control radiotherapy

[69]. Some studies also reported long-term remission with the combined approach of irradiation with chemotherapy in selected patients [60].

3.6.2 Ewing's sarcoma

Ewing's sarcoma, first described by James Ewing in 1921, includes "classic" Ewing's sarcoma of bone, extraskeletal Ewing's sarcoma, small cell tumor of the thoracopulmonary region (Askin tumor), and soft-tissue-based primitive neuroectodermal tumors (PNETs). The PNETs show morphological features similar to those of small round cell sarcomas [76–79].

Ewing's sarcoma is characterized by the fusion of the EWS gene (*EWSR1*) on chromosome 22q12 with various members of the ETS gene family (*FLI1*, *ERG*, *ETV1*, *ETVR*, and *FEV*). The *EWS-FLI1* fusion gene is recognized in nearly 85% of patients with Ewing's sarcoma [80]. Ewing's sarcoma also appears to highly express the cell surface glycoprotein MIC2 (CD99) [81]. The expression of CD99 may play a role in distinguishing Ewing's sarcoma from other small round cell tumors, although it is not specific for these tumors [82].

Based on the data from the SEER registry, the incidence of Ewing's sarcoma is about one case per 1 million per year in the United States. The median age of patients with Ewing's sarcoma is 15 years, and more than 50% of patients are adolescents [83]. Ewing's sarcoma patients show a mild male predominance [84]. The incidence of Ewing's sarcoma in the United States is nine times greater in Caucasians than in African Americans [85].

The most common primary sites of Ewing's sarcoma are the lower extremities (41%), pelvis (26%), chest wall (16%), upper extremities (9%), and spine (6%). When Ewing's sarcomas occur in the long bones, they arise most commonly in the diaphysis. This diaphyseal predilection for Ewing's sarcoma differs from that of OS, which arises most frequently in the metaphyseal region of a long bone.

Pain and swelling are the most common symptoms. Many patients first present with pain, which initially may be intermittent and worse at night. Pathologic fracture is uncommon. In patients with locally advanced or metastatic disease, tumor growth is often accompanied by fever, or a chronic inflammatory state manifested by anemia, leukocytosis, or an elevated erythrocyte sedimentation rate. Most patients have a palpable, tender mass. Dilated veins over the tumor may appear in some cases (Figs. 3.5 and 3.6),

The radiographic appearance of Ewing's sarcoma is variable. However, it most often shows a clearly aggressive radiographic appearance (Fig. 3.7). It is often quite large on initial presentation and has ill-defined margins. Over 80% of Ewing's sarcomas involve the soft tissues adjacent to the bone upon their initial presentation. The most common radiographic pattern is one of permeative or lytic destruction. The

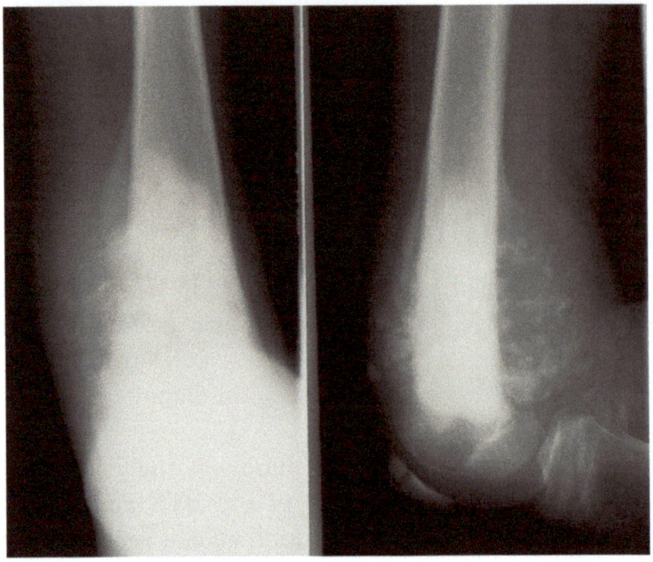

Figure 3.5 Osteosarcoma of the distal femur, demonstrating dense tumor bone formation and a sunburst pattern of periosteal reaction. *http://www.rad.washington.edu/academics/academic-sections/msk/teaching-materials/online-musculoskeletal-radiology-book/periosteal-reaction.*

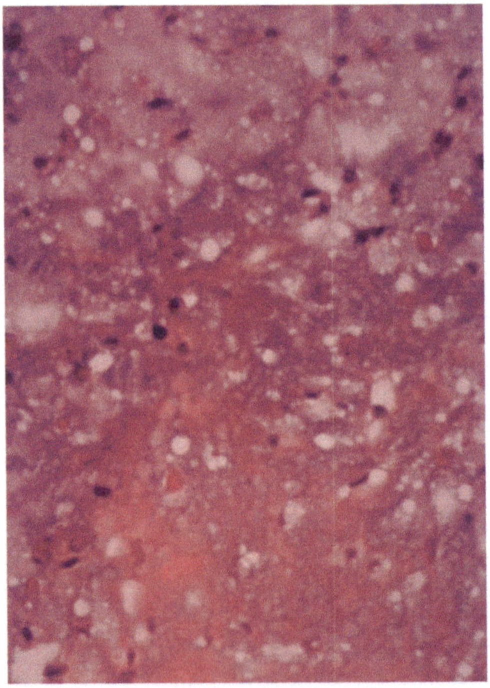

Figure 3.6 This is a medium-power picture of a chondroblastic osteosarcoma. One can see the dark-staining nuclei of tumor cells distributed in an irregular manner in a background matrix material. In some areas the background matrix is dense and very pink, typical of osteoid. In the other half of the picture the background matrix is pale, slightly bubbly, in appearance and bluish gray in color. This is more typical of chondroid matrix. (Hematoxylin and eosin $\times 20$.) *Downloaded from Bonetumor.org on 1 June 2016.*

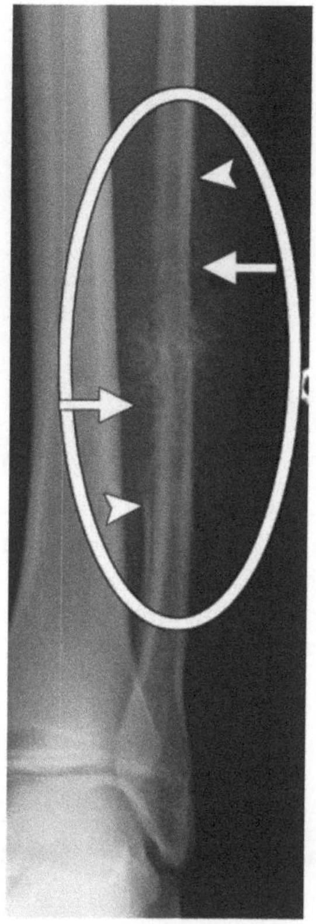

Figure 3.7 The plain film shows a permeative lytic bone lesion in the distal fibular diaphysis (white oval) with aggressive hair-on-end ("sunburst") periosteal reaction (arrows) and Codman triangles (arrowheads). *From: Murphey MD, et al. From the radiologic pathology archives: Ewing sarcoma family of tumors: radiologic-pathologic correlation. Radiographics 2013;33(3):803–31.*

periosteum is gradually elevated by the tumor, breaks through the cortex, and produces the characteristic multiple layers of subperiosteal reactive new bone ("onion skin appearance"). Sclerosis also occurs in some cases, due to stimulation of new bone formation by the tumor [63,86].

The use of CT and MR imaging studies are essential components of the evaluation in suspected Ewing's sarcoma. These two imaging studies provide accurate determination of both intraosseous tumor extension and soft tissue involvement. They help the surgeon determine whether the neurovascular bundle is involved by the tumor, which is critical to making a surgical plan.

Histologically, Ewing's sarcoma consists of small cells with a high nuclear to cytoplasmic ratio (Fig. 3.8). The cytoplasm is scant, eosinophilic, and usually contains glycogen. The nuclei are round, with finely dispersed chromatin, and one or more tiny nucleoli. Ewing's sarcoma does not produce any matrix. This tumor usually undergoes

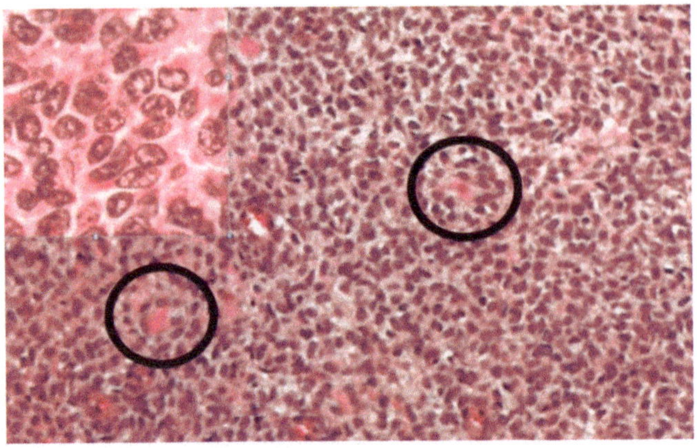

Figure 3.8 Photomicrograph (original magnification, ×250; hematoxylin-eosin (H-E) stain) demonstrates monotonous round blue cells typical of Ewing sarcoma. There is mild pseudorosette formation (circles). Inset (upper left corner) (original magnification, ×450) reveals typical indistinct cell membranes, indented nuclei, and scant cytoplasm. *From: Murphey MD, et al. From the radiologic pathology archives: Ewing sarcoma family of tumors: radiologic-pathologic correlation. Radiographics 2013;33(3):803–31.*

necrosis, and the residual viable cells show a "peritheliomatous" or a perivascular distribution. The cell membrane expresses CD99, a 32-kDa cell surface glycoprotein encoded by the *MIC2* gene. Based on the degree of neuroectodermal differentiation, the tumor cells may also express neuron-specific enolase (NSE), synaptophysin, and S-100 protein. Antibody against FLI1, which is centered in the nucleus of the tumor cells, has been shown to be specific for Ewing's sarcoma. As there are other types of small round cell tumors, including non-Hodgkin's lymphoma, neuroblastoma, rhabdomyosarcoma, mesenchymal chondrosarcoma, retinoblastoma (Rb), and desmoplastic small round cell tumor, a panel of immunohistochemical stains is necessary to reach a final diagnosis. For Ewing's sarcoma and primitive neuroectodermal tumor, CD99, FLI1, and NSE would be positive. Non-Hodgkin's lymphoma would express the lymphoid markers, i.e., CD45RB, CD3, CD20, and TdT. Neuroblastoma would be positive for neuroendocrine markers (synaptophysin, chromogranin). Rhabdomyosarcoma would be positive for skeletal muscle markers, e.g., desmin, myogenin, myo-D1, and myoglobin. Synovial sarcoma would also express pancytokeratins, EMA, BCL2, and calponin [87,88].

The local control therapies for patients with Ewing's sarcoma include surgery and/or radiotherapy. There are no randomized studies that directly compare these two treatment methods to each other. Generally speaking, wide (R0) resection is preferred for patients with surgically accessible and resectable tumors. Radiotherapy may be added after inadequate resection, in cases involving poor responders to chemotherapy, or in surgically resected tumors that have excessively narrow surgical margins. Ewing's sarcoma is sensitive to radiotherapy, and the radiation doses range from 36 to 60 Gray (Gy).

There are two irradiation techniques commonly used for patients with Ewing's sarcoma, including definitive radiotherapy for local control and pre- or postoperative adjuvant radiotherapy. Definitive radiotherapy aims to destroy all viable tumor cells and is performed on patients with tumors not amenable to surgical resection with wide (R0) margins. After radiotherapy for a tumor that was deemed unresectable, it sometimes becomes possible to resect the tumor with a wide margin [89–92].

With the use of neoadjuvant and adjuvant chemotherapy, the 5-year survival rate has improved from less than 10% to about 50–70% for patients with Ewing's sarcoma [63]. VAC/IE (vincristine, doxorubicin, and cyclophosphamide alternating with ifosfamide and etoposide) is the preferred regimen for patients with localized disease, whereas VadrialC (vincristine, doxorubicin, and cyclophosphamide) is the preferred regimen for patients with metastatic disease [92]. Neoadjuvant chemotherapy before local treatment is used to shrink the tumor and increase the possibility of resecting the tumor with a wide margin. Adjuvant chemotherapy (after surgical or radiotherapy control of the primary tumor) is performed for the purpose of improving the overall survival rate and relapse-free survival rate [92].

3.6.3 Chondrosarcoma

Chondrosarcomas are a heterogeneous group of neoplasms that have in common the production of cartilage matrix by the tumor cells [93]. Conventional chondrosarcoma of bone accounts for 85% of all chondrosarcomas. Other types of chondrosarcoma include clear cell, dedifferentiated, myxoid, and mesenchymal. Collectively, these four subtypes account for approximately 10–15% of all chondrosarcomas [94,95]. The majority of conventional chondrosarcomas are primary neoplasms (often centrally located) that originate from previously normal-appearing bone that was preformed from cartilage. A minority of chondrosarcomas are secondary lesions that develop from previous benign tumors such as enchondromas. These enchondromas can be solitary or multiple (Ollier disease). Multiple enchondromas that occur together with hemangiomas (Maffucci syndrome) have a higher risk of malignant transformation to chondrosarcoma and merit enhanced scrutiny. Chondrosarcoma can also arise from the cartilage cap of an osteochondroma [92].

The etiology of chondrosarcoma is still unclear, but about half of chondrosarcoma cases are related to isocitrate dehydrogenase (IDH1 or IDH2) mutations [92]. The estimated incidence of chondrosarcoma in the United States is 1 case in 200,000 people per year. The mean age at the time of diagnosis is 51 years, and approximately 60% of patients are in their fourth, fifth, and sixth decades of life [63,96]. The sex distribution shows a slight male predominance (55%) [96].

The tumor location is most commonly classified as appendicular (44.5%), followed by axial (31.1%), and then by soft tissue (9.6%) [96]. The pelvis and the proximal femur are the most common primary sites [92].

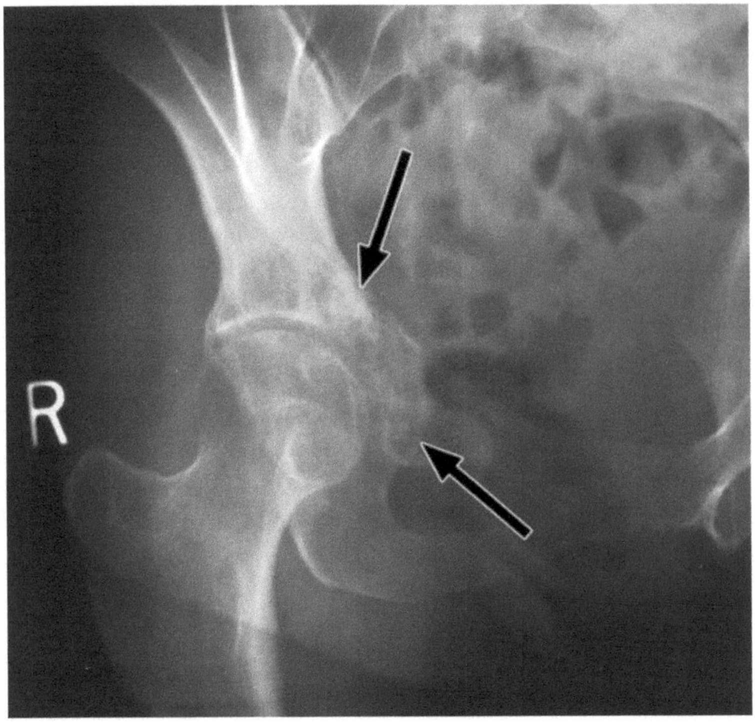

Figure 3.9 Anteroposterior hip radiograph shows subtle sclerosis caused by chondroid matrix mineralization and bone destruction of the ilium and iliopectineal line cortex lesion center at the previous site of the triradiate cartilage (arrows). *From: Murphey MD, et al. From the archives of the AFIP: imaging of primary chondrosarcoma: radiologic-pathologic correlation. Radiographics 2003;23 (5):1245–78.*

Symptoms of chondrosarcoma are usually mild, and patients may have had symptoms for many years before seeking treatment. The most common symptoms are pain and local swelling, but are not specific. Pathologic fracture may be the presenting symptom. An osteochondroma may undergo malignant transformation after being quiescent for decades.

The radiographic appearance of chondrosarcoma varies according to the subtypes (Fig. 3.9). Plain radiography can show both the location of the tumor and its cartilaginous nature. Central chondrosarcoma is the most frequent type of lesion. The lytic lesion commonly appears well-defined, associated with endosteal scalloping, and either cortical thinning or thickening. The intralesional calcifications may be punctate, flocculent, or have a ring-like pattern. In high-grade tumors (myxoid, dedifferentiated, and mesenchymal chondrosarcoma), the lesion margins are ill-defined (moth-eaten or permeative appearance) and some of these lesions lack calcifications. Some aggressive chondrosarcomas may have large associated soft tissue masses.

It is difficult to make a distinction between an enchondroma and a central grade I chondrosarcoma by imaging studies. Cartilaginous tumors that occur in the axial skeleton (centrally located tumors) and that are larger than 5 cm in their greatest dimension are likely to be malignant [97]. Cortical remodeling, thickening, and periosteal reaction are radiographic clues that are associated with malignant cartilage tumors, and that help make a distinction between enchondroma and central grade I chondrosarcoma.

The CT scan is useful to show the bone destruction and the small calcifications that occur in chondrosarcoma, especially for the lesions in the pelvis and other flat bones. The MRI helps to determine the extent of both the medullary tumor involvement and the soft-tissue mass. MRI shows a lobulated lesion with low or intermediate signal intensity on T1-weighted images and high signal intensity on T2-weighted images [98].

Conventional chondrosarcomas are all histologically similar to each other. They are classified into three different grades, which are currently the best predictors of the clinical behavior of these tumors. Grade I chondrosarcomas have low cellularity with an abundant hyaline cartilage matrix, and they rarely metastasize. Grade II chondrosarcomas have an intermediate level of cellularity between grade I and grade III chondrosarcomas, and mitoses are present histologically. Grade III chondrosarcomas are highly cellular with a mucomyxoid matrix and the presence of frequent mitoses. The metastasis rate for grade II and grade III chondrosarcomas ranges from 40% to 70%. Approximately 13% of recurrent chondrosarcomas show a trend toward a higher grade of malignancy than the primary tumor from which they arose, which demonstrates that chondrosarcomas have the potential to dedifferentiate [99,100].

Surgical resection with tumor-free (R0) wide margins on the resected specimen provides the only chance for cure in grade II and grade III nonmetastatic chondrosarcomas. Wide resection with tumor-free (R0) margins is also preferred for patients with large tumors and pelvic lesions, regardless of the histological grade. This surgical decision-making strategy has led to an event-free survival rate and an overall survival rate in patients who have chondrosarcomas located in the axial skeleton and pelvic girdle that is higher compared to patients who had intralesional curettage of those tumors. In patients with low-grade extrapelvic chondrosarcoma (grade I), extensive intralesional curettage followed by local adjuvant treatment (e.g., phenolization or liquid nitrogen cryosurgery) has shown satisfactory local control, and serves as an alternative to wide resection in low-grade extrapelvic chondrosarcomas [92].

Although chondrosarcoma is relatively radioresistant, radiation therapy can be considered for patients with unresectable tumors or after incomplete resections [95]. Radiation therapy can be classified as either curative radiotherapy or palliative radiotherapy. Curative radiotherapy is used for patients who have undergone an incomplete resection (R1 or R2 margins on the resected specimen) and for whom the treatment goal is to achieve optimum local control. Radiation doses greater than 60 Gy are often required to achieve local control of these tumors. The delivery of such a high dose using conventional photon radiation therapy is often difficult for tumor beds that are near critical structures, especially for those originating in the skull base and axial skeleton. Proton beam radiation therapy, when compared to conventional photon radiation therapy, allows a higher dose of radiation to be delivered directly to where it needs to be, while sparing healthy tissues and critical areas of the body that are near the tumor. Proton therapy alone or in combination with photon therapy has shown good local control in patients with skull base and upper cervical spine chondrosarcomas [92]. There are also other particle therapy methods, such as carbon ions, that have been utilized in the treatment of chondrosarcoma, with the same advantages that proton therapy offers.

Palliative radiotherapy is considered for patients with unresectable tumors, especially when the tumor is the mesenchymal subtype of chondrosarcoma, as these tumors are more radiosensitive compared to other chondrosarcoma subtypes. A study from MD Anderson showed that five of 11 patients treated with radiation therapy alone were well controlled [101].

Generally speaking, traditional chemotherapy is not effective in chondrosarcoma. Although there have been reports in the literature which suggest that chemotherapy could improve the survival rate of patients with mesenchymal or dedifferentiated chondrosarcomas, there are also reports that suggest that there is no advantage to its use in these patients. The National Comprehensive Cancer Network (NCCN) guidelines suggest that patients with mesenchymal chondrosarcoma can be treated in the same manner as Ewing's sarcoma patients, and that patients with dedifferentiated chondrosarcoma can be treated in the same manner as those with OS.

3.7 SUMMARY AND FUTURE DIRECTIONS

Despite the significant improvement in both diagnostic and therapeutic modalities for the treatment of bone disorders, there are still some issues that need to be solved. Novel drugs and effective delivery systems for metabolic diseases and bone cancers, optimum tissue engineering materials for bone defect repair, and effective agents for degenerative diseases are urgently needed.

The treatments that are currently available for osteoporosis are effective. However, some of the drugs are limited by their side effects, concurrent patient comorbidities, and long-term patient compliance. New drugs with higher efficacy, less side effects, and more convenient administration need to be developed. The more convenient formulations include oral calcitonin, odanacatib (an oral antiresorptive cathepsin K inhibitor), and oral parathyroid hormone. Their efficacy and safety profiles still need confirmation. Physiologically, osteoclastic and osteoblastic functions are coupled with bidirectional communication between these two cell types. Traditional antiresorptive drugs can reduce osteoclast viability. Therefore, osteoblastic bone formation is also inhibited due to a lack of communication between osteoblasts with the treated, nonviable osteoclasts. Uncoupling antiresorptive drugs suppress osteoclast activity rather than osteoclast viability, allowing physiological communication between osteoclasts and osteoblasts. This class of antiresorptive drugs preserves osteoblastic bone formation [102]. These novel drugs target specific pathways in osteoclasts, and include catepsin K inhibitors, c-Src kinase inhibitors, integrin antagonists, inhibitors of the acidification process within the resorption lacunae, and glucagon-like peptides. The clinical effects of these drugs are still under investigation [103,104].

Paget's disease manifests an increased bone remodeling rate and an uncoupling of bone resorption from bone formation during that remodeling. Thus, drugs that target osteoclasts have been used for its treatment. The RANKL/RANK/OPG system is known to act on osteoclast formation and activity. Drugs that affect this system, such as denosumab (a human monoclonal antibody against RANKL) and osteoprotegerin, have been investigated for their effect in the treatment of Paget's. Their long-term safety and efficacy are still under investigation in large clinical trials. Although the current treatment of existing Paget's disease is effective, it would be a reasonable goal to work toward preventing Paget's in populations that are at increased risk for its occurrence. For example, prophylactic treatment might be recommended for people who have *SQTSM1* gene mutations. People with this mutation are at high risk for the development of Paget's disease in the future.

As the traditional chemotherapy regimens for bone cancers reached a plateau phase in the 1980s, further research on novel therapeutic modalities and more target-selective agents for sarcoma treatment is a current unmet need. For example, although multiple therapeutic modalities have been used for patients with recurrent or metastatic Ewing's sarcoma, these patients still have a poor prognosis, with their 5-year survival remaining less than 25%. Novel treatment strategies for OS include drug-delivery systems, immunotherapeutic agents, molecular strategies that target specific signaling pathways, and manipulation of the tumor microenvironment [84,105–108].

There are several promising therapeutic targets for treatment strategies to improve local tumor control and patient survival. Therapies that target the EWS-FLI1 genetic abnormalities are crucial, but are still at an early stage. The development of inhibitors of EWS-FLI1 transcription factor (mithramycin, ET-743) require the development of pharmacodynamic assays to correlate drug exposure with EWS-FLI1 blockade. Meanwhile, it is necessary to find a more effective way to use agents that inhibit important pathways associated with EWS-FLI1 such as the IGF pathway, epigenetic pathways, and pathways associated with the DNA damage repair such as poly(ADP-ribose) polymerase (PARP). Given the multiplicity of EWS-FLI1 targets and signaling pathway redundancies, inhibition of growth factor receptors and downstream pathways might be helpful to overcome resistance.

The current treatment results for patients with nonresectable metastatic tumors are far from satisfactory; future work should focus on promising agents and effective agent-delivery systems. Several agents, such as 17-DMAG (heat shock protein 90 inhibitor), Oncostatin (a proapoptotic, cytostatic cytokine), Apo2L/TRAIL (recombinant human apoptosis ligand 2/tumor necrosis factor-related apoptosis-inducing ligand) have been shown to have an effect on chondrosarcoma [109,110]. There are other promising agents that target IDH1/IDH2 (isocitrate dehydrogenase 1/2), BCL-2 (B-cell lymphoma-2 protein), COX-2 (cyclooxygenase 2), IHH (Indian hedgehog), ER (estrogen receptor), PDGFR-α (platelet-derived growth factor receptor α), integrins, and PTHLH (parathyroid hormone-like hormone) [95]. However, the above agents are still at very early stages of development. The low vascular penetration and abundant matrix surrounding the tumor cells in cartilaginous tumors make it difficult to deliver effective chemotherapeutic agents throughout these sarcomas.

The current treatment options for DDDs often involve attempts to relieve symptoms by removing the affected intervertebral disc, and then performing a reconstruction with either a fusion procedure or an artificial disc replacement. The disc is incapable of repairing itself, and heals injuries with scar tissue rather than reconstituting its normal anatomy. Some emerging methods to promote the process of disc repair are currently under development. These include cell therapy (including stem cells), and tissue engineering strategies to reconstitute normal disc anatomy and function [111]. Treatment via cell therapy is somewhat limited by the number of autologous disc cells available for expansion, and either cell transformation or infection during that culture expansion of the initial autologous disc cell population. The use of stem cells appears more attractive, as it has the advantage of a sufficient source of stem cells for expansion [112]. Tissue engineering of the disc is also under development for the treatment of DDD. Tissue engineering can target the repair or regeneration of one or more disc tissues (i.e., nucleus pulposus, annulus fibrosus, and cartilage endplate). There has also been progress made in generating a composite tissue-engineered intervertebral disc with integration of all three of its components [113].

OA is not a curable disease, and the current treatment options focus on pain relief and functional improvement of the affected joints. The development of effective agents that will prevent, slow down, or reverse the OA disease process is an unmet clinical need.

Bone can repair and regenerate itself in many cases. However, in fractures with large segmental bone defects, bone healing and regeneration often fail. The materials used for the reconstruction of segmental skeletal defects include autografts (bone transplanted from the same person), allografts (bone transplanted from another human being), xenografts (bone transplanted from a different species), and tissue engineering biomaterials. Each of these choices has advantages and disadvantages. Autografts are the "gold standard" material used for bone grafting and provide the osteogenic (may contain cells that secrete new bone matrix), osteoinductive (contain the growth and differentiation factors that direct the osteoblasts to make new bone), and osteoconductive (serve as a scaffold for the formation of new bone) characteristics necessary for bone regeneration [114]. The main disadvantages of bone autografts include donor site morbidity, pain, and risks, such as major vessel or visceral injuries during autograft harvesting [115]. Allografts and xenografts are alternative choices for bone grafting. However, they have the disadvantages of lacking osteogenicity, osteoinductivity, and the rare, but possible, transmission of diseases [116].

For these reasons, tissue engineering materials have been under development for several years to provide potential alternative options for the regeneration of bone in segmental skeletal defects. The purpose of these bone tissue engineering materials is to increase the osteogenicity, osteoinductivity, and osteoconductivity of the bone grafts, and concomitantly to decrease the disadvantages of the traditional grafts. Tissue engineering involves the combination of scaffolds, growth factors, and cells [117]. Scaffolds provide a surface on which the cells can attach and express their physiologic function. The scaffolds can be biologic (natural or organic) or synthetic (artificial) materials. Scaffold design focuses on the development of materials that have good biocompatibility, controllable biodegradation, sufficient strength, osteoconductivity, and osteoinductivity. Growth factors also play an important role in the bone healing process. They modulate proliferation and differentiation of the osteoblasts. Growth factors such as vascular endothelial growth factor (VEGF), transforming growth factor-beta (TGF-β), platelet-derived growth factor (PDGF), bone morphogenic proteins (BMPs), and insulin-like growth factor (IGF) are present in the bone matrix and are expressed during bone healing. Although there is much work to be done, including regulatory requirements, human and animal studies, commercialization issues, and physician acceptance of novel treatment options, tissue engineering is a promising field in the future of bone healing and regeneration [116].

REFERENCES

[1] Claus-Peter Adler FS, Steel J, Feldmann F, Dahlin Bone DC. Diseases: macroscopic, histological, and radiological diagnosis of structural changes in the skeleton. Berlin: Springer; 2000.

[2] Allan Praemer SF, Dorothy P. Rice. Musculoskeletal conditions in the United States. 1 ed Park Ridge, IL: Amer Acad of Orthopaedic Surgeons; 1992.

[3] Woolf AD. The bone and joint decade 2000–2010. Ann Rheum Dis 2000;59:81–2.

[4] Burden of Musculoskeletal Diseases in the United States: Prevalence, Societal and Economic Cost. 1 ed: American Academy of Orthopaedic Surgeons; 2008.

[5] "Bone Health and Osteoporosis, A Report of the Surgeon General". Office of the Surgeon General. Rockville, MD; 2004.

[6] Consensus NIH. Development panel on osteoporosis prevention, diagnosis, and therapy, March 7-29, 2000: highlights of the conference. South Med J 2001;94:569–73.

[7] Looker AC, Dawson-Hughes B, Tosteson AN, Johansson H, Kanis JA, Melton III LJ. Hip fracture risk in older US adults by treatment eligibility status based on new National Osteoporosis Foundation guidance. Osteoporos Int 2011;22:541–9.

[8] Lane NE. Epidemiology, etiology, and diagnosis of osteoporosis. Am J Obstet Gynecol 2006;194: S3–11.
[9] Edward F, McCarthy MD, Frassica FJ. Pathology of bone and joint disorders with clinical and radiographic correlation. 1st edition Philadelphia, PA: Saunders; 1998.
[10] Prevention and management of osteoporosis. World Health Organ Tech Rep Ser. 2003;921:1–164, back cover.
[11] Management of osteoporosis in postmenopausal women: 2010 position statement of The North American Menopause Society. Menopause. 2010;17:25–54; quiz 5–6.
[12] Schuiling KD, Robinia K, Nye R. Osteoporosis update. J Midwifery Womens Health 2011;56:615–27.
[13] Tinetti ME. Clinical practice. Preventing falls in elderly persons. N Engl J Med 2003;348:42–9.
[14] Watts NB, Lewiecki EM, Miller PD, Baim S. National osteoporosis foundation 2008 clinician's guide to prevention and treatment of osteoporosis and the World Health Organization Fracture Risk Assessment Tool (FRAX): what they mean to the bone densitometrist and bone technologist. J Clin Densitom 2008;11:473–7.
[15] Helfrich MH, Hobson RP, Grabowski PS, Zurbriggen A, Cosby SL, Dickson GR, et al. A negative search for a paramyxoviral etiology of Paget's disease of bone: molecular, immunological, and ultrastructural studies in UK patients. J Bone Miner Res 2000;15:2315–29.
[16] Friedrichs WE, Reddy SV, Bruder JM, Cundy T, Cornish J, Singer FR, et al. Sequence analysis of measles virus nucleocapsid transcripts in patients with Paget's disease. J Bone Miner Res 2002;17:145–51.
[17] Janssens K, Van Hul W. Molecular genetics of too much bone. Hum Mol Genet 2002;11:2385–93.
[18] Barker DJ, Chamberlain AT, Guyer PB, Gardner MJ. Paget's disease of bone: the Lancashire focus. Br Med J 1980;280:1105–7.
[19] Altman RD, Bloch DA, Hochberg MC, Murphy WA. Prevalence of pelvic Paget's disease of bone in the United States. J Bone Miner Res 2000;15:461–5.
[20] Wermers RA, Tiegs RD, Atkinson EJ, Achenbach SJ, Melton III LJ. Morbidity and mortality associated with Paget's disease of bone: a population-based study. J Bone Miner Res 2008;23:819–25.
[21] van Staa TP, Selby P, Leufkens HG, Lyles K, Sprafka JM, Cooper C. Incidence and natural history of Paget's disease of bone in England and Wales. J Bone Miner Res 2002;17:465–71.
[22] Siris ES. Paget's disease of bone. J Bone Miner Res 1998;13:1061–5.
[23] Maldague B, Malghem J. Dynamic radiologic patterns of Paget's disease of bone. Clin Orthop Relat Res 1987;126–51.
[24] Singer F. 2000. Paget's disease of bone. In: De Groot LJ, Beck-Peccoz P, Chrousos G, Dungan K, Grossman A, Hershman JM, et al., editors. Endotext [Internet]. South Dartmouth, MA: MDText. com, Inc.
[25] Griz L, Fontan D, Mesquita P, Lazaretti-Castro M, Borba VZ, Borges JL, et al. Diagnosis and management of Paget's disease of bone. Arq Bras Endocrinol Metabol 2014;58:587–99.
[26] Monfort J, Sala DR, Romero AB, Duro JC, Maymo J, Carbonell J. Epidemiological, clinical, biochemical, and imaging characteristics of monostotic and polyostotic Paget's disease. Bone 1999;24:13S–14SS.
[27] Chambers TJ, Magnus CJ. Calcitonin alters behaviour of isolated osteoclasts. J Pathol 1982;136:27–39.
[28] Walsh JP, Ward LC, Stewart GO, Will RK, Criddle RA, Prince RL, et al. A randomized clinical trial comparing oral alendronate and intravenous pamidronate for the treatment of Paget's disease of bone. Bone 2004;34:747–54.
[29] Deyo RA, Mirza SK, Martin BI. Back pain prevalence and visit rates: estimates from U.S. national surveys, 2002. Spine (Phila Pa 1976) 2006;31:2724–7.
[30] Freburger JK, Holmes GM, Agans RP, Jackman AM, Darter JD, Wallace AS, et al. The rising prevalence of chronic low back pain. Arch Intern Med 2009;169:251–8.
[31] Luo XM, Pietrobon R, Sun SX, Liu GG, Hey L. Estimates and patterns of direct health care expenditures among individuals with back pain in the United States. Spine 2004;29:79–86.

[32] Hadjipavlou AG, Tzermiadianos MN, Bogduk N, Zindrick MR. The pathophysiology of disc degeneration: a critical review. J Bone Joint Surg Br 2008;90:1261–70.
[33] Chou R, Qaseem A, Snow V, Casey D, Cross Jr. JT, Shekelle P, et al. Diagnosis and treatment of low back pain: a joint clinical practice guideline from the American College of Physicians and the American Pain Society. Ann Intern Med 2007;147:478–91.
[34] Khadilkar A, Milne S, Brosseau L, Robinson V, Saginur M, Shea B, et al. Transcutaneous electrical nerve stimulation (TENS) for chronic low-back pain. Cochrane Database Syst Rev 2005; CD003008.
[35] Yokoyama M, Sun X, Oku S, Taga N, Sato K, Mizobuchi S, et al. Comparison of percutaneous electrical nerve stimulation with transcutaneous electrical nerve stimulation for long-term pain relief in patients with chronic low back pain. Anesth Analg 2004;98:1552–6. table of contents.
[36] Roger Chou M. Subacute and chronic low back pain: surgical treatment; 2015.
[37] Maroon JC. Current concepts in minimally invasive discectomy. Neurosurgery 2002;51:S137–45.
[38] Carette S, Fehlings MG. Clinical practice. Cervical radiculopathy. N Engl J Med 2005;353:392–9.
[39] Lawrence RC, Felson DT, Helmick CG, Arnold LM, Choi H, Deyo RA, et al. Estimates of the prevalence of arthritis and other rheumatic conditions in the United States. Part II. Arthritis Rheum 2008;58:26–35.
[40] Michael JW, Schluter-Brust KU, Eysel P. The epidemiology, etiology, diagnosis, and treatment of osteoarthritis of the knee. Dtsch Arztebl Int 2010;107:152–62.
[41] McAlindon TE, Bannuru RR, Sullivan MC, Arden NK, Berenbaum F, Bierma-Zeinstra SM, et al. OARSI guidelines for the non-surgical management of knee osteoarthritis. Osteoarthritis Cartilage 2014;22:363–88.
[42] Richmond J, Hunter D, Irrgang J, Jones MH, Levy B, Marx R, et al. Treatment of osteoarthritis of the knee (nonarthroplasty). J Am Acad Orthop Surg 2009;17:591–600.
[43] Henry A. Arthroscopy of the knee joint. Guys Hosp Rep 1972;121:25–30.
[44] Outerbridge RE. The etiology of chondromalacia patellae. J Bone Joint Surg Br 1961;43-B:752–7.
[45] Magnuson PB. The classic: joint debridement: surgical treatment of degenerative arthritis. Clin Orthop Relat Res 1974;4–12.
[46] Hangody L, Rathonyi GK, Duska Z, Vasarhelyi G, Fules P, Modis L. Autologous osteochondral mosaicplasty. Surgical technique. J Bone Joint Surg Am 2004;(86-A Suppl. 1):65–72.
[47] Corso P, Finkelstein E, Miller T, Fiebelkorn I, Zaloshnja E. Incidence and lifetime costs of injuries in the United States. Inj Prev 2006;12:212–18.
[48] Beveridge M, Howard A. The burden of orthopaedic disease in developing countries. J Bone Joint Surg Am 2004;86-A:1819–22.
[49] Campbell's ST C. Operative orthoaedics. 10 ed St Louis, MO: Mosby-Year Book; 2003.
[50] Whiteing NL. Fractures: pathophysiology, treatment and nursing care. Nurs Stand 2008;23:49–57 quiz 8, 60.
[51] Siegel R, Ma J, Zou Z, Jemal A. Cancer statistics. CA Cancer J Clin 2014;64:9–29.
[52] Jo VY, Fletcher CD. WHO classification of soft tissue tumours: an update based on the 2013 (4th) edition. Pathology 2014;46:95–104.
[53] Gorlick R. Current concepts on the molecular biology of osteosarcoma. Cancer Treat Res 2009;152:467–78.
[54] Luetke A, Meyers PA, Lewis I, Juergens H. Osteosarcoma treatment—where do we stand? A state of the art review. Cancer Treat Rev 2014;40:523–32.
[55] Entz-Werle N, Schneider A, Kalifa C, Voegeli AC, Tabone MD, Marec-Berard P, et al. Genetic alterations in primary osteosarcoma from 54 children and adolescents by targeted allelotyping. Br J Cancer 2003;88:1925–31.
[56] Mirabello L, Troisi RJ, Savage SA. Osteosarcoma incidence and survival rates from 1973 to 2004: data from the Surveillance, Epidemiology, and End Results Program. Cancer 2009;115:1531–43.
[57] Osteosarcoma. American Cancer Society; 2015.
[58] Geller DS, Gorlick R. Osteosarcoma: a review of diagnosis, management, and treatment strategies. Clin Adv Hematol Oncol 2010;8:705–18.

[59] Bielack SS, Kempf-Bielack B, Delling G, Exner GU, Flege S, Helmke K, et al. Prognostic factors in high-grade osteosarcoma of the extremities or trunk: an analysis of 1,702 patients treated on neoadjuvant cooperative osteosarcoma study group protocols. J Clin Oncol 2002;20:776−90.
[60] Ozaki T, Flege S, Liljenqvist U, Hillmann A, Delling G, Salzer-Kuntschik M, et al. Osteosarcoma of the spine: experience of the Cooperative Osteosarcoma Study Group. Cancer 2002;94:1069−77.
[61] Clark JC, Dass CR, Choong PF. A review of clinical and molecular prognostic factors in osteosarcoma. J Cancer Res Clin Oncol 2008;134:281−97.
[62] Jawad MU, Cheung MC, Clarke J, Koniaris LG, Scully SP. Osteosarcoma: improvement in survival limited to high-grade patients only. J Cancer Res Clin Oncol 2011;137:597−607.
[63] Krishnan Unni K. MBBS CYIM. Dahlin's bone tumors general aspects and data on 10,165 cases. 6th ed Philadelphia, PA: Wolters Kluwer; 2009.
[64] Marulanda GA, Henderson ER, Johnson DA, Letson GD, Cheong D. Orthopedic surgery options for the treatment of primary osteosarcoma. Cancer Control 2008;15:13−20.
[65] Bacci G, Ferrari S, Lari S, Mercuri M, Donati D, Longhi A, et al. Osteosarcoma of the limb. Amputation or limb salvage in patients treated by neoadjuvant chemotherapy. J Bone Joint Surg Br 2002;84:88−92.
[66] Mavrogenis AF, Abati CN, Romagnoli C, Ruggieri P. Similar survival but better function for patients after limb salvage versus amputation for distal tibia osteosarcoma. Clin Orthop Relat Res 2012;470:1735−48.
[67] Aksnes LH, Bauer HC, Jebsen NL, Folleras G, Allert C, Haugen GS, et al. Limb-sparing surgery preserves more function than amputation: a Scandinavian sarcoma group study of 118 patients. J Bone Joint Surg Br 2008;90:786−94.
[68] Jaffe N. Osteosarcoma: review of the past, impact on the future. The American experience. Cancer Treat Res 2009;152:239−62.
[69] Errani C, Longhi A, Rossi G, Rimondi E, Biazzo A, Toscano A, et al. Palliative therapy for osteosarcoma. Expert Rev Anticancer Ther 2011;11:217−27.
[70] Grimer RJ, Taminiau AM, Cannon SR. Surgical outcomes in osteosarcoma. J Bone Joint Surg Br 2002;84:395−400.
[71] Allison DC, Carney SC, Ahlmann ER, Hendifar A, Chawla S, Fedenko A, et al. A meta-analysis of osteosarcoma outcomes in the modern medical era. Sarcoma 2012;2012:704872.
[72] Carrle D, Bielack SS. Current strategies of chemotherapy in osteosarcoma. Int Orthop 2006;30:445−51.
[73] Bleher EA. Is there a rational role for radiotherapy in the treatment of osteosarcoma? Cancer Treat Res 1993;62:379−81.
[74] Dincbas FO, Koca S, Mandel NM, Hiz M, Dervisoglu S, Secmezacar H, et al. The role of preoperative radiotherapy in nonmetastatic high-grade osteosarcoma of the extremities for limb-sparing surgery. Int J Radiat Oncol Biol Phys 2005;62:820−8.
[75] Tatezaki S. Systematic multi-modal treatment of osteosarcoma, with special reference to the role of fast neutron radiotherapy. Nihon Seikeigeka Gakkai Zasshi 1979;53:831−46.
[76] Ewing J. Classics in oncology. Diffuse endothelioma of bone. James Ewing. Proceedings of the New York Pathological Society, 1921. CA Cancer J Clin 1972;22:95−8.
[77] Angervall L, Enzinger FM. Extraskeletal neoplasm resembling Ewing's sarcoma. Cancer 1975;36:240−51.
[78] Askin FB, Rosai J, Sibley RK, Dehner LP, McAlister WH. Malignant small cell tumor of the thoracopulmonary region in childhood: a distinctive clinicopathologic entity of uncertain histogenesis. Cancer 1979;43:2438−51.
[79] Jaffe R, Santamaria M, Yunis EJ, Tannery NH, Agostini Jr. RM, Medina J, et al. The neuroectodermal tumor of bone. Am J Surg Pathol 1984;8:885−98.
[80] Delattre O, Zucman J, Melot T, Garau XS, Zucker JM, Lenoir GM, et al. The Ewing family of tumors—a subgroup of small-round-cell tumors defined by specific chimeric transcripts. N Engl J Med 1994;331:294−9.
[81] Ambros IM, Ambros PF, Strehl S, Kovar H, Gadner H, Salzer-Kuntschik M. MIC2 is a specific marker for Ewing's sarcoma and peripheral primitive neuroectodermal tumors. Evidence for a common histogenesis of Ewing's sarcoma and peripheral primitive neuroectodermal tumors from MIC2 expression and specific chromosome aberration. Cancer 1991;67:1886−93.

[82] Olsen SH, Thomas DG, Lucas DR. Cluster analysis of immunohistochemical profiles in synovial sarcoma, malignant peripheral nerve sheath tumor, and Ewing sarcoma. Mod Pathol 2006;19:659–68.
[83] Kim SY, Tsokos M, Helman LJ. Dilemmas associated with congenital ewing sarcoma family tumors. J Pediatr Hematol Oncol 2008;30:4–7.
[84] Hense HW, Ahrens S, Paulussen M, Lehnert M, Jurgens H. [Descriptive epidemiology of Ewing's tumor—analysis of German patients from (EI)CESS 1980-1997]. Klin Padiatr 1999;211:271–5.
[85] Jawad MU, Cheung MC, Min ES, Schneiderbauer MM, Koniaris LG, Scully SP. Ewing sarcoma demonstrates racial disparities in incidence-related and sex-related differences in outcome: an analysis of 1631 cases from the SEER database, 1973-2005. Cancer 2009;115:3526–36.
[86] Maygarden SJ, Askin FB, Siegal GP, Gilula LA, Schoppe J, Foulkes M, et al. Ewing sarcoma of bone in infants and toddlers. A clinicopathologic report from the Intergroup Ewing's Study. Cancer 1993;71:2109–18.
[87] Folpe AL, Hill CE, Parham DM, O'Shea PA, Weiss SW. Immunohistochemical detection of FLI-1 protein expression: a study of 132 round cell tumors with emphasis on CD99-positive mimics of Ewing's sarcoma/primitive neuroectodermal tumor. Am J Surg Pathol 2000;24:1657–62.
[88] Desai SS, Jambhekar NA. Pathology of Ewing's sarcoma/PNET: current opinion and emerging concepts. Indian J Orthop 2010;44:363–8.
[89] Ozaki T. Diagnosis and treatment of Ewing sarcoma of the bone: a review article. J Orthop Sci 2015;20:250–63.
[90] Jurgens H, Exner U, Gadner H, Harms D, Michaelis J, Sauer R, et al. Multidisciplinary treatment of primary Ewing's sarcoma of bone. A 6-year experience of a European Cooperative Trial. Cancer 1988;61:23–32.
[91] Paulussen M, Craft AW, Lewis I, Hackshaw A, Douglas C, Dunst J, et al. Results of the EICESS-92 study: two randomized trials of Ewing's sarcoma treatment - Cyclophosphamide compared with ifosfamide in standard-risk patients and assessment of benefit of etoposide added to standard treatment in high-risk patients. J Clin Oncol 2008;26:4385–93.
[92] Bone Cancer, NCCN clinical practice guidelines in oncology; 2015.
[93] Hanson CA, Morice WG. The clinical and laboratory approach to the CD5/CD10 negative B-cell chronic lymphoproliferative leukemias. Am J Hematol 2008;83:347–8.
[94] Mankin HJ, Cantley KP, Lippiello L, Schiller AL, Campbell CJ. The biology of human chondrosarcoma. I. Description of the cases, grading, and biochemical analyses. J Bone Joint Surg Am 1980;62:160–76.
[95] Gelderblom H, Hogendoorn PC, Dijkstra SD, van Rijswijk CS, Krol AD, Taminiau AH, et al. The clinical approach towards chondrosarcoma. Oncologist 2008;13:320–9.
[96] Giuffrida AY, Burgueno JE, Koniaris LG, Gutierrez JC, Duncan R, Scully SP. Chondrosarcoma in the United States (1973 to 2003): an analysis of 2890 cases from the SEER database. J Bone Joint Surg Am 2009;91:1063–72.
[97] Geirnaerdt MJ, Hermans J, Bloem JL, Kroon HM, Pope TL, Taminiau AH, et al. Usefulness of radiography in differentiating enchondroma from central grade 1 chondrosarcoma. AJR Am J Roentgenol 1997;169:1097–104.
[98] Varma DG, Ayala AG, Carrasco CH, Guo SQ, Kumar R, Edeiken J. Chondrosarcoma: MR imaging with pathologic correlation. Radiographics 1992;12:687–704.
[99] Bjornsson J, McLeod RA, Unni KK, Ilstrup DM, Pritchard DJ. Primary chondrosarcoma of long bones and limb girdles. Cancer 1998;83:2105–19.
[100] Evans HL, Ayala AG, Romsdahl MM. Prognostic factors in chondrosarcoma of bone: a clinicopathologic analysis with emphasis on histologic grading. Cancer 1977;40:818–31.
[101] McNaney D, Lindberg RD, Ayala AG, Barkley Jr. HT, Hussey DH. Fifteen year radiotherapy experience with chondrosarcoma of bone. Int J Radiat Oncol Biol Phys 1982;8:187–90.
[102] Rachner TD, Khosla S, Hofbauer LC. Osteoporosis: now and the future. Lancet 2011;377:1276–87.
[103] Rejnmark L, Mosekilde L. New and emerging antiresorptive treatments in osteoporosis. Curr Drug Saf 2011;6:75–88.
[104] Brandi ML. Current treatment approaches for Paget's Disease of Bone. Discov Med 2010;10:209–12.

[105] Chou AJ, Geller DS, Gorlick R. Therapy for osteosarcoma: where do we go from here? Paediatr Drugs 2008;10:315−27.
[106] Hattinger CM, Pasello M, Ferrari S, Picci P, Serra M. Emerging drugs for high-grade osteosarcoma. Expert Opin Emerg Drugs 2010;15:615−34.
[107] van Oosterwijk JG, Anninga JK, Gelderblom H, Cleton-Jansen AM, Bovee JV. Update on targets and novel treatment options for high-grade osteosarcoma and chondrosarcoma. Hematol Oncol Clin North Am 2013;27:1021−48.
[108] Grignani G, Palmerini E, Dileo P, Asaftei SD, D'Ambrosio L, Pignochino Y, et al. A phase II trial of sorafenib in relapsed and unresectable high-grade osteosarcoma after failure of standard multimodal therapy: an Italian Sarcoma Group study. Ann Oncol 2012;23:508−16.
[109] Workman P, Burrows F, Neckers L, Rosen N. Drugging the cancer chaperone HSP90: combinatorial therapeutic exploitation of oncogene addiction and tumor stress. Ann N Y Acad Sci 2007;1113:202−16.
[110] Pacey S, Wilson RH, Walton M, Eatock MM, Hardcastle A, Zetterlund A, et al. A phase I study of the heat shock protein 90 inhibitor alvespimycin (17-DMAG) given intravenously to patients with advanced solid tumors. Clin Cancer Res 2011;17:1561−70.
[111] Hughes SP, Freemont AJ, Hukins DW, McGregor AH, Roberts S. The pathogenesis of degeneration of the intervertebral disc and emerging therapies in the management of back pain. J Bone Joint Surg Br 2012;94:1298−304.
[112] Steck E, Bertram H, Abel R, Chen BH, Winter A, Richter W. Induction of intervertebral disc-like cells from adult mesenchymal stem cells. Stem Cells 2005;23:403−11.
[113] Kandel R, Roberts S, Urban JP. Tissue engineering and the intervertebral disc: the challenges. Eur Spine J 2008;17(Suppl. 4):480−91.
[114] Athanasiou VT, Papachristou DJ, Panagopoulos A, Saridis A, Scopa CD, Megas P. Histological comparison of autograft, allograft-DBM, xenograft, and synthetic grafts in a trabecular bone defect: an experimental study in rabbits. Med Sci Monitor 2010;16:Br24−31.
[115] Ehrler DM, Vaccaro AR. The use of allograft bone in lumbar spine surgery. Clin Orthop Relat Res 2000;38−45.
[116] Oryan A, Alidadi S, Moshiri A, Maffulli N. Bone regenerative medicine: classic options, novel strategies, and future directions. J Orthop Surg Res 2014;9:18.
[117] Lee KW, Wang SF, Fox BC, Ritman EL, Yaszemski MJ, Lu LC. Poly(propylene fumarate) bone tissue engineering scaffold fabrication using stereolithography: effects of resin formulations and laser parameters. Biomacromolecules 2007;8:1077−84.

CHAPTER 4

Implants for Joint Replacement of the Hip and Knee

J. Gallo[1], E. Gibon[2] and S.B. Goodman[2]
[1]Palacky University, Olomouc, Czech Republic
[2]Stanford University, Stanford, CA, United States

Contents

4.1 HISTORICAL PERSPECTIVE

Total joint replacements (TJRs) of the hip and knee are arguably the most cost-effective operations in all of surgery. Joint replacement surgery is time-proven for relieving pain and restoring more normal function in centers worldwide. TJRs were first perfected and subsequently implanted in Europe and America in the late 1960s and 1970s by Sir John Charnley, Mr. Robin Ling, and Dr. Maurice Muller (hip), and by Dr. John Insall and Mr. Michael Freeman (knee), amongst others. Current total hip and knee replacements using modern designs and materials, and with appropriate patient selection and surgical technique have satisfactory outcomes that last for 15 years or more in the majority of patients [1–7]. However, this outcome has not come without much research and development, as well as some successes and failures. Indeed, different implants still demonstrate a variable degree of durability [8].

Treatments for arthritis of the hip were very primitive prior to the seminal work of Sir John Charnley, who is known as the father of joint replacement. Prior to Charnley's work, debilitating hip arthritis was treated by protected weight-bearing with walking aids, intermittent traction, realignment osteotomy of the proximal femur, excision arthroplasty, interposition arthroplasty, or unipolar arthroplasty [9]. These treatments and operations generally failed to relieve pain and improve function because they did not address the fact that the arthritis affected both acetabular and femoral cartilage, the reconstructions were biomechanically suboptimal and used inferior materials, or deep infection subsequently occurred (the reader should be mindful of the fact that these surgeries were performed before the modern era of antibiotics). Wood, ivory, rubber, glass, allogenic and xenogenic tissues, and other materials were used as implants and interpositional prostheses. Metallic unipolar implants which were anchored in the femur, such as the Moore and Thompson prostheses (normally used for the treatment of femoral neck fractures) fared somewhat better, although pain relief and functional improvement were unpredictable due to acetabular cartilage erosion and inability to restore femoral offset and limb length.

Charnley and his team faced the daunting task of devising a device to replace the degenerated hip joint with a functional, biomechanically sound prosthesis that was durable and infection-free. This challenge was eventually met (after some major setbacks), and the prosthesis was designated as the low-friction arthroplasty (LFA) [10]. Charnley's LFA and subsequent advancements in the field have become known as the operation of the 20th century [11]. Charnley's approach was to use a one-piece stainless steel femoral stem containing a small 22.25 mm head that was cemented into the proximal femur using polymethylmethacrylate (PMMA) as a grout (the latter was suggested to Charnley by a dental chemist, Dennis Smith). On the acetabular side, a high-density polyethylene liner was cemented into the acetabulum that was previously reamed to expose the underlying cancellous bone. At first, Charnley had chosen a different polymer, poly-tetra-fluor-ethylene (Fluon), however, the tribological characteristics of this material were inferior and led to rapid generation of wear particles and a florid foreign body response. The eventual LFA using high-density polyethylene was designed to have low frictional torque, thereby minimizing wear and implant loosening. Charnley emphasized precise preoperative planning and surgical technique, and reconstruction of the normal biomechanics of the hip. To minimize infection, his team worked in a special enclosure with laminar flow within the operating room, and the surgeons wore body exhaust suits so as to not contaminate the wound. Once perfected, Charnley's results were no less than spectacular, and have been replicated worldwide. Indeed his prosthesis and concepts are still regarded as the gold standard with which to compare. Successful long-term results with greater than 25 years of service with this prosthesis are still being reported [12–14].

Despite the successes of Charnley's LFA, problems began to surface. Others altered the original concept in less than favorable ways [8]. Prostheses with suboptimal metallurgy and design broke; those with sharp edges fractured the bone cement during intermittent loading, which led to prosthesis loosening and so called "cement disease," i.e., a foreign body response to particulate cement debris leading to bone destruction (osteolysis). Larger femoral heads articulating with conventional (sterilized by irradiation in air) polyethylene lead to increased volumetric polyethylene wear and periprosthetic osteolysis due to the biological reaction to plastic debris. Infection was still a major problem, often necessitating removal of the prosthesis. Advancements made during the last 25 years have included the use of prophylactic antibiotics to mitigate prosthetic infection, the use of modern metallic alloys including cobalt chrome and titanium alloys, improved prosthetic design, meticulous preoperative planning and surgical technique, and more recently, modularity of components and alternative bearing surfaces.

Today's hip implants are both cemented and cementless, depending on the surgeon's choice. If cemented, meticulous technique includes pressurization of the cement into a clean and dry bone bed, with centralization of the prosthesis to help ensure a uniform cement mantle. A homogeneous polymer with minimal stress-concentrating inclusions is obtained by using vacuum mixing or centrifugation. The cement is delivered to the intended area using a special cement gun, and the cement is pressurized with special instrumentation.

Cementless hip implants are favored by many, and facilitate modularity to accommodate different patients' anatomical variations and provide exchangeability of worn parts. Bone and fibrous tissue ingrowth/ongrowth is obtained by press fitting the device into a bone bed that has been precisely prepared, prosthesis coatings and surface roughening, and additional flanges, screws, and other appendages on the surface of the prosthesis. Cementless implants are particularly useful in younger patients with good bone stock, and in revision cases in which modularity is often desired.

In the 1980s and 1990s, the major problem with total hip arthroplasty (THA) was wear of the polyethylene and periprosthetic osteolysis due to an inflammatory reaction to polyethylene wear debris. This spawned the introduction of new technologies to limit wear. However, alternative bearing surfaces for hip replacement have generated much controversy [15,16]. Whereas the new crosslinked polyethylene components have proven clinically to decrease wear and osteolysis, so-called hard-on-hard bearings including metal-on-metal (MoM) and ceramic-on-ceramic (CoC) have faced numerous setbacks [17]. The MoM articulations were supposed to demonstrate minimal wear due to fluid film lubrication. However, breakdown of lubrication, inadequate prosthesis designs, and suboptimal implant positioning have been associated with the generation of metallic particles and ions that are toxic to bone and soft tissue [18]. CoC bearings have demonstrated other problems including poor designs, inadequate seating of modular components, chipping, striped wear, squeaking, and breakage [19]. For the most part, the gold standard is currently a metal or ceramic on polyethylene articulation. However, new problems continue to arise: excessive metal debris is generated at modular junctions (such as with modular head—stem and stem—neck articulations), further complicating matters. There is also controversy regarding the use of large femoral heads, although the dislocation rate has dramatically decreased with their use [20].

Total knee replacement (TKR) has also had a somewhat difficult past. The original designs for TKR did not take into account that the knee is more complicated than the hip joint, i.e., that the knee is not a simple hinge and depends on soft tissues including muscles, tendons, and ligaments for guided motion and stability. Whereas the hip joint is a simple ball and socket which rotates, the knee undergoes bending, sliding, and rotation. Most of the original knee replacements were poorly designed, retained the cruciate and collateral ligaments, and were more of a simple resurfacing operation. The prostheses did not reestablish the complex kinematics of the knee joint. On the other hand, highly constrained knees including hinges demanded extensive exposure and used long stems; these implants often became infected, loosened early, or broke because of the limited unforgiving soft tissue envelope around the knee (as opposed to the extensively muscled hip girdle), and the high stresses placed on the implants and interfaces. The forebearers of modern Western implants were first designed at the Hospital for Special Surgery in New York (total condylar prosthesis, Insall Burstein prosthesis), in Boston (Duopatellar and Kinematic prostheses), and in London (Freeman Swanson prosthesis) in the 1970s and onwards. These implants utilized more modern alloys and were cemented in place. Some retained the posterior cruciate ligament (PCL), whereas others sacrificed it. The anterior cruciate ligament was uniformly sacrificed. As the kinematics of the knee were better understood, designs were perfected and the condylar type prosthesis, with/without retention of the PCL, was redesigned for better stability throughout a limited but functional range of motion (ROM). One important advancement was the introduction of the posterior stabilized knee, which substituted the PCL for a post and cam mechanism, facilitating femoral rollback and more normal knee kinematics. Both cruciate sacrificing and substituting designs have had great long-term success, with fixed and mobile bearings [6,7,21,22]. Although some have dabbled in cementless knee implant designs, the vast majority of knee replacements are still cemented.

Some of the newer concepts in TKR include anatomical rather than symmetrical femoral components, femoral components that provide alternatives for specific populations such as those with smaller proportions or female patients, younger more active patients, those that require more flexion than conventional knee replacements (so-called high flexion TKRs), etc. [23–28]. In addition, TKAs with different kinematics have been designed, recognizing that femoral rollback is more accentuated on the lateral compared to the medial side [29]. Newer instrumentation that purportedly helps components to be placed more reproducibly (such as with surgical navigation) and custom jigs and implants based on advanced imaging methods are also recently introduced innovations [24,30–33]. The introduction of crosslinked polyethylene, vitamin E-doped polyethylene, surface coatings, and newer ceramic materials is controversial. Whether these innovations decrease complication rates, and improve long-term outcome and patient satisfaction is to be determined.

4.2 DESIGN AND MATERIAL ISSUES, CLINICAL OUTCOME

4.2.1 Current bearing materials in hip and knee replacement

THA was originally designed for elderly patients with limited life span [10]. When the procedure was extended to younger, more active patients, polyethylene wear and periprosthetic osteolysis became major issues limiting the durability of THA [34,35]. To address these issues, THAs with alternative bearing surfaces to metal-on-conventional polyethylene (MoP) were introduced [15,16,35]. These bearings were invented ostensibly to mitigate wear and therefore provide a smaller particle load to the body, leading to less osteolysis. The three major types of bearings introduced include: (1) metal or ceramic on highly crosslinked polyethylene (XLPE); (2) CoC; and (3) MoM.

4.2.1.1 New polyethylenes

Metallic or ceramic femoral heads articulating with an acetabular component made of XLPE have been one of the most important advances in THA. With over 10 years of data from numerous centers worldwide, this bearing couple has proved to be safe, effective, and durable, at least into the second decade of use [36–45]. Whether the stem is cemented or cementless, remarkably less polyethylene wear has been demonstrated. Wear rates of HLPE are approximately 5–10 times less than that noted with conventional polyethylene. In fact, a clear-cut case of periprosthetic osteolysis of an articulation in which XLPE has been used has not been reported. However, the use of larger femoral heads may lead to increased volumetric wear of even XLPE, so that further follow-up into the second and third decades after implantation is indicated [44]. If the XLPE is melted at high temperatures to quench the residual free radicals associated with sterilization by irradiation, the fatigue properties and strength of the resulting material are reduced compared to conventional polyethylene. Thus, with improper placement of the hip components with edge loading, or with the use of thin unsupported polyethylene usually articulating with a larger femoral head, fracture of the plastic has been encountered [46–48]. This has emphasized the tradeoffs and choices that have to be made with regard to conventional versus XLPE with respect to the mechanical properties, wear, and oxidation resistance [49]. Newer polyethylene bearings incorporating multiple cycles of increased pressure and heating below the melting point, or the addition of vitamin E or other free radical scavengers have shown great promise [38,50,51].

4.2.1.2 Ceramic-on-ceramic bearings

Ceramic bearings have been used extensively in France, Japan, Korea, and, to a lesser degree, in other geographic locations worldwide including the United States [52–54]. These bearings have numerous advantages including very low friction, high wear resistance, few wear particles generated, low incidence of osteolysis, and the possibility of larger femoral heads being used for enhanced stability [16,19,55,56]. Previous issues with femoral head breakage are rare with modern composite ceramics [57,58]. However, other issues have arisen including difficulties with acetabular cup assembly with incomplete seating, liner canting and dissociation, liner chipping, and fracture. If the components are not precisely implanted, there can be edge loading with striped wear, and even squeaking with some implants due to faulty lubrication at the bearing surface. These bearings are also more expensive than others currently used. Furthermore, there is no conclusive evidence that modern hard-on-hard bearings including CoC bearings are more durable than bearings using XLPE, or even conventional polyethylene [59,60]. The proponents of CoC bearings emphasize their use in younger patients whose physical activities involve repetitive impact loading such as running, skiing, etc.

4.2.1.3 Metal-on-metal bearings

Perhaps the most controversial bearing couple for THA involves MoM articulations. These bearings were thought to provide very low friction and wear, allowing a greater breadth of physical activity and the use of larger femoral heads for enhanced stability [15,56,59,61]. The articulation is dependent on fluid film lubrication to maintain the very low wear rate. Although some implants have functioned admirably, others have failed due to breakdown of fluid film lubrication, resulting in the generation of small nanoparticulates and ions [62]. In some cases, this has led to patients complaining of feelings of ratcheting and squeaking, pain, and poor hip function. Excessive production of metallic by-products has been associated with adverse local tissue reactions (ALTRs), immune reactions, and the formation of masses called pseudotumors [63,64]. These phenomena are the result of a hypersensitivity type IV immune reaction to metallic debris and ions, which can attach to plasma proteins forming haptens, and extensive necrosis of bone and surrounding soft tissue [18]. For MoM resurfacing arthroplasty, risk factors for the above include female sex, small-sized implants, bilateral replacements, obesity, and suboptimal implant alignment with edge loading. Some of the problems associated with MoM bearings are related to faulty design [65]. Because of the above issues, the number of resurfacing arthroplasties and THAs with MoM components has dramatically decreased over the last 5 years [15,16,60].

4.2.2 Cemented hip arthroplasty

Cemented THA means that both components are fixed to the bone bed by acrylic bone cement, whereas hybrid THA means that only one of the two components is fixed to the bone by acrylic bone cement. Usually the cup is cementless and the stem is cemented, but it can be also the reverse situation with cemented cup and cementless stem.

Since the time of Sir John Charnley to the beginning of the 21st century, a cemented THA has been considered as the gold standard; however, in the last decade the clinical position of this combination has declined even in the countries that had been assumed to be the traditional pillars for cemented THAs. In this section we will discuss current information relevant to cemented THA.

4.2.2.1 Acrylic bone cement: Polymethylmethacrylate

PMMA is a thermoplastic polymer, widely used in orthopedics for its strong mix of mechanical and biological properties. The history of development of PMMA for orthopedic surgery [66], as well as its biologic and biomechanical properties, are described elsewhere [67].

Commercially available PMMAs are marketed as a two-component product consisting of the polymer powder component and liquid methyl methacrylate. They all differ in their precise chemical formulation and composition, resulting in different properties such as viscosity, heat, and mechanics [68]. Generally, PMMA is strong in compression, and it can relax during a period of unloading (self-protection), but it is relatively weak in tension and bending. In addition, it exhibits fatigue changes after a long period of use [69].

4.2.2.2 Firmness and durability of implant–cement composite

The peak hip forces have been reported with values ranging from 2.4 to 4.1 times body weight recorded during gait [70]. Specific activities like alpine skiing can produce joint contact forces equivalent to up to 7.8 times body weight [71]. It is also estimated that several million work-cycles have to be expected in THA each year [72]. Thus the mechanical strength and resistance to fatigue are critical parameters for long-term success of the surgical procedure.

Based on extensive experimental research and analysis of clinical data, there is clear evidence that the cement–implant composite is highly resistant and durable, and thus appropriate for THA [73]. However, every surgeon has to know the key steps of optimal operative technique in order to prevent premature failure of cemented THA. Principally the longevity of fixation of a cemented implant depends on three interfaces (i.e., bone-to-cement, within the cement itself, cement-to-implant). Each of these contributes to the overall durability of the system but, in turn, the weakness of one of them can induce mechanical failure of the whole system. In this line, the bone–cement interface requires particular attention because vital bone surrounding the cement surface undergoes remodeling, thus reducing the total contact between bone and PMMA, which can eventually lead to weakening of the interface [74].

4.2.2.3 Material and design of cemented implants

Polyethylenes are the only biomaterial used in cemented cups. The metal-backed concept used for cementless implants has not been shown to offer any advantage for cemented cups and has been abandoned.

In terms of optimizing the cement mantle around a cup, several strategies have been proposed from the time of Charnley. The oldest innovation lies in the use of flanged or unflanged designs. The former restricts the leakage of PMMA during cup insertion and can increase the pressure inside PMMA. In fact, some studies demonstrate higher pressures in cement and greater intrusion of PMMA into the spongy bone compared to unflanged cups [75]. However, others have emphasized the role of preinsertion pressurization and other factors related to cement and the cementing technique [76]. Therefore, the only advantage of the flange might lie in the avoidance of the cup to "bottom out," i.e., have no cement at all medially. A number of other design and material changes continue in progress in cemented cups, including the new highly crosslinked polyethylenes.

Metallic stems for cemented THA are generally made from stainless steel or cobalt–chromium alloy. A large variety of cemented stem designs have been available in clinical practice differing in shape, length, and surface roughness (pretreatment). Huiskes et al. proposed two opposing principles of stem design fixation and retention defined as "shape closed fixation" and "force closed fixation" [77]. The former depends on the shape of the implant and on a firm bond between the implant surface and surrounding cement offering an immediate interlock and preventing subsidence. The latter is ideally polished and straight tapered from top to bottom achieving the interlock gradually in relation to implant load and creep of PMMA. The advantage of the polished tapered stem is that it can—in contrast to a composite beam—restore a more stable configuration repeatedly in its lifetime of use. Long-term studies show continual subsidence of this type of stem without risk for premature loosening [78]. In addition, a highly polished surface prevents excessive interface abrasion that could lead to generation of metallic by-products (metallosis). As a result, some stems like the Exeter [79] or MS-30 [80] present very good long-term survivorship in comparison to stems intended to be fixed more by "shape closed fixation."

4.2.2.4 Cementing technique during THA

An optimal cementing technique is the key prerequisite for long-term stability of a cemented THA. Because cementing is a multistep process, there are multiple opportunities for mistakes. All surgeons agree that sound, continual, and a well-anchored cemented interface is of paramount importance, but surgeons widely differ in the manner as to how this is achieved. As a result, this is the most important source for heterogeneity in meta-analysis and systematic reviews.

Cementing is considered "good" when a cement mantle is *continuous and of particular thickness* covering the whole fixation surface of a cemented component (Fig. 4.1). In addition, there should be specific *density and depth of cement intrusions* into the optimally prepared bone bed [81]. In this line, a sclerotic polished bone bed is not suitable for cementing, and should be addressed whenever possible.

To date there is relatively strong evidence for a third-generation cement technique (Fig. 4.2) in combination with vacuum mixing as the standard to be undertaken. This decreases the porosity of PMMA compared with hand mixing and improves the mechanical strength [82]. On the other hand, some authors dispute that vacuum mixing leads to a decrease in overall porosity in cemented stems [83]. Data from implant registries will definitively determine the true contribution of vacuum mixing techniques to the long-term survivorship of cemented THAs. The list of basic requirements for an optimal cementing technique in THA is shown in Table 4.1.

4.2.2.5 Clinical evidence for cemented THA

The position of a therapy in the armamentarium of therapeutic interventions is determined by the strength of evidence coming from methodologically sound clinical

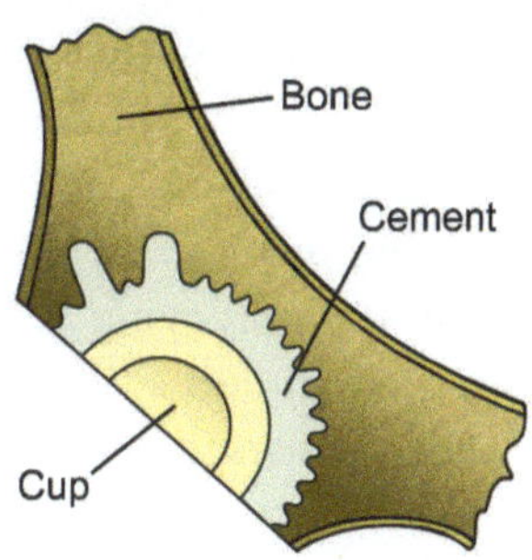

Figure 4.1 Basic prerequisite for a stable bone–cement–implant interface is a continuous and thick cement mantle with a set of dense intrusions of PMMA into the bone bed augmented by several keyholes.

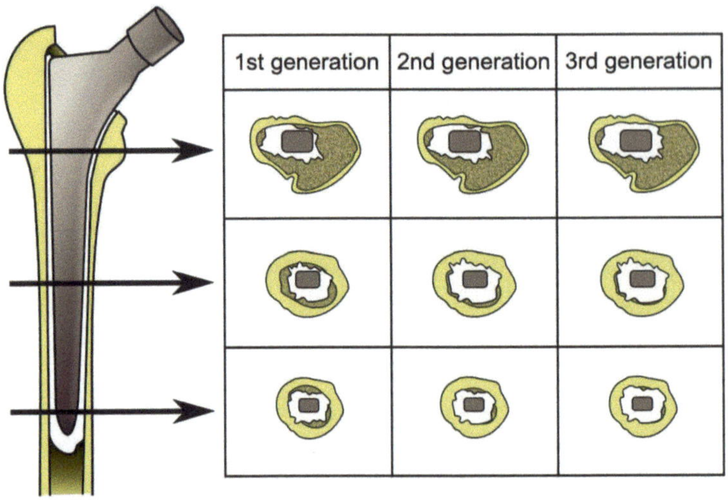

Figure 4.2 Newer generations of cementing techniques improve the quality of cement mantle, especially in terms of symmetry, continuousness, thickness, and decrease in porosity. (A) Cementing of first generation; (B) cementing of second generation; (C) cementing of third generation *Adapted from Breusch S, Malchau H, eds. The well-cemented total hip arthroplasty. Theory and practice. Berlin: Springer; 2005. ISBN 3-540-24197-3.*

studies. Patients as well as other stakeholders usually have two basic requirements. The first is related to the effect size of a treatment, and the second is how long the achieved effect will last (durability of the effect). For the first requirement, specific outcomes tool, including currently popular "patient-reported outcome measures" are used. With regard to the second requirement, surgeons rely on the Kaplan–Meier method of estimating survivorship at the specific time elapsed from the surgery. However, this method is now subject to strong criticism, especially for how it handles patients that die at some point during a study's follow-up period. It is obvious that death precludes future implant failure. That is why the Kaplan–Meier method overestimates the likelihood of implant failure if a substantial proportion of the patients enrolled in the study at its beginning die during the follow-up. To address this problem a competing-risks analysis has been introduced [84]. However, there is still a paucity of studies with long-term follow-up employing competing-risks analysis.

Table 4.2 demonstrates that the best studies available for cemented THA meet the NICE criteria [85]. In addition, recent systematic reviews and meta-analyses were not able to detect a significant difference between cemented and cementless THAs in terms of survivorship. This conclusion is particularly strong in relation to the care of elderly patients [86,87] and specifically for cemented stems [73].

Table 4.1 Overview of basic requirements for cementing technique in THA

Acetabulum	**Bone bed preparation**
Cement mantle should be continuous, at least 1.5–2 mm thick and intrusion should be 5–6 mm	a. Meticulous removal of all soft tissues, including debridement of bone cysts (larger should be grafted by bone from the femoral head); b. Reaming should be done with the goal to preserve at least part of the subchondral plate; c. Acetabular parts with sclerosis should be treated with multiple small anchorage holes (4.5–6 mm drilling; some surgeons use in addition keyholes with a diameter 10–12 mm and depth of 6–10 mm); d. The use of pulsatile lavage to cleanse the detritus and blood. Cementing technique a. Reducing bleeding by hypotensive anesthesia and/or hydrogen peroxide, solution of adrenaline, tranexamic acid, etc.; b. Mixing the PMMA according to manufacturer's manual (the same is valid for the femoral portion); c. Pressurization of PMMA with a provisional or standard pressurizer; d. Insertion of a polyethylene cup with moderate pressure and in optimal position.
Femur Continuous cement mantle should be of a minimum thickness of 2 mm; proximally the mantle should be even thicker (3–5 mm)	Bone bed preparation a. Progressive broaching to stably fit the largest size broach; trial reduction; b. Meticulous removal of all soft, bone detritus from the femoral canal. Cementing technique a. Placement of a distal plug (cement restrictor) at an adequate depth allowing 1.5–2 cm cement mantle distal to the tip of the stem; b. Cleansing of the detritus by pulsatile lavage; c. Both decreasing bleeding and drying the femoral canal via hydrogen peroxide or packing the canal with epinephrine-soaked gauze; d. Retrograde cement application via cement gun; e. Slow pressurization of PMMA with provisional or standard pressurizer; f. Insertion of a stem with a distal (and proximal if available) centralizer in optimal position.

Table 4.2 Examples of the best available survivorship data for cemented THA

Author	Implant	*N*	Age	Gender	FU_{MIN}	Surv.	95% CI	End point
Berry et al. [88]	Charnley cup + stem	2000	63.5	50.2% female	25 years	77.5% at 25 years	74.9–80.3%	Revision for any reason
Brigstocke et al. [80]	MS-30 stem	55	59	43.7% female	10 years	100% at 10 years	NA	Revision for any reason
Aubault et al. [89]	Zimmer PF cup + stem	83	66	42.5% female	10 years	98.3% at 10 years	NA	Revision for any reason
Martin et al. [90]	Charnley cup + stem	109	<50	NA	20 years	81% at 20 years	73–87%	Revision for aseptic loosening
Martin et al. [90]	Charnley cup + stem	649	≥50	NA	20 years	95% at 20 years	93–97%	Revision for aseptic loosening
Clauss et al. [91]	Müller straight stem	165	Average 69	42.4% female	20 years	81% at 20 years	76–86%	Revision of stem for any reason
de Jong et al. [92]	Weber cup	287	65.3	73.4% female	10 years	99.1% at 10 years	97.9–100%	Revision for aseptic loosening
Thomsen et al. [93]	Exeter (cup + stem)	200	71 (26–90)	52% female	18 years	73% at 18 years	49–89%	Revision for any reason
Thomsen et al. [93]	Exeter (cup + stem)	200	71 (26–90)	52% female	18 years	84% for stem/76% for cup at 18 years	68–96%/ 61–92%	Revision for aseptic loosening of the stem/cup
Wroblewski et al. [94]	Charnley cup + stem	1434	41 (12–51)	61.2% female	11 years	93.7% at 11 years	92.3–95.0%	Revision for any indication
Nich et al. [95]	Charnley–Kerboull	122	50.8 (21–85)	27.1% female	10 years	89.8% at 15 years	81.7–97.9%	Revision for aseptic loosening

Age is reported as the mean; *N*, number; FU_{MIN}, minimum length of follow-up; Surv, survivorship; CI, confidence interval.

Additional evidence for cemented THA comes from arthroplasty registries that are considered the most powerful tool for information concerning the clinical performance of implants. Registries use large numbers of patients and robust statistics (for instance the Cox's multiple regression model) allowing a number of adjustments made for potential differences between compared groups. Table 4.3 shows registry-based data for cemented THA. When data for cemented and cementless THAs from four Nordic registries were compared, the survival of cemented implants for THA was higher than that of cementless implants in patients aged 65 years or older [96].

Should only implants with a proven track record be used in clinical practice? Interestingly, in the United Kingdom 24% (57/235) of all hip replacement implants available to surgeons have no evidence of clinical effectiveness [99]. This percentage may be even higher in other countries.

4.2.2.6 Clinical evidence for partially cemented THA (cementless cup-cemented stem)

Recent studies have suggested that the cup is the weak link, which compromises the survivorship of a cemented THA [12,100,101]. Thus some surgeons have believed for more than three decades that the optimal solution could be a combination of advantages of cementless cups and cemented stems [102]. However, the key step is to choose the optimal implant combination, i.e., the best cup and the best stem. The survivorship data illustrating this concept are shown in Table 4.4.

4.2.2.7 Current indications for cemented or partially cemented THA

There is little agreement on the specific indications related exclusively to cemented THA. Some surgeons believe it would be a better choice than cementless THA in cases of inflammatory arthropathies, osteopenia/osteoporosis, protrusio deformities, and perhaps also in patients with radiation necrosis of the pelvis. With regard to the latter diagnosis, it is important to emphasize the necessity to produce a firm foundation such as with a reconstruction cage before cementing the cup.

There is intermediate to strong evidence that in elderly patients, the long-term outcomes of cemented THAs are better in comparison to cementless ones [96]. On the other hand, there are centers that use cementless THAs with predictable outcomes also in patients older than 75 years. Cost may play a role in decision-making because cementless implants are substantially more expensive in comparison to cemented ones.

4.2.2.8 Conclusion

Cemented THA is still a viable option despite the great progress achieved with cementless implants. At least for elderly patients (75 years and above) and some specific indications, the cemented THAs remain a reliable choice under the assumption that an appropriate technique and implants are used.

Table 4.3 Data from registries describing the role of cemented THA (endpoint = revision for any reason); age is reported as the mean

Registry	*N* (C/NC)	% of C in all THA	Age	Surv. at 10 years	95% CI
RIPO (2000–2011)	3894/40,378	9.6%	66.9 (16–101)	93.6% at 12 years	91.9–95.3%
SHAR (1999–2013)	110,633	>66%	>70 years	94.4%	94.1–94.7%
AOJR (1999–2013)	NA	8.4%	NA	94.0%	93.6–94.5%
NZJR (1999–2013)	6290/4261	37.7%	NA	94.5%	NA
FAR [97]	3811/464	79. 8%	82 (80–102)	97.4%	96.9–98.0%*
[96]	40,202/35,092	44.3%	55–64	92.2%	91.8–92.5%
[96]	96,346/26,940	68.9%	65–74	93.8%	93.6–94.0%
[96]	96,055/9422	81.9%	≥75	95.9%	95.8–96.1%
[98]	6824/16,407	23.1%	<55	90.2%	NA

N, number; C, cemented THA; NC, noncemented THA; Surv., survivorship of cemented THA; CI, confidence interval; RIPO, Regional Register of Orthopedic Prosthetic Implantology (Report of R.I.P.O.; https://ripo.cineca.it/pdf/report_2012_en_rev1.pdf); SHAR, Swedish Hip Arthroplasty Register (Annual Report 2013; http://www.shpr.se/Libraries/Documents/AnnualReport_2013-04-1_1.sflb.ashx); AOJR, Australian Orthopaedic Association National Joint Replacement Registry (Annual Report 2014; https://aoanjrr.dmac.adelaide.edu.au/documents/10180/172286/Annual%20Report%202014); NZJR, The New Zealand Joint Registry (see attachment 13.5.15); *, the survival without revision was calculated using cumulative incidence function (competing risks survival analysis); FAR, Finnish Arthroplasty Register (Annual Report 2014).

However, in contrast to available data, cemented implants are under strong criticism, especially for the acetabulum. As a result, the use of cemented cups has substantially decreased in many countries; e.g., in the United States cemented cups are rare today despite the fact that the evidence in the literature against their usage is weak or none existent [96,108]. Cemented stems are still used by some orthopedic surgeons due to identified benefits and low cost, at least under specific clinical conditions [109].

4.2.3 Cementless hip arthroplasty

The first total hip arthroplasties (THAs) were cemented using PMMA. The first modern cementless THAs appeared in the 1980s and have continued to develop over the last four decades. Surgeons now have at their disposal a wide choice of different implants, surfaces, and coatings.

Regarding the cementless femoral stem, the surface can be peened, ridged, fluted, porous coated, or the implant surface can be covered with a three-dimensional,

Table 4.4 Examples of studies reporting data on survivorship of partially cemented THA

Author	Implant	*N*	Age	Gender	FU_{MIN}	Surv.	95% CI	End point
Berger et al. [103]	Harris-Galante-I-Precoat	150	39–85	66.7% female	7 years	96.9% at 10 years	95.4–98.4%	Revision, radiographic loosening
Clohisy et al. [104]	Harris-Galante (+screws)–Precoat, Zimmer	100	45–87	51.2% female	7 years	96% at 10 years	93–98%	Revision for any reason
Kim et al. [105]	Duraloc 100 –Charnley Elite	64	43.4	21.8% female	8 years	98% at 9.4 years	93–100%	Revision for any reason
Firestone et al. [106]	Harris-Galante-II-Iowa	149	32–87	63.6% female	10 years	95.3% at 10 years	91.3–99.3%	Revision for any reason
DHAR (1995–2010)	Mallory-Head – Exeter	2258	NA	NA	10 years	95.8% at 10 years	94.7–96.9%	Revision for any reason
SHAR 2004–2013	NA	2778	60–69	NA	NA	91.8% at 10 years	89.5–94.2%	Revision for any reason
NJR [107]	Trident- Exeter V40	15,740	68	60.8% female	NA	98.44% at 5 years	98.11–98.77%	Revision for any reason

Age is reported as the mean; *N*, number; FU_{MIN}, minimum length of follow-up; Surv., survivorship; CI, confidence interval; DHAR, Danish Hip Arthroplasty Register (Annual Repord 2011; http://www.dhr.dk/Ny%20mappe/rapporter/DHR%20Aarsrapport_2011%20t_web.pdf); SHAR, Swedish Hip Arthroplasty Register (Annual Report 2013; http://www.shpr.se/Libraries/Documents/AnnualReport_2013-04-1_1.sflb.ashx); NJR, National Joint Registry of England, Wales and Northern Ireland.

trabecular bone-like layer or a bioactive coating (e.g., hydroxyapatite). The shape may be straight, anatomic, or patient-specific. The large range of surface choices applies to the acetabular cup as well. Additional stabilization of the cup can be achieved with spikes, ridges, screws, etc. Moreover, the cup can be either impacted directly or screwed into place using large surface threads.

Cementless components for THA have the advantage of avoiding the use of cement, which could fail (leading to loss of fixation), and produce particles and third body wear. Cementless THAs allow biologic incorporation of the implant to the host via ingrown/ongrown bone. This biologic incorporation of the prosthesis, also known as osseointegration can be compared to the bone-healing process following a fracture.

The first implants were designed to create a mechanical interlock with the host bone. This was achieved through surface treatments such as porous coating, roughening, etching, flutes, or lattice layers. Mechanical fixation along the entire length of the stem led to adverse bone remodeling (i.e., loss of bone) proximally, also referred to as stress shielding. Partially coated stems, especially noncircumferential coatings allowed the ingress of polyethylene wear particles from the articulation, resulting in a high rate of osteolysis associated with this type of implant [110,111]. Furthermore, a fibrous layer between the bone and the implant often developed due to inadequate stability of the prosthesis.

The more recent use of titanium alloy implants with titanium surface coating, or bioactive hydroxyapatite coating has led to implants capable of osseointegration. The bone ingrowth phenomenon is a biologic process similar to primary fracture healing; hydroxyapatite coating functions as an osteoinductive scaffold that is replaced, with time, by mature bone. This prevents the migration of wear debris that could trigger a periprosthetic osteolysis.

Preoperative templating allows the size of the implant, the level of the cut at the femoral neck and the length of the neck (standard or lateralized) to be anticipated.

The template and the preoperative X-rays should be at the same magnification to allow for accurate planning:

- The acetabular implant should be between 40 and 45 degrees of the line joining the two acetabular teardrops. The cup size is templated so that the acetabular implant is covered by the acetabular roof.
- The femoral implant is templated to fit the femoral metaphysis and proximal shaft, as well as determining femoral offset and neck length.

Properly sized and implanted cementless THAs have excellent primary mechanical stability within bone and can support physiologic loads. Their behavior with the host bone is dependent on their initial stability and surface contact, and subsequent bone and fibrous tissue ingrowth/ongrowth. Alternatively, implants with a bioactive surface such as a hydroxyapatite coating facilitate a direct link to the host bone. Studies have shown durability of these implants with survivorship up to 95% at 15 years [112,113].

Many retrieval studies have been performed to understand the mechanism of success and failure of cementless THA. Retrievals of Harris-Galante I acetabular cups after at a mean of 11 years reported by Urban et al. [114] found that the mean extent of bone ingrowth was 33%. However, they identified pelvic granulomas in more than one-third of the specimens and found a significant correlation between granuloma size and decreasing patient age. Sychterz et al. [115] reported an average of 35% of available surface with bone ingrowth in femoral components and an average of 32% for the acetabular component. von Knoch et al. [116] analyzed the migration of polyethylene wear debris around cementless femoral stems. They showed that a complete circumferential porous-coated surface could prevent distal migration of polyethylene particles, however the bone ingrown surface ranged from 5% to 80% of the implant circumference. Surprisingly, McAuley et al. [117] found that extensively porous coated stems had less bone loss on average than proximally coated stem. Differences in stem design, and the location and amount of various coatings have a major effect on subsequent bone remodeling [118]. Characterization of wear particles around failed revised hip arthroplasties disclosed that most of the particles (>90%) are submicron in size with a mean number of particles of 1.7 billion per gram of tissue [119].

4.2.4 Cemented total knee replacement

The number of primary total knee arthroplasties (TKAs) is projected to grow by 673% by 2030 [120]. A TKA can be fully cemented (femoral, tibial, and patellar implants), cementless (none of the implants are cemented), or hybrid.

Cementation of knee implants gives immediate initial implant fixation. Preparation of the bone is critical prior to cementation. In an in vitro study, van de Groes et al. [121] have shown all of the periosteum should be removed from the anterior surface of the cortical bone on the femur. They also recommended to drill small holes through the cortex below the anterior flange of the femoral implant for optimal fixation of the component. Maistrelli et al. [122] have shown that pulsed lavage significantly increases the penetration of the cement on both the femoral and tibial sides. Lutz et al. [123] compared three different methods to cement the tibial implants: with a pressurized cement gun, a cement syringe, and by hand. Their results showed that when a cement gun or syringe was used, the depth of the cement penetration was significantly higher and there was a significant reduction in radiolucent lines when compared to cement applied by hand. Moreover, no difference was found between pressurized gun and cement syringe.

Early application of cement onto the cut bone surface refers to use of the cement when it is in a more liquid state; late application refers to use of cement in a more doughy state. Silverman et al. [124] concluded that the doughy phase of the cement allows deeper penetration of the cement, thereby providing a stronger cement—bone interphase, using a cadaver model. They also found that continuous application of pressure to the components after applying the cement improved interdigitation compared to direct impaction only. Continuous application of pressure gives more time for the cement to penetrate into the interstices of cancellous bone. Walker et al. [125] have shown that the ideal depth of cement penetration is 3—4 mm, and that depths greater that 5 mm increase the potential risk of thermal necrosis of the underlying bone.

Whether to cement the stem plus undersurface of the tibial tray, or only the undersurface of the tibial tray alone is controversial. In an interesting study comparing long-term results of these techniques (surface cementation vs full cementation), Schlegel et al. [126] have shown no significant difference in terms of survivorship. Bohm et al. [127] have shown that the use of antibiotic-loaded bone cement does not increase the risk for revision due to mechanical loosening either.

The following table sums up the key points of cemented TKA (Table 4.5).

Cementless TKA is a less frequently used option for implant fixation. Several studies have been performed to compare cemented versus cementless TKA. Wang et al. [128] showed no significant difference in survival rates in their meta-analysis between cemented and cementless TKRs. Even in young patients (younger than 55 years old), Kim et al. [129] found no difference in the outcome of these techniques either.

4.3 CURRENT CRITICAL ISSUES

4.3.1 Introduction of new technologies to orthopedics

New technologies are vital to orthopedic surgery. Many of these devices have revolutionized orthopedic clinical care, including the treatment of fractures and nonunions (e.g., with plates, screws, intramedullary rods, and external fixation devices), joint replacements (hip, knee, shoulder, and other joints), arthroscopic procedures, spinal instrumentation devices (for deformities, fracture stabilization, artificial discs), bone graft substitutes, and many others. However, the processes by which devices, drugs, biologics, and combination products are introduced to the American orthopedic marketplace have come under recent scrutiny [130]. The majority of devices in orthopedic surgery gain approval through the FDA 510(k) process, which specifies that the device is substantially equivalent to a preexisting or predicate, previously approved device [18,131]. The new device is labeled as Class II, and exhibits moderate, controlled risk when used in patients. Class II devices are subject to general controls

Table 4.5 Key points regarding cementing of TKA

Technique	Recommendations	Author
Preparation of the bone	Remove all the periosteum	van de Groes et al. [121]
Type of lavage	Pulsed lavage	Maistrelli et al. [122]
Cement application	Pressurized gun or syringe	Lutz et al. [123]
Timing of application of bone cement	Dough phase + continuous pressure	Silverman et al. [124]
Cement penetration	3–4 mm is optimal	Walker et al. [125]
Cement the tibial baseplate only or also cement the tibial stem	Not necessary to cement the stem	Schlegel et al. [126]
Effect of antibiotic-loaded cement on mechanical loosening	No difference versus antibiotic-free cement	Bohm et al. [127]

(similar to low-risk Class I devices), as well as special controls that are more relevant to the function and use of that specific device. Examples of Class II devices include conventional hip and knee joint replacements. Class II devices and products often require biomechanical, material, and biological data that demonstrate substantial equivalence to a device that is already approved by the FDA. In general, this process has worked quite well for patients, surgeons, manufacturers, and the marketplace in general. Some Class II devices and all Class III devices are subject to the general and special controls, similar to Class II devices, but in addition, Class III devices must demonstrate that they are safe and effective in patients. This necessitates conducting an approved clinical trial under an Investigational Device Exemption (IDE). The bench testing and clinical data are then presented to the FDA to support a Premarket Approval Application (PMA). Rarely, some Class II and III devices that are used in less than 4000 cases per year are reviewed by the FDA for a Human Device Exemption (HDE). This designation is requested in very special situations; devices given an HDE designation are subject to general and special controls and have demonstrated that the potential benefits outweigh the risks with high probability.

Although this governmental device approval system seems logical, there are dissenters on both sides of the debate [132–135]. Manufacturers may feel that the current regulatory pathways are too onerous, expensive, time-consuming, and withhold innovative products from needing patients for too long. Governmental agencies such as the FDA are overburdened; yet still this agency attempts to hold the highest of standards to maintain safety and effectiveness for products that cross their desk. The public, including payers, doctors, and patients all want cost-effective implants and drugs that are not only safe and efficacious, but also readily available and cost-effective. Thus there are many stakeholders in the debate on orthopedic innovation, who seem to have specialized positions and needs [136].

Several recent implants and biologics have fueled the controversy concerning the governmental approval process, and in particular the concept of substantial equivalence. MoM and CoC bearings for total hip replacement were supposedly the answer to the higher wear rates seen in younger patients with MoP articulations [16]. However, as outlined previously, both MoM and CoC hard bearings have demonstrated unanticipated issues and adverse events. For example, some MoM bearings have been associated with the development of increased numbers of small nano-sized particles and ions, which have led to immune reactions, extensive local bone and soft tissue destruction, and pseudotumor formation [15,18,137]. Revision surgeries for these cases are more complex, with poorer outcomes and higher complication rates, compared to MoP revision cases. CoC bearings have their own issues including striped wear, chipping and breakage, incomplete seating of the acetabular ceramic insert, as well as squeaking [55]. On the contrary, XLPE for hip replacement has been a major success story, with over a decade of positive demonstrated outcomes in patients, with proven low wear rates and essentially no osteolysis [41,42,138]. A new systematic review concluded that five so-called recently introduced "advances" in joint replacement prosthetic devices have limited peer-reviewed evidence of superiority and, in some cases, have demonstrated inferiority compared to more conventional devices [139]. Although it is difficult to discern how an individual prosthesis will function in any specific patient, clearly, extensive preclinical and short-term clinical studies may not adequately predict how a prosthesis will function in the long term in an individual. In this respect, long-term surveillance including the timely reporting of adverse events, and the use of databases and registries is of paramount importance so as to avoid painful and costly revision surgeries.

The same case can be made for the use of biologics. Given the recent controversies concerning the adequacy and veracity of the clinical studies in determining the safety and efficacy of Bone Morphogenetic Protein-2 (BMP-2) for spine fusion, continued vigilance and oversight are necessary to protect the public from the overenthusiastic use of new devices and biologics [140]. Reservations concerning the use of other biologics and cellular product has also been raised [141,142].

Various frameworks have been proposed to address how new technologies should be introduced into surgical practice to improve outcomes, mitigate adverse events, and maximize cost-effectiveness. The IDEAL protocol developed by a conglomerate of surgical specialists and epidemiologists outlines a framework for innovation and evaluation of new surgical technologies. The stages include formulation of an innovative idea and preclinical testing, development of this idea by surgeon innovators in limited clinical situations, exploration and usage of the technology by many surgeons in clinical trials and in more community scenarios, assessment of outcomes of the device which is now widely used, and long-term evaluation and surveillance using databases, registries, and other means [143,144]. Innovation in surgery must be based on sound scientific evidence including preclinical data, well-designed clinical trials, informed consent, appropriate control groups and defined outcome parameters with sufficient follow-up with documentation of adverse events; potential conflicts of interest, surgeon bias, and marketing influences should not cloud the emphasis on safety and efficacy [145,146]. Hospitals have a corporate responsibility to ensure that the surgeon and surgical team have the necessary qualifications, competency, and proficiency to perform the procedure [147]. Various authors and associations have opined on different protocols and structures to bring new orthopedic products to the marketplace [148,149]. Some have outlined a stepwise method of introducing new devices, emphasizing randomized clinical trials, multicenter studies, and comprehensive national and international registries to document outcome and complications [150]. Others have suggested a gradual introduction of new orthopedic implants beginning with centers with special expertise in the area, and infrastructure to adequately gather and assess the clinical data accrued [151]. Ultimately, it is the medical practitioner who must decide when and how to use a new approved device, biologic, or drug using their best medical knowledge and judgment, in conjunction with a fully informed patient [152].

4.3.2 Younger more active patient population

Despite the progress in the field of biomaterials, surgical technique, and patient education, young age and high level of physical activity are still a challenge for THA/TKA because these patients often try to return to their previous activity level. Both young age and high activity levels compromise the survival of THAs/TKAs, mainly because of repetitive high-load cycles during which bearing and fixation surfaces as well as host tissues are gradually damaged. While in older patients the modern THAs/TKAs often serve for their lifetime, younger more active patients have substantially increased risk of premature failure of THAs/TKAs, requiring at least one to two reoperations during their lifetime.

High-risk younger patients often have the following characteristics: age of 40 years and younger, a wide range of physically demanding activities, on average 15,000 steps per day (i.e., above 5 million steps per year).

To address challenges related to younger and more active patients several strategies have been proposed including more strict indications for THA/TKA, bone-sparing surgical technique, special design, and material options.

4.3.2.1 Indications

The indications for THA/TKA in younger more active patients are the same as those in older less active patients: disabling pain, functional handicap, and poor quality of life due to the affected joint.

However, in younger active patients the tendency to postpone the indication for THA/TKA should be straightforward. Surgeon experience and familiarity with alternative treatment strategies and a thorough balance of the benefits and risks are important. The more severe the clinical and radiographic picture of the affected joint, the easier is the decision for arthroplasty for both the patient and the surgeon.

Firstly, alternative strategies including joint-preserving operations may "buy time" for the affected hip joint [153]. Such surgery can facilitate the maintenance of a higher level of sporting activity postoperatively without a risk for damage of a THA/TKA [154]. There is some evidence that these requirements could be fulfilled for postdysplastic sequelae [155,156] and osteonecrosis of the hip [157]. An osteotomy of the knee is the most viable surgical alternative supported by strong and long-term clinical evidence [158]. In addition, the osteotomy can be combined with a chondroplasty of the damaged articular surface and/or reconstruction of the cruciate ligament [159]. Regardless of the type of intervention, the alternative surgery should not compromise the future THA/TKA [160].

Secondly, Charnley tested the optimal candidacy for THA by the "pseudoarthrosis test" [161]. He told the patient to imagine he or she underwent THA that subsequently failed and no further reconstruction was possible. Therefore, the patient would end with resection arthroplasty for the remaining lifetime, and the question was whether this was acceptable for him/her in comparison to the original (evaluated) preoperative status. However, the clinical utility of the test was not determined as well as its social, ethical, psychological, and cognitive ramifications. Furthermore, many young patients' views are focused on their present pain and limitations, not the future, which to them may be unpredictable.

The postoperative activity level of a potential candidate can be estimated roughly using a specific activity score [162] or indirectly by including gender, primary diagnosis, number of other affected joints, or other signs like cognitive and neuromotor functions (dysfunctions) into the analysis. There is an intermediate to strong correlation between the preoperative condition of the musculoskeletal system and the postoperative level of activity in younger patients [163]. Young patients with diagnoses other than osteoarthritis tend to have lower levels of postoperative activity. In the context of aseptic loosening, male sex (OR, 1.39; 95% CI 1.22–1.58; $P = 0.001$) and high activity level (University of California Los Angeles (UCLA) activity score ≥ 8 points; OR, 4.24; 95% CI 2.46–7.31; $P = 0.001$) create the highest risk combination [164].

However, only some patients are likely to return to high levels of physical activity after surgery [163]. The primary diagnosis influences the survivorship of THA/TKA in younger patients. Patients with systemic inflammatory diseases are often precluded from a substantial increase of activity postoperatively due to multiple joint involvement, muscle and ligament damage, modifications in neural-motor function, and perhaps, also due to adaptation of cognitive functions on the diseased status. Osteonecrosis of the femoral head (OFH) is a frequent indication for THA and these patients frequently partake in increased physical activity after surgery. However, OFH increases the risk of a future revision in a complex way (see below). Table 4.6 shows outcomes of THA in younger patients.

4.3.2.2 Surgical technique

There is no single surgical approach devoted specifically to younger active patients. Mini-invasive surgery may be preferred to limit soft tissue dissection, however, this can be a problem in athletic men and some deformities associated with the primary diagnosis (dysplasia, posttraumatic arthritis, etc.).

At the site of the knee, meticulous operative technique is essential in influencing survival and satisfaction after TKA. Computer-assisted TKA reduces the variability in implant placement compared to surgery performed without computer navigation but has not been shown to affect the clinical outcome [32]. Patient-specific instrumentation has been introduced in order to further individualize TKA surgery. Several tools like navigation or robotic surgery are also available to improve placement of the cup at the site of THA [174]. The reason for these technologies is to optimize implant position and minimize premature failure requiring revision surgery.

4.3.2.3 Design and material options

For THA, the majority of surgeons favor cementless implants combined with modern bearing surfaces in younger and active patients. Cemented THA implants are selected only for patients with poor bone quality or problems potentially interfering with osseointegration. However, these are not usually highly active patients. Importantly, when studies published before 1988 and thereafter were compared, there was demonstrated improvement in radiographic outcomes and survivorship of THA in the later studies using all techniques [175].

At the site of the cup, hemispherical, screwed, or expansive shells made predominantly of commercially pure and titanium alloys, less frequently cobalt—chrome alloys, are evidence-based. Up to now Ti-6Al-4V alloy has been the most frequent substrate but new alloys substituting vanadium with other less toxic metals are ongoing. A thin-walled shell is of concern assuming heavy mechanical loads experienced with THA over many years, although data substantiating this concern are not present.

At the site of the femoral component, several traditional stems can be recommended with one exception: extensively porous coating stems. The latter have strong evidence in terms of survivorship in the general population but they induce stress

Table 4.6 Examples of studies showing the durability of THA/TKA in younger patients

Authors	Location	Diagnosis	*N*	Age (years)	Implants	FU	Survivorship
Tai et al. [165]	Knee	OA	82/118	50.7 (32–55)	Cementless, HAC	7.9 (5–12.5)	92.1% at 10 yrs (CI 82.3–97.3)
Nizard et al. [166]	Hip	OFH	64/NA	23.4 ± 5 (13–30)	Ceramic	6.9 (1–26.5)	85.7% at 15 yrs
Bisschop et al. [167]	Knee	Mix	31/39	52.6 (21–60)	Cemented, monoblock tibial component	12.8 (2.1–21.6)	89.7% at a mean FU of 12.8 yrs
Julin et al. [168]	Knee	Mix	NA/1,748	< 55 yrs	Mix	3.9 (1–8)	92% at 5 yrs (CI 89.7–93.3)
Odland et al. [169]	Knee	OA	59/67	48.5 (28.2–55.6)	Cemented, modular	12.4 (9.9–18.4)	78.5% ± 16% at 10 yrs 69% ± 16% at 15 yrs
Swarup et al. [170]	Hip	JRA	56/97	22 (SD 7.2)	32% C-stem 4% C-cup	12.3 (1.67–22.9)	96% at 5 yrs (CI 92–100) 84% at 10 yrs (CI 73–94) 62% at 15 yrs (CI 51–74) 50% at 20 yrs (CI 37–64)
Goodman et al. [171]	Hip	JRA	15/24	35 (21–3)	Cemented and cementless	10 (5–19)	83% at 10 yrs
Imbuldeniya et al. [172]	Hip	PD	25/30	47 (23–89)	Cementless	18.7 (15.8–21.8)	86% at 10 yrs (CI 77.5–94.5) 81% at 15 yrs (CI 60.1–92.3) 28% at 20 yrs (CI 13.3–41.8)
Cruz-Pardos et al. [173]	Hip	PD	NA/50	NA	Ceramic	5 (5–10)	83.9% at 10 yrs 80.1% at 15 yrs
Nizard et al. [166]	Hip	Trauma	18/NA	23.4 ± 5 (13–30)	Ceramic	6.9 (1–6.5)	65.5% at 14 yrs
Long et al. [5]	Knee	OA	88/114	51 (22–55)	Cemented, PS		70.1% at 30 yrs (CI 57.1–79.9)# 55.0% at 30 yrs (CI 34.9–71.2)*

N, number of cases (patients/hips or knees); yrs, years; FU, follow-up; OA, osteoarthritis; CI, 95% confidence interval; HAC, hydroxyapatite-coated; OFH, osteonecrosis of the femoral head; NA, not available; JRA, juvenile rheumatoid arthritis; PD, postdysplastic hip; PS, posterior stabilized; #, survival rate for TKA surviving without revision for any cause; *, overall patient survival rate.

shielding and are difficult to revise. With the thought of more durable implants and greater expectations in younger patients, so-called more conservative femoral replacements have been designed. They should minimize stress-shielding, protect the bone stock of the proximal femur as much as possible, and offer easier conditions during reoperation [176]. However, there is still relatively low evidence that this concept is appropriate for patients with highly vigorous activity [177].

There is still a continuing debate concerning which specific treatment of the outer surface of a cementless implant (Table 4.7) is associated with increased survivorship. Generally, surface modifications can be distinguished into:

- Chemical or physical alterations of the existing surface (e.g., grit-blasting);
- Coating the existing surface with a material of different composition (e.g., hydroxyapatite coating, sintering);
- Creating surface textures or patterns on the existing surface by a different technology [178].

Based on the available literature, no particular preferences are known in relation to younger and highly active patients.

Modular components were introduced into clinical practice in order to fit the commercially manufactured THA as much as possible to a particular patient's anatomy and biomechanics. They enable specific adjustment of femoral offset, anteversion/retroversion, and femoral length. However, modularity is also of concern, especially in younger active patients. With the expected time in service these components can be associated with corrosion and fretting resulting in ALTRs to THA. In addition, long-term data demonstrating the advantage of modular components in young active patients are missing.

Modern wear-resistant bearing materials are strongly recommended in younger active patients [181]. One of the most promising is CoC pairing but this can be prone to striped wear and rim-fracture. A large ceramic head could at least partially eliminate this by extending the zone of safe motion. Unpleasant squeaking can also occur in THA with ceramic bearings, and there is also a concern about the risk for fracture (despite that the risk is low, i.e., approximately 1 in 75,000 in the latest generation of ceramic). A recent study revealed a higher risk for revision for any reason in combination CoC in comparison to MoP at 9 years postoperatively [182]. Alternatively the combinations of metallic or ceramic heads with modern polyethylene liners are still widely used in younger and active patients.

TKAs are made of standard metallic alloys like THA (i.e., stainless steel, cobalt—chrome—molybdenum alloy, Ti-6Al-4V, new generation of titanium alloys, tantalum for trabecular metal). In the case of proven metal allergy, a specific knee implant made of cobalt—chrome or titanium alloys with surface masking could be indicated. Surface masking is achieved via titanium or zirconium nitride coatings. Another option is oxidized zirconium (Oxinium). It is a metal component in which the surface is

Table 4.7 Examples of technologies developed for an improvement of bone–implant interface

Technology	Features	Clinical evidence
Titanium vacuum plasma spray (VPS); also cancellous structured titanium technique	A set of techniques ensuring high levels of purity, firm adhesion strength, required roughness, and porosity microstructure (different pore sizes, porosity levels, etc.) ME (GPa) = 106–115 Average pore size = up to 500 μm Porosity (%) = 50–60 Coefficient of friction = NA	Strong clinical evidence, more than 25 years in practice
CPT fiber metal technology (wire mesh)	Molding and sintering short Ti metal fibers fabricate this porous aggregate ME (GPa) = 106–115 Pore sizes = 100–400 μm Porosity (%) = 40–50 Coefficient of friction = 0.63	Strong clinical evidence, more than 25 years in practice *Disadvantage:* fragmentation of fiber mesh was observed in older designs in the second decade
Co–Cr alloy with a Co–Cr beaded surface	Fabrication process begins with the production of spherical Co–Cr beads; these are then sintered to the implant substrate ME (GPa) = 210 Average pore size = 100–400 μm Porosity (%) = 30–50 Coefficient of friction = 0.53	More than 20 years in clinical practice Concerns with stress shielding and thigh pain after THA
Sprayed hydroxyapatite (HA)	A set of different coating methods (plasma spraying, laser ablation, ion beam-assisted deposition, hot isostatic pressing, electrophoretic deposition, dip coating, etc.) Thickness = from 70 to 100 μm Bonding strength (MPa) = 13–20 ME (GPa) = 80 Pore size = up to 200 μm Porosity (%) = different (11–70) Coefficient of friction = NA	More than 25 years in clinical practice Note the vital role of HA coating stability and the underlying surface texture

(*Continued*)

Table 4.7 (Continued)

Technology	Features	Clinical evidence
Trabecular metal technology	Tantalum with up to 80% porosity, nearly 100% open-pore structure	More than 12 years in clinical practice
Biofoam (Wright Medical, Arlington, TN)	Titanium-based metallic foam with open-cell structure; optimal for rapid bony ingrowth ME (GPa) = 2.7 Average pore size = 530 μm Porosity (%) = 60–70 Coefficient of friction = NA	Limited clinical experience
Tritanium (Stryker, Mahwah, NJ)	Titanium open-cell, highly porous, three-dimensional coating/material ME (GPa) = NA Average pore size = 546 μm Porosity (%) = 72 Coefficient of friction = 1.01	Limited clinical experience
Gription (DePuy, Warsaw, IN)	Ultraporous, supertextured, CPT coating material combining macro- and microtexture approaches to improve conditions for bone ingrowth. ME (GPa) = NA Average pore size = 300 μm Porosity (%) = 63 Coefficient of friction = 1.2	Limited clinical experience
StikTite (Smith and Nephew, Memphis, TN)	Titanium-based, open-cell, highly porous metallic coating ME (GPa) = NA Average pore size = 200 μm Porosity (%) = 60 Coefficient of friction = 0.9 (cortical bone), 1.4 (cancellous bone)	Limited clinical experience

ME, modulus of elasticity; CPT, commercially pure titanium; Co–Cr, cobalt–chrome; NA, not applicable.
Sources: Almost all data were retrieved from Frank RM, Fabi D, Levine BR. Modern porous coatings in orthopaedic applications. In: Nazarpour S, editor. Thin films and coatings in biology. Dordrecht: Springer; 2013. p. 69–104 [179] and Bose S, Tarafder S, Bandyopadhyay A. Hydroxyapatite coatings for metallic implants. In: Mucalo M, editor. Hydroxyapatite (HAp) for biomedical applications. Cambridge: Woodhead Publishing Elsevier Ltd.; 2015. p. 143–58 [180].

transformed into a ceramic layer serving also as a barrier. Pure ceramic femoral components can be used as an alternative option. Similarly to the case of THA, no particular preferences are known in relation to younger and highly active patients.

A number of design variations of TKA have been developed. They differ basically in terms of fixation (cemented vs cementless), PCL preservation/nonpreservation (bicruciate TKA exists in clinical practice too), kinematic concepts, type of bearings (all-poly, modular designs) or whether the bearing surface is firmly fixed to the tibial component or not (mobile vs fixed in modular components). The most common bearing surface has been metal-on-noncrosslinked polyethylene and the advantage of crosslinked over noncrosslinked polyethylenes has to be demonstrated. The superiority of mobile bearing designs over the fixed ones has not been as well demonstrated to date. Some investigators believe that younger active patients should be treated within the concept of a high-performance TKA that has been proposed to address expectations of younger and very active patient population. Accordingly, the joint must "feel" normal, it should allow participation in a wide range of activities including high-impact sports, and it must demonstrate long-term durability [183]. On the other hand, some surgeons even claim that it is unclear whether younger patients noticed whether they had received the newer type of TKA [184].

In conclusion, currently it is not clear which available design is the most appropriate for young more active patients, and further research in this field is warranted. It is also necessary to examine, among others, whether the technological progress (and associated costs) is followed by a substantial increase in the patient-reported outcomes and survivorship (cost-effectiveness of a new approach) [185].

4.3.3 Prosthetic joint infection

Prosthetic joint infection (PJI) is a disastrous complication for a patient requiring reoperations almost always including removal of the original implants and long-term administration of antibiotics. Despite the fact that modern therapeutic guidelines are applied, some patients still end without a functional joint and for a minority of them, a salvage procedure such as fusion or amputation is the last choice. Therapy of PJI is associated with a strong psychological and social burden as well as with enormous financial costs [186]. Some studies concern the interrelation between PJI and an increased mortality rate [187].

Precise data on incidence of PJI in THA and TKA are missing. Current estimates suggest that up to 2.2% of primary hip and knee arthroplasties are complicated by PJI [188]. There is also growing evidence that arthroplasty registries underestimate the true numbers of PJI [189]. Other studies show that the numbers are on the rise [190]. As a result, PJI is the leading cause of revision surgery during the early postoperative period both at the sites of hip and knee [191].

Staphylococci and gram-positive pathogens generally are the leading cause of both surgical site infections (SSIs) and PJIs [188]. In relation to biomaterials, the *biofilm-based concept of PJI* is dominating. Importantly, the prevalence of multiresistant strains among causative agents in SSIs and PJIs is increasing [192,193].

4.3.3.1 Prevention of PJI

All reasons mentioned above justify the implementation of strong preventative measures. Strategies relying on decreased bacterial load and creating bacteria-free environment around an implant during the perioperative period are widely implemented in clinical practice. There is also sufficient evidence supporting systemic and in some cases local antibiotic prophylaxis [194]. Attempts at formulating evidence-based standards for good clinical practice in orthopedic operating rooms have been utilized [195]. However, it is clear that not all patients avoid PJI. This gives rise to two crucial questions: First is who are the patients at risk? Second, will it be possible to interrupt events leading to PJI in patients at risk?

Theoretically all patients undergoing total joint arthroplasty are at risk for PJI. As a result, one could argue that all patients should benefit from implants coated with a proven antiinfective surface. On the other hand, the risk for PJI is not homogeneously distributed among arthroplasty patients: it is stratified into the specific groups [196]. Therefore, it might be convincing to implant "biofilm-resistant" implants only in patients at increased risk of PJI. This opens a very difficult problem on how to identify these patients. However, neither an "antiinfective" implant nor a validated tool for screening patients for increased risk of PJI does currently exist.

An implant surface-based strategy has to fulfill a number of very strict criteria related to both the implant mission and to antiinfective efficiency [197]. A wide spectrum of substances and technological approaches has been proposed and tested for antibacterial features. A change in the surface chemistry of the bulk implant can be achieved either by chemically or physically altering the surface layer in the existing biomaterial (e.g., nanopatterning of titanium surface). A different method involves coating the existing surface with a new thin layer having a different composition (e.g., antibiotics, other antimicrobial compounds bound to the substrate) [198].

Antiinfective surfaces can employ *antiadhesive properties, contact killing, and elution of antimicrobial agent*. They should cover a wide spectrum of potential pathogens rather than only a specific set of them. In terms of functionality, one may choose to divide surfaces into *monofunctional* (i.e., only antiinfective) and *multifunctional*. The latter are expected to target multiple biological tasks simultaneously (Fig. 4.3). *Smart surface* is designed to be a self-responsive multitask micromachine that releases antimicrobial as well as other substances after stimulation by microbial/nonmicrobial signals.

Some *antiadhesive surface* treatment technologies are very effective in vitro; however, this approach also has several important limitations including those related to host cell attachment to an implant surface. Several studies have investigated the efficacy of surfaces coated with *covalently linked antibiotics* [199]. Clinical effectiveness of such implants is most likely limited to infections caused by bacteria that are sensitive to the specific antibiotic that has been coupled. *Nonantibiotic surface* technologies offer wider antibacterial coverage. These can employ *metals* (silver, zinc, copper, zirconium, etc.), *nonmetal elements* (e.g., selenium), *organic substances* (antibiotics, antiinfective peptides, chitosan, and other substances), and *their combinations* (e.g., silver—vancomycin conjugate) [200,201].

Silver is the most prevalent metal used in biomedical applications [202]. Initial clinical experiences with galvanic silver treatment of implants have been promising. On the other hand, argyria has been concerned especially in relation to large implants coated with silver [203]. Taken together, further studies with longer follow-up are required before a definitive conclusion.

Examination of global grants and published studies on this topic suggests a striking discrepancy between proposed strategies of antibacterial surface treatment and little progress made in the translation of the aforementioned modalities into clinically useful technologies. Barriers to translational medicine in this arena are most likely related to economic, medical-legal, and biotechnological issues [204].

4.3.3.2 Diagnostics

To detect a disease we need the definition of a particular target (here PJI) and a validated diagnostic strategy. Infection can be defined as a result of complex interactions

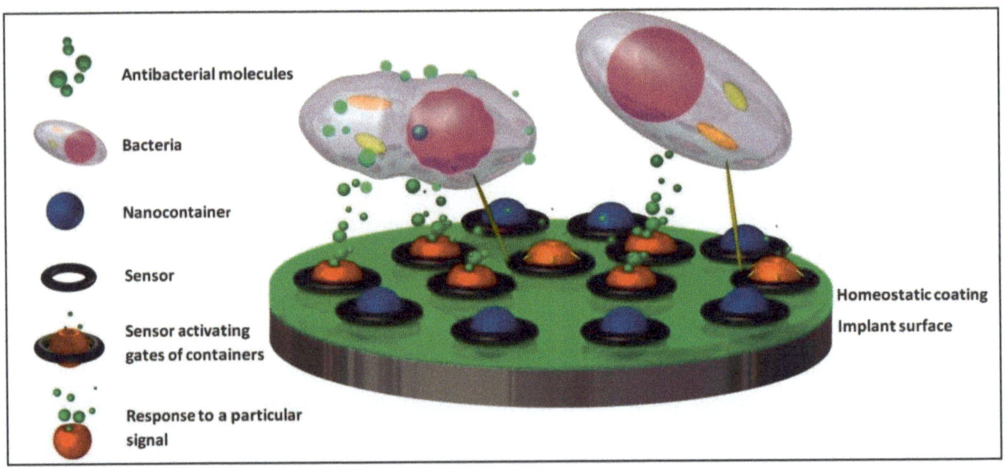

Figure 4.3 Concept of the smart surface strategy in the protection of total joint arthroplasty; molecules releasing from bacteria activate sensors on the implant surface which in turn trigger the release of antibacterial substances (e.g., bactericidal, phenotype modifying, interfering with quorum-sensing).

Table 4.8 Definition of PJI according to MSIS (Musculoskeletal Infection Society) [205]

1. There is a sinus tract communicating with the prosthesis; *or*
2. A pathogen is isolated by culture from at least two separate tissue or fluid samples obtained from the affected prosthetic joint; *or*
3. Three of the following five criteria exist:
   a. Elevated serum erythrocyte sedimentation rate (ESR) and serum C-reactive protein (CRP) concentration
   b. Elevated synovial leukocyte count *or* + + result on leukocyte esterase test strip
   c. Elevated synovial neutrophil percentage (PMN%)
   d. Isolation of a microorganism in one culture or periprosthetic tissue or fluid, *or*
   e. Greater than five neutrophils per high-power field in five high-power fields observed from histologic analysis of periprosthetic tissue at 400 × magnification.

between bacteria (fungi) and host tissues resulting in a destabilization of periimplant environment by infective inflammation and implant failure. As a result, the diagnosis requires: (1) evidence of bacteria (fungi); (2) evidence of host antibacterial (antifungal) response; and (3) evidence of clinical failure. Table 4.8 shows one of the latest definitions for diagnosing PJI.

To date a number of diagnostic methods/strategies have been validated for the purpose of PJI diagnosing. Samples of any possible origin (joint fluid, periprosthetic tissues, implant surface) can be investigated by culture and nonculture methods. Improvement of culture is related to automated BACTEC blood culture bottle methods [206]. Good laboratory practice with prolonged cultivation periods and procedures strictly oriented at biofilm are important [207]. The most exciting progress has been observed in the field of molecular diagnostics. These methods are based either on detection of bacterial nucleic acids (proteins) or specific biomarkers in the joint fluid. Recent meta-analysis calculated the likelihood ratios for both the sonication fluid culture (LR + =17.2; 95% CI 7.6–38.7; LR− =0.21; 95% CI 0.17–0.27) [208] and PCR methods in PJI (LR + =9.1; 95% CI 4.6–18.2; LR− =0.16; 95% CI 0.10–0.25) [209]. The place for nucleic acid–based methods is probably reserved for patients who have known reasons interfering with culture methods. These are especially patients with a pretest administration of antibiotic.

A new set of molecular markers of antibacterial response includes molecules such as defensins, neutrophil elastase 2 (ELA-2), bactericidal/permeability-increasing protein (BPI), and neutrophil gelatinase-associated lipocalin (NGAL) that combine optimal sensitivity and specificity [210].

An important issue is when to adopt specific diagnostic tests in the patients with a variety of symptoms and clinical courses [211]. When considering infection, experts on infection, informatics, and decision-making must develop a rational and probabilistic algorithm for indications of diagnostic tests [212]. First-line tests should be cheap

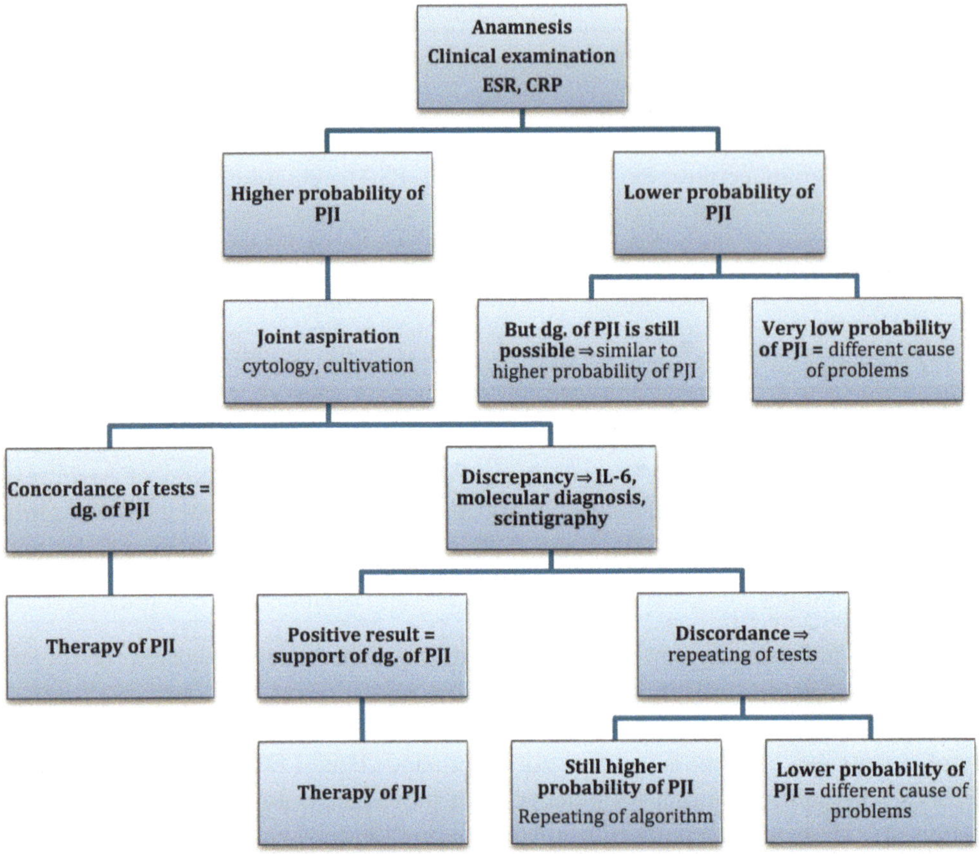

Figure 4.4 Diagnostic approach to detection/exclusion of PJI; *ESR*, erythrocyte sedimentation rate; *CRP*, C reactive protein; *PJI*, prosthetic joint infection; *dg.*, diagnosis; *IL-6*, interleukin 6.

and very sensitive (have very low rate of false-negative results). When the posttest clinical probability is still not proven after first-line tests, then there is a place for second-line tests to validate/exclude the PJI diagnosis (Fig. 4.4). Finally, a "diagnostic calculator" could be useful [213]. However, this has to be thoroughly validated before implementation into the practice.

4.3.3.3 Treatment

Generally, surgery is the most reliable approach to PJI. Conservative treatment is reserved only for patients that cannot undergo an operation. Recent data show that the differences in outcomes of one- versus two-stage surgery are smaller than previously thought [214].

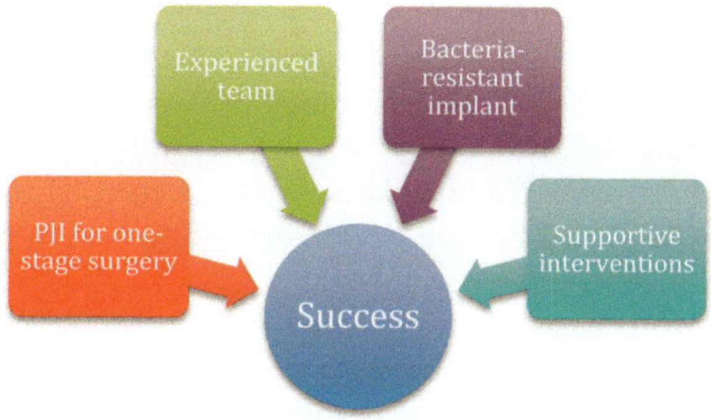
Experienced team
Bacteria-resistant implant
PJI for one-stage surgery
Supportive interventions
Success

Figure 4.5 Conditions underlying the success of one-stage surgery.

The critical step is now to define optimal candidates for one-stage reimplantation. There are characteristics related to a patient's general and local health status (especially soft tissues, type of inflammation) and those related to causative agent(s). The latter would induce a proposal of rational and effective antibacterial treatment. The second essential step is to train the surgical teams with respect to success and prevention of avoidable harm. The third step might lie in the use of an implant with strong antiinfective surface activity as soon as it will be available. Finally, interventions affecting immune responsiveness, supporting of homeostatic, and antiinflammatory mechanisms may be justified to eradicate PJI completely and in the long-term perspective (Fig. 4.5).

Theoretically, an antibiofilm approach might be used in patients with a stable implant. With regard to the type of host–infection interrelationship, perhaps those with low-grade infection would be more suitable than those with a dramatically appearing clinical picture. A number of strategies have been tested [215]. However, no one approach is favored in clinical practice.

4.3.4 Wear and osteolysis

Periprosthetic osteolysis refers to progressive insidious bone resorption associated at first with a well-functioning THA or TKA; later the implant loses its stable bone bed required for optimal function, and aseptic loosening occurs. From the clinical point of view, it is important to note that aseptic loosening often develops without symptoms. From an epidemiological point of view, aseptic loosening together with osteolysis and other wear-related problems is the most frequent late reason for the first reoperation in both THA [216] and TKA [191]. The more severe the bone defects, the more difficult revision surgery is. In addition, clinical outcome and survivorship in such difficult cases can be compromised. Research on the mechanisms of wear and pathophysiology of osteolysis is of paramount importance and well justified with this in mind.

4.3.4.1 Wear of prosthetic surfaces

The artificial implants for weight-bearing joints were originally intended as low-friction arthroplasties, with low levels of removal of material (generally called debris) from the softer bearing surfaces during each step. Historically, ultrahigh-molecular-weight polyethylene (UHMWPE) articulating against a metallic surface (counterpart) was the most commonly used bearing couple exhibiting a wide range of wear rates from 0.01 to several millimeters per year.

Wherever there exists relative motion between two materials in contact with one another, there will be wear. Generally, wear is a function of motion, load-bearing material properties, and lubrication. Under ideal conditions the lubricating film separates the two articulating bearing surfaces ("elastohydrodynamic mode of lubrication") mitigating wear [217]. However, it is neither easy nor predictable to create such an optimal biotribological situation in each patient after THA or TKA surgery for a substantial time of implant service. Analyses of retrieved polyethylenes do not support the existence of continual elastohydrodynamic lubrication and demonstrate some degree of wear damage. Thus, most THAs work in the mixed lubrication mode, which leads to wear commonly observed on the articulating surfaces. Rules controlling the lubrication in TKA are less clear.

Currently, four major wear mechanisms are distinguished: (1) *adhesion*; (2) *abrasion*; (3) *surface fatigue*; and (4) *tribochemical reactions* [218] that contribute differently in THA compared to TKA. Importantly, in modular implants adhesive and abrasive wear can occur on the articular and backside surfaces. On the other hand, plastic deformation of polyethylene has not been traditionally included into the mechanisms of wear because it is not associated with a material removal.

At the site of THA, McKellop proposed four modes of wear in an attempt to characterize potential mechanisms behind [219]: (1) *intended wear* when two bearing surfaces are in contact with each other and are moving under load in the manner intended by the designers, surfaces are damaged by adhesion; (2) *nonintended wear from articulating bearing surface against a nonbearing surface* as, for instance, after complete wear through the liner; (3) *third-body wear* with the primary bearing surfaces articulating with each other, but with abrasive third-body particles interposed; and (4) *wear from articulating of two nonbearing surfaces* against each other under load like in the case of backside wear or neck-rim impingement.

At the site of knee implants, polyethylene wear occurs through the same mechanisms but the account each of them has on total wear is different in comparison to THA. Specific components of wear have been described like *surface deformation, third body debris, scratching, burnishing, delamination, pitting, abrasion* [220], or *rim fracture*. Particular attention has been devoted to backside wear analysis in modular implants and tibial post damage in posterior stabilized designs [221].

However, wear is not the only source of particles (ions) liberated from an implant surface. The other important mechanism is *corrosion leading to metal ion release.* Prosthetic particles/ions generated via any of the above-mentioned mechanisms are the most important end product in relation to osteolysis and aseptic loosening development. The reason is that their parameters, e.g., their size, total amount, and other characteristics like immunologic and chemical reactivity strongly *influence the host response.*

4.3.4.2 Periprosthetic osteolysis

Willert and Semlitsch were the first to introduce the concept of aseptic loosening and osteolysis as a result of periprosthetic tissue reaction to large amounts of prosthetic wear microparticles [222]. The term "particle disease" was coined by Harris to focus attention on the importance of particles generated by a prosthesis for induction of host response [223]. Recently, Konttinen introduced the term "ion disease" to emphasize the role of soluble debris in the mechanisms underlying osteolysis and aseptic loosening [224].

The key concept in particle and ion disease is that very small prosthetic particles (micrometers and less in size) together with soluble ions interact with host proteins and periprosthetic cells to express proinflammatory/pro-osteoclastic cytokines and other substances that orchestrate increased accumulation/activity/survival of osteoclasts, and inhibit the osteogenic activity of osteoblasts. As a result, bone resorption predominates over osteogenesis at the level of the bone multicellular units around the implant, leading eventually to macroscopic bone defects. The degree of bone loss according to this concept is a function of the number and depth of deregulated resorption sites [225].

The expansion of particle and ion disease across the prosthetic joint is facilitated by joint fluid that is abundantly synthesized by synovial-like membrane composed of macrophages and fibroblasts. Accordingly, joint fluid washes the prosthetic by-products from the articulating surfaces and transports them together with signaling and non-signaling molecules to adjacent bone sites. For this reason, particle and ion disease can extend to new sites, contributing in this way to an overall expansion of osteolysis and weakening of the bone–implant interface (the effective joint space concept) [226]. In addition, compressed joint fluid can also induce direct bone resorption, and thus contribute to overall bone loss [227].

Currently, a number of studies give strong experimental evidence that *prosthetic particles can activate surface/intracellular innate immune receptors* of macrophages/fibroblasts and other resident cells. Particles coated by diverse host proteins including complement are endocytosed or stimulate innate immunity cells via surface receptors [224]. To determine the reactivity of distinct prosthetic by-products (either wear or corrosive) methods for analyzing in vitro their

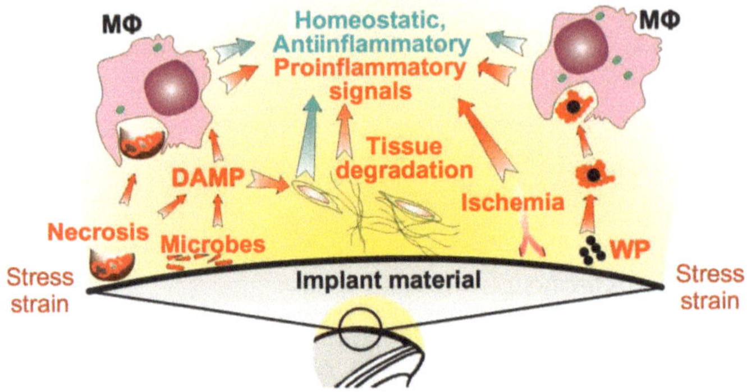

Figure 4.6 Concept of periprosthetic osteolysis as a result of dynamic interrelationships between inflammatory and homeostatic mechanisms in the periprosthetic tissues; this concept can, among others, explain heterogeneity observed among the clinical cases; *DAMP*, danger/damage-associated molecular patterns; *MΦ*, macrophage before functional polarization; *WP*, wear particles. *Courtesy of Milan Raška.*

functional biologic activity have been proposed [228]. These studies have shown a much stronger biologic response to debris in the submicrometer size range [229,230]. With regard to the biomaterial origin, polyethylene particles appear to be biologically more active than titanium and ceramic particles [231]. In fact, the particles of different biomaterial origin can stimulate the innate immune cells in a synergistic fashion. Some investigators also noticed that the expression of proinflammatory cytokines and chemokines was increased when particles were contaminated with endotoxin in comparison to experiments with endotoxin-free samples [232].

In response, the stimulated cells activate foreign body response pathways according to a program inherent for this type of reaction and under tight supervision of homeostatic regulations working in a particular tissue (Fig. 4.6). Among the first molecules that are detected after activation of tissue cells by prosthetic particles are IL-1β and IL-18, both released from NALP3 inflammasome [233] and some chemokines (e.g., MCP-1, MIP-1α, IL-8). The latter molecules attract new monocytes from the bloodstream to a place around total joint arthroplasty, perhaps in an attempt to resolve the foreign body reaction [234] (Fig. 4.6).

Simultaneously with the recruitment of new innate immune cells into the periprosthetic tissues an inflammatory pathway network is activated and perpetuated [235]. The inflammatory pathways are tightly conjoined with *a network of osteoclastogenic pathways* which explains the "biological arm" of periprosthetic osteolysis [236]. Moreover, the prosthetic by-products (particles, ions) can simultaneously suppress the

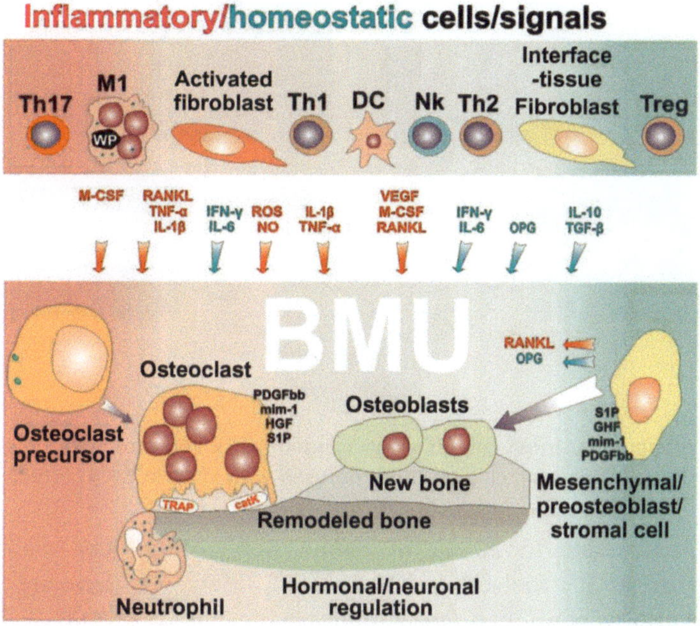

Figure 4.7 Bone multicellular unit (BMU) is a place where the homeostatic tools have to neutralize the pressure of damage pathways associated with total joint arthroplasty service. If the adaptation to this load is successful, the periprosthetic bone remodels in a normal (regular) way. In the opposite case, increased osteoclast maturation/activity/survival leads to increased resorption without adequate bone formation. Osteolysis is excessive bone resorption running in a large number of neighboring BMUs. *catK*, cathepsin K; *DC*, dendritic cells; *HGF*, hepatocyte growth factor—perhaps one of the coupling factors; IFN-γ, IL-1β, -6, 10, M-CSF, mim-1, TGF-β, TNF-α, VEGF, examples of cytokines regulating the response to prosthetic by-products (inflammatory in red; antiinflammatory or homeostatic in blue); *M1*, classically activated macrophages; *NK*, natural killers; *PDGFbb*, platelet derived growth factor-bb secreted by preosteoclasts to promote angiogenesis; *RANKL/OPG*, key molecules regulating maturation of osteoclasts; *ROS*, reactive oxygen species; *S1P*, sphingosine-1-phoshate; *Th1*, *Th17*, proinflammatory cells; *TRAP*, tartarate-resistant acid phosphatase; *Treg*, regulatory T cells and *Th1*, *Th2* cells, type 1 T helper and type 2 T helper cells. *Courtesy of Milan Raška.*

number and function of the osteoblastic cell line [237]. As a result, the bone-multicellular units around an implant are imbalanced (Fig. 4.7).

Another very important source of periprosthetic inflammatory inducers is tissue ischemia and cell necrosis resulting from chronic particle and ion load, nonresolved inflammation, unfavorable mechanical conditions, and repetitive joint fluid waves associated with use of the limb [225]. However, to date a number of mechanisms/pathways still remain to be elucidated.

Engh et al. estimated that both wear and patient propensity to osteolysis might together account for 53% of the variance in total area of osteolysis [238]. Clinically, the high-volume producers of prosthetic particles are at higher risk for development

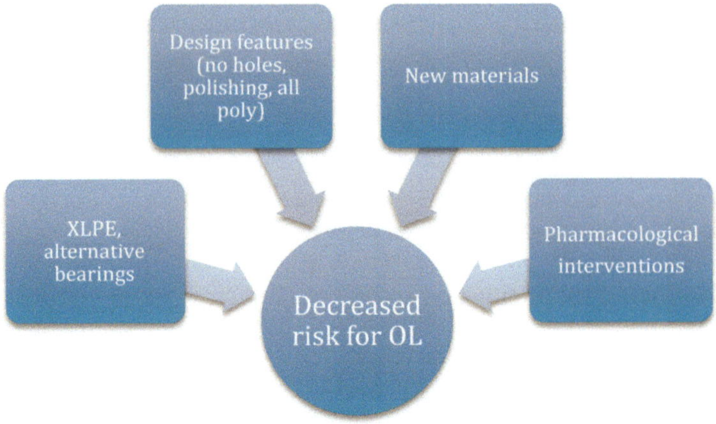

Figure 4.8 List of potential interventions decreasing the risk for osteolysis development; *XLPE*, highly crosslinked polyethylenes including those diffused with vitamin E; *OL*, osteolysis.

of osteolysis and aseptic loosening in comparison to the low-volume producers (concept of "particles as a fuel of particle disease"). However, there are many patients that escape the above-mentioned fate despite having the same type of THA or TKA with comparable alignment and physical activity as those who demonstrated osteolysis. This fact points to much more effective control of the foreign body response in the tissues of these patients or existence of individual susceptibility to development of an adverse host response in those that exhibit osteolysis. In relation to the latter, a genetic predisposition to inflammation or in the field of regulation of the bone multicellular unit was examined [239,240]. However, to date the data are inconclusive, and further research is highly expected in this field.

4.3.4.3 Strategies aimed at diminishing the risk for osteolysis and aseptic loosening

Several strategies have been implemented in clinical practice (Fig. 4.8). Recently, conventional UHMWPE was replaced by more wear-resistant XLPE *and alternative bearing materials* predominantly at the site of the hip with significantly reduced wear rates in comparison to conventional UHMWPE. However, even when the loss of material is in the order of tenths of millimeters, the total number of polymer particles can achieve the order of hundreds of trillions under assumption these are on the nanoscale [241]. This could at least in part explain an increased inflammatory reaction observed in vivo in XLPE with vitamin E (i.e., due to the smaller size and greater amount) [242]. On the other hand, at least one study did not observe increased osteolytic potential in vitamin E diffused XLPE [243] and also clinical studies with longer follow-up show that the survivorship increased and frequency of osteolysis have substantially decreased even in younger and more active patients [181,244]. The evidence for

CoC THA is strong, but many surgeons still hesitate to use this bearing couple, perhaps due to concerns related to squeaking, striped wear, chipping and fracture, and cost.

In comparison to THA, the advantages of newer bearings for TKA have not been clearly demonstrated [245]. In order to avoid backside wear in TKA several design changes have been introduced. The most influential one of them seems to be an improvement of the locking mechanism and polished trays [221]. For at least some group of patients the solution could lie in using all-polyethylene TKA instead of metal-backed modular design [246].

Osteolysis is a disease caused by access of pro-osteolytic pathways to the bone bed [247]. A number of modern technologies have been proposed and tested to improve osseointegration of implants [248]. The key is to maintain a vital and osteolysis-resistant bone bed for several decades postoperatively. Today it is, however, evident that even the implants with hydroxyapatite coating cannot compensate for high wear rate and/or other design/material flaws facilitating the development of osteolysis in the long-term perspective [249].

In relation to corrosion of vulnerable parts of orthopedic implants several strategies have been proposed to eliminate this complication. These vary from small improvements in the design (e.g., via changes in shape, tolerances of modular interfaces) across modern metallurgical processes leading to coverage of the most loaded surfaces with specific super-resistant layer(s) of appropriate materials with a barrier function to the development of completely new "antiallergic" biomaterials [250].

Numerous studies have examined the possibility of inhibiting the inflammatory and pro-osteolytic pathways pharmacologically [251]. Despite the fact that none of the described experimental strategies has achieved clinical usage to date, it may be that the patients with stable implants could benefit from that approach in the future. With all innovations, their clinical, biomaterial, and biological performances have to be carefully assessed and validated.

4.3.5 Hip: Other concerns (dislocation, big heads, alternative bearing surfaces, head–neck taper interface)

4.3.5.1 Dislocation

Dislocation is an extremely painful complication. It remains among the most frequent complications of primary and revision THA. Despite the fact that not all dislocations are included in the registries because some of them are treated conservatively, it still is the second or third most common reason for reoperation, and the leading cause of failure during the first 5 years postoperatively in revision THA [252]. The cumulative risk of redislocation and rerevision for all reasons was 34.5% and 45.9% at 15 years, respectively, in one study [253].

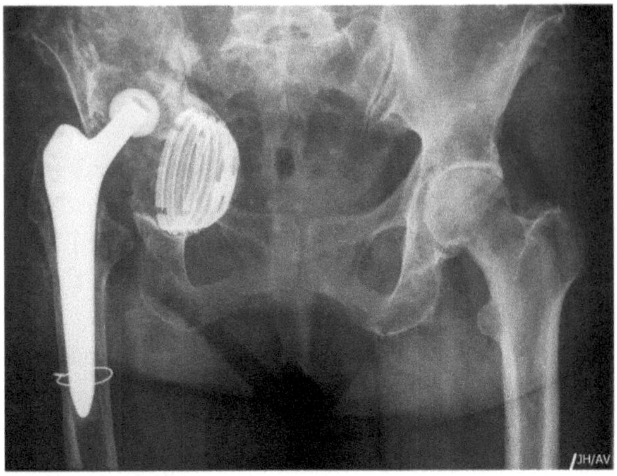

Figure 4.9 An example of late dislocation of the right THA observed 12 years postoperatively.

The position of a dislocated femoral head (type of dislocation) is determined using history ("conditions related to the dislocation"), radiographic examination (the true lateral view centered on the cup), and confirmed by the mechanism of reduction.

4.3.5.2 Prevention

Most dislocations occur within 3 months postoperatively and the risk for dislocation decreases with follow-up. Late dislocations are often associated with excessive polyethylene wear or with aseptic loosening of the cup (Fig. 4.9). Thus, the primary subject for preventative measures is focused on early dislocation.

Prevention of dislocation is based on understanding of pathogenetic mechanisms [254]. These can be divided into explainable and "idiopathic" (to date the reasons for dislocation are not known). A classic example of the explainable and modifiable factors is orientation of the cup. The most frequently cited is the safe zone (such configuration that offers the highest stability of THA) by Lewinnek et al. [255] recommending 40 ± 10 degrees of inclination and 15 ± 10 degrees of anteversion for a cup. However, many patients do not experience either subluxation or dislocation even when the cup is out of the proposed Lewinnek range. Thus the majority of cases are the result of a combination of several risk factors contributing to the dislocating mechanism (Table 4.9).

A number of strategies have been proposed in order to decrease the risk for dislocation. The most reasonable is to recognize preoperatively the specific risks in each patient. Based on this assessment, the surgical and implant-related factors could be individualized (Table 4.9). However, to date we are not aware of a validated and systematically used predictive approach (Table 4.10).

Table 4.9 Risk factors associated with THA dislocation

Source	Factors
Patient	Conditions leading to muscle weakness and/or imbalance (including a hypermobile hip)
	Altered mental status (alcoholism and drug dependencies, other cognitive causes such as inability to follow recommendations after THA)
Surgeon's experience	Component positioning
	Postoperative soft-tissue tension
	Surgical approach
	Implant parameters
	Impingement unrelated to a pathologic position of the implants

Table 4.10 List of preventative measures that should contribute to a decrease of the risk for dislocation

Strategy	
Surgical technique	A lower risk for dislocation has been observed in anterior and lateral approaches compared to the posterior approach. Regardless of a particular approach the key step is meticulous reconstruction of soft tissues
	Specific techniques have been introduced to strengthen the posterior (posterior soft tissue repair) and anterolateral (modified anterolateral approach for stable hip) structures
	Removal of sources of impingement
Implant placement	Cup placement in the safe zone, restoration (increase) of femoral offset. Navigation/robotics could possibly assist in the placement of the cup into the safe zone
Testing stability of THA	Careful assessment of an impingement and soft tissue laxity, examination of the maximum range of motion in all planes and their combinations (especially maximum flexion, adduction, and inner rotation) with trial components
Implant choice	Proper restoration of femoral neck length and offset, larger femoral heads, liners with elevated rim, dual-mobility THA
Surgeon's experience	Critical despite that a direct association between dislocation and a surgeon's scope and length of practice has not been detected
Education about the risk of dislocation	Written/video presentations containing of a list of do's and don'ts (including elevated toilet seats, using a sock aid, bath safety aids, etc.)

4.3.5.3 Treatment of dislocated THA

Patients with acute early dislocation of THA should be treated emergently regardless of pathology causing the dislocation. After a successful reduction, the leading

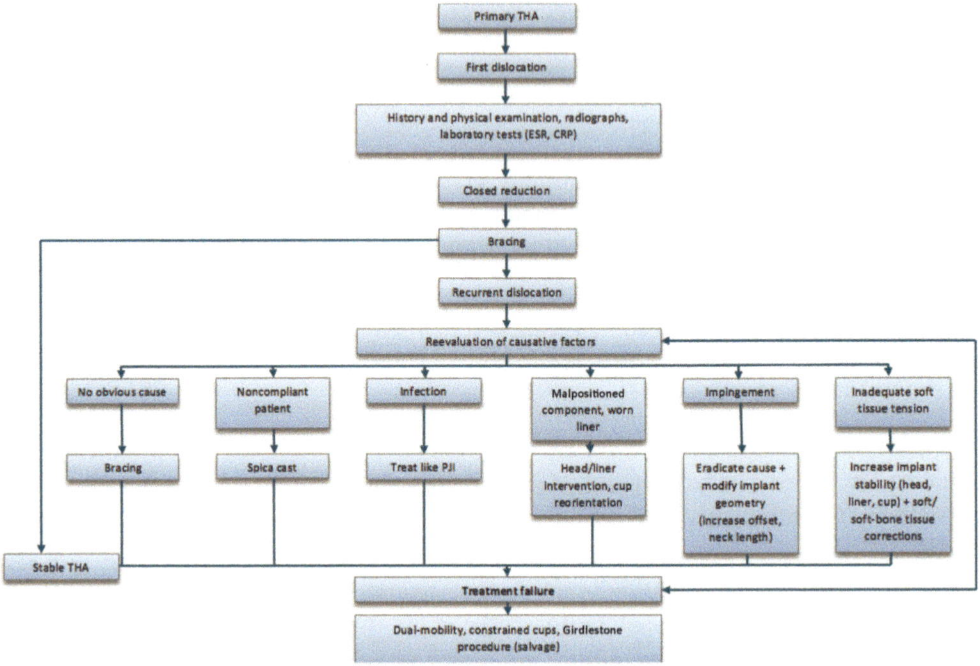

Figure 4.10 Algorithm for treatment of dislocations of THA; *ESR*, erythrocyte sedimentation rate; *CRP*, C reactive protein; *PJI*, prosthetic joint infection.

pathology underlying a dislocation and the best approach to management should be analyzed and managed.

The choice of approach depends on the stability of THA (tested immediately after reduction), time elapsing from the previous surgery, the understanding of the true cause of dislocation, and on the order of dislocation (first vs recurrent). Thorough clinical examination, radiography, and less frequently CT examination are performed.

After the first event of dislocation that occurs within a year postoperatively in a patient whose cognitive functions are normal, components well positioned and without soft-tissue pathology, the hip can be braced for 3–6 months. Patients with malposition of the implants, loose soft tissues, those with recurrent dislocations, and late dislocations are usually indicated for operative intervention (Fig. 4.10). This should address the recognized causative factors.

4.3.5.4 Modular component exchange

In the case of modular cup, one can use a liner with elevated rim. It increases the "jump distance" before the femoral head dislocates. In nonmodular cups the same effect can be achieved by the technique of fixing a wedge of polyethylene to a particular part of the cup [256]. This is placed in the direction of dislocation in order to increase the

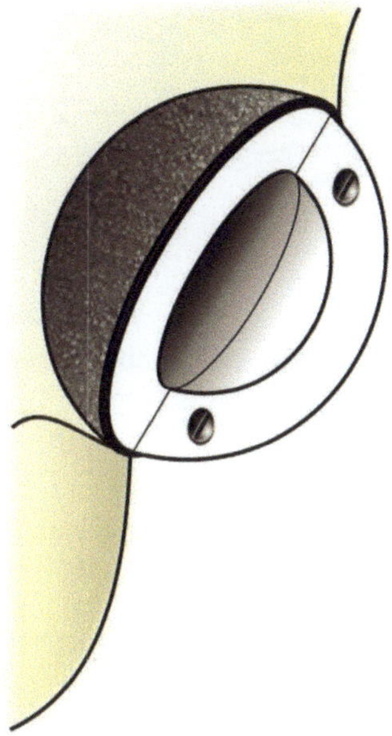

Figure 4.11 Olerud's principle of increasing of the jump distance by screwing a wedge of polyethylene to the original polyethylene.

"jump distance" (Fig. 4.11). Despite their effectiveness in terms of reducing the risk for redislocation the polyethylene lip augmentation devices can be exposed to high mechanical stresses (as well as liners with elevated rims to some degree).

Recently emphasized is the usage of large femoral heads (with or without increased neck length) in order to stabilize the hip. They function on the principle of optimization of the head–neck ratio to increase the ROM before impingement. This could be an appropriate solution in the case that the metallic shell and/or the stem are well fixed and oriented. However, a large head cannot compensate for a malposition, impingement, or hyperlaxity of soft tissues.

4.3.5.5 Reorientation of THA

Malpositioned implants should undergo reoperation. Besides the correct implant placement, the surgeon should also consider a contribution of a cup with elevated rim, larger head, proper length of the stem neck to the stability of THA, and carefully restore the tension of soft tissue.

4.3.5.6 Improvement of abductor moment

There is strong clinical evidence for a substantial role of abductor muscles in the stability of a hip after THA [257]. That is why the stability cannot be often achieved when the hip abductors are dysfunctional [258]. Several reconstruction techniques

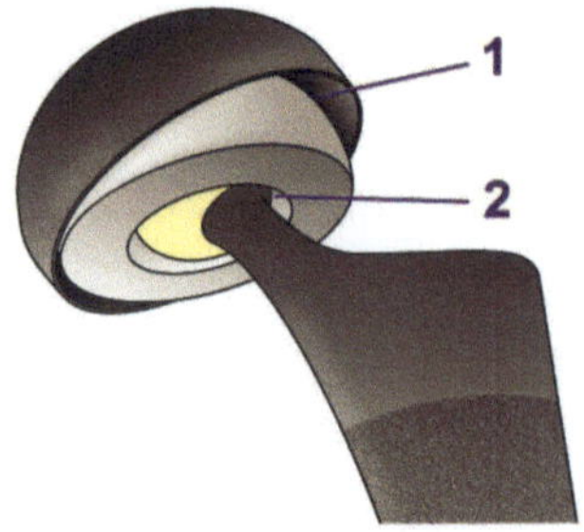

Figure 4.12 Schematic depiction of the dual-mobility cup; *1*, first articulation; *2*, second articulation.

Table 4.11 Results for dual-mobility cup used in patients with primary and revision THA

Author	DMC	*N* (pts)	Dislocation rate	FU (months)
Langlais et al. [261]	Medial cup (France)	85	1.1%	36 (24–60)
Guyen et al. [262]	Saturne (France)	54	5.5%	48 (26.4–81.6)
Hamadouche et al. [263]	Medial cup (France)	51	4%	22 (6–63)
Leiber-Wackenheim et al. [264]	Novae cup (UK)	59	1.7%	96 (72–132)
Schneider et al. [265]	Novae cup (UK)	96	10.4%	40.8 (1–100.8)
Civinini et al. [266]	Avantage (Biomet, USA)	33#	0%	39.6 (24–60)
Hailer et al. [267]	Avantage (Biomet, USA)	228	2%	24 (0–72)
Combes et al. [268]	Hemispherical DMC	2179*	0.88%	84
Philippot et al. [269]	Novae cup (UK)	163#	3.7%	64
Mohammed et al. [270]	Novae cup (UK)	41	0%	22 (6–63)

DMC, dual-mobility cup; *N*, number; pts, patients; FU, follow-up; #, reoperations for any reason were included; *, primary THA were included.

have been proposed to restore the function including trochanteric advancement and usage of tendon allograft as a sling.

4.3.5.7 Dual-mobility cups

Another approach to treatment of recurrent instability of THA is the use of dual-mobility or tripolar cups. The dual-mobility cup uses two articular surfaces within the range of a "single" cup [259]. A regular-size femoral head component articulates

Table 4.12 Clinical results of several constrained cups used for recurrent instability

Author	Implant	*N* (pts/hips)	Rate of failure	FU (months)
Bremner et al. [272]	Stryker Howmedica Osteonics	100 THAs	6%#	123.6 (74–164)*
Shapiro et al. [273]	Omnifit (Osteonics)	87 THAs	2.4% redislocation 8.2% revision	58 (36–89)
Shrader et al. [274]	PSL acetabular shell (Howmedica, Rutherford, New Jersey)	110 THAs	0% redislocation, 2% subluxation; 8% revision for other reasons	38.4 (24–96)
Berend et al. [275]	S-ROM Poly-Dial (JMP) RingLoc I (Biomet) Osteonics (Osteonics)	138	28.9% recurrent dislocation	31.3 (0.5–136.3)
Della Valle et al. [276]	Duraloc (J + J)	51	16% redislocation	44 (24–81)
Noble et al. [277]	4 designs	57 THAs	51% (overall)	36
Andersen et al. [278]	Trilogy (Zimmer)	32	12% redislocation	21.6 (3–63)

N, number; pts, patients; FU, follow-up; #, including the failure of constrained acetabular component; *, average time to failure (range).

within a larger size polyethylene liner while this larger diameter polyethylene moves against a metallic cup fixed to the acetabular bone (Fig. 4.12).

A number of studies (Table 4.11) demonstrate the efficacy of dual-mobility THAs in terms of lower dislocation rate without a negative impact on survivorships of the implants even in high-risk patients [260]. On the other hand, it was also emphasized repeatedly that dual-mobility cups should not compensate for technical errors. Furthermore, dissociation of the components requiring further surgery has been described.

4.3.5.8 Constrained liners

Constrained devices prevent the dislocation by locking the femoral head inside the cup. Multiple authors have reported the efficacy of this solution to achieve a stable THA [271]. However, this device leads to excessive loading transmitted from the locking mechanism to the implant and thus to the bone–implant interface. Therefore, studies with longer follow-ups report an increased rate of mechanical failure, reoperations, and a limited range of motion. In addition, the results differ according to manufacturer and the reported group; thus not all the devices offer the same probability of success (Table 4.12).

Taken together, orthopedic surgeons should be aware of the potential risk for complications in these implants, and use constrained cups only when there is no other viable option available.

4.3.5.9 Large femoral heads

Currently, THA with a large head is used with increasing frequency [279]. Large femoral heads are those of 36 mm and larger. They can be made of metal and ceramic; the counterpart can be made of polyethylene or ceramic material. The metallic liner has been virtually abandoned due to a high rate of failure reported for the large head MoM THA [280]. A very specific approach is dual-mobility THA, also offering a combination with big head.

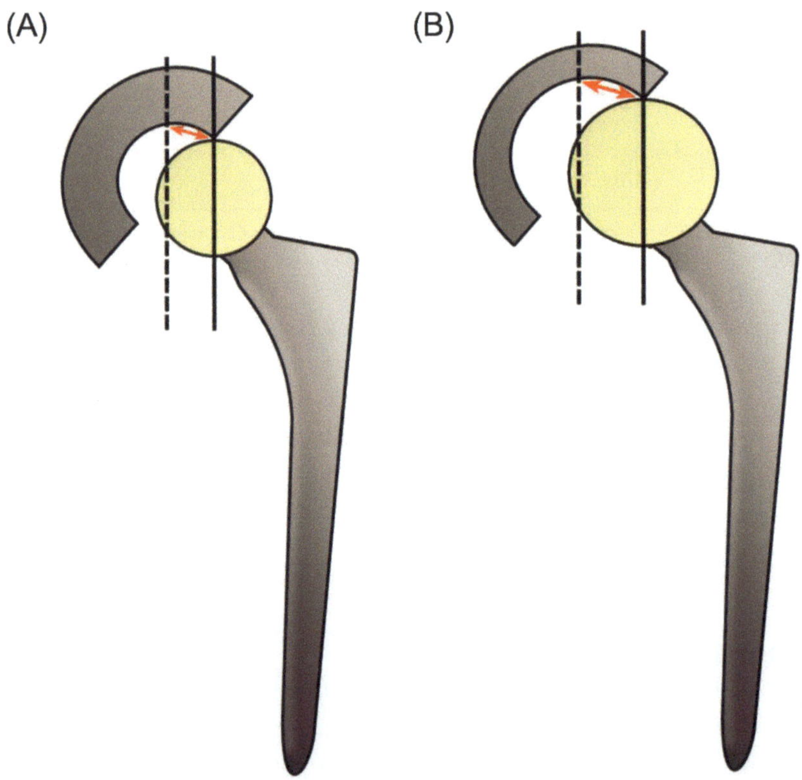

Figure 4.13 A larger femoral head increases the jump distance, on the other hand a larger diameter means a longer sliding distance; (A) articulation with a smaller head; (B) with a larger head.

Larger femoral heads do not improve the functional outcome in THA [281] and also range of motion seems to be comparable with standard head sizes [282]. Their use is primarily motivated by increased stability of THA (Fig. 4.13), and thus a decreased risk of dislocation [283].

4.3.5.10 Concerns related to large femoral heads

The problem is that the big heads require thinner polyethylene liners in comparison to smaller heads. In some patients, this may be associated with a risk for fractures of the polyethylene, and increased wear and/or premature degradation caused by excessive strain generated inside the material [284]. As a result, further studies are required to determine a minimum thickness acceptable for XLPE followed by exclusion of "risk size combinations" from clinical practice.

Larger femoral heads ("larger diameter = longer sliding distance") may cause higher volumetric wear despite the fact that only modern extremely polished heads (either metal or ceramic) are paired with XLPE or ceramic cups, i.e., highly wear-resistant materials. Accordingly, some studies report that the wear rate in the modern metal-on-polyethylene combination is higher in pairs with larger heads [285]. On the other hand, at least one study demonstrated comparable wear rate when thin (3.8 mm) and thick (7.9 mm) XLPE liners were tested under ideal conditions [286]. Because of the relative paucity of relevant clinical studies with longer follow-up [44], this concern remains.

Large heads have large frictional torque and larger bending moments on the femoral trunnion, and in this manner they may contribute to pathology at this junction including corrosion [287]. To confirm or reject this theory, other studies are needed examining the true size of the problem in clinical practice.

Some patients report anterior hip and groin pathology including pseudotumor formation in MoM THAs [288]. Others can suffer from anterior pain induced at least in part by an interaction between a large head and the iliopsoas tendon and/or a part of the rectus femoris muscle [289].

4.3.5.11 Alternative bearing surfaces

The term alternative bearing refers to combinations with the materials of other than polyethylene origin. A number of studies demonstrate that articulating (bearing) pairs like CoC or MoM have a significantly lower wear rate in comparison to pairs containing polyethylene cup [219].

The idea behind the more frequent implementation of alternative bearings into clinical practice in the last two decades is to avoid periprosthetic osteolysis, to delay the processes leading to aseptic loosening, and thus to prolong the survivorship of THA. It is expected that THA with alternative bearing surfaces should offer a significantly lower wear rate under the same or even higher load.

4.3.5.12 Ceramic-on-ceramic

Modern ceramic for THA is extremely hard and scratch-resistant. It also has extraordinary tribological features like a very low coefficient of friction. There is growing evidence that CoC THAs can achieve impressive survivorship at both 10 and 15 years follow-up based on individual studies including nonrandomized studies [19]. A lower rate of periprosthetic osteolysis and aseptic loosening has also been reported for these implants even in younger patients. However, a recent systematic review and meta-analysis of randomized trials do not find superiority of CoC over ceramic-on-polyethylene bearings in terms of radiolucent line formation, osteolysis, aseptic loosening, and reoperation rate [290].

Concerns are still related to squeaking (up to 30%), a specific type of wear (e.g., rim wear, stripe wear), and perhaps to the risk of ceramic component fracture (it may be about 0.02% even with delta ceramic) [291].

4.3.5.13 Metal-on-metal

Despite the fact that very low wear rate was observed in modern MoM THA, a MoM THA are very controversial and has been abandoned by most surgeons because of severe adverse events that have been associated with metallic by-products. Wear rates of less than 1 mm^3 per million work cycles are reported [292]. However, almost all metal particles are of nanometer size and are readily transported away from a joint. An excessive load of cobalt–chrome nanoparticles in the periprosthetic tissues induces a spectrum of cytotoxic (necrosis), inflammatory, and allergic reactions [293]. A concern is also related to a long-term increase in the levels of cobalt, chromium, and also other metals in the blood with potential systemic effects.

Taken together, currently MoM has been rejected by the majority of surgeons because of an increased risk of development of an adverse reaction to metal debris.

4.3.5.14 Ceramic-on-metal

This combination has been introduced in order to combine advantages of basic pair combinations (i.e., CoC and MoM) and also to diminish disadvantages related to them. Therefore, the ceramic-on-metal THA articulates a thin metal acetabular shell containing a metal liner with a ceramic head. Some studies show a wear rate comparable with MoM; others emphasize the about zero risk for a metal liner fracture as well as the possibility to use a larger head in a wider range of cups. The latter is due to the fact that a metallic liner can be thinner than a ceramic one. The use of metal bearing is also associated with a release of metal wear debris in patients having this bearing [294]. In addition, preliminary studies have not reported acceptable outcomes [295]. As a result, this combination should still be considered as clinically unproven.

4.3.5.15 New materials

Wear resistance can be improved by applying a diamond-like coating (DLC) layer on the traditional/new nonceramic material. The deposition of DLC increases wear resistance, improves the lubrication in THA, prevents corrosion, and it is also highly biocompatible [296]. Bearings treated with DLC are increasingly utilized to extend bearing life even in extreme industry applications. Clinically tested were combinations of femoral heads with DLC articulating against the polyethylene cups [297]. However, the evidence for their clinical usage is still insufficient.

4.3.5.16 Carbon-fiber-reinforced polyaryletheretherketone

Carbon-fiber-reinforced polyaryletheretherketone (CFR-PEEK) has been widely tested in vitro showing promising tribological (two orders of magnitude less wear than the control), mechanical, and biological properties [298]. In THA and TKA (UKA) usage with a metallic or ceramic counterface is intended. However, at least one study reported that PEEK particles induced higher amounts of inflammatory cytokines compared to polyethylene particles [299]. In spite of supporting literature for the use of CFR-PEEK in orthopedics [300], the evidence for their use in THA bearings is still insufficient.

Also other carbon—carbon composite materials have been tested and demonstrated a low wear rate in vitro, and low specific biological activity has been observed for their wear debris [301]. However, there is no clinical experience available to date.

4.3.5.17 Head—Neck taper interface damage

Modularity as a concept for THA was proposed and patented in the 1970s. During the 1980s this concept has increased dramatically and now it is considered an inevitable part of modern THA. The current potential of modularity enables surgeons to optimize THA reconstruction in terms of stability, biomechanics, and kinematics. It also offers a valuable tool for the solution of leg-length discrepancy. However, theoretically, with increasing number of parts constituting the prosthesis the risk of failure increases.

Here we will address only the head—neck taper junction as the most frequent example of modern modular THA. It consists of the femoral stem trunnion (stem taper) and a taper inside the femoral ball head. Regardless of the diameter of the head or the neck length, the precise matching of both components is crucial. The interface between the trunnion and head surfaces is force-fit ("taper locking") and in this way it is extremely tight while exposed to chronic stress and strain. Generally, this trunnion can be damaged by mechanically assisted crevice corrosion, when a wide range of the shape and structure damage was observed in retrieved femoral components [302]. Interestingly, there is growing awareness that the pathology of the trunnion interface can significantly contribute to ALTR, [303].

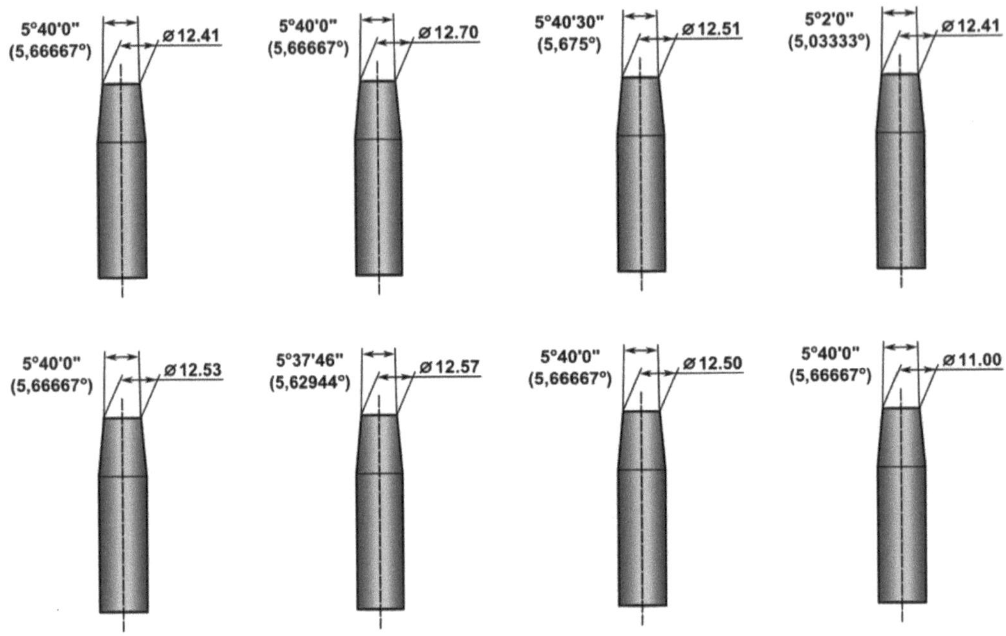

Figure 4.14 Trunnion parameters can differ among the manufacturers even for the same specification. *From: Scheuber LF, Usbeck S, Petkow F. The taper in hip arthroplasty: what does the surgeon have to pay attention to? CeraNews 2014;2014(1):18.*

4.3.5.18 What is clear?

The modular taper interface enables the pairing of materials of the same (metal with metal) or different (ceramic with metal) type without the risk of premature failure.

Together with head parameters trunnion parameters such as length, diameter, or taper angle contribute to the head–neck taper interface characteristics (Fig. 4.14). These influence the size and distribution of forces at the interface. A combination of bigger heads with a decreased trunnion size should be carefully monitored [287].

Unfortunately, the effort to standardize the taper parameters of trunnions has not been successful. Trunnions differ in terms of geometry, structure, and surface properties. Neither the neck length (either expressed as S, M, L, XL, or in millimeters) is the same when comparing the products of different manufacturers. As a result, surgeons have to face the reoperation of a stable stem with a nonstandard taper specification or known specification that is not available at the time of reoperation. Moreover, even when the specification of a taper is 12/14, this does not automatically mean that one can use a head with a 12/14 specification [304]. Under such conditions, it is important to respect the manufacturer's instructions. On the other hand, all the stakeholders have to place increasing pressure on all manufacturers to unify key parameters.

4.3.6 Other issues with TKA (malalignment, stiffness, allergy, patient satisfaction)

TKA is a cost-effective procedure to relieve pain and restore the patient's mobility and function. Orthopedic surgeons have helped design knee implants that are now safe, effective, and durable. Survivorship studies have reported revision-free success ranging from 81.7% to 98.14% after 15 or more years [305–307]. Studies focusing on THA have similar results with survivorship after 15 years being above 90% [308,309]. Although TKAs are expected to improve the patient's quality of life, some patients remain with some degree of pain after the procedure. Nashi et al. [310] reported that 31.1% and 28.9% of patients describe a residual knee pain at 1 and 2 years, respectively, after TKA. Interestingly, patients experience more pain after TKA compared to THA, with a prevalence of up to 20% with long-term pain [311,312].

Stiffness after knee replacement is usually defined as >10 degrees of extension deficit and/or <95 degrees of flexion in the first 6 weeks after surgery [313]. Stiffness, also known as arthrofibrosis, is reported to be a common reason for reoperation after TKA [314]. Several factors affect the postoperative range of motion including preoperative range of motion, body habitus, component alignment, oversized implants, heterotopic ossification, patellofemoral dysfunction, poor control of perioperative pain, complex regional pain syndrome, and others. The cause of the stiffness should be investigated before starting any invasive treatment. When no obvious reason related to a surgical procedure is diagnosed, then stiffness is first treated by pain control and intense physical therapy. When physical therapy fails then manipulation under anesthesia (MUA) is an alternative. The incidence of MUA has been reported as 1.3–13.5% [313,315–317]. The best time to perform MUA is still under debate. Some authors recommend manipulation within 2 weeks postoperatively [318], whereas others advocate MUA after the third week [319]. However, Daluga et al. have shown that early manipulation (within the first 3 weeks) is associated with better results than late manipulation (3 weeks to 3 months) [320]. MUA is not a straightforward procedure and must be performed carefully. MUA may have serious and detrimental complications such as femoral supracondylar fracture, extensor mechanism injury, wound dehiscence, or hemarthrosis. Ultimately, if the stiffness is not resolved through MUA, alternative options are arthroscopic release or open surgery with or without associated further procedures (changing of implants, new bone cuts, soft tissue releases).

Component malposition or malalignment can be defined as abnormal positioning or rotation of one or more components, causing pain abnormal kinematics or maltracking. Femoral and tibial components should be placed in slight external rotation (ER). The degree of rotation can be assessed intraoperatively using known landmarks, or with computer-assisted surgery. With a preoperative varus deformity, the femoral component should be placed in about 3 degrees of ER, whereas with a valgus

Table 4.13 Reasons for revision TKA

Country	Three most common reasons	Authors
USA	Infection, mechanical loosening, implant failure	Bozic et al. [322] Le et al. [323] Siqueira et al. [324]
Netherlands	Mechanical loosening, infection, malposition	van Kempen et al. [325]
Japan	Mechanical loosening, infection, wear/osteolysis	Kasahara et al. [326]

Table 4.14 Reasons for litigation after TKA

Country	Three most frequent medicolegal claims	Authors
USA	Nerve injury, limb-length discrepancy, infection	McGrory et al. [327]
UK	Infection, technical error, alleged negligence	McWilliams et al. [328]
France	Infection, neurological deficit, unsatisfactory result	Gibon et al. [329]

deformity, slightly more ER is recommended [321]. Regarding the tibial component, ER is important as it improves patellar tracking and decreases the risk of patellar subluxation/dislocation. Evaluation of the position of the knee components may be delineated postoperatively with the use of CT scanning. However, the exact landmarks to use on these scans are controversial.

The reasons for knee revision are numerous, and dependent on the date and country of origin of the report (Table 4.13).

The reasons for litigation and malpractice claims after knee arthroplasty vary depending on the country of origin of the study (Table 4.14).

4.3.7 Patients with severe bone-related comorbidities (elderly patients with osteoporosis, patients with rheumatic diseases, osteonecrosis of the femoral head, chronic renal osteopathy, Paget disease)

A myriad of factors contribute to eventual loosening and a majority are perhaps unknown. Moreover, it appears that the causative factors are different for each patient. Based on the occurrence of known risk factors, one can distinguish between *patients with a more favorable prognosis* for prosthetic durability and *those with an unfavorable prognosis* for THA [330]. The former are those of female sex, multiple joint involvement, bilateral hip disease, and patients who are less active and lightweight. The latter include men with unilateral osteoarthritis or traumatic arthritis, heavy laborers, athletes, and also patients with compromised bone structure/metabolism around an implant (poor bone bed = poor prognosis for THA). A similar concept may be introduced for TKA despite the fact that our knowledge is less clear than in the case of THA.

4.3.7.1 Osteoporosis

In relation to THA, severe osteoporosis could lead to mechanical failure of the bone–implant interface as the bone quality, including basic mechanical features, is compromised. Studies report poor retention of osteosynthetic devices in the osteoporotic proximal femurs [331]. The same is perhaps relevant also in the case of TKA. On the other hand, these patients do not increase the activity significantly after the surgery, which could at least in part compensate for the suboptimal bone quality. As a result, the association between osteoporotic bone and premature aseptic loosening can be demonstrated with the case of cementless cups that are relatively prone to early migration in older patients. The evidence for aseptic loosening in cementless stems in the same age group is somewhat weaker [332].

4.3.7.1.1 Indication for THA/TKA

Osteoporosis is not a contraindication to THA/TKA itself. People suffering from a wide range of bone metabolic diseases are indicated for THA/TKA at the time when an alternative viable therapeutic option is not available. If arthroplasty is the best choice then it is necessary to know whether THA or hemiarthroplasty, which type of fixation (cemented or cementless), and what are the recommended parameters of bearing surfaces. In addition, optimal postoperative care for elderly patients has to be defined, including a strategy targeting osteoporosis.

4.3.7.1.2 Design and material options

Even osteoporotic bone is able to cooperate with cementless implant surfaces under specific conditions [333]. There are also clinical studies for cementless THA in elderly patients [334] but the problem is that preoperatively it is not easy to identify in whom the cementless surface will work. In addition, individual studies and data from the hip arthroplasty registries support the use of cemented over the cementless THAs in elderly patients [96,97]. As a result, in patients with severe osteoporosis, a cemented implant is the method of choice at both the acetabular and femoral sites. A cemented hemiarthroplasty is a valuable and cost-effective choice in elderly patients with a limited life expectancy. When the acetabulum is affected severely or fractured, it may be necessary to reconstruct the bed for a cup using an acetabular cage [335].

At the knee, cemented TKA is the method of choice [336]. In the case of severely affected bone bed at the distal femur or proximal tibia, a stem with or without an augmenting sleeve can be used to transmit the load to a stronger bone segment.

4.3.7.2 Systemic inflammatory diseases

Chronic inflammatory hip and knee arthritis develops within a range of systemic inflammatory diseases, including autoimmune diseases (e.g., rheumatoid arthritis). For this highly heterogeneous group of diseases, inflammation is a central component contributing to development of both organ and tissue damage [337]. In the cases of rheumatoid arthritis and systemic lupus erythematosus, the probability of developing inflammatory hip disease is relatively high [338]. But the incidence and prevalence (between 0.4% and 1%) are much higher in the former; therefore, many more candidates for THA are patients with rheumatoid arthritis than those with systemic lupus erythematosus. The same is true for the knee.

For a rheumatic joint a combination of alignment abnormalities and/or deformities with periarticular osteoporosis, bone erosions, and joint space narrowing is due to chronic inflammation and dysregulation of immune system [339]. Progressive inflammatory and bone-resorptive hip/knee disease leads eventually to severe secondary osteoarthritis requiring THA/TKA. In relation to both THA/TKA, the key question is whether these pathways will contribute to the host response to implants and especially to its by-products.

4.3.7.2.1 Design and material options

Both the cemented and cementless THA can be used in these patients offering similar survival of primary THA compared to that in patients with idiopathic osteoarthritis [340]. One particular study supports even the use of a short metaphyseal stem [341] while the evidence for the use of resurfacing hip arthroplasty in patients with rheumatoid arthritis is insufficient. With regard to bearing surfaces, the decision-making should be similar to that in other patients.

A cemented TKA is the proven method of choice. In relation to cruciate ligament retention, a posterior stabilized implant may have an advantage at least in some patients but the difference is not significant [21]. The mobile bearing TKA may have similar effects on knee compared to a fixed bearing one [342]. In the case of severely damaged bone bed at the distal femur or proximal tibia, a stem with or without an augmenting sleeve can be used to solve bone defects and transmit the load to a stronger bone segment.

Patients with rheumatoid arthritis could have an increased risk of aseptic loosening, PJI, and periprosthetic fractures compared to osteoarthritis. If this is true, then these patients should be treated with implants covered ideally by multifunctional surfaces containing the antiinflammatory and bone-homeostatic components together with antibacterial agents (Fig. 4.3). However, these implants are unavailable now.

4.3.7.2.2 Evidence for THA/TKA

In patients with systemic inflammatory hip disease both the cemented [343] and cementless [344] THAs can be implanted with predictable long-term survival.

Systematic reviews are also available in support of TKA in patients with rheumatoid arthritis [342]. It seems even that patients with rheumatoid arthritis show better outcomes than those with osteoarthritis in terms of pain relief and satisfaction [345].

On the other hand, the overall risk of PJI is increased in patients with rheumatoid arthritis compared to patients with primary osteoarthritis [346]. A recent review revealed an increased risk for proximal femur fracture occurring either intraoperatively or postoperatively in rheumatic patients [347]. In addition, these patients with at least 10 years of follow-up are at higher risk for TKA component-loosening and periprosthetic fractures [348].

4.3.7.3 Osteonecrosis of the hip

Osteonecrosis of the femoral head (OFH) is a disabling disease affecting young and middle-aged patients. It is a relatively common condition with a strong tendency to progress to end-stage osteoarthritis.

The pathogenesis of the disease is still not fully elucidated but the key findings of focal intravascular thrombosis that affects the terminal arterioles, and postsinusoidal venules is generally accepted. Obliteration of the microcirculation at the large segments of femoral head (acetabulum) together with bone marrow edema causes an increased intraosseous pressure compromising the subchondral bone microcirculation, and thus vitality. This eventually leads to ischemic death of subchondral bone and the development of advanced osteoarthritis requiring THA [349].

The key question is whether the bone disease inducing the need for THA continues after the surgery or not with the former being a potential risk for long-term survival of the bone–implant interface. OFH can be associated with a known disease or without a clear predisposition. Based on this, one can distinguish between idiopathic and secondary osteonecrosis with a known underlying disease (Table 4.15).

Table 4.15 Classification of osteonecrosis of the hip according to risk factors with estimated influence on the bone–implant interface

Type of ON	Type of pathology	Examples	Estimated impact on BII
Idiopathic	True pathology is unknown	All cases without a listed pathology below	–
Secondary	Direct bone insult	Trauma, radiation, chemotherapy, Caisson disease, Gaucher disease	Trauma – Others +
	Indirect influence—modifiable or temporal	Associated with excessive alcohol and smoking, corticosteroid use, pregnancy, etc.	Cessation could lead to normal bone remodeling
	Indirect influence—nonmodifiable or constant	Coagulopathies, inflammatory bowel disease, organ transplants, sickle cell disease, systemic lupus erythematosus, etc.	+

ON, osteonecrosis; BII, bone–implant interface; –, the underlying pathology probably does not continue in effect; +, the underlying pathology could probably continue in effect.

4.3.7.3.1 Indication for THA

Patients with OFH are generally younger than those indicated for primary osteoarthritis, and some may have had previous hip-preserving surgery. The indication for THA should be always weighed against the expected risk for complications that could be increased at least in some kinds of secondary osteonecrosis.

In the future, potential information from imaging and/or laboratory studies (markers from serum, synovial fluid, etc.) could be made available to modify preoperatively the surgeon's decision-making when contemplating THA in these patients. Arlot et al. examined bone samples obtained by bone biopsy from patients suffering from OFH [350]. The underlying pathology was chronic steroids and alcoholism in the majority of cases. The authors revealed a dysfunction in the osteoblastic new bone apposition, and thus a decrease in bone formation. Another study demonstrated that the zone affected by ischemic dysfunction could extend several centimeters below the lesser trochanter [351]. To date no noninvasive method is available to identify patients with a poor or good prognosis for THA.

4.3.7.3.2 Design and material option

The surgeon faces many challenges during operation of an osteonecrotic hip in terms of bone quality (from an extremely poor bone with large bone defects to sclerotic bone), bone deformity, and/or occurrence of osteosynthetic or other (e.g., tantalum implants) materials. However, to date there are no data favoring a specific THA in hips affected with osteonecrosis. In other words, all the implants that function well in osteoarthritic hips can achieve reliable long-term outcomes also in patients with osteonecrosis.

Special attention is required of acetabular involvement and specifically that caused by irradiation. In that particular case the use of cementless implant is associated with an increased risk of premature aseptic loosening. Thus, some authors recommend using a reinforcement cage and a cemented cup [352].

4.3.7.3.3 Evidence for THA

Despite the fact that the risk for reoperation is still increased in patients with OFH compared to primary osteoarthritis, the results of THA in these patients have improved over the past decades [353]. According to a recent study reporting data for patients with follow-up between 0 and 16 years [354], the unadjusted and adjusted risks of revision were higher in the patients with necrosis than in those with primary osteoarthritis (adjusted RR = 1.3, CI 1.1–1.4). Surprisingly, age-stratified analyses showed that the unadjusted and adjusted risks of revision were similar when patients of age under 50 years were compared.

In relation to the fixation of THA the decision should be made with regard to outcomes reported for a particular type of osteonecrosis. A proven cementless implant

Table 4.16 Risk of prosthetic joint infections and mortality rate in patients with chronic renal failure who underwent THA

Author	*N* (hips/pts)	PJI (hips in pts)	Reoperation rate for all indications (hips in pts)	Mortality	Note
Naito et al. [356]	17/15	2/17 (11.8%) in 1/15 (6.7%)	0	6.7%	All patients in this study were hemodialyzed Mean age 61, mean follow-up 8.6 years. Failure rate 35%, 0 reoperation due to poor general condition and unwillingness
Lieberman et al. [357]	46/30	4/46 (8.7%) in 4/30 (13.3%)	4/46 (8.7%) in 4/30 (13.3%)	4/30 (13.3%) related to THA; total of 8/30 (26.7%)	Mean follow-up was 54 months
Sakalkale et al. [358]	15/12	2/15 (13.3%) in 2/12 (16.7%)	3/15 (20%) in 3/12 (25%)	1/12 (8.33%) related to THA; total of 7/12 (58%)	Mean age 57 years, mean follow-up 64 months. Two hips were reoperated due to infection, one due to aseptic loosening
Nagoya et al. [359]	11/7	0%	1/11 (9.1%) in 1/7 (14.3%)	2/7 (28.6%)	Mean age 42, mean follow-up 99 months. All deaths were unrelated to THA
Shrader et al. [360]	45/37	2/45 (4.3%) in 2/37 (5.4%)	14/45 (31.1%) in 13/37 (35.1%)	11/37 (29.7%)	Mean age 67 in dialysis group, mean follow-up 6 years. Mean age 46 in transplant group, mean follow-up 11 years
Miric et al. [355]	1269 pts	9/1269 (0.7%) including surgical site infection	18/1269 (1.4%)	50/1269 (3.9%)	In comparison to control group, only, readmission rate within 90 days was different, adjusted HR = 1.37 (1.06–1.78)

N, number; pts, patients; PJI, prosthetic joint infection; HR, hazard ratio.

seems to be a better choice than a cemented implant in idiopathic, traumatic, and some other types of osteonecrosis with a less compromised bone bed, especially when it is combined with modern bearing surfaces. On the other hand, the cemented or partially cemented THA should be carefully weighed in inflammatory, tumor, or metabolic hip osteonecrosis.

4.3.7.4 Renal osteopathy

A relatively rare indication to THA is osteonecrosis associated with chronic renal diseases. The renal osteopathy influences the bone metabolism, thus it potentially compromises the bone–implant parameters necessary for long-term functioning of THA. An associated comorbidity contributes to an increased risk for complications such as PJI and mortality (Table 4.16). The risk for a complication as well as the readmission rate depend on the particular type of chronic renal disease [355]. There is also a great difference when comparing patients on dialysis and those who have undergone a renal transplant, with the former having a much poorer prognosis.

4.3.7.4.1 Design and material option

Patients with chronic renal failure undergoing THA/TKA are undoubtedly the ideal candidates for implants having surface functionalities with a strong antiinfective and bone-preserving (stimulating) coating. Currently cementless THA is generally used in younger patients after successful transplantation with a good estimation of life expectancy while those with a poorer prognosis and dialyzed are treated with a cemented THA and TKA.

4.3.7.4.2 Evidence for THA/TKA

There is limited evidence in terms of long-term survivorship of THA in patients with chronic renal osteopathy despite the fact that at least one study reports excellent survivorship (98.8 $\pm$ 2.2% at 10 years) for the cemented THA [361]. As a result, these patients have to be carefully considered for THA/TKA. Collaboration and coordination with the nephrology service are important to mitigate complications and maximize outcome.

4.3.7.5 Paget disease

Paget disease is a bone disease combining signs of increased bone resorption, formation, and remodeling which leads to deformities of the hip joint. It is relatively common in Europe among those of Anglo-Saxon ancestry; it affects about 1% of the US population over the age of 40, and it is very rare in Africa and Asia. However, the incidence of the disease has been decreasing in recent decades.

The pathogenesis is not fully elucidated. To date, it is postulated that a viral agent or another environmental agent in combination with individual susceptibility could underlie an excessive number and activity of osteoclasts and osteoblasts [362]. For hip, the development of varus femoral deformity in combination with a sclerotic canal, and acetabular protrusio is a typical finding [363].

Surgeons should be aware of the risk of increased intraoperative bleeding. In addition, the degree of femoral and acetabular deformity together with the local bone status have to be taken into the preoperative planning.

4.3.7.5.1 Design and material option

The most favorable fixation method of THA has yet to be determined. Bowing of the femur may require femoral osteotomy to allow placement of cementless stem. Acetabular protrusio is better to be treated using a large cementless cup anchored to the acetabular wall in combination with bone grafting of the bottom. In some cases of severe protrusio, acetabular cages are a more viable option in combination with a cemented cup.

4.3.7.5.2 Evidence for THA/TKA

There are several studies reporting good long-term survivorship in the cemented (98% at 10 years; 95% confidence interval = 95–100%) [364] and cementless THA [365] used in Paget's hip disease.

At least one study supports the usage of cemented TKA in patients with Paget disease [366].

4.4 FUTURE TRENDS AND NEXT-GENERATION DEVICES

As outlined above, in general, total joint replacements (TJRs) is a very successful surgical procedure that continues to improve the quality of life of millions of patients worldwide. The clinical survivorship is quite remarkable; most modern implants are routinely lasting into the second or third decades of use, and some even longer. This statement is made on a backdrop of two important considerations. First, patients are living longer and more active lives. Therefore the TJRs currently performed are expected to be more durable, and therefore be in situ for a more extended period of time. Second, joint replacements are being implanted in younger patients with greater expectations of high physical performance. These patients often aspire to do impact-loading sports such as running and skiing again, and will do so whether or not they are admonished to avoid these activities. This fact presents a dilemma. The patient has definite desires and wishes to lead a fully active life, without restrictions. The surgeon would like a satisfied patient, who has a pain-free, well-functioning joint replacement with a satisfactory stable range of motion, without infection, loosening, or other complication. Thus the patient, surgeon, and implant manufacturer as well as payers, hospitals, and government agencies must walk a fine line together to ensure that safe and efficacious implants are produced and appropriately implanted and maintained, so that patient satisfaction is optimized at a reasonable cost to society.

Thus, the concept of joint replacement must be improved in the future to address these higher expectations. Some issues to address are outlined below.

4.4.1 Improved patient selection

Patient selection is an important aspect of undergoing joint replacement surgery. Frank discussions must be undertaken between surgeons and patients preoperatively concerning the goals and limitations of current implants. Higher-risk patients, such as those with complex medical issues (diabetes, chronic heart disease, kidney failure, significant neurological disease, obesity, etc.), need to have their health issues optimized preoperatively; higher rates of complications postoperatively need to be anticipated and clearly explained to the patient preoperatively. Patients with musculoskeletal deformities near the proposed joint replacement may require multistaged procedures, special instrumentation, and implants. One good example is the conversion of a failed fracture fixation device to total hip replacement in the elderly patient with numerous medical comorbidities.

4.4.2 Improved surgical technique and instrumentation

In the United States and other countries worldwide, many of the joint replacements are performed by surgeons who are general orthopedic surgeons and not subspecialists. Much of their knowledge base is derived from their orthopedic residency, journals, instructional courses, and their implant manufacturer representative. Newer simpler techniques of implantation of joint replacements must address these facts. Recently introduced concepts such as surgical navigation using computers, patient-specific instruments, and others have made their way into some practices, however these innovations are often cumbersome, labor-intensive, necessitate further preoperative imaging, and expensive. Furthermore, the clinical outcomes have not been demonstrated to be superior to the use of conventional instruments in "good hands." These innovations need to be improved and high-level, evidence-based studies need to validate their use and cost.

4.4.3 Improved implant design

More recently, a plethora of new implants have flooded the orthopedic marketplace. As outlined above, new implants should be evidence-based and fulfill a definite need in the marketplace that currently available implants do not fulfill. There are protocols and governmental agencies presently in place in the United States and other countries for how this might be accomplished. However, these mechanisms of approval should be carefully scrutinized and reevaluated at regular intervals to help ensure that the best implants reach the marketplace and are followed carefully with appropriate surveillance mechanisms. All of this has to be accomplished without stifling innovation.

National implant registries, as well as governmental- and manufacturer-supported adverse event reporting are important mechanisms that help determine the safety and efficacy of different implant systems. These should be supported and the findings publicized in a quick and transparent manner.

There is a need for different implant systems for different patient subgroups. A new, high-impact-resisting knee replacement targeted for younger active patients is not necessary for much older, more sedentary individuals. Implant—patient matching could potentially optimize the patient's and surgeon's goals with implant characteristics in a cost-effective fashion. This pertains also to the different anatomical variations observed around the hip and knee. For example, it is only recently that femoral components for hip replacement have had the capability of reestablishing femoral offset and tissue tension without having to overlengthen the limb.

4.4.4 Improved bearing surfaces

Issues related to bearing surfaces have been discussed in detail above. Suffice it to say that newer bearing surfaces are needed that will withstand normal physiologic loads without excessive wear or deformation. Furthermore, the by-products from wear must be limited, nontoxic, easily dealt with by the body's normal biological mechanisms, and not lead to adverse events such as chronic inflammation, osteolysis, tissue necrosis, or allergic responses.

4.4.5 Improving implant integration and avoiding infection

Specific biological situations present great challenges for the orthopedic surgeon. For example, in hip revision situations using cementless implants, osseointegration may be difficult to achieve if the bone stock is deficient or of poor quality. Mechanical or biological implant surface coatings may facilitate this goal. In addition, as infection is a major source of implant failure leading to further surgery and often removal of the implant, new methods to avoid this dreaded complication are needed. This may entail systemic or local treatments delivered to the patient or implant. Questions related to how this should be accomplished are under current investigation.

4.5 CONCLUSION

It should be remembered that joint replacement is one of the greatest innovations of all time. The operation generally provides pain-free ambulation and function for many years. Yet, there is still room for improvement in this currently health-conscious environment. It behooves surgeons, manufacturers, payers, hospitals, and governmental agencies to collaborate with the public to continue to provide safe and effective implants for joint replacement at a reasonable cost.

REFERENCES

[1] Tsertsvadze A, Grove A, Freeman K, Court R, Johnson S, Connock M, et al. Total hip replacement for the treatment of end stage arthritis of the hip: a systematic review and meta-analysis. PLoS One 2014;9:e99804.

[2] Corten K, Bourne RB, Charron KD, Au K, Rorabeck CH. What works best, a cemented or cementless primary total hip arthroplasty?: minimum 17-year followup of a randomized controlled trial. Clin Orthop Relat Res 2011;469:209–17.

[3] Corten K, Bourne RB, Charron KD, Au K, Rorabeck CH. Comparison of total hip arthroplasty performed with and without cement: a randomized trial. A concise follow-up, at twenty years, of previous reports. J Bone Joint Surg Am 2011;93:1335–8.

[4] Shan L, Shan B, Suzuki A, Nouh F, Saxena A. Intermediate and long-term quality of life after total knee replacement: a systematic review and meta-analysis. J Bone Joint Surg Am 2015;97:156–68.

[5] Long WJ, Bryce CD, Hollenbeak CS, Benner RW, Scott WN. Total knee replacement in young, active patients: long-term follow-up and functional outcome: a concise follow-up of a previous report. J Bone Joint Surg Am 2014;96:e159.

[6] Ritter MA. The Anatomical Graduated Component total knee replacement: a long-term evaluation with 20-year survival analysis. J Bone Joint Surg Br 2009;91:745–9.

[7] Abram SG, Nicol F, Hullin MG, Spencer SJ. The long-term outcome of uncemented Low Contact Stress total knee replacement in patients with rheumatoid arthritis: results at a mean of 22 years. Bone Joint J 2013;95-B:1497–9.

[8] Keurentjes JC, Pijls BG, Van Tol FR, Mentink JF, Mes SD, Schoones JW, et al. Which implant should we use for primary total hip replacement? A systematic review and meta-analysis. J Bone Joint Surg Am 2014;96(Suppl. 1):79–97.

[9] Hernigou P. Earliest times before hip arthroplasty: from John Rhea Barton to Themistocles Gluck. Int Orthop 2013;37:2313–18.

[10] Charnley J. Low friction arthroplasty of the hip. New York, NY: Springer-Verlag; 1979.

[11] Learmonth ID, Young C, Rorabeck C. The operation of the century: total hip replacement. Lancet 2007;370:1508–19.

[12] Warth LC, Callaghan JJ, Liu SS, Klaassen AL, Goetz DD, Johnston RC. Thirty-five-year results after Charnley total hip arthroplasty in patients less than fifty years old. A concise follow-up of previous reports. J Bone Joint Surg Am 2014;96:1814–19.

[13] Goto E, Teranishi T, Tsuji M, Ando M. Long-term clinical results of Charnley total hip arthroplasty using a matte satin-finished stem: a 30-year average follow-up study. J Orthop Sci 2014;19:959–64.

[14] Lampropoulou-Adamidou K, Georgiades G, Vlamis J, Hartofilakidis G. Charnley low-friction arthroplasty in patients 35 years of age or younger. Results at a minimum of 23 years. Bone Joint J 2013;95-B:1052–6.

[15] Rajpura A, Kendoff D, Board TN. The current state of bearing surfaces in total hip replacement. Bone Joint J 2014;96-B:147–56.

[16] Kamath AF, Prieto H, Lewallen DG. Alternative bearings in total hip arthroplasty in the young patient. Orthop ClinNorth Am 2013;44:451–62.

[17] Zywiel MG, Sayeed SA, Johnson AJ, Schmalzried TP, Mont MA. Survival of hard-on-hard bearings in total hip arthroplasty: a systematic review. Clin Orthop Relat Res 2011;469:1536–46.

[18] Gill HS, Grammatopoulos G, Adshead S, Tsialogiannis E, Tsiridis E. Molecular and immune toxicity of CoCr nanoparticles in MoM hip arthroplasty. Trends Mol Med 2012;18:145–55.

[19] Gallo J, Goodman SB, Lostak J, Janout M. Advantages and disadvantages of ceramic on ceramic total hip arthroplasty: a review. Biomed Pap Med Fac Univ Palacky Olomouc Czech Repub 2012;156:204–12.

[20] Cooper HJ, Della Valle CJ. Large diameter femoral heads: is bigger always better? Bone Joint J 2014;96-B:23–6.
[21] Verra WC, van den Boom LG, Jacobs W, Clement DJ, Wymenga AA, Nelissen RG. Retention versus sacrifice of the posterior cruciate ligament in total knee arthroplasty for treating osteoarthritis. Cochrane Database System Rev 2013;10:CD004803.
[22] Callaghan JJ, Wells CW, Liu SS, Goetz DD, Johnston RC. Cemented rotating-platform total knee replacement: a concise follow-up, at a minimum of twenty years, of a previous report. J Bone Joint Surg Am 2010;92:1635–9.
[23] van der Voort P, Pijls BG, Nouta KA, Valstar ER, Jacobs WC, Nelissen RG. A systematic review and meta-regression of mobile-bearing versus fixed-bearing total knee replacement in 41 studies. Bone Joint J 2013;95-B:1209–16.
[24] Thienpont E, Fennema P, Price A. Can technology improve alignment during knee arthroplasty. Knee 2013;20(Suppl. 1):S21–8.
[25] Arirachakaran A, Wande T, Pituckhanotai K, Predeeprompan P, Kongtharvonskul J. Clinical outcomes after high-flex versus conventional total knee arthroplasty. Knee Surg Sports Traumatol Arthrosc 2015;23(6):1610–21.
[26] Jiang Y, Yao JF, Xiong YM, Ma JB, Kang H, Xu P. No superiority of high-flexion vs standard total knee arthroplasty: an update meta-analysis of randomized controlled trials. J Arthroplasty 2015;30 (6):980–6.
[27] Naziri Q, Pivec R, Harwin SF, Costa CR, Johnson AJ, Bonutti PM, et al. Surg Technol Int 2012;22:272–84.
[28] Higuera CA, Deirmengian C. The new technologies in knee arthroplasty. J Clin Rheumatol 2012;18:345–8.
[29] Fitch DA, Sedacki K, Yang Y. Mid- to long-term outcomes of a medial-pivot system for primary total knee replacement: a systematic review and meta-analysis. Bone Joint Res 2014;3:297–304.
[30] Sassoon A, Nam D, Nunley R, Barrack R. Systematic review of patient-specific instrumentation in total knee arthroplasty: new but not improved. Clin Orthop Relat Res 2015;473:151–8.
[31] Voleti PB, Hamula MJ, Baldwin KD, Lee GC. Current data do not support routine use of patient-specific instrumentation in total knee arthroplasty. J Arthroplasty 2014;29:1709–12.
[32] Clayton AW, Cherian JJ, Banerjee S, Kapadia BH, Jauregui JJ, Harwin SF, et al. Does the use of navigation in total knee arthroplasty affect outcomes? J Knee Surg 2014;27:171–5.
[33] Burnett RS, Barrack RL. Computer-assisted total knee arthroplasty is currently of no proven clinical benefit: a systematic review. Clin Orthop Relat Res 2013;471:264–76.
[34] Dumbleton JH, Manley MT, Edidin AA. A literature review of the association between wear rate and osteolysis in total hip arthroplasty. J Arthroplasty 2002;17:649–61.
[35] Schmalzried TP, Shepherd EF, Dorey FJ, Jackson WO, dela Rosa M, Fa'vae F, et al. The John Charnley Award. Wear is a function of use, not time. Clin Orthop Relat Res 2000;381:36–46.
[36] Gordon AC, D'Lima DD, Colwell Jr. CW. Highly cross-linked polyethylene in total hip arthroplasty. J Am Acad Orthop Surg 2006;14:511–23.
[37] Jacobs CA, Christensen CP, Greenwald AS, McKellop H. Clinical performance of highly cross-linked polyethylenes in total hip arthroplasty. J Bone Joint Surg Am 2007;89:2779–86.
[38] Dion NT, Bragdon C, Muratoglu O, Freiberg AA. Durability of highly cross-linked polyethylene in total hip and total knee arthroplasty. Orthop Clin North Am 2015;46:321–7.
[39] Shen C, Tang ZH, Hu JZ, Zou GY, Xiao RC, Yan DX. Does cross-linked polyethylene decrease the revision rate of total hip arthroplasty compared with conventional polyethylene? A meta-analysis. Orthop Traumatol Surg Res 2014;100:745–50.
[40] Callary SA, Solomon LB, Holubowycz OT, Campbell DG, Munn Z, Howie DW. Wear of highly crosslinked polyethylene acetabular components. Acta Orthop 2015;86:159–68.
[41] Kurtz SM, Gawel HA, Patel JD. History and systematic review of wear and osteolysis outcomes for first-generation highly crosslinked polyethylene. Clin Orthop Relat Res 2011;469:2262–77.
[42] Babovic N, Trousdale RT. Total hip arthroplasty using highly cross-linked polyethylene in patients younger than 50 years with minimum 10-year follow-up. J Arthroplasty 2013;28:815–17.
[43] Garvin KL, White TC, Dusad A, Hartman CW, Martell J. Low wear rates seen in THAs with highly crosslinked polyethylene at 9 to 14 years in patients younger than age 50 years. Clin Orthop Relat Res 2015;473:3829–35.

[44] Lachiewicz PF, Soileau ES, Martell JM. Wear and osteolysis of highly crosslinked polyethylene at 10 to 14 years: the effect of femoral head size. Clin Orthop Relat Res 2016;474(2):365–71.
[45] Glyn-Jones S, Thomas GE, Garfjeld-Roberts P, Gundle R, Taylor A, McLardy-Smith P, et al. The John Charnley award: highly crosslinked polyethylene in total hip arthroplasty decreases long-term wear: a double-blind randomized trial. Clin Orthop Relat Res 2015;473:432–8.
[46] Waewsawangwong W, Goodman SB. Unexpected failure of highly cross-linked polyethylene acetabular liner. J Arthroplasty 2012;27(323):e321–4.
[47] Tower SS, Currier JH, Currier BH, Lyford KA, Van Citters DW, Mayor MB. Rim cracking of the cross-linked longevity polyethylene acetabular liner after total hip arthroplasty. J Bone Joint Surg Am 2007;89:2212–17.
[48] Furmanski J, Anderson M, Bal S, Greenwald AS, Halley D, Penenberg B, et al. Clinical fracture of cross-linked UHMWPE acetabular liners. Biomaterials 2009;30:5572–82.
[49] Atwood SA, Van Citters DW, Patten EW, Furmanski J, Ries MD, Pruitt LA. Tradeoffs amongst fatigue, wear, and oxidation resistance of cross-linked ultra-high molecular weight polyethylene. J Mech Behav Biomed Mater 2011;4:1033–45.
[50] Gascoyne TC, Petrak MJ, Turgeon TR, Bohm ER. Wear of a sequentially annealed polyethylene acetabular liner. Acta Orthop 2014;85:470–3.
[51] Oral E, Muratoglu OK. Vitamin E diffused, highly crosslinked UHMWPE: a review. Int Orthop 2011;35:215–23.
[52] Hannouche D, Zaoui A, Zadegan F, Sedel L, Nizard R. Thirty years of experience with alumina-on-alumina bearings in total hip arthroplasty. Int Orthop 2011;35:207–13.
[53] D'Antonio JA, Capello WN, Naughton M. Ceramic bearings for total hip arthroplasty have high survivorship at 10 years. Clin Orthop Relat Res 2012;470:373–81.
[54] Yoon HJ, Yoo JJ, Yoon KS, Koo KH, Kim HJ. Alumina-on-alumina THA performed in patients younger than 30 years: a 10-year minimum followup study. Clin Orthop Relat Res 2012;470:3530–6.
[55] Jeffers JR, Walter WL. Ceramic-on-ceramic bearings in hip arthroplasty: state of the art and the future. J Bone Joint Surg Br 2012;94:735–45.
[56] Shetty V, Shitole B, Shetty G, Thakur H, Bhandari M. Optimal bearing surfaces for total hip replacement in the young patient: a meta-analysis. Int Orthop 2011;35:1281–7.
[57] Barrack RL, Burak C, Skinner HB. Concerns about ceramics in THA. Clin Orthop Relat Res 2004;429:73–9.
[58] Massin P, Lopes R, Masson B, Mainard D, French H, Knee S. Does Biolox Delta ceramic reduce the rate of component fractures in total hip replacement? Orthop Traumatol Surg Res 2014;100: S317–21.
[59] Mihalko WM, Wimmer MA, Pacione CA, Laurent MP, Murphy RF, Rider C. How have alternative bearings and modularity affected revision rates in total hip arthroplasty? Clin Orthop Relat Res 2014;472:3747–58.
[60] Milosev I, Kovac S, Trebse R, Levasic V, Pisot V. Comparison of ten-year survivorship of hip prostheses with use of conventional polyethylene, metal-on-metal, or ceramic-on-ceramic bearings. J Bone Joint Surg Am 2012;94:1756–63.
[61] Bozic KJ, Browne J, Dangles CJ, Manner PA, Yates Jr. AJ, Weber KL, et al. Modern metal-on-metal hip implants. J Am Acad Orthop Surg 2012;20:402–6.
[62] Fehring KA, Fehring TK. Modes of failure in metal-on-metal total hip arthroplasty. Orthop Clin North Am 2015;46:185–92.
[63] Bauer TW, Campbell PA, Hallerberg G, Biological Working G. How have new bearing surfaces altered the local biological reactions to byproducts of wear and modularity? Clin Orthop Relat Res 2014;472:3687–98.
[64] Berry DJ, Abdel MP, Callaghan JJ, Members of the Clinical Research G. What are the current clinical issues in wear and tribocorrosion? Clin Orthop Relat Res 2014;472:3659–64.
[65] Langton DJ, Jameson SS, Joyce TJ, Gandhi JN, Sidaginamale R, Mereddy P, et al. Accelerating failure rate of the ASR total hip replacement. J Bone Joint Surg Br 2011;93:1011–16.
[66] Smith DC. The genesis and evolution of acrylic bone cement. Orthop Clin North Am 2005;36:1–10.

[67] Kuehn KD, Ege W, Gopp U. Acrylic bone cements: composition and properties. Orthop Clin North Am 2005;36:17–28.
[68] Arora M, Chan EK, Gupta S, Diwan AD. Polymethylmethacrylate bone cements and additives: a review of the literature. World J Ortho 2013;4:67–74.
[69] Lee C. Properties of bone cement: the mechanical properties of PMMA bone cement. In: Breusch SMH, editor. The well-cemented total hip arthroplasty Theory and practice. Berlin: Springer; 2005. p. 60–78.
[70] Li J, Redmond AC, Jin Z, Fisher J, Stone MH, Stewart TD. Hip contact forces in asymptomatic total hip replacement patients differ from normal healthy individuals: Implications for preclinical testing. Clin Biomech (Bristol, Avon) 2014;29:747–51.
[71] van den Bogert AJ, Read L, Nigg BM. An analysis of hip joint loading during walking, running, and skiing. Med Sci Sports Exerc 1999;31:131–42.
[72] Schmalzried TP, Szuszczewicz ES, Northfield MR, Akizuki KH, Frankel RE, Belcher G, et al. Quantitative assessment of walking activity after total hip or knee replacement. J Bone Joint Surg Am 1998;80:54–9.
[73] Bedard NA, Callaghan JJ, Stefl MD, Liu SS. Systematic review of literature of cemented femoral components: what is the durability at minimum 20 years followup? Clin Orthop Relat Res 2015;473:563–71.
[74] Miller MA, Eberhardt AW, Cleary RJ, Verdonschot N, Mann KA. Micromechanics of postmortem-retrieved cement-bone interfaces. J Orthop Res 2010;28:170–7.
[75] Shelley P, Wroblewski BM. Socket design and cement pressurisation in the Charnley low-friction arthroplasty. J Bone Joint Surg Br 1988;70:358–63.
[76] Bhattacharya R, Attar FG, Green S, Port A. Comparison of cement pressurisation in flanged and unflanged acetabular cups. J Orthop Surg Res 2012;7:5.
[77] Huiskes R, Verdonschot N, Nivbrant B. Migration, stem shape, and surface finish in cemented total hip arthroplasty. Clin Orthop Relat Res 1998;355:103–12.
[78] Nieuwenhuijse MJ, Valstar ER, Kaptein BL, Nelissen RG. The Exeter femoral stem continues to migrate during its first decade after implantation: 10-12 years of follow-up with radiostereometric analysis (RSA). Acta Orthop 2012;83:129–34.
[79] Ling RS, Charity J, Lee AJ, Whitehouse SL, Timperley AJ, Gie GA. The long-term results of the original Exeter polished cemented femoral component: a follow-up report. J Arthroplasty 2009;24:511–17.
[80] Brigstocke GH, Mitchell PA, Rosson JW. Total hip arthroplasty with the MS-30 polished surface cemented stem: a single surgeon consecutive series study at 10 year follow-up. Eur J Orthop Surg Traumatol 2014;24:63–6.
[81] Janssen D, van Aken J, Scheerlinck T, Verdonschot N. Finite element analysis of the effect of cementing concepts on implant stability and cement fatigue failure. Acta Orthop 2009;80:319–24.
[82] Mau H, Schelling K, Heisel C, Wang JS, Breusch SJ. Comparison of various vacuum mixing systems and bone cements as regards reliability, porosity and bending strength. Acta Orthop Scand 2004;75:160–72.
[83] Messick KJ, Miller MA, Damron LA, Race A, Clarke MT, Mann KA. Vacuum-mixing cement does not decrease overall porosity in cemented femoral stems: an in vitro laboratory investigation. J Bone Joint Surg Br 2007;89:1115–21.
[84] Biau DJ, Latouche A, Porcher R. Competing events influence estimated survival probability: when is Kaplan-Meier analysis appropriate? Clin Orthop Relat Res 2007;462:229–33.
[85] Roberts VI, Esler CN, Harper WM. What impact have NICE guidelines had on the trends of hip arthroplasty since their publication? The results from the Trent Regional Arthroplasty Study between 1990 and 2005. J Bone Joint Surg Br 2007;89:864–7.
[86] Pakvis D, van Hellemondt G, de Visser E, Jacobs W, Spruit M. Is there evidence for a superior method of socket fixation in hip arthroplasty? A systematic review. Int Orthop 2011;35:1109–18.
[87] Stea S, Comfort T, Sedrakyan A, Havelin L, Marinelli M, Barber T, et al. Multinational comprehensive evaluation of the fixation method used in hip replacement: interaction with age in context. J Bone Joint Surg Am 2014;96(Suppl. 1):42–51.

[88] Berry DJ, Harmsen WS, Cabanela ME, Morrey BF. Twenty-five-year survivorship of two thousand consecutive primary Charnley total hip replacements: factors affecting survivorship of acetabular and femoral components. J Bone Joint Surg Am 2002;84-A:171–7.

[89] Aubault M, Druon J, Le Nail L, Rosset P. Outcomes at least 10 years after cemented PF(R) (Zimmer) total hip arthroplasty: 83 cases. Orthop Traumatol Surg Res 2013;99:S235–9.

[90] Martin CT, Callaghan JJ, Gao Y, Pugely AJ, Liu SS, Warth LC, et al. What can we learn from 20-year followup studies of hip replacement? Clin Orthop Relat Res 2016;474(2):402–7.

[91] Clauss M, Luem M, Ochsner PE, Ilchmann T. Fixation and loosening of the cemented Muller straight stem: a long-term clinical and radiological review. J Bone Joint Surg Br 2009;91:1158–63.

[92] de Jong PT, de Man FH, Haverkamp D, Marti RK. The long-term outcome of the cemented Weber acetabular component in total hip replacement using a second-generation cementing technique. J Bone Joint Surg Br 2009;91:31–6.

[93] Thomsen PB, Dalsgaard J, Vainorius D, Hansen TB. Acceptable long-term results after Boneloc hip arthroplasty. Dan Med J 2013;60:A4671.

[94] Wroblewski BM, Siney PD, Fleming PA. Charnley low-frictional torque arthroplasty in patients under the age of 51 years. Follow-up to 33 years. J Bone Joint Surg Br 2002;84:540–3.

[95] Nich C, Courpied JP, Kerboull M, Postel M, Hamadouche M. Charnley-Kerboull total hip arthroplasty for osteonecrosis of the femoral head a minimal 10-year follow-up study. J Arthroplasty 2006;21:533–40.

[96] Makela KT, Matilainen M, Pulkkinen P, Fenstad AM, Havelin L, Engesaeter L, et al. Failure rate of cemented and uncemented total hip replacements: register study of combined Nordic database of four nations. BMJ 2014;348:f7592.

[97] Jamsen E, Eskelinen A, Peltola M, Makela K. High early failure rate after cementless hip replacement in the octogenarian. Clin Orthop Relat Res 2014;472:2779–89.

[98] Pedersen AB, Mehnert F, Havelin LI, Furnes O, Herberts P, Karrholm J, et al. Association between fixation technique and revision risk in total hip arthroplasty patients younger than 55 years of age. Results from the Nordic Arthroplasty Register Association. Osteoarthritis Cartilage 2014;22:659–67.

[99] Kynaston-Pearson F, Ashmore AM, Malak TT, Rombach I, Taylor A, Beard D, et al. Primary hip replacement prostheses and their evidence base: systematic review of literature. BMJ 2013;347: f6956.

[100] Hirose S, Otsuka H, Morishima T, Sato K. Outcomes of Charnley total hip arthroplasty using improved cementing with so-called second- and third-generation techniques. J Orthop Sci 2012;17:118–23.

[101] Klapach AS, Callaghan JJ, Goetz DD, Olejniczak JP, Johnston RC. Charnley total hip arthroplasty with use of improved cementing techniques: a minimum twenty-year follow-up study. J Bone Joint Surg Am 2001;83-A:1840–8.

[102] Harris WH, Maloney WJ. Hybrid total hip arthroplasty. Clin Orthop Relat Res 1989;249:21–9.

[103] Berger RA, Kull LR, Rosenberg AG, Galante JO. Hybrid total hip arthroplasty: 7- to 10-year results. Clin Orthop Relat Res 1996;333:134–46.

[104] Clohisy JC, Harris WH. Primary hybrid total hip replacement, performed with insertion of the acetabular component without cement and a precoat femoral component with cement. An average ten-year follow-up study. J Bone Joint Surg Am 1999;81:247–55.

[105] Kim YH, Kook HK, Kim JS. Total hip replacement with a cementless acetabular component and a cemented femoral component in patients younger than fifty years of age. J Bone Joint Surg Am 2002;84-A:770–4.

[106] Firestone DE, Callaghan JJ, Liu SS, Goetz DD, Sullivan PM, Vittetoe DA, et al. Total hip arthroplasty with a cemented, polished, collared femoral stem and a cementless acetabular component. A follow-up study at a minimum of ten years. J Bone Joint Surg Am 2007;89:126–32.

[107] Jameson SS, Mason JM, Baker PN, Jettoo P, Deehan DJ, Reed MR. Factors influencing revision risk following 15 740 single-brand hybrid hip arthroplasties: a cohort study from a National Joint Registry. J Arthroplasty 2013;28:1152–9.

[108] Toossi N, Adeli B, Timperley AJ, Haddad FS, Maltenfort M, Parvizi J. Acetabular components in total hip arthroplasty: is there evidence that cementless fixation is better? J Bone Joint Surg Am 2013;95:168–74.
[109] Griffiths EJ, Stevenson D, Porteous MJ. Cost savings of using a cemented total hip replacement: an analysis of the National Joint Registry data. J Bone Joint Surg Br 2012;94:1032–5.
[110] Engh CA, Massin P, Suthers KE. Roentgenographic assessment of the biologic fixation of porous-surfaced femoral components. Clin Orthop Relat Res 1990;257:107–28.
[111] Engh CA, Hooten JP, Zettl-Schaffer KF, Ghaffarpour M, McGovern TF, Macalino GE, et al. Porous-coated total hip replacement. Clin Orthop Relat Res 1994;298:89–96.
[112] Furlong RJ, Osborn JF. Fixation of hip prostheses by hydroxyapatite ceramic coatings. J Bone Joint Surg Br 1991;73:741–5.
[113] D'Antonio JA, Capello WN, Jaffe WL. Hydroxylapatite-coated hip implants. Multicenter three-year clinical and roentgenographic results. Clin Orthop Relat Res 1992;285:102–15.
[114] Urban RM, Hall DJ, Della Valle C, Wimmer MA, Jacobs JJ, Galante JO. Successful long-term fixation and progression of osteolysis associated with first-generation cementless acetabular components retrieved post mortem. J Bone Joint Surg Am 2012;94:1877–85.
[115] Sychterz CJ, Claus AM, Engh CA. What we have learned about long-term cementless fixation from autopsy retrievals. Clin Orthop Relat Res 2002;405:79–91.
[116] von Knoch M, Engh CA, Sychterz CJ, Willert HG. Migration of polyethylene wear debris in one type of uncemented femoral component with circumferential porous coating: an autopsy study of 5 femurs. J Arthroplasty 2000;15:72–8.
[117] McAuley JP, Sychterz CJ, Engh CA. Influence of porous coating level on proximal femoral remodeling. A postmortem analysis. Clin Orthop Relat Res 2000;371:146–53.
[118] Maloney WJ, Sychterz C, Bragdon C, McGovern T, Jasty M, Engh CA, et al. The Otto Aufranc Award. Skeletal response to well fixed femoral components inserted with and without cement. Clin Orthop Relat Res 1996;333:15–26.
[119] Maloney WJ, Smith RL, Schmalzried TP, Chiba J, Huene D, Rubash H. Isolation and characterization of wear particles generated in patients who have had failure of a hip arthroplasty without cement. J Bone Joint Surg Am 1995;77:1301–10.
[120] Kurtz S, Ong K, Lau E, Mowat F, Halpern M. Projections of primary and revision hip and knee arthroplasty in the United States from 2005 to 2030. J Bone Joint Surg Am 2007;89:780–5.
[121] van de Groes SaW, de Waal Malefijt MC, Verdonschot N. Influence of preparation techniques to the strength of the bone-cement interface behind the flange in total knee arthroplasty. Knee 2013;20:186–90.
[122] Maistrelli GL, Antonelli L, Fornasier V, Mahomed N. Cement penetration with pulsed lavage versus syringe irrigation in total knee arthroplasty. Clin Orthop Relat Res 1995;312:261–5.
[123] Lutz MJ, Pincus PF, Whitehouse SL, Halliday BR. The effect of cement gun and cement syringe use on the tibial cement mantle in total knee arthroplasty. J Arthroplasty 2009;24:461–7.
[124] Silverman EJ, Landy DC, Massel DH, Kaimrajh DN, Latta LL, Robinson RP. The effect of viscosity on cement penetration in total knee arthroplasty, an application of the squeeze film effect. J Arthroplasty 2014;29:2039–42.
[125] Walker PS, Soudry M, Ewald FC, McVickar H. Control of cement penetration in total knee arthroplasty. Clin Orthop Relat Res 1984;185:155–64.
[126] Schlegel UJ, Bruckner T, Schneider M, Parsch D, Geiger F, Breusch SJ. Surface or full cementation of the tibial component in total knee arthroplasty: a matched-pair analysis of mid- to long-term results. Arch Orthop Trauma Surg 2015;135:703–8.
[127] Bohm E, Zhu N, Gu J, de Guia N, Linton C, Anderson T, et al. Does adding antibiotics to cement reduce the need for early revision in total knee arthroplasty? Clin Orthop Relat Res 2014;472:162–8.
[128] Wang H, Lou H, Zhang H, Jiang J, Liu K. Similar survival between uncemented and cemented fixation prostheses in total knee arthroplasty: a meta-analysis and systematic comparative analysis using registers. Knee Surg Sports Traumatol Arthrosc 2014;22:3191–7.
[129] Kim Y-H, Park J-W, Lim H-M, Park E-S. Cementless and cemented total knee arthroplasty in patients younger than fifty five years. Which is better? Int Orthop 2014;38:297–303.

[130] Cigada A, Cotogno G, Chiesa R. The ceramic-on-metal coupling in total hip replacements for young patients: a review study. J Appl Biomater Biomech 2011;9:2–10.

[131] Sheth U, Nguyen NA, Gaines S, Bhandari M, Mehlman CT, Klein G. New orthopedic devices and the FDA. J Long Term Eff Med Implants 2009;19:173–84.

[132] Kramer DB, Xu S, Kesselheim AS. How does medical device regulation perform in the United States and the European union? A systematic review. PLoS Med 2012;9:e1001276.

[133] Kramer DB, Xu S, Kesselheim AS. Regulation of medical devices in the United States and European Union. N Engl J Med 2012;366:848–55.

[134] Curfman GD, Redberg RF. Medical devices--balancing regulation and innovation. N Engl J Med 2011;365:975–7.

[135] Gelberman RH, Samson D, Mirza SK, Callaghan JJ, Pellegrini Jr. VD. Orthopaedic surgeons and the medical device industry: the threat to scientific integrity and the public trust. J Bone Joint Surg Am 2010;92:765–77.

[136] de Ana FJ, Umstead KA, Phillips GJ, Conner CP. Value driven innovation in medical device design: a process for balancing stakeholder voices. Ann Biomed Eng 2013;41:1811–21.

[137] Willert HG, Buchhorn GH, Fayyazi A, Flury R, Windler M, Koster G, et al. Metal-on-metal bearings and hypersensitivity in patients with artificial hip joints. A clinical and histomorphological study. J Bone Joint Surg Am 2005;87:28–36.

[138] Khatod M, Cafri G, Namba RS, Inacio MC, Paxton EW. Risk factors for total hip arthroplasty aseptic revision. J Arthroplasty 2014;29:1412–17.

[139] Nieuwenhuijse MJ, Nelissen RG, Schoones JW, Sedrakyan A. Appraisal of evidence base for introduction of new implants in hip and knee replacement: a systematic review of five widely used device technologies. BMJ 2014;349:g5133.

[140] Carragee EJ, Hurwitz EL, Weiner BK. A critical review of recombinant human bone morphogenetic protein-2 trials in spinal surgery: emerging safety concerns and lessons learned. Spine J 2011;11:471–91.

[141] Hsu WK, Mishra A, Rodeo SR, Fu F, Terry MA, Randelli P, et al. Platelet-rich plasma in orthopaedic applications: evidence-based recommendations for treatment. J Am Acad Orthop Surg 2013;21:739–48.

[142] Moraes VY, Lenza M, Tamaoki MJ, Faloppa F, Belloti JC. Platelet-rich therapies for musculoskeletal soft tissue injuries. Cochrane Database Syst Rev 2014;4:CD010071.

[143] Ergina PL, Barkun JS, McCulloch P, Cook JA, Altman DG, Group I. IDEAL framework for surgical innovation 2: observational studies in the exploration and assessment stages. BMJ 2013;346: f3011.

[144] McCulloch P, Altman DG, Campbell WB, Flum DR, Glasziou P, Marshall JC, et al. No surgical innovation without evaluation: the IDEAL recommendations. Lancet 2009;374:1105–12.

[145] Hofbauer M, Muller B, Murawski CD, Karlsson J, Fu FH. Innovation in orthopaedic surgery as it relates to evidence-based practice. Knee Surg Sports Traumatol Arthrosc 2013;21:511–14.

[146] Sussman MD. Ethical requirements that must be met before the introduction of new procedures. Clin Orthop Relat Res 2000;378:15–22.

[147] Bal BS, Brenner LH. Physician competence and skill part I: the role of hospital corporate liability. Clin Orthop Relat Res 2014;472:1089–92.

[148] Schemitsch EH, Bhandari M, Boden SD, Bourne RB, Bozic KJ, Jacobs JJ, et al. The evidence-based approach in bringing new orthopaedic devices to market. J Bone Joint Surg Am 2010;92:1030–7.

[149] Wright JG, Weinstein S. The innovation cycle: a framework for taking surgical innovation into clinical practice. J Bone Joint Surg Am 2013;95:e164.

[150] Malchau H, Bragdon CR, Muratoglu OK. The stepwise introduction of innovation into orthopedic surgery: the next level of dilemmas. J Arthroplasty 2011;26:825–31.

[151] Zywiel MG, Johnson AJ, Mont MA. Graduated introduction of orthopaedic implants: encouraging innovation and minimizing harm. J Bone Joint Surg Am 2012;94:e158.

[152] Buch B. FDA medical device approval: things you didn't learn in medical school or residency. Am J Orthop (Belle Mead NJ) 2007;36:407–12.

[153] Leunig M, Ganz R. The evolution and concepts of joint-preserving surgery of the hip. Bone Joint J 2014;96-B:5–18.
[154] Ettinger M, Berger S, Floerkemeier T, Windhagen H, Ezechieli M. Sports activity after treatment of residual hip dysplasia with triple pelvic osteotomy using the tonnis and kalchschmidt technique. Am J Sports Med 2015;43:715–20.
[155] Fukui K, Kaneuji A, Sugimori T, Ichiseki T, Matsumoto T. Does rotational acetabular osteotomy affect subsequent total hip arthroplasty? Arch Orthop Trauma Surg 2015;135:407–15.
[156] Hashemi-Nejad A, Haddad FS, Tong KM, Muirhead-Allwood SK, Catterall A. Does Chiari osteotomy compromise subsequent total hip arthroplasty? J Arthroplasty 2002;17:731–9.
[157] Issa K, Johnson AJ, Naziri Q, Khanuja HS, Delanois RE, Mont MA. Hip osteonecrosis: does prior hip surgery alter outcomes compared to an initial primary total hip arthroplasty? J Arthroplasty 2014;29:162–6.
[158] Brouwer RW, Huizinga MR, Duivenvoorden T, van Raaij TM, Verhagen AP, Bierma-Zeinstra SM, et al. Osteotomy for treating knee osteoarthritis. Cochrane Database Syst Rev 2014;12.
[159] Li Y, Zhang H, Zhang J, Li X, Song G, Feng H. Clinical outcome of simultaneous high tibial osteotomy and anterior cruciate ligament reconstruction for medial compartment osteoarthritis in young patients with anterior cruciate ligament-deficient knees: a systematic review. Arthroscopy 2015;31:507–19.
[160] Badawy M, Fenstad AM, Indrekvam K, Havelin LI, Furnes O. The risk of revision in total knee arthroplasty is not affected by previous high tibial osteotomy. Acta Orthop 2015;1–6.
[161] Halley DK, Charnley J. Results of low friction arthroplasty in patients thirty years of age or younger. Clin Orthop Relat Res 1975;112:180–91.
[162] Malcolm TL, Szubski CR, Nowacki AS, Klika AK, Iannotti JP, Barsoum WK. Activity levels and functional outcomes of young patients undergoing total hip arthroplasty. Orthopedics 2014;37: e983–992.
[163] Keeney JA, Nunley RM, Baca GR, Clohisy JC. Are younger patients undergoing THA appropriately characterized as active? Clin Orthop Relat Res 2015;473:1083–92.
[164] Cherian JJ, Jauregui JJ, Banerjee S, Pierce T, Mont MA. What host factors affect aseptic loosening after THA and TKA? Clin Orthop Relat Res 2015;473(8):2700–9.
[165] Tai CC, Cross MJ. Five- to 12-year follow-up of a hydroxyapatite-coated, cementless total knee replacement in young, active patients. J Bone Joint Surg Br 2006;88:1158–63.
[166] Nizard R, Pourreyron D, Raould A, Hannouche D, Sedel L. Alumina-on-alumina hip arthroplasty in patients younger than 30 years old. Clin Orthop Relat Res 2008;466:317–23.
[167] Bisschop R, Brouwer RW, Van Raay JJ. Total knee arthroplasty in younger patients: a 13-year follow-up study. Orthopedics 2010;33:876.
[168] Julin J, Jamsen E, Puolakka T, Konttinen YT, Moilanen T. Younger age increases the risk of early prosthesis failure following primary total knee replacement for osteoarthritis. A follow-up study of 32,019 total knee replacements in the Finnish Arthroplasty Register. Acta Orthop 2010;81:413–19.
[169] Odland AN, Callaghan JJ, Liu SS, Wells CW. Wear and lysis is the problem in modular TKA in the young OA patient at 10 years. Clin Orthop Relat Res 2011;469:41–7.
[170] Swarup I, Lee YY, Christoph EI, Mandl LA, Goodman SM, Figgie MP. Implant survival and patient-reported outcomes after total hip arthroplasty in young patients with juvenile idiopathic arthritis. J Arthroplasty 2015;30:398–402.
[171] Goodman SB, Hwang K, Imrie S. High complication rate in revision total hip arthroplasty in juvenile idiopathic arthritis. Clin Orthop Relat Res 2014;472:637–44.
[172] Imbuldeniya AM, Walter WL, Zicat BA, Walter WK. Cementless total hip replacement without femoral osteotomy in patients with severe developmental dysplasia of the hip: minimum 15-year clinical and radiological results. Bone Joint J 2014;96-B:1449–54.
[173] Cruz-Pardos A, Garcia-Rey E, Ortega-Chamarro J, Castro-Garcia F. Alumina-on-alumina hip replacement in developmental dysplasia of the hip. Hip Int 2010;20(Suppl. 7):S94–101.
[174] Elmallah RK, Cherian JJ, Jauregui JJ, Padden DA, Harwin SF, Mont MA. Robotic-arm assisted surgery in total hip arthroplasty. Surg Technol Int 2015;26:283–8.

[175] Adelani MA, Keeney JA, Palisch A, Fowler SA, Clohisy JC. Has total hip arthroplasty in patients 30 years or younger improved? A systematic review. Clin Orthop Relat Res 2013;471:2595–601.
[176] Khanuja HS, Banerjee S, Jain D, Pivec R, Mont MA. Short bone-conserving stems in cementless hip arthroplasty. J Bone Joint Surg Am 2014;96:1742–52.
[177] Goebel D, Schultz W. The Mayo cementless femoral component in active patients with osteoarthritis. Hip Int 2009;19:206–10.
[178] Ratner BD, Hoffman AS. Physicochemical surface modification of materials used in medicine. In: Ratner BDH, Hoffman AS, Schoen FJ, Lemons JE, editors. Biomaterials science an introduction to materials in medicine. 3rd ed. Oxford: Academic Press; 2013. p. 259–76.
[179] Frank RM, Fabi D, Levine BR. Modern porous coatings in orthopaedic applications. In: Nazarpour S, editor. Thin films and coatings in biology. Dordrecht: Springer; 2013. p. 69–104.
[180] Bose S, Tarafder S, Bandyopadhyay A. Hydroxyapatite coatings for metallic implants. In: Mucalo M, editor. Hydroxyapatite (HAp) for biomedical applications. Cambridge: Woodhead Publishing Elsevier Ltd; 2015. p. 143–58.
[181] Keeney JA, Martell JM, Pashos G, Nelson CJ, Maloney WJ, Clohisy JC. Highly cross-linked polyethylene improves wear and mid-term failure rates for young total hip arthroplasty patients. Hip Int 2015;25:435–41.
[182] Varnum C, Pedersen AB, Kjaersgaard-Andersen P, Overgaard S. Comparison of the risk of revision in cementless total hip arthroplasty with ceramic-on-ceramic and metal-on-polyethylene bearings. Acta Orthop 2015;86(4):477–84.
[183] Ilalov K, Cohn RM, Slover J. High-performance total knee replacement. Bull Hosp Jt Dis 2013;71:79–88.
[184] Nunley RM, Nam D, Berend KR, Lombardi AV, Dennis DA, Della Valle CJ, et al. New total knee arthroplasty designs: do young patients notice? Clin Orthop Relat Res 2015;473:101–8.
[185] Gioe TJ, Sharma A, Tatman P, Mehle S. Do "premium" joint implants add value?: analysis of high cost joint implants in a community registry. Clin Orthop Relat Res 2011;469:48–54.
[186] Kurtz SM, Lau E, Watson H, Schmier JK, Parvizi J. Economic burden of periprosthetic joint infection in the United States. J Arthroplasty 2012;27:61–5.
[187] Zmistowski B, Karam JA, Durinka JB, Casper DS, Parvizi J. Periprosthetic joint infection increases the risk of one-year mortality. J Bone Joint Surg Am 2013;95:2177–84.
[188] Tande AJ, Patel R. Prosthetic joint infection. Clin Microbiol Rev 2014;27:302–45.
[189] Witso E. The rate of prosthetic joint infection is underestimated in the arthroplasty registers. Acta Orthop 2015;86(3):277–8.
[190] Dale H, Hallan G, Hallan G, Espehaug B, Havelin LI, Engesaeter LB. Increasing risk of revision due to deep infection after hip arthroplasty. Acta Orthop 2009;80:639–45.
[191] Thiele K, Perka C, Matziolis G, Mayr HO, Sostheim M, Hube R. Current failure mechanisms after knee arthroplasty have changed: polyethylene wear is less common in revision surgery. J Bone Joint Surg Am 2015;97:715–20.
[192] Aggarwal VK, Bakhshi H, Ecker NU, Parvizi J, Gehrke T, Kendoff D. Organism profile in periprosthetic joint infection: pathogens differ at two arthroplasty infection referral centers in Europe and in the United States. J Knee Surg 2014;27(5):399–406.
[193] Lutro O, Langvatn H, Dale H, Schrama JC, Hallan G, Espehaug B, et al. Increasing resistance of coagulase-negative staphylococci in total hip arthroplasty infections: 278 THA-revisions due to infection reported to the norwegian arthroplasty register from 1993 to 2007. Adv Orthop 2014;2014:580359.
[194] Jamsen E, Furnes O, Engesaeter LB, Konttinen YT, Odgaard A, Stefansdottir A, et al. Prevention of deep infection in joint replacement surgery. Acta Orthop 2010;81:660–6.
[195] Ricciardi BF, Bostrom MP, Lidgren L, Ranstam J, Merollini KM, W-Dahl A. Prevention of surgical site infection in total joint arthroplasty: an international tertiary care center survey. HSS J 2014;10:45–51.
[196] Jamsen E, Nevalainen P, Eskelinen A, Huotari K, Kalliovalkama J, Moilanen T. Obesity, diabetes, and preoperative hyperglycemia as predictors of periprosthetic joint infection: a single-center

analysis of 7181 primary hip and knee replacements for osteoarthritis. J Bone Joint Surg Am 2012;94:e101.
[197] Gallo J, Holinka M, Moucha CS. Antibacterial surface treatment for orthopaedic implants. Int J Mol Sci 2014;15:13849–80.
[198] Ratner BD, Hoffman AS. Physicochemical surface modifications of materials used in medicine. In: Ratner BD, Hoffman AS, Schoen FJ, Lemons JE, editors. Biomaterials science: an introduction to materials in medicine. Waltham, MA: Academic Press (Elsevier); 2013. p. 259–76.
[199] Antoci Jr. V, King SB, Jose B, Parvizi J, Zeiger AR, Wickstrom E, et al. Vancomycin covalently bonded to titanium alloy prevents bacterial colonization. J Orthop Res 2007;25:858–66.
[200] Varisco M, Khanna N, Brunetto PS, Fromm KM. New antimicrobial and biocompatible implant coating with synergic silver-vancomycin conjugate action. ChemMedChem 2014;9:1221–30.
[201] Campoccia D, Montanaro L, Arciola CR. A review of the biomaterials technologies for infection-resistant surfaces. Biomaterials 2013;34:8533–54.
[202] Brennan SA, Ni Fhoghlu C, Devitt BM, O'Mahony FJ, Brabazon D, Walsh A. Silver nanoparticles and their orthopaedic applications. Bone Joint J 2015;97-B:582–9.
[203] Glehr M, Leithner A, Friesenbichler J, Goessler W, Avian A, Andreou D, et al. Argyria following the use of silver-coated megaprostheses: no association between the development of local argyria and elevated silver levels. Bone Joint J 2013;95-B:988–92.
[204] Grainger DW, van der Mei HC, Jutte PC, van den Dungen JJ, Schultz MJ, van der Laan BF, et al. Critical factors in the translation of improved antimicrobial strategies for medical implants and devices. Biomaterials 2013;34:9237–43.
[205] Springer BD. The diagnosis of periprosthetic joint infection. J Arthroplasty 2015;30(6):908–11.
[206] Minassian AM, Newnham R, Kalimeris E, Bejon P, Atkins BL, Bowler IC. Use of an automated blood culture system (BD BACTEC) for diagnosis of prosthetic joint infections: easy and fast. BMC Infect Dis 2014;14:233.
[207] Trampuz A, Piper KE, Jacobson MJ, Hanssen AD, Unni KK, Osmon DR, et al. Sonication of removed hip and knee prostheses for diagnosis of infection. N Engl J Med 2007;357:654–63.
[208] Zhai Z, Li H, Qin A, Liu G, Liu X, Wu C, et al. Meta-analysis of sonication fluid samples from prosthetic components for diagnosis of infection after total joint arthroplasty. J Clin Microbiol 2014;52:1730–6.
[209] Qu X, Zhai Z, Li H, Li H, Liu X, Zhu Z, et al. PCR-based diagnosis of prosthetic joint infection. J Clin Microbiol 2013;51:2742–6.
[210] Deirmengian C, Kardos K, Kilmartin P, Cameron A, Schiller K, Parvizi J. Diagnosing periprosthetic joint infection: has the era of the biomarker arrived? Clin Orthop Relat Res 2014;472:3254–62.
[211] Nodzo SR, Bauer T, Pottinger PS, Garrigues GE, Bedair H, Deirmengian CA, et al. Conventional diagnostic challenges in periprosthetic joint infection. J Am Acad Orthop Surg 2015;23(Suppl):S18–25.
[212] Della Valle C, Parvizi J, Bauer TW, Dicesare PE, Evans RP, Segreti J, et al. Diagnosis of periprosthetic joint infections of the hip and knee. J Am Acad Orthop Surg 2010;18:760–70.
[213] Romano CL, Romano D, Bonora C, Degrate A, Mineo G. Combined Diagnostic Tool for joint prosthesis infections. Infez Med 2009;17:141–50.
[214] Haddad FS, Sukeik M, Alazzawi S. Is single-stage revision according to a strict protocol effective in treatment of chronic knee arthroplasty infections? Clin Orthop Relat Res 2015;473:8–14.
[215] McConoughey SJ, Howlin R, Granger JF, Manring MM, Calhoun JH, Shirtliff M, et al. Biofilms in periprosthetic orthopedic infections. Future Microbiol 2014;9:987–1007.
[216] Bozic KJ, Kamath AF, Ong K, Lau E, Kurtz S, Chan V, et al. Comparative epidemiology of revision arthroplasty: failed THA poses greater clinical and economic burdens than failed TKA. Clin Orthop Relat Res 2015;473:2131–8.
[217] Di Puccio F, Mattei L. Biotribology of artificial hip joints. World J Orthop 2015;6:77–94.
[218] Wimmer MA, Laurent MP. Tribology of the artificial hip joint. In: Berry DJ, Lieberman JR, editors. Surgery of the hip. Philadelphia, PA: Elsevier Saunders; 2013. p. 35–53.

[219] McKellop HA. The lexicon of polyethylene wear in artificial joints. Biomaterials 2007;28:5049–57.
[220] Hood RW, Wright TM, Burstein AH. Retrieval analysis of total knee prostheses: a method and its application to 48 total condylar prostheses. J Biomed Mater Res 1983;17:829–42.
[221] Abdel MP, Gesell MW, Hoedt CW, Meyers KN, Wright TM, Haas SB. Polished trays reduce backside wear independent of post location in posterior-stabilized TKAs. Clin Orthop Relat Res 2014;472:2477–82.
[222] Willert HG, Semlitsch M. Reactions of the articular capsule to wear products of artificial joint prostheses. J Biomed Mater Res 1977;11:157–64.
[223] Harris WH. Osteolysis and particle disease in hip replacement. A review. Acta Orthop Scand 1994;65:113–23.
[224] Konttinen YT, Pajarinen J, Takakubo Y, Gallo J, Nich C, Takagi M, et al. Macrophage polarization and activation in response to implant debris: influence by "particle disease" and "ion disease". J Long Term Eff Med Implants 2014;24:267–81.
[225] Gallo J, Goodman SB, Konttinen YT, Raska M. Particle disease: biologic mechanisms of periprosthetic osteolysis in total hip arthroplasty. Innate Immun 2013;19:213–24.
[226] Schmalzried TP, Jasty M, Harris WH. Periprosthetic bone loss in total hip arthroplasty. Polyethylene wear debris and the concept of the effective joint space. J Bone Joint Surg Am 1992;74:849–63.
[227] Aspenberg P, van der Vis H. Fluid pressure may cause periprosthetic osteolysis. Particles are not the only thing. Acta Orthop Scand 1998;69:1–4.
[228] Fisher J, Bell J, Barbour PS, Tipper JL, Matthews JB, Besong AA, et al. A novel method for the prediction of functional biological activity of polyethylene wear debris. Proc Inst Mech Eng H 2001;215:127–32.
[229] Green TR, Fisher J, Stone M, Wroblewski BM, Ingham E. Polyethylene particles of a 'critical size' are necessary for the induction of cytokines by macrophages in vitro. Biomaterials 1998;19:2297–302.
[230] Baxter RM, MacDonald DW, Kurtz SM, Steinbeck MJ. Characteristics of highly cross-linked polyethylene wear debris in vivo. J Biomed Mater Res B Appl Biomater 2013;101:467–75.
[231] Catelas I, Jacobs JJ. Biologic activity of wear particles. Instr Course Lect 2010;59:3–16.
[232] Greenfield EM, Beidelschies MA, Tatro JM, Goldberg VM, Hise AG. Bacterial pathogen-associated molecular patterns stimulate biological activity of orthopaedic wear particles by activating cognate Toll-like receptors. J Biol Chem 2010;285:32378–84.
[233] Maitra R, Clement CC, Scharf B, Crisi GM, Chitta S, Paget D, et al. Endosomal damage and TLR2 mediated inflammasome activation by alkane particles in the generation of aseptic osteolysis. Mol Immunol 2009;47:175–84.
[234] Gibon E, Yao Z, Rao AJ, Zwingenberger S, Batke B, Valladares R, et al. Effect of a CCR1 receptor antagonist on systemic trafficking of MSCs and polyethylene particle-associated bone loss. Biomaterials 2012;33:3632–8.
[235] Lin TH, Tamaki Y, Pajarinen J, Waters HA, Woo DK, Yao Z, et al. Chronic inflammation in biomaterial-induced periprosthetic osteolysis: NF-kappaB as a therapeutic target. Acta Biomater 2014;10:1–10.
[236] Purdue PE, Crotti TN, Shen Z, Swantek J, Li J, Hill J, et al. Comprehensive profiling analysis of actively resorbing osteoclasts identifies critical signaling pathways regulated by bone substrate. Sci Rep 2014;4:7595.
[237] O'Neill SC, Queally JM, Devitt BM, Doran PP, O'Byrne JM. The role of osteoblasts in periprosthetic osteolysis. Bone Joint J 2013;95-B:1022–6.
[238] Engh CA, Ho H, Powers CC, Huynh C, Beykirch SE, Hopper Jr. RH. Osteolysis propensity among bilateral total hip arthroplasty patients. J Arthroplasty 2011;26:555–61.
[239] Greenfield EM. Do genetic susceptibility, toll-like receptors, and pathogen-associated molecular patterns modulate the effects of wear? Clin Orthop Relat Res 2014;472(12):3709–17.
[240] Del Buono A, Denaro V, Maffulli N. Genetic susceptibility to aseptic loosening following total hip arthroplasty: a systematic review. Br Med Bull 2012;101:39–55.

[241] Gallo J, Slouf M, Goodman SB. The relationship of polyethylene wear to particle size, distribution, and number: a possible factor explaining the risk of osteolysis after hip arthroplasty. J Biomed Mater Res B Appl Biomater 2010;94:171–7.
[242] Huang CH, Lu YC, Chang TK, Hsiao IL, Su YC, Yeh ST, et al. In vivo biological response to highly cross-linked and vitamin e-doped polyethylene-a particle-Induced osteolysis animal study. J Biomed Mater Res B Appl Biomater 2016;104:561–7.
[243] Bichara DA, Malchau E, Sillesen NH, Cakmak S, Nielsen GP, Muratoglu OK. Vitamin E-diffused highly cross-linked UHMWPE particles induce less osteolysis compared to highly cross-linked virgin UHMWPE particles in vivo. J Arthroplasty 2014;29:232–7.
[244] Kim YH, Park JW, Kulkarni SS, Kim YH. A randomised prospective evaluation of ceramic-on-ceramic and ceramic-on-highly cross-linked polyethylene bearings in the same patients with primary cementless total hip arthroplasty. Int Orthop 2013;37:2131–7.
[245] Kim YH, Park JW. Comparison of highly cross-linked and conventional polyethylene in posterior cruciate-substituting total knee arthroplasty in the same patients. J Bone Joint Surg Am 2014;96:1807–13.
[246] Voigt J, Mosier M. Cemented all-polyethylene and metal-backed polyethylene tibial components used for primary total knee arthroplasty: a systematic review of the literature and meta-analysis of randomized controlled trials involving 1798 primary total knee implants. J Bone Joint Surg Am 2011;93:1790–8.
[247] Manley MT, D'Antonio JA, Capello WN, Edidin AA. Osteolysis: a disease of access to fixation interfaces. Clin Orthop Relat Res 2002;405:129–37.
[248] Lewallen EA, Riester SM, Bonin CA, Kremers HM, Dudakovic A, Kakar S, et al. Biological strategies for improved osseointegration and osteoinduction of porous metal orthopedic implants. Tissue Eng Part B Rev 2015;21:218–30.
[249] Gallo J, Havranek V, Zapletalova J. Risk factors for accelerated polyethylene wear and osteolysis in ABG I total hip arthroplasty. Int Orthop 2010;34:19–26.
[250] Sorensen PA, Kiil S, Dam-Johansen K, Weinell CE. Anticorrosive coatings: a review. J Coat Technol Res 2009;6:135–76.
[251] Goodman SB, Gibon E, Pajarinen J, Lin TH, Keeney M, Ren PG, et al. Novel biological strategies for treatment of wear particle-induced periprosthetic osteolysis of orthopaedic implants for joint replacement. J R Soc Interface 2014;11:20130962.
[252] Bozic KJ, Kamath AF, Ong K, Lau E, Kurtz S, Chan V, et al. Comparative epidemiology of revision arthroplasty: failed THA poses greater clinical and economic burdens than failed TKA. Clin Orthop Relat Res 2014;473(6):2131–8.
[253] Jo S, Jimenez Almonte JH, Sierra RJ. The cumulative risk of re-dislocation after revision THA performed for instability increases close to 35% at 15 years. J Arthroplasty 2015;30(7):1177–82.
[254] Berry DJ. Dislocation. In: Steinberg ME, Garino JP, editors. Revision total hip arthroplasty. Philadelphia, PA: Lippincott Williams & Wilkins; 1999. p. 463–81.
[255] Lewinnek GE, Lewis JL, Tarr R, Compere CL, Zimmerman JR. Dislocations after total hip-replacement arthroplasties. J Bone Joint Surg Am 1978;60:217–20.
[256] Olerud S, Karlstrom G. Recurrent dislocation after total hip replacement. Treatment by fixing an additional sector to the acetabular component. J Bone Joint Surg Br 1985;67:402–5.
[257] Woo RY, Morrey BF. Dislocations after total hip arthroplasty. J Bone Joint Surg Am 1982;64:1295–306.
[258] Rogers M, Blom AW, Barnett A, Karantana A, Bannister GC. Revision for recurrent dislocation of total hip replacement. Hip Int 2009;19:109–13.
[259] Philippot R, Camilleri JP, Boyer B, Adam P, Farizon F. The use of a dual-articulation acetabular cup system to prevent dislocation after primary total hip arthroplasty: analysis of 384 cases at a mean follow-up of 15 years. Int Orthop 2009;33:927–32.
[260] Epinette JA, Beracassat R, Tracol P, Pagazani G, Vandenbussche E. Are modern dual mobility cups a valuable option in reducing instability after primary hip arthroplasty, even in younger patients? J Arthroplasty 2014;29:1323–8.

[261] Langlais FL, Ropars M, Gaucher F, Musset T, Chaix O. Dual mobility cemented cups have low dislocation rates in THA revisions. Clin Orthop Relat Res 2008;466:389–95.
[262] Guyen O, Pibarot V, Vaz G, Chevillotte C, Bejui-Hugues J. Use of a dual mobility socket to manage total hip arthroplasty instability. Clin Orthop Relat Res 2009;467:465–72.
[263] Hamadouche M, Biau DJ, Huten D, Musset T, Gaucher F. The use of a cemented dual mobility socket to treat recurrent dislocation. Clin Orthop Relat Res 2010;468:3248–54.
[264] Leiber-Wackenheim F, Brunschweiler B, Ehlinger M, Gabrion A, Mertl P. Treatment of recurrent THR dislocation using of a cementless dual-mobility cup: a 59 cases series with a mean 8 years' follow-up. Orthop Traumatol Surg Res 2011;97:8–13.
[265] Schneider L, Philippot R, Boyer B, Farizon F. Revision total hip arthroplasty using a reconstruction cage device and a cemented dual mobility cup. Orthop Traumatol Surg Res 2011;97:807–13.
[266] Civinini R, Carulli C, Matassi F, Nistri L, Innocenti M. A dual-mobility cup reduces risk of dislocation in isolated acetabular revisions. Clin Orthop Relat Res 2012;470:3542–8.
[267] Hailer NP, Weiss RJ, Stark A, Karrholm J. Dual-mobility cups for revision due to instability are associated with a low rate of re-revisions due to dislocation: 228 patients from the Swedish. Hip Arthroplasty Register. Acta Arthop 2012;83:566–71.
[268] Combes A, Migaud H, Girard J, Duhamel A, Fessy MH. Low rate of dislocation of dual-mobility cups in primary total hip arthroplasty. Clin Orthop Relat Res 2013;471:3891–900.
[269] Philippot R, Meucci JF, Boyer B, Farizon F. Modern dual-mobility cup implanted with an uncemented stem: about 100 cases with 12-year follow-up. Surg Technol Int 2013;23:208–12.
[270] Mohammed R, Hayward K, Mulay S, Bindi F, Wallace M. Outcomes of dual-mobility acetabular cup for instability in primary and revision total hip arthroplasty. J Orthop Traumatol 2015;16:9–13.
[271] Berend KR, Sporer SM, Sierra RJ, Glassman AH, Morris MJ. Achieving stability and lower-limb length in total hip arthroplasty. J Bone Joint Surg Am 2010;92:2737–52.
[272] Bremner BR, Goetz DD, Callaghan JJ, Capello WN, Johnston RC. Use of constrained acetabular components for hip instability: an average 10-year follow-up study. J Arthroplasty 2003;18:131–7.
[273] Shapiro GS, Weiland DE, Markel DC, Padgett DE, Sculco TP, Pellicci PM. The use of a constrained acetabular component for recurrent dislocation. J Arthroplasty 2003;18:250–8.
[274] Shrader MW, Parvizi J, Lewallen DG. The use of a constrained acetabular component to treat instability after total hip arthroplasty. J Bone Joint Surg Am 2003;85-A:2179–83.
[275] Berend KR, Lombardi Jr. AV, Mallory TH, Adams JB, Russell JH, Groseth KL. The long-term outcome of 755 consecutive constrained acetabular components in total hip arthroplasty examining the successes and failures. J Arthroplasty 2005;20:93–102.
[276] Della Valle CJ, Chang D, Sporer S, Berger RA, Rosenberg AG, Paprosky WG. High failure rate of a constrained acetabular liner in revision total hip arthroplasty. J Arthroplasty 2005;20:103–7.
[277] Noble PC, Durrani SK, Usrey MM, Mathis KB, Bardakos NV. Constrained cups appear incapable of meeting the demands of revision THA. Clin Orthop Relat Res 2012;470:1907–16.
[278] Andersen AV, Kjersgaard AG, Solgaard S. Trilogy-constrained acetabular component for recurrent dislocation. ISRN Orthop 2013;2013:629201.
[279] Lehil MS, Bozic KJ. Trends in total hip arthroplasty implant utilization in the United States. J Arthroplasty 2014;29:1915–18.
[280] Tanne JH. FDA warns about metal-on-metal hip replacements. BMJ 2013;346:f429.
[281] Allen CL, Hooper GJ, Frampton CM. Do larger femoral heads improve the functional outcome in total hip arthroplasty? J Arthroplasty 2014;29:401–4.
[282] Penny JO, Ovesen O, Varmarken JE, Overgaard S. Similar range of motion and function after resurfacing large-head or standard total hip arthroplasty. Acta Orthop 2013;84:246–53.
[283] Howie DW, Holubowycz OT, Middleton R, Large Articulation Study G. Large femoral heads decrease the incidence of dislocation after total hip arthroplasty: a randomized controlled trial. J Bone Joint Surg Am 2012;94:1095–102.
[284] Johnson AJ, Loving L, Herrera L, Delanois RE, Wang A, Mont MA. Short-term wear evaluation of thin acetabular liners on 36-mm femoral heads. Clin Orthop Relat Res 2014;472:624–9.

[285] Zietz C, Fabry C, Middelborg L, Fulda G, Mittelmeier W, Bader R. Wear testing and particle characterisation of sequentially crosslinked polyethylene acetabular liners using different femoral head sizes. J Mater Sci Mater Med 2013;24:2057–65.
[286] Kelly NH, Rajadhyaksha AD, Wright TM, Maher SA, Westrich GH. High stress conditions do not increase wear of thin highly crosslinked UHMWPE. Clin Orthop Relat Res 2010;468:418–23.
[287] Lavernia CJ, Iacobelli DA, Villa JM, Jones K, Gonzalez JL, Jones WK. Trunnion-head stresses in THA: are big heads trouble? J Arthroplasty 2015;30(6):1085–8.
[288] Bosker BH, Ettema HB, van Rossum M, Boomsma MF, Kollen BJ, Maas M, et al. Pseudotumor formation and serum ions after large head metal-on-metal stemmed total hip replacement. Risk factors, time course and revisions in 706 hips. Arch Orthop Trauma Surg 2015;135:417–25.
[289] Browne JA, Polga DJ, Sierra RJ, Trousdale RT, Cabanela ME. Failure of larger-diameter metal-on-metal total hip arthroplasty resulting from anterior iliopsoas impingement. J Arthroplasty 2011;26(978):e975–978.
[290] Si HB, Zeng Y, Cao F, Pei FX, Shen B. Is a ceramic-on-ceramic bearing really superior to ceramic-on-polyethylene for primary total hip arthroplasty? A systematic review and meta-analysis of randomised controlled trials. Hip Int 2015;5(3):191–8.
[291] Senturk U, Perka C. Ceramic-on-Ceramic Bearings in Total Hip Arthroplasty (THA). Z Orthop Unfall 2015;153:198–202.
[292] Fisher J. Bioengineering reasons for the failure of metal-on-metal hip prostheses: an engineer's perspective. J Bone Joint Surg Br 2011;93:1001–4.
[293] Haddad FS, Thakrar RR, Hart AJ, Skinner JA, Nargol AV, Nolan JF, et al. Metal-on-metal bearings: the evidence so far. J Bone Joint Surg Br 2011;93:572–9.
[294] Cadossi M, Mazzotti A, Baldini N, Giannini S, Savarino L. New couplings, old problems: is there a role for ceramic-on-metal hip arthroplasty? J Biomed Mater Res B Appl Biomater 2016;104:204–9.
[295] Hill JC, Diamond OJ, O'Brien S, Boldt JG, Stevenson M, Beverland DE. Early surveillance of ceramic-on-metal total hip arthroplasty. Bone Joint J 2015;97-B:300–5.
[296] Alakoski E, Tiainen VM, Soininen A, Konttinen YT. Load-bearing biomedical applications of diamond-like carbon coatings—current status. Open Orthop J 2008;2:43–50.
[297] Hauert R, Falub CV, Thorwarth G, Thorwarth K, Affolter C, Stiefel M, et al. Retrospective lifetime estimation of failed and explanted diamond-like carbon coated hip joint balls. Acta Biomater 2012;8:3170–6.
[298] Kurtz SM. Nevelos. J. Arthroplasty bearing surfaces. PEEK biomaterials handbook. Oxford: PDL Elsevier; 2012. p. 261–76.
[299] Lorber V, Paulus AC, Buschmann A, Schmitt B, Grupp TM, Jansson V, et al. Elevated cytokine expression of different PEEK wear particles compared to UHMWPE in vivo. J Mater Sci Mater Med 2014;25:141–9.
[300] Li CS, Vannabouathong C, Sprague S, Bhandari M. The use of carbon-fiber-reinforced (CFR) PEEK material in orthopedic implants: a systematic review. Clin Med Insights Arthritis Musculoskelet Disord 2015;8:33–45.
[301] Howling GI, Ingham E, Sakoda H, Stewart TD, Fisher J, Antonarulrajah A, et al. Carbon-carbon composite bearing materials in hip arthroplasty: analysis of wear and biological response to wear debris. J Mater Sci Mater Med 2004;15:91–8.
[302] Esposito CI, Wright TM, Goodman SB, Berry DJ, Clinical B, Bioengineering Study Groups from Carl TBW. What is the trouble with trunnions? Clin Orthop Relat Res 2014;472:3652–8.
[303] Khair MM, Nam D, DiCarlo E, Su E. Aseptic lymphocyte dominated vasculitis-associated lesion resulting from trunnion corrosion in a cobalt-chrome unipolar hemiarthroplasty. J Arthroplasty 2013;28(196):e111–194.
[304] Werner PH, Ettema HB, Witt F, Morlock MM, Verheyen CC. Basic principles and uniform terminology for the head-neck junction in hip replacement. Hip Int 2015;25:115–19.
[305] Epinette JA, Manley MT. Hydroxyapatite-coated total knee replacement: clinical experience at 10 to 15 years. J Bone Joint Surg Br 2007;89:34–8.

[306] Attar FG, Khaw F-M, Kirk LMG, Gregg PJ. Survivorship analysis at 15 years of cemented press-fit condylar total knee arthroplasty. J Arthroplasty 2008;23:344–9.
[307] Melton JTK, Mayahi R, Baxter SE, Facek M, Glezos C. Long-term outcome in an uncemented, hydroxyapatite-coated total knee replacement: a 15- to 18-year survivorship analysis. J Bone Joint Surg Br 2012;94:1067–70.
[308] McLaughlin JR, Lee KR. The outcome of total hip replacement in obese and non-obese patients at 10- to 18-years. J Bone Joint Surg Br 2006;88:1286–92.
[309] El Masri F, Kerboull L, Kerboull M, Courpied JP, Hamadouche M. Is the so-called 'French paradox' a reality?: long-term survival and migration of the Charnley-Kerboull stem cemented line-to-line. J Bone Joint Surg Br 2010;92:342–8.
[310] Nashi N, Hong CC, Krishna L. Residual knee pain and functional outcome following total knee arthroplasty in osteoarthritic patients. Knee Surg Sports Traumatol Arthrosc 2014;23(6):1841–7.
[311] Wylde V, Hewlett S, Learmonth ID, Dieppe P. Persistent pain after joint replacement: prevalence, sensory qualities, and postoperative determinants. Pain 2011;152:566–72.
[312] Beswick AD, Wylde V, Gooberman-Hill R, Blom A, Dieppe P. What proportion of patients report long-term pain after total hip or knee replacement for osteoarthritis? A systematic review of prospective studies in unselected patients. BMJ Open 2012;2(1):e000435.
[313] Yercan HS, Sugun TS, Bussiere C, Ait Si Selmi T, Davies A, Neyret P. Stiffness after total knee arthroplasty: prevalence, management and outcomes. Knee 2006;13:111–17.
[314] Zmistowski B, Restrepo C, Kahl LK, Parvizi J, Sharkey PF. Incidence and reasons for nonrevision reoperation after total knee arthroplasty. Clin Orthop Relat Res 2011;469:138–45.
[315] Kim J, Nelson CL, Lotke PA. Stiffness after total knee arthroplasty. Prevalence of the complication and outcomes of revision. J Bone Joint Surg Am 2004;86-A:1479–84.
[316] Mauerhan DR, Mokris JG, Ly A, Kiebzak GM. Relationship between length of stay and manipulation rate after total knee arthroplasty. J Arthroplasty 1998;13:896–900.
[317] Rubinstein RA, DeHaan A. The incidence and results of manipulation after primary total knee arthroplasty. Knee 2010;17:29–32.
[318] Fox JL, Poss R. The role of manipulation following total knee replacement. J Bone Joint Surg Am 1981;63:357–62.
[319] Esler CN, Lock K, Harper WM, Gregg PJ. Manipulation of total knee replacements. Is the flexion gained retained? J Bone Joint Surg Br 1999;81:27–9.
[320] Daluga D, Lombardi AV, Mallory TH, Vaughn BK. Knee manipulation following total knee arthroplasty. Analysis of prognostic variables. J Arthroplasty 1991;6:119–28.
[321] Aglietti P, Sensi L, Cuomo P, Ciardullo A. Rotational position of femoral and tibial components in TKA using the femoral transepicondylar axis. Clin Orthop Relat Res 2008;466:2751–5.
[322] Bozic KJ, Kurtz SM, Lau E, Ong K, Chiu V, Vail TP, et al. The epidemiology of revision total knee arthroplasty in the United States. Clin Orthop Relat Res 2009;468:45–51.
[323] Le DH, Goodman SB, Maloney WJ, Huddleston JI. Current modes of failure in TKA: infection, instability, and stiffness predominate. Clin Orthop Relat Res 2014;472:2197–200.
[324] Siqueira MB, Klika AK, Higuera CA, Barsoum WK. Modes of failure of total knee arthroplasty: registries and realities. J Knee Surg 2015;28:127–38.
[325] van Kempen RWTM, Schimmel JJP, van Hellemondt GG, Vandenneucker H, Wymenga AB. Reason for revision TKA predicts clinical outcome: prospective evaluation of 150 consecutive patients with 2-years followup. Clin Orthop Relat Res 2013;471:2296–302.
[326] Kasahara Y, Majima T, Kimura S, Nishiike O, Uchida J. What are the causes of revision total knee arthroplasty in Japan? Clin Orthop Relat Res 2013;471:1533–8.
[327] McGrory BJ, Bal BS, York S, Macaulay W, McConnell DB. Surgeon demographics and medical malpractice in adult reconstruction. Clin Orthop Relat Res 2009;467:358–66.
[328] McWilliams AB, Douglas SL, Redmond AC, Grainger AJ, O'Connor PJ, Stewart TD, et al. Litigation after hip and knee replacement in the National Health Service. Bone Joint J 2013;95-B:122–6.
[329] Gibon E, Farman T, Marmor S. Knee arthroplasty and lawsuits: the experience in France. Knee Surg Sports Traumatol Arthrosc 2015;23:3723–8.

[330] Babis GCM, Morrey BF, Trousdale RT. The young patient: indications and results. In: Morrey BF, Berry DJ, editors. Joint replacement arthroplasty. Philadelphia, PA: Lippincott Williams and Wilkins, a Wolters Kluwer business; 2011. p. 537−49.
[331] Kammerlander C, Erhart S, Doshi H, Gosch M, Blauth M. Principles of osteoporotic fracture treatment. Best Pract Res Clin Rheumatol 2013;27:757−69.
[332] Russell LA. Osteoporosis and orthopedic surgery: effect of bone health on total joint arthroplasty outcome. Curr Rheumatol Rep 2013;15:371.
[333] Piarulli G, Rossi A, Zatti G. Osseointegration in the elderly. Aging Clin Exp Res 2013;25(Suppl. 1): S59−60.
[334] Neumann D, Dueckelmann L, Thaler C, Dorn U. Revision total hip arthroplasty using a cementless tapered revision stem in patients with a mean age of 82 years. Int Orthop 2012;36:961−5.
[335] Rickman M, Young J, Trompeter A, Pearce R, Hamilton M. Managing acetabular fractures in the elderly with fixation and primary arthroplasty: aiming for early weightbearing. Clin Orthop Relat Res 2014;472:3375−82.
[336] Spinarelli A, Petrera M, Vicenti G, Pesce V, Patella V. Total knee arthroplasty in elderly osteoporotic patients. Aging Clin Exp Res 2011;23:78−80.
[337] Brasenger Jr. RD. Clinical features of rheumatoid arthritis. In: Hochberg MC, Silman AJ, Smolen JS, Weinblatt ME, Weisman MH, editors. Rheumatology. Philadelphia, PA: Mosby Elsevier; 2011. p. 829−37.
[338] Görtz S, Fricka KB, Bugbee WD. The hip. In: Hochberg MC, Silman AJ, Smolen JS, Weinblatt ME, Weisman MH, editors. Rheumatology. 5th ed. Philadelphia, PA: Mosby Elsevier; 2011. p. 719−28.
[339] Jung SM, Kim KW, Yang CW, Park SH, Ju JH. Cytokine-mediated bone destruction in rheumatoid arthritis. J Immunol Res 2014;2014:263625.
[340] Rud-Sorensen C, Pedersen AB, Johnsen SP, Riis AH, Overgaard S. Survival of primary total hip arthroplasty in rheumatoid arthritis patients. Acta Orthop 2010;81:60−5.
[341] Bause L. Short stem total hip arthroplasty in patients with rheumatoid arthritis. Orthopedics 2015;38:S46−50.
[342] Hofstede SN, Nouta KA, Jacobs W, van Hooff ML, Wymenga AB, Pijls BG, et al. Mobile bearing vs fixed bearing prostheses for posterior cruciate retaining total knee arthroplasty for postoperative functional status in patients with osteoarthritis and rheumatoid arthritis. Cochrane Database Syst Rev 2015;2:CD003130.
[343] Zwartele R, Poll RG. Cemented total hip arthroplasty in rheumatoid arthritis. A systematic review of the literature. Hip Int 2013;23:111−22.
[344] Zwartele RE, Witjes S, Doets HC, Stijnen T, Poll RG. Cementless total hip arthroplasty in rheumatoid arthritis: a systematic review of the literature. Arch Orthop Trauma Surg 2012;132:535−46.
[345] Judge A, Arden NK, Cooper C, Kassim Javaid M, Carr AJ, Field RE, et al. Predictors of outcomes of total knee replacement surgery. Rheumatology 2012;51:1804−13.
[346] Schrama JC, Espehaug B, Hallan G, Engesaeter LB, Furnes O, Havelin LI, et al. Risk of revision for infection in primary total hip and knee arthroplasty in patients with rheumatoid arthritis compared with osteoarthritis: a prospective, population-based study on 108,786 hip and knee joint arthroplasties from the Norwegian Arthroplasty Register. Arthritis Care Res 2010;62:473−9.
[347] Sidler-Maier CC, Waddell JP. Incidence and predisposing factors of periprosthetic proximal femoral fractures: a literature review. Int Orthop 2015;39:1673−82.
[348] Lee JK, Kee YM, Chung HK, Choi CH. Long-term results of cruciate-retaining total knee replacement in patients with rheumatoid arthritis: a minimum 15-year review. Can J Surg 2015;58:193−7.
[349] van der Jagt D, Mokete L, Pietrzak J, Zalavras CG, Lieberman JR. Osteonecrosis of the femoral head: evaluation and treatment. J Am Acad Orthop Surg 2015;23:69−70.
[350] Arlot ME, Bonjean M, Chavassieux PM, Meunier PJ. Bone histology in adults with aseptic necrosis. Histomorphometric evaluation of iliac biopsies in seventy-seven patients. J Bone Joint Surg Am 1983;65:1319−27.

[351] Calder JD, Pearse MF, Revell PA. The extent of osteocyte death in the proximal femur of patients with osteonecrosis of the femoral head. J Bone Joint Surg Br 2001;83:419–22.
[352] Felden A, Vaz G, Kreps S, Anract P, Hamadouche M, Biau DJ. A cemented acetabular component with a reinforcement cross provides excellent medium-term fixation in total hip arthroplasty after pelvic irradiation. Bone Joint J 2015;97-B:177–84.
[353] Johnson AJ, Mont MA, Tsao AK, Jones LC. Treatment of femoral head osteonecrosis in the United States: 16-year analysis of the Nationwide Inpatient Sample. Clin Orthop Relat Res 2014;472:617–23.
[354] Bergh C, Fenstad AM, Furnes O, Garellick G, Havelin LI, Overgaard S, et al. Increased risk of revision in patients with non-traumatic femoral head necrosis. Acta Orthop 2014;85:11–17.
[355] Miric A, Inacio MC, Namba RS. The effect of chronic kidney disease on total hip arthroplasty. J Arthroplasty 2014;29:1225–30.
[356] Naito M, Ogata K, Shiota E, Nakamoto M, Goya T. Hip arthroplasty in haemodialysis patients. J Bone Joint Surg Br 1994;76:428–31.
[357] Lieberman JR, Fuchs MD, Haas SB, Garvin KL, Goldstock L, Gupta R, et al. Hip arthroplasty in patients with chronic renal failure. J Arthroplasty 1995;10:191–5.
[358] Sakalkale DP, Hozack WJ, Rothman RH. Total hip arthroplasty in patients on long-term renal dialysis. J Arthroplasty 1999;14:571–5.
[359] Nagoya S, Nagao M, Takada J, Kuwabara H, Kaya M, Yamashita T. Efficacy of cementless total hip arthroplasty in patients on long-term hemodialysis. J Arthroplasty 2005;20:66–71.
[360] Shrader MW, Schall D, Parvizi J, McCarthy JT, Lewallen DG. Total hip arthroplasty in patients with renal failure: a comparison between transplant and dialysis patients. J Arthroplasty 2006;21:324–9.
[361] Goffin E, Baertz G, Rombouts JJ. Long-term survivorship analysis of cemented total hip replacement (THR) after avascular necrosis of the femoral head in renal transplant recipients. Nephrol Dial Transplant 2006;21:784–8.
[362] Galson DL, Roodman GD. Pathobiology of Paget's disease of bone. J Bone Metab 2014;21:85–98.
[363] Singer F. In: De Groot LJ, Beck-Peccoz P, Chrousos G, Dungan K, Grossman A, Hershman JM, et al., editors. Paget's disease of bone. South Dartmouth (MA): Endotext; 2000.
[364] Sochart DH, Porter ML. Charnley low-friction arthroplasty for Paget's disease of the hip. J Arthroplasty 2000;15:210–19.
[365] Imbuldeniya AM, Tai SM, Aboelmagd T, Walter WL, Walter WK, Zicat BA. Cementless hip arthroplasty in Paget's disease at long-term follow-up (average of 12.3 years). J Arthroplasty 2014;29:1063–6.
[366] Gabel GT, Rand JA, Sim FH. Total knee arthroplasty for osteoarthrosis in patients who have Paget disease of bone at the knee. J Bone Joint Surg Am 1991;73:739–44.

CHAPTER 5

Material and Mechanobiological Considerations for Bone Regeneration

B.S. Klosterhoff[1], S. Nagaraja[2], J.J. Dedania[2], R.E. Guldberg[1] and N.J. Willett[1,3,4]
[1]Georgia Institute of Technology, Atlanta, GA, United States
[2]Center for Devices and Radiological Health, Silver Spring, MD, United States
[3]Emory University, Decatur, GA, United States
[4]Atlanta Veteran's Affairs Medical Center, Decatur, GA, United States

Contents

5.1 INTRODUCTION

Bone defects due to traumatic injury, tumor resection, and congenital or degenerative anatomical deformities present clinicians with a challenging condition and strikingly limited treatment options to achieve successful patient outcomes. Simple fractures are typically able to heal without surgical administration of implants, fixation devices, or osteoinductive biologics. In contrast, large, segmental bone defects or geometrically complex fractures require intervention to augment, coordinate and sustain the body's endogenous healing response to span the void with functional load-bearing tissue [1]. In addition to the physiological challenge of synthesizing enough tissue to fill the large bone void, regeneration is often complicated further by insufficient vascular infiltration in central regions of the defect, resulting in inadequate delivery of nutrients required for mineralization. The annual rate of fracture occurrences in the United States alone exceeds 12 million, and researchers estimate that up to 10% result in nonunion depending on the anatomical site [2,3]. The consequences of nonunion to the patient are debilitating, often requiring numerous revision surgeries and resulting in chronic pain and disability.

Currently, the gold standard for the treatment of large bone defects is to harvest an autologous bone graft for implantation into the defect site. Autografts possess intrinsic stores of native osteogenic cells, growth factors, and extracellular matrix (ECM). They also exhibit low immunogenicity. However, autografting approaches have inherent limitations, including limited tissue availability, incongruent graft geometry, donor site morbidity, and poor integration at the defect site. This can ultimately result in delayed or chronic nonunion and lasting pain at the injury or donor site. Persistent donor site pain at the iliac crest has been reported with conflicting accounts of prevalence. One prospective study reported that 16.5% of 110 patients experience donor site pain after 1 year, while another study reported that 18.7% of 87 patients report donor site pain at 2 years postoperation [4,5]. However, a more recent prospective study indicates that autografts from the iliac crest result in persistent pain in only 2% of 92 patients treated for nonunion or delayed union [6]. The procurement of autograft also adds socioeconomic burden and patient risk associated with an additional surgical procedure. The reamer-irrigator-aspirator (RIA) system has been adopted as a relatively less invasive graft harvesting technique compared to the iliac crest and can obtain large volumes (30–90 cm^3) of morselized intramedullary bone [7–9]. However, the morselized tissue obtained from RIA requires supplementation with fixation or a structural implant at load-bearing injury sites. A 2014 survey of 379 clinicians on nonunion and segmental defect treatment established that 92% use autografts. Surgeons identified all graft harvest techniques they utilize in practice, with 50.9% using RIA and 49.9% using the anterior iliac crest [9].

Allograft bone specimens harvested from donors or cadavers are another frequently utilized treatment option for large bone defect repair. However, allografts have their own limitations, including poor functional integration and remodeling as well as increased chance of immune rejection or disease transmission. A clinical study of allograft procedures between the middle femur and middle tibia of pediatric patients found that 37% of the treatments were failures, with disabling outcomes including fracture, nonunion, and amputation occurring [10]. The threat of disease transmission is another potential, though relatively rare, risk of allogeneic grafts. The transmission risks of human immunodeficiency virus (HIV), hepatitis C, and hepatitis B are estimated to be 1:1,500,000, 1:60,000, and 1:100,000, respectively [11]. To mitigate immune rejection and disease transmission risks, the vast majority of bone allografts are devitalized by freeze-dried processing, eliminating the osteogenic potential of the implant [12]. The bone allograft banking industry is well established in the United States and Europe. However, in many Asian countries, including China, tissue banking and allografting is much less prevalent due to negative cultural views on the reuse of human tissue. Reliance on donor bank supply as well as the additional costs to screen donors and preserve harvested tissue are notable shortcomings to allograft treatment strategies which are fundamentally impossible to overcome.

Underscoring the clinical dependence on autologous and allogeneic treatment approaches, bone is currently the second most common tissue transplant, behind blood, with an estimated 2.2 million annual incidences of bone grafting procedures worldwide and 500,000 occurring in the United States alone [13,14]. Bone defect repair in the United States is a $2.5 billion industry, and continues to grow rapidly in step with rising clinical demand. Aging domestic and global populations have motivated estimates that clinical interventions for bone defect repair will double by 2020 [15]. Accordingly, there is an urgent need for novel tissue-engineered bone graft substitutes with enhanced osteogenic potential to alleviate clinical reliance on autologous and allogeneic grafting procedures and to improve long-term patient outcomes.

In order to heal critically sized defects, tissue-engineered graft substitutes must impart a suitable biochemical, microstructural, and mechanical environment to facilitate recruitment of mesenchymal progenitor cells from neighboring tissues to the bone void and direct the cells down an osteogenic lineage. Additionally, infiltration of the bone void with a functional neovascular network is critical for nutrient delivery, waste clearance, and callus mineralization to occur. Mesenchymal stem cells (MSCs) stored in the periosteum, surrounding tissue, and bone marrow are exquisitely sensitive to mechanical perturbations imposed by their surrounding microenvironment. It has been clearly established that traction forces formed by MSC adhesion with their underlying substrate microarchitecture influence cell signaling pathways that regulate differentiation, proliferation, and chemotaxis [16—18]. Likewise, the rate, directionality, and branching of angiogenic microvessels by endothelial cells is regulated by mechanical strain [19—21]. In the context of load-bearing orthopedic tissues such as bone, potentially large-magnitude or high-frequency external mechanical forces are transmitted directly to surrounding cells by deformation of the substrate matrix. Accordingly, bone graft substitute mechanical properties, such as elastic modulus, maintain a critical role in cellular mechanotransduction and are fundamental design features which dictate the migration, lineage, and growth of mesenchymal progenitors and neovascular networks. Thus, it is essential that novel bone graft substitutes are designed, fabricated, and administered with rigorous consideration for the complex relationships between construct material properties and the transmission of local mechanobiological cues to the regenerative niche.

Remarkably, a consensus in the field on even an approximate range of suitable bone implant stiffness has not been reached. Consequently, there is a continuum of graft substitute stiffnesses under active investigation encompassing seven orders of magnitude, from 2.6 kPa for highly compliant and viscous hydrogels to 410 GPa for stiff ceramic oxides like alumina [22,23]. However, the diversity of bone graft substitutes can roughly be delineated by two distinct categories with different design rationales: (1) relatively compliant scaffolds or constructs, often loaded with bioactive osteoinductive molecules such as recombinant human bone morphogenic protein 2 or 7 (rhBMP-2, rhBMP-7), which are intended to degrade as newly formed bone bridges the defect to bear load; and (2) stiff implants whose primary function is to promote osseointegration with the mineralized boundaries of the defect and remain as a long-term load-bearing surrogate.

Supplementary fixation devices are another crucial aspect regulating the mechanics of large bone defect regeneration, particularly at the early stages of healing. Fixation devices impose mechanical boundary conditions on the defect by governing the magnitude and direction of physiological load share transmitted to the regenerating tissue. Defined fixation schemes must be carefully balanced to prevent excessive interfragmentary motion known to inhibit initial osteogenesis, or at the other extreme, prolonged stress-shielding which can produce newly regenerated bone with inferior load-bearing architecture and fragile mechanical characteristics. Therefore, a robustly engineered large bone defect therapy is comprised of a bone void-filling construct and adjuvant fixation which together provide a controlled mechanical environment on the healing tissue to promote osteogenesis and ultimately aid in the restoration of bone function.

The purpose of this chapter is to examine the state of biomaterial platforms for the treatment of bone defects and to motivate dialog to define appropriate mechanobiological criteria for future bone graft substitute research and development. First, a brief summary of the physiological process of bone regeneration is outlined. Second, material approaches for bone graft substitutes including FDA device classifications and testing considerations are reviewed. Finally, we review in vitro and in vivo evidence elucidating how bone regeneration is regulated by the mechanical environment across multiple length scales.

5.2 PHYSIOLOGY OF BONE REGENERATION

Bone possesses an extraordinary capacity for endogenous healing. It is typically able to recover biomechanical competence after injury through a coordinated healing response. The progression of bone regeneration is a transient and spatially heterogeneous process characterized by rapid morphogenesis of numerous tissue phenotypes over days, weeks, and months after the initial insult. In the case of critically sized defects, the intrinsic regenerative potential of the native tissue is insufficient to completely heal the injury. Thus, effectively designed clinical interventions must leverage stages of the bone-healing process to enhance either bridging of the defect or surface integration with the surrogate implant to form a mechanically competent composite structure. This dynamic regenerative process is commonly delineated into four major phases (and associated timelines) of tissue formation: (1) inflammation and hematoma (hours and days); (2) soft callus (days and weeks); (3) immature bone (weeks and months); and (4) bone remodeling (months and years) [24]. However, it should be noted that spatiotemporal variability is common in the healing of large bone defects, and different phases occur simultaneously within a fracture zone as dictated by the local biophysical and biochemical conditions of the cellular niche. In this section, the characteristic physiology of bone regeneration will be reviewed, and the critical regulatory role of biomechanics on tissue differentiation, neovascularization, and inflammation will be motivated briefly before receiving a more targeted review in Sections 5.4 and 5.5.

5.2.1 Inflammation and hematoma

Whether a defect is created by a controlled surgical technique or due to a traumatic injury, the fracture inflicts damage on cells of the bone, periosteum, and neighboring tissues, including rupture of surrounding vasculature. Tissue destruction initiates a cascade of acute inflammatory signals which mark the beginning of the regenerative process [25,26]. Disruption of nearby blood vessels quickly floods the defect zone with clotting blood and results in the formation of a hematoma. Interrupted circulation results in localized hypoxia, and the hematoma is characterized by low oxygen tension, acidic pH, and high lactate concentration [27]. The hematoma is also rich with neutrophils, macrophages, and other immune cells found in the peripheral blood supply as well as the bone marrow of long bones [26,28]. The inflammatory signals facilitate coagulation in response to hypoxia and concurrently activate this dense population of immune cells to secrete important molecular factors which mediate early stages of necrotic tissue clearance, ECM production of granulation tissue, angiogenesis, and MSC recruitment [27]. Critical signaling molecules within the early hematoma include inflammatory cytokines like tumor necrosis factor alpha (TNF-α), interleukins 1 and 6 (IL-1 and IL-6), macrophage colony-stimulating factor (M-CSF), receptor activator of nuclear factor κB ligand (RANKL), and the enzyme cyclooxygenase-2 (COX-2) [29,30]. Expression of osteoinductive BMP family members as well as proangiogenic factors including hypoxia-inducible factor alpha

(HIF-1α) and its downstream partner vascular endothelial growth factor (VEGF) are also upregulated in the fracture hematoma [27,31]. Underscoring its vital role as the foundational scaffold for fracture healing, removal of the hematoma delays fracture repair, while excision and subcutaneous implantation of the hematoma elicits ectopic bone formation [32,33].

While an initial inflammatory response is critical to successful bone regeneration, excessive or chronic inflammation counteracts the aforementioned beneficial aspects and can attenuate healing [25]. In traumatic injuries which result in open fractures or composite tissue trauma, associated surges in systemic inflammation are thought to inhibit bone formation and increase the risk of reoperation [34]. Biomechanical conditions are also influential on the degree of magnitude and duration of inflammation in the defect zone. Relatively large-magnitude mechanical strain within the hematoma as a result of poor implant stability or flexible fixation increases and prolongs the presence of cytotoxic immune cells and ultimately leads to delayed healing or nonunion [26,35,36]. The threshold delineating positive and negative levels of inflammation is multifactorial and thus difficult to define [25]. It is also important to note that the majority of available literature on early stages of bone healing is concentrated on simple transverse fractures, and the initial phase of large bone defect repair is not well characterized. Future research on the interplay between defect type, mechanical stability, and patient comorbidities on early inflammation will greatly enhance the data available to develop personalized clinical strategies for healing more complex bone defect injuries.

5.2.2 Soft callus and neovascularization

As peripheral cells from the circulation, periosteum, surrounding tissue, and bone marrow begin to infiltrate the hematoma, a soft callus of granulation tissue is formed. The granulation tissue primarily consists of an immature fibrous matrix. Neovascularization of the granulation tissue is promoted by local diffusion of hypoxic paracrine factors. Nascent vessel formation proceeds through vasculogenesis, in which immature angioblasts form de novo primitive vessels, and angiogenesis, where the preexisting intact vasculature sprouts, branches and remodels to extend the functional vessel network [37]. Increased arterial blood flow also occurs by radial growth of intact vessels, known as arteriogenesis [38]. Functional vascularization within the hematoma is crucial to deliver oxygen and nutrients for MSC proliferation and maturation, and for waste removal. HIF-1α-induced VEGF expression is the most well characterized molecular pathway stimulating angiogenesis into the defect space. Inhibition of VEGF reduced callus vascularization and impaired bone healing in the mouse, while administration of VEGF enhanced mineralized callus volume in a critically sized rabbit defect model [39].

Unsurprisingly, new vessel growth is highly dependent on biomechanical boundary conditions imposed on the regenerating tissue in vivo. In a rodent critically sized segmental defect model, uniaxial compressive load transfer at the onset of injury dramatically attenuated vessel ingrowth and connectivity within the defect zone, resulting in nonunion. Interestingly, compressive loading after initial stabilization of the defect by bridging with immature mineralized tissue reduced vascular connectivity but increased vascular thickness and bone volume, indicating that mechanical loading may disrupt small vessels while stimulating arteriogenesis of large vessels and deposition of new bone [40]. The specific influences of mechanics on vascular ingrowth will be discussed in greater detail in Sections 5.4 and 5.5.

5.2.3 Immature bone

Increases in local oxygen tension and pH buffering due to capillary infiltration within the granulation tissue-filled callus coincide with differentiation of recruited MSCs into osteogenic and chondrogenic phenotypes [41–43]. As MSCs mature, mineralization of the callus occurs primarily through two mechanisms: intramembranous (primary) or endochondral (secondary) ossification. Intramembranous ossification takes place by direct deposition and mineralization of osteoid matrix along a front propagating from peripheral intact bone. In endochondral ossification, a cartilage intermediary replaces the soft callus of granulation tissue before chondrocyte hypertrophy and mineralization occurs. Endochondral ossification proceeds over a longer timescale than intramembranous ossification, and leverages the low oxygen demand of native cartilage better suited for avascular environments [44]. Thus, endochondral ossification is prevalent in callus regions which are slow to restore sufficient vascularization such as central portions of large bone defects [45].

The linkage of angiogenesis with osteogenesis is well demonstrated at the molecular scale, and their physiological roles cannot be decoupled [31,39]. VEGF expression and sufficient oxygen tension promote chemotaxis of MSCs and subsequent adoption of an osteoblastic phenotype [46,47]. Likewise, BMP-2, 4, and 6 promote differentiation of MSCs into osteoblasts, and these newly osteogenic cells simultaneously enhance secretion of VEGF in a differentiation-dependent fashion [48,49]. This osteogenic–angiogenic coupling is hypothesized to promote paracrine signaling to nearby endothelial cells which support increased vascular capacity along newly formed mineralization fronts.

Newly differentiated osteoblasts maintain sensitivity to local oxygen tension. Experimental evidence has demonstrated that type I collagen (Col I) matrix synthesis, as well as osteocalcin (OC) and alkaline phosphatase (ALP) activity is suppressed in hypoxic conditions [50–52]. If deficient vascularization and hypoxia persist within the defect space, bone regeneration cannot occur regardless of the healing mechanism and nonunion will be established [39,53]. Stimulation of sufficient vascularization remains a critical obstacle to the successful treatment of large bone defects, open fractures, and polytraumatic injuries [44,54].

Mechanobiological cues are known to direct the evolution of the fracture callus and ultimately the healing outcome of bone regeneration [55]. Highlighting the role of local mechanics on healing, both intramembranous and endochondral mechanisms of mineralization can occur simultaneously within a single healing defect as dictated by the mechanical conditions of the microenvironment [56]. In regions of high mechanical stability, intramembranous ossification is predominant, while larger magnitude strain typically stimulates endochondral ossification. Fibrocartilage, as well as connective and adipose tissue, is formed and tends to persist in regions of excessive strain and may lead to chronic nonunion.

5.2.4 Bone remodeling

The transition of soft callus to immature, woven bone ensues by rapid deposition and mineralization of type I collagen in a random, isotropic fashion [57]. This disorganized phenotype lacks the robust and spatially optimized mechanical characteristics of mature bone, but is typically adequate to bear physiological loads due to hypertrophy of the woven bone callus. Structural homeostasis is restored by remodeling of the tissue micro- and macrostructure, which occurs over months and years after the original insult. Mechanically driven remodeling increases the alignment of the collagen matrix with principal loading directions and initiates resorption of mechanically superfluous ectopic bone [57]. In the diaphysis of long bones, reestablishment of the intramedullary canal and formation of bone marrow occurs over time.

Conversely, prolonged stress-shielding by supplementary fixation after the defect is bridged can slow mechanically driven remodeling [58,59]. In addition to fixation, the bone graft substitute is an important factor in long-term function even after defect bridging is achieved. Sustained stress-shielding in very stiff implants has long been known to cause implant loosening and failure due to bone resorption at the implant—tissue interface. This effect is still an important challenge to longevity in load-bearing implants designed to remain in vivo for many years [60]. Thus, it is critical that both short- and long-term mechanical conditions within the healed tissue are considered when selecting a bone defect treatment approach, particularly in the case of prosthetic implants where the healed tissue must function as a composite of dissimilar materials for decades.

In this section, the complex physiological mechanisms and clinical challenges of successful bone regeneration were reviewed. Basic concepts of the interactions between biomechanical stimuli and key aspects of healing including inflammation, neovascularization, and osteogenesis were introduced. In the following sections, the state of the art in clinical and preclinical bone implants will be reviewed, with an emphasis on their respective mechanical properties.

5.3 MECHANICAL PROPERTIES OF MATERIALS FOR BONE REGENERATION

The field of bone tissue engineering and regenerative medicine has remained a highly active area of research for decades, and much progress has been made toward understanding the pathophysiology and treatment of large defects. However, a distinct clinical need remains for improved therapeutics and engineered scaffolds to reduce clinical reliance on grafting procedures and to decrease the significant rate of persistent non-union. Notably, a rigorous definition of engineering criteria and functional properties of an ideal graft substitute has not been recognized in the field. In Fig. 5.1, a plot of elastic modulus versus yield or failure strength is depicted to illustrate the vast range of mechanical properties reported in the literature. This fact highlights both the successes and challenges of large bone defect treatment, as many disparate construct approaches have exhibited some degree of success in clinical or preclinical studies, but few if any graft substitute materials have established the robust and consistent positive healing outcomes needed to target future work in the field. Table 5.1 is included as a reference of key mechanical properties (strength, elastic modulus, and fracture toughness)

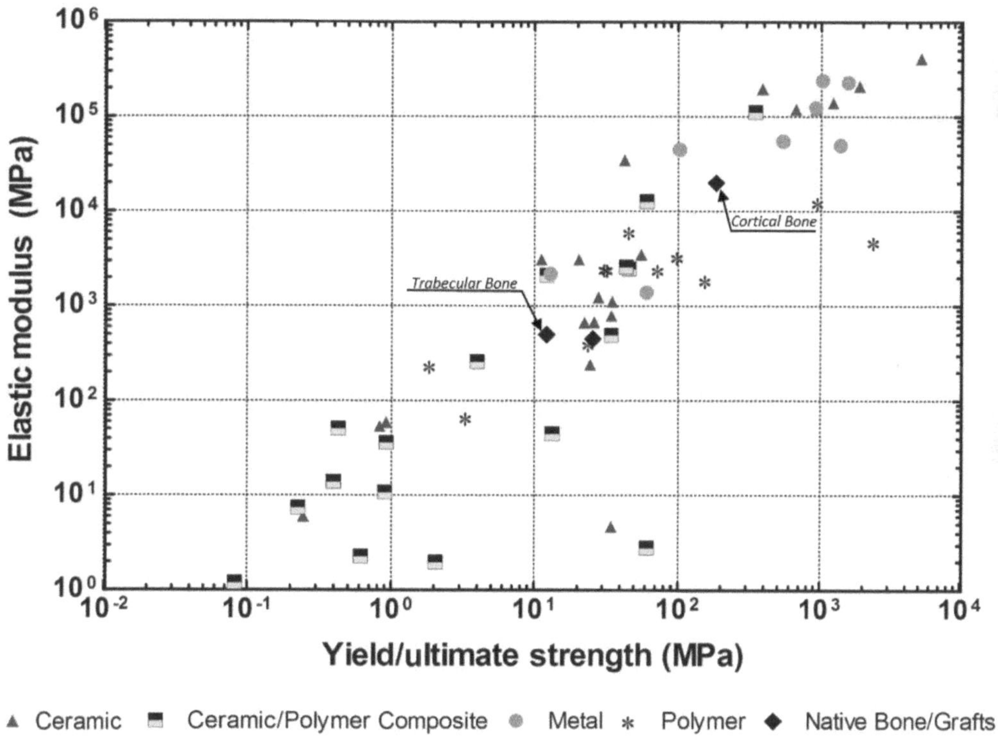

Figure 5.1 Elastic modulus versus yield or ultimate strength of bone scaffold materials (Refs. [23,61–75]).

Table 5.1 Mechanical properties of materials and scaffolds for bone defect treatment—additional references for table not already cited in text [301–310]

Material	Preparation	Porosity (%)	Yield/ultimate strength (MPa)	Elastic modulus (MPa)	Fracture toughness (MPa $\cdot \sqrt{m}$)	Refs.
Ceramic						
Alumina	Bulk		3000–5000	380,000–410,000	3–6	[23]
Bioglass	Bulk		42	35,000	2	[66]
Bioglass	Bulk		800–1200	40,000–140,000	2	[23]
Bioglass	Paste		47.3			[64]
Bioglass-Silicon nitride	Bulk		383	197,000	4.4	[66]
Calcium phosphate	Paste	46	6.3–34	3.6–4.7		[74]
Calcium phosphate	Paste		0.24	6		[64]
Calcium phosphate	Paste		0.81	54		[64]
Calcium phosphate	Paste		14–24	125–240		[74]
Calcium phosphate	Paste		25.6	674		[64]
Calcium phosphate	Paste		34	790		[64]
Calcium phosphate	Paste	30–40	35–55	2500–3500		[74]
Calcium phosphate	Bulk		450–650	90,000–120,000	1.2	[23]
Calcium phosphate	Paste		14–24			[64]
Calcium phosphate	Scaffold		0.8–342			[150]
Calcium phosphate	Paste		23–55			[74]
Calcium phosphate	Paste		15.1			[75]
Calcium phosphate	Paste		4			[75]
Calcium sulfate	Scaffold		0.6–0.9	59		[74]
Calcium sulfate	Paste		21.8	665		[64]
Calcium sulfate	Paste		9.9			[75]
Calcium sulfate	Paste		52.9			[75]
Calcium sulfate	Paste		0.6			[74]
Coral exoskeleton (Calcium carbonate)	Scaffold	61–74	2.6–12.1			[154]
HA	Scaffold	41	34.4	1110		[23]
HA	Scaffold	41	27.4	1240		[23]

(Continued)

Table 5.1 (Continued)

Material	Preparation	Porosity (%)	Yield/ultimate strength (MPa)	Elastic modulus (MPa)	Fracture toughness ($MPa \cdot \sqrt{m}$)	Refs.
HA	Scaffold		1–11	200–3100		[67]
HA	Scaffold	60–80	1–20	20–3100		[74]
HA	Bulk		300–900	80,000–120,000	0.6–1	[23]
HA	Paste		3.8			[75]
SiO_2 glass	Bulk			70,000	0.7–0.8	[23]
Zirconia	Bulk		1850	195,000-210,000	5–8	[23]
			Composite			
Bioglass-Collagen	Hydrogel			0.13–0.28 (storage)		[302]
Bioglass-Collagen-Phosphatidylserine	Scaffold	75.4	1.5			[301]
Bioglass-PDLLA	Scaffold	5–29	0.07–0.08	0.65–1.2		[63]
Bioglass-PGA	Scaffold		0.5–2 (tensile)	0.5–2 (tensile)		[65]
Bioglass-PGS	Scaffold	> 90	0.4–1			[65]
Bioglass-PLGA	Scaffold	75	0.42	51		[63]
Bioglass-PLLA	Scaffold	77–80	1.5–3.9	137–260		[63]
Bioglass-Stainless steel	Scaffold		290–339	83,000–112,000		[66]
Calcium Phosphate-Chitosan gelatin	Scaffold		0.32–0.88	3.94–10.88		[63]
Calcium Phosphate-PLGA	Scaffold	75		65		[63]
Calcium Carbonate-PLLA	Scaffold			3500–6000		[65]
HA-Chitosan-PLGA	Scaffold		43 (flexural)	2600		[65]
HA-Chitosan	Scaffold		12 (flexural)	2150		[65]
HA-Collagen	Scaffold	~0	34–60	0.44–2.8		[63]
HA-Collagen-PLLA	Scaffold	80	1.9–13	20–45		[73]
HA-PCL	Scaffold		0.1–0.6	0.6–2.3		[69]
HA-PCL	Scaffold	81	0.8–0.9	26.4–36.2		[176]
HA-PCL	Bulk		24.6–33.7	311–498		[176]
HA-PDLLA	Scaffold		45 (flexural)	1750–2470		[65]

(Continued)

Table 5.1 (Continued)

Material	Preparation	Porosity (%)	Yield/ultimate strength (MPa)	Elastic modulus (MPa)	Fracture toughness (MPa · $\sqrt{m}$)	Refs.
HA-PLGA	Scaffold	81–91	0.07–0.22	2–7.5		[63]
HA-PLGA	Scaffold			1100		[65]
HA-PLLA	Scaffold	85–96	0.39	10–14		[63]
HA-PLLA	Scaffold		50–60 (flexural)	6400–12,800		[65]
HA-Silk	Scaffold		0.121–0.251			[304]
Magnesium Calcium phosphate-Gelatin Sponge	Scaffold	33–50		2–4.75		[303]
Metal						
CoCrMo alloys	Bulk		900–1540	220,000–230,000	100	[61]
Magnesium	Bulk		65–100	41,000–45,000	15–40	[139]
NiTi	Bulk		1355	30,000–50,000	30–60	[61]
Stainless steel-316	Bulk		540–1000	240,000	100	[61]
Tantalum	Scaffold	75–85	60	1400		[124]
Tantalum	Scaffold	66–88	4–12.7	373–2200		[308]
TiNb	Bulk			60,000–85,000		[62]
Titanium alloys	Bulk		900	105,000–125,000	80	[61]
TNZT	Bulk		530	55,000		[62]
Polymer						
Alginate	Hydrogel			0.025–0.05 (shear)		[305]
Collagen	Hydrogel			0.75 (storage)		[302]
Collagen-GAG	Scaffold		0.176–0.229			[306]
Hyaluronic acid-fibronectin	Hydrogel			0.0025–0.0026		[307]
PCL	Scaffold	38–55	2–3.2	52–67		[70]
PCL	Scaffold		23	400		[63]
PDLLA	Scaffold		29–150	1900		[63]
PEEK	Scaffold	67 (at surface)	71.1 (tensile)	2450 (tensile)		[174]

(Continued)

Table 5.1 (Continued)

Material	Preparation	Porosity (%)	Yield/ultimate strength (MPa)	Elastic modulus (MPa)	Fracture toughness (MPa · $\sqrt{m}$)	Refs.
PEEK	Bulk		96.1 (tensile)	3340 (tensile)		[174]
PEU-peptide linked	Scaffold		43–45 (tensile)	4400–6100 (tensile)		[71]
PGA	Scaffold		350–920	12,500		[63]
PLAGA	Scaffold		1.8 (tensile)	237		[72]
PLLA	Scaffold		28–2300	4800		[63]
PMMA	Paste		88.5			[75]
Silk	Scaffold			25		[309]
Starch	Scaffold		25.03–31.50 (tensile)	1620–2470 (tensile)		[68]
UHMWPE	Bulk		20–30 (tensile)	1000–2500 (tensile)		[310]
Native Bone/Grafts						
Cortical bone	Bulk		130–180	12,000–20,000	6–8	[78,79]
Trabecular bone	Bulk		4–12	100–500		[79]
Demineralized cortical bone	Bulk		15–25 (tensile)	275–450 (tensile)		[90]

reported in the literature for a majority of materials investigated and used clinically to treat bone defects. Examination of Fig. 5.1 and Table 5.1 makes it easy to see that a clear consensus has yet to be established.

Graft substitutes are often described by their innate capacity to promote osteogenic, osteoinductive or osteoconductive healing mechanisms. Osteogenic constructs and grafts possess an intrinsic store of osteoblasts or MSCs which secrete and mineralize de novo bone ECM. Osteoinductivity is defined as the ability to stimulate osteogenesis through the recruitment and differentiation of immature MSCs into osteoblasts in the defect zone. Osteoconductivity is the ability for new bone to grow on the surface of a graft substitute, which is essential to support mineral infiltration into the central region of large defects as well as for osseointegration [76]. Osseointegration is defined as direct contact at the interface of regenerated bone and an implant. Osseointegration is vital to successfully anchor long-term graft substitutes [77]. From an engineering standpoint, countless biochemical, architectural, and physical factors determine a graft substitute's capacity for these four basic modes of bone regeneration.

Among the many critical parameters of a bone graft substitute, the mechanical properties play a fundamental role in the healing outcome. In particular, both bulk (intensive) and apparent (extensive) mechanical parameters, such as elastic modulus and construct stiffness, are critical to endogenous cell migration, proliferation, and differentiation within the defect. Additionally, material failure strength and fracture toughness are important constraints for nonresorbing constructs or implants, since they must be sufficiently durable to bear load past the initial healing phase. From a design perspective, both material and processing techniques of a successful bone graft substitute must be selected with intent to confer appropriate biomechanical characteristics for the duration of the projected graft substitute lifecycle.

Construct material approaches can roughly be divided into basic five material classes: (1) grafts, (2) metals, (3) ceramics, (4) polymers, and (5) composites. Each material class comprises many formulations and fabrication strategies which significantly alter construct mechanical properties. Thus, there is a high degree of variability within, as well as significant overlap between approaches (see Fig. 5.1). In this section, basic mechanical properties of clinical and preclinical bone graft substitutes published in the literature will be reviewed, with a critical focus on their respective advantages and limitations.

5.3.1 Native bone and grafts

The final objective of any bone regeneration treatment strategy is to bridge a volumetric defect with a material that has similar structural-functional properties as the original tissue. Thus, the mechanical properties of bone must be well understood.

Bone is an anisotropic and heterogeneous nanocomposite. In long bones, such as the femur, cortical bone exhibits a modulus of approximately 20 GPa in the longitudinal direction and 12 GPa in the transverse direction [78,79]. The compressive and tensile strengths of cortical bone are typically between 130–180 MPa and 50–151 MPa, respectively, dependent on the anatomical site and the circumstance of the individual [79]. The complex microarchitecture of trabecular bone makes it a challenging material to characterize mechanically. Acoustic and nanoindentation experiments demonstrate that the intrinsic elastic modulus of trabecular bone is quite close to cortical bone: between 6.9 and 18.1 GPa [80,81]. However, mainly due to its porosity at the apparent level, trabecular bone possesses a significantly lower apparent modulus and compressive strength, ranging between 100–500 MPa and 4–12 MPa, respectively [79]. Some additional important mechanical properties of intact cortical and trabecular bone are presented in Table 5.1.

The first reported instance of bone grafting was by Job van-Meek'ren, a Dutch surgeon, in 1668 [82]. Van-Meek'ren successfully implanted a canine xenograft to treat a defect in the skull of a soldier. Over 250 years later, autologous bone grafting was reported by Fred Albee, who harvested a graft from the tibia for spinal fusion [83]. As discussed in the Introduction, autologous and allogeneic grafts have numerous limitations, yet they remain the clinical standard for large bone defect treatment. Autografts in particular have distinct advantages as they stimulate each of the three basic osteogenic, osteoconductive, and osteoinductive regeneration mechanisms thanks to their intrinsic supply of native bone cells, collagen-mineral matrix, and noncollagenous proteins [84,85]. Allografts are typically devoid of cells to prevent immunogenic effects, but still exhibit varying degrees of osteoinductive and osteoconductive properties, depending on how they are processed.

From a strictly mechanical standpoint, intact autografts and structural allografts provide nearly equivalent microstructural and apparent physical properties as the native bone they replace. Nonstructural formulations of autografts and allografts are also used extensively. In nonstructural allografts, the tissue is first morselized into small chips or blocks of cortical bone, cancellous bone, or a combination of the two. Some morselized allograft products are then embedded in a gel-like carrier to provide shape, while others are simply rehydrated as unincorporated fragments prior to implantation. Obviously, morselized grafts do not possess a high apparent stiffness compared to intact grafts, but the fragments act as a microstructural substrate for invading progenitor cells with similar properties to bone. To enhance stability of the structural implants, morsel impaction techniques may be utilized as in total hip replacements, but graft strength remains a concern in load-bearing sites [86,87].

Other common allogeneic graft preprocessing procedures include demineralization, freezing, freeze-drying, and gamma irradiation sterilization. Demineralization through submersion in an acidic solution is a commonly used allograft preparation technique that is hypothesized to enhance bone formation by improving accessibility and diffusion of internal noncollagenous proteins including BMP and other growth factors typically embedded in mineral phases [88,89]. However, demineralized bone matrices possess substantially reduced mechanical properties compared to autograft tissue. Tensile tests have demonstrated that demineralization of unmorselized human and bovine cortical bone specimens reduced their elastic modulus by approximately 25-fold (to 275–450 MPa), and reduced ultimate strength by at least half (to 15–25 MPa) [90].

Allogeneic graft specimens are typically deep-frozen or lyophilized to enhance shelf-life at tissue banks. The mechanical properties of fresh-frozen samples are preserved after thawing and rehydration, but freeze-dried specimens exhibit increased brittleness and reduced strength in torsion [91]. Up to eight additional freeze–thaw cycles have been shown to have no effect on mechanical properties of cadaveric fibular allograft specimens [92]. Gamma irradiation, commonly used to sterilize allogeneic graft specimens, further reduces lyophilized tissue strength and work to failure by over 40% and 70%, respectively [93].

Long-term mechanical competency of allografts has also been shown to be inconsistent in clinical evaluations. Rates of allograft fracture incidence in one clinical study were found to be nearly 16% [94]. To elucidate the mechanisms of allograft failure, an evaluation of failed allografts revealed degraded mechanical properties and bone mineral density, as well as increased susceptibility to microfracture when compared to nonimplanted allograft specimens [95].

5.3.2 Metals

Metallic implants and instrumentation have long been utilized for arthroplasties and for the surgical management of fractures and large bone defects. The first reported uses of metal implants in orthopedics were for fracture fixation. While reports of fracture stabilization with metal wires date back to the latter half of the 1700s, it was the Scottish surgeon, Sir William Arbuthnot Lane, who made significant contributions to develop and popularize internal fracture fixation techniques with steel plates and screws from 1893 to 1914 [96–98]. Since then, the use of metallic implants has been widely adapted to a vast array of orthopedic surgery applications including prosthetic hip and knee joints, spinal fusion cages, and bone graft substitutes. Metallic implants or scaffolds are particularly desirable for load-bearing applications due to their high mechanical stiffness, strength, fracture toughness, and resilience. These characteristics reduce the risk of implant failure (see bulk material properties of metals in Table 5.1). In addition, the relatively low cost and ease of processing metals facilitates device translation to the clinic. In particular, stainless steel (SS), titanium (Ti), and cobalt–chromium (Co–Cr) alloys gained prominence in the clinic due to their superior corrosion resistance compared to other common engineering metals.

Traditional metallic implants are nondegradable. Consequently, the primary goal of the implanted construct is to form a robust physical connection at the interfaces of the defect. In the context of large bone defects, the vast majority of metallic bone graft substitutes investigated in preclinical models and utilized in the clinic possess some level of porosity or surface modification to enhance osseointegration at the defect boundaries or throughout its entirety. The literature on the effects of numerous surface functionalization techniques and porous architectures is extensive and outside the scope of this chapter. However, these implant design parameters are critical factors independent of the selected material which can be leveraged to drastically alter the micro- or macromechanical environment conferred by metal implant devices [99–103]. Many excellent articles review the topic of implant porosity and surface modifications are available in the literature. We refer readers interested in the topic to a few reviews in particular [101,104,105].

Porous titanium scaffolds, cages, and meshes are a particularly well-established example of a metallic construct utilized clinically for the treatment of numerous types of large bone defects, particularly in craniomaxillofacial reconstructive and spinal fusion procedures [106–109]. The use of titanium and its alloys has become relatively commonplace due to its higher strength-to-density ratio (specific strength), lower modulus, and superior biocompatibility in comparison to cobalt and stainless steel-based materials [61,110]. Titanium constructs are osteoconductive and porous structures that exhibit integration with native tissue and cells without extensive fibrous encapsulation [111,112]. To impart osteoinductive properties to titanium implants, they are frequently augmented with autogenous or allogeneic bone or rh-BMP2 [113–115].

Traditional approaches to metallic implants are intended to remain in the defect and not degrade. Consequently, they must bear mechanical loads for the duration of the implant lifetime. The characteristic strength and resilience of stainless steel, cobalt–chromium, and titanium are well-suited to fulfill this functional criterion. While adequate mechanical properties are critical, the moduli of traditional metals are substantially higher, often over an order of magnitude, than native cortical bone. Thus, there are broad concerns on the long-term effects of heterogeneous stress distributions resulting from extremely stiff, nonresorbing metallic implants. Sustained stress-shielding is known to result in resorption of adjacent bone tissue, which can cause implant loosening or failure and impaired biomechanical function of the bone, particularly in total joint arthroplasty [60,116].

Due to long-term stress-shielding concerns, increasing focus has been shifted to the development of material, architectural, and processing modifications to produce more compliant metal scaffolds with mechanical properties closer to native bone. Novel techniques have also been investigated with the intent to confer osteoinductive and degradable properties to metallic implants. Contemporary material approaches include porous tantalum, titanium alloys such as shape-memory nickel–titanium, as well as magnesium [62]. Advanced processing approaches include hierarchically structured scaffolds produced by additive manufacturing and highly porous metallic foams formed by expansion of pressurized bubbles or powder sintering [117–119].

Porous tantalum was developed in the early 2000s to reduce the very high density of bulk tantalum, which had prohibited its use as a large bone graft substitute or joint prosthesis [120]. Porous tantalum exhibits similar osteoconductivity and biocompatibility characteristics as titanium [121,122]. Notably, the modulus of porous tantalum is substantially lower than titanium and its alloys (see Table 5.1), while maintaining sufficient strength to bear physiological loads [123]. Thus, tantalum scaffolds are hypothesized to improve stress homogeneity at the bone–scaffold interface, although strong clinical evidence of this proposed phenomenon has not been demonstrated [124]. Selective laser sintering (SLS) additive manufacturing techniques have been leveraged to develop porous tantalum scaffolds with a unit cell architecture, controlled pore and strut sizes, and high (80%) bulk porosity [125]. While preclinical development and clinical utilization of porous tantalum scaffolds and prostheses have drastically increased since their introduction, high raw material and processing expenses remain a significant obstacle to widespread use of porous tantalum [125].

Nickel–titanium (NiTi) alloys are superelastic materials which exhibit shape-memory behavior, permitting elastic recovery of strains up to 10% [126,127]. NiTi has garnered attention in the orthopedics field for several decades because it possesses an elastic modulus that is nearly equivalent to cortical bone while maintaining an ultimate tensile strength comparable to stainless steel [61,128] (see Table 5.1). Fully porous NiTi scaffolds have demonstrated promising short-term host cell and tissue responses in vitro and in vivo [129,130]. However, long-term in vivo biocompatibility data have not sufficiently addressed concerns of toxicity and carcinogenicity due to nickel ion release and accumulation. This has posed a significant impediment to clinical implementation of large volume scaffolds or implants in the United States and Europe; and consequently NiTi has primarily been used for bone suture anchors and nonorthopedic applications such as vascular stents [131–134]. A recently developed intramedullary nail system for ankle fusion is one of the first examples of an orthopedic fixation device utilizing NiTi in a major structural role, though the majority of its surface is housed within a titanium cylinder [135]. To mitigate cytotoxicity risks, recent research has focused on nickel-free shape-memory alloys as well as novel NiTi surface modification techniques to reduce corrosive release of nickel [129,130,136,137].

As mentioned earlier, two of the most significant drawbacks to the majority of metals in bone tissue engineering are their disproportionately high mechanical stiffness compared to native bone, and their lack of degradability. Taken together, these characteristics require metal bone graft substitutes to be durable enough to survive decades of load-bearing service in vivo without shielding mechanical stress from adjacent tissue. This dichotomy is a difficult engineering challenge to balance in the design of metallic bone graft substitutes, particularly when compared to more compliant and/or degradable ceramics, polymers, or composites. Due to these shortcomings in most metals, magnesium is an intriguing biomaterial for orthopedic tissue engineering applications. It possesses a relatively compliant elastic modulus (approximately 40 GPa) closer to native cortical bone compared to the preceding metals, but retains superior strength and toughness compared to most ceramics and polymers (see Table 5.1) [61]. In addition, magnesium is naturally found in high concentrations in the human body, is efficiently degraded at physiological salinity by oxidation-reduction reactions, and is excreted safely as an oxide in the urine [138,139]. These properties indicate magnesium could be a promising bone graft substitute for regenerative applications where the implant is intended to initially stabilize the defect and degrade during new bone bridging.

A significant obstacle preventing clinical utilization of magnesium is precisely tuning the degradation rate to account for the high spatiotemporal variability in the regenerative response of the host bone. Additionally, deficient vascularization and waste transport are typical in large bone defects, and thus can slow the clearance of hydrogen gas produced by magnesium oxidation. Consequently, formation of hydrogen gas pockets has been reported in the literature [140]. Degradability and hydrogen gas production rate can be modulated by alloying magnesium with other elements including zinc, manganese, calcium, aluminum, and rare earth elements [140–143]. However, the in vivo release kinetics and solubility of corrosion products from magnesium alloys are not well studied.

5.3.3 Ceramics

The inorganic mineral hydroxyapatite (HA) is the primary constituent of bone, comprising approximately 65% of tissue volume. HA imparts high mechanical stiffness and strength in compression, and serves as a hydrophilic substrate which promotes cellular adhesion and migration. Ceramic fillers for large bone defects have been utilized for over a century. The first reported treatment of a bone defect with calcium sulfate, commonly known as plaster of Paris, was first reported in 1892 by Dressman [144]. Since then, numerous natural and synthetic ceramic formulations have been explored and widely utilized in the clinic. General beneficial characteristics of ceramics include analogous elastic modulus to native bone and strong surface osteoconductivity, which promotes robust tissue infiltration, osseointegration, and growth. There are a variety of both natural and synthetic ceramic materials utilized in the clinic which can be implemented in several preparations including pastes, powders, and solid or porous blocks. Ceramic bone graft substitute materials can broadly be categorized as calcium phosphates, corals, calcium sulfates, bioglasses, and crystalline oxides. Generally speaking, many pure ceramic bone graft substitute materials possess a bulk elastic modulus comparable to intact cortical and trabecular bone and good strength in compression.

However, pure ceramics exhibit inferior strength in tension and shear as well as brittle failure behavior. Consequently, ceramic bone graft substitutes have lower toughness and fatigue strength than metals when subjected to more complex and physiologically relevant loading patterns.

The calcium phosphate family is a mineral classification consisting primarily of calcium ions and ortho- or metaphosphates, and may also include hydrogen or hydroxide ions [63]. There are an array of calcium phosphate compounds utilized as bone graft substitute materials including β-tricalcium phosphate (β-TCP), biphasic calcium phosphate (BCP), calcium carbonate, β-calcium pyrophosphate (β-CPP), octacalcium phosphate (OCP), dicalcium phosphate (DCP), and HA [63]. The published mechanical properties of selected preclinical and commercially available calcium phosphates are also tabulated in Table 5.1. The degradation products of calcium phosphates are generally noncytotoxic. While crystalline HA implants degrade very slowly, β-TCP implants readily degrade, often within months of surgical administration [145]. BCPs consisting of different ratios of HA and β-TCP have been developed to permit tunable degradation kinetics [145]. Additionally, ECM adhesion proteins and cell adhesion transmembrane receptors including fibronectin and integrins are known to readily adsorb to HA surfaces, providing an osteoconductive scaffold interface [146]. The favorable surface chemistry characteristics of calcium phosphates have also been leveraged to bind and release drugs or growth factors, such as the bisphosphonate alendronate, with a sustained release profile [147,148].

Calcium phosphate scaffolds with a wide range of pore sizes and architectures have been developed. For example, macroporous (250–350 μm pore sizes) scaffolds have been fabricated with or without the addition of micropores (2–8 μm pore sizes), allowing independent control of tissue-level and cell-level environments at the scaffold interface [149]. However, the stiffness and strength of calcium phosphates decreases rapidly with the addition of microporosity, decreasing 46% and 15%, respectively [149]. The brittle characteristics of calcium phosphates are a key drawback to their clinical use. Regrettably, mechanical properties of calcium phosphates under cyclic loading such as fracture toughness and fatigue life are rarely reported in the literature, so their functional limits are not well characterized [150]. Thus, the vast majority of calcium phosphates have limited applicability in load-bearing sites when compared to more durable metals.

Bone graft substitutes derived from coral exoskeleton are an example of a naturally derived ceramic biomaterial utilized clinically since 1979 [151]. Corals share many favorable characteristics with calcium phosphates including good osteoconductivity, highly interconnected porosity, degradability, and straightforward preparation for delivering biologics or cells [152,153]. Common coral species utilized for graft substitution include those with a $CaCO_3$-based skeleton, such as *Acropora*, *Porites*, and *Goniopora*. While the species are of similar origin, a comparative study showed drastic differences in compressive strength, porosity, and permeability between the corals. *Goniopora* exhibited the largest porosity as well as similar permeability and compressive strength to trabecular bone, indicating certain coral species are more favorable for clinical application [154].

Calcium sulfate, better known as plaster of Paris, is the oldest reported ceramic bone graft substitute [144]. As a low-cost, readily biodegradable material, calcium sulfate is often indicated as a bone filler for stable defects like metaphyseal voids [155]. Calcium sulfate is commonly prepared as an injectable paste, formable putty, or solid pellets and used as a delivery vehicle for antibiotics to mitigate the risk of infection at the injury site. A prospective study of 109 patients with bone defects treated with calcium sulfate alone or in combination with bone marrow aspirate, DBM, or autograft showed that 99% of the calcium sulfate was cleared from the defect within 6 months [64,156]. Functional mechanical loading can be used to improve synchronization of bone regeneration with calcium degradation in mechanically stable defects. A metaphyseal drill hole defect model in the rat femur demonstrated that treadmill walking simultaneously accelerated bone growth and calcium sulfate degradation in the defect space [157]. Biomechanical testing confirmed a significant improvement in femur strength relative to nonexercising controls. While the mechanical properties (see Table 5.1) and rapid degradation kinetics of calcium sulfate are inadequate for use as the sole implant material in unconfined defects and certainly unstable nonunions, it remains a cost-effective filler when used in conjunction with other biomaterials.

Bioactive glasses (bioglasses) are an additional family of ceramic materials exhibiting favorable osteoconductivity, degradability, and well-characterized processing techniques which allow for precise control of scaffold architecture, porosity, degradation kinetics, and surface chemistry [158]. While numerous bioglass preparations have been developed, they consist of the same primary components, mainly SiO_2, Na_2O, CaO, and P_2O_5. The strength and fracture toughness of select bioglasses are reported as superior to calcium phosphates, but they still do not achieve the same fracture toughness performance as common orthopedic metals (see Table 5.1). Thus, bioglasses share many of the same limitations as calcium phosphates for mechanically demanding applications. Established fabrication processes allow for rapid construction of bioglasses with tailored chemical compositions and degradation rates of soluble ionic products such as Si, Ca, P, Na, and AgO_2 to elicit distinct biological responses [159,160]. Notably, osteoinductive properties have been conferred to bioglasses by seeding silicon ions on the scaffold surface [161].

Alumina and zirconia are stiff, high-strength, wear-resistant crystalline oxides. Thanks to these properties, alumina and zirconia have been utilized as ceramic heads in total hip replacement for decades [162–164]. To leverage the high-strength and stiffness of these materials, highly porous (sometimes exceeding 90% porosity) alumina and zirconia foams have been investigated as bone graft substitutes [165,166].

Although increasing porosity certainly reduces the apparent stiffness of the scaffold, the effect of the supraphysiological elastic modulus of these materials on the function of adhered cells is not well understood. The importance of substrate modulus on MSC function is reviewed in more detail in Section 5.4.2. Alumina and zirconia are considered relatively inert and they do not elicit a strong biological response or integrate well with the host tissue [167]. Consequently, their utility as a bone graft substitute is limited. To address this limitation and augment the bioactivity of zirconia and alumina scaffolds, HA surface coatings have been explored. A zirconia–HA composite scaffold exhibited a sevenfold improvement in strength over pure HA as well as a significant increase in ALP activity of cultured human osteosarcoma cells compared to pure zirconia [167]. Composite ceramic–metal scaffolds have continued to grow as a promising avenue to overcome inherent limitations of individual materials. Composite designs consisting of multiple material classes will be discussed in Section 5.3.5.

5.3.4 Polymers

Natural and synthetic polymers have been explored as regenerative scaffolds to take advantage of their good biocompatibility and ductility as well as the wide range of porosities, degradation rates, and mechanical properties available. Natural polymers include type I collagen (Col I), silk, chitosan, alginate, and hyaluronic acid. Col I is the primary organic component of bone, and thus exhibits excellent biocompatibility. Bovine-derived Col I sponges are a popular surgical material for a wide range of applications, including as a rapidly degraded delivery vehicle of rhBMP-2 for select spine fusion, fracture, and craniomaxillofacial procedures. Similarly, the vast majority of natural polymer scaffolds are intended to serve as degradable carriers for biomolecule or cell delivery, which provide osteoinductive or osteogenic healing cues. Alginate, silk, collagen, chitosan, and hyaluronic acid hydrogel preparations have all been developed [168–171]. Hydrogels are an easily injectable scaffold that can provide sustained release of biologics [171]. As a result, natural polymers occupy a unique space in bone regeneration research as a nonload-bearing carrier for therapeutics. To impart weight-bearing functionality, natural polymers are often incorporated into composites with stronger materials to improve scaffold mechanical properties and slow degradation (see Section 5.3.5).

Synthetic polymers investigated to treat bone defects include polylactic acid (PLA), polyglycolic acid (PGA), poly(lactic-*co*-glycolic acid) (PLGA), polycaprolactone (PCL), poly(methyl methacrylate) (PMMA), polydiaxanone (PDS), poly(propylene fumarate) (PPF), polyanhdrides, polyether ether ketone (PEEK), and ultrahigh-molecular-weight polyethylene (UHMWPE). PLA, PGA, PLGA, and PCL are all rigid aliphatic polyesters that are naturally biodegraded, with PGA being the most quickly degraded and PCL lasting up to 2–3 years in vivo [65,172]. Common fabrication techniques for polymer scaffolds include solvent casting and leaching, electrospinning, and 3-D printing. Polyesters are the most widely investigated synthetic polymers for bone regeneration. The elastic moduli of these materials can approach 4.8 GPa for PLA and 12.5 GPa for PGA (see Table 5.1) [63]. However, the surfaces of these polymers are all hydrophobic and consequently they do not support cell adhesion and tissue integration without incorporation of hydrophilic copolymers or ceramics. Likewise, the rest of the preceding synthetic polymers exhibit poor osteoconductivity compared to ceramics.

PEEK and UHMWPE are nondegrading, high-strength, wear-resistant polymers commonly utilized as joint replacement components and interbody cages in spine fusion [62,173]. While PEEK and UHMWPE, as well as many of the other previously mentioned synthetic polymers, exhibit similar mechanical properties to native bone in bulk, their mechanical properties decrease rapidly with the addition of porosity. This is a significant obstacle for degradable porous scaffolds intended to promote perfusion and tissue infiltration into the defect, as well as for the osseointegration of long-term load-bearing implants like spine cages. To address this limitation, the fabrication of PEEK implants with a thin layer of porosity at the surface has been developed. This approach is intended to promote osseointegration at the polymer—tissue interface while maintaining bulk strength of the implant. In vivo application in a rodent segmental defect showed improved mineral apposition at the implant surface compared to smooth PEEK [174]. Continued research to optimize bioactivity, surface chemistry, and scaffold architecture is needed to exploit the favorable mechanical characteristics of both degradable and nondegradable polymeric bone graft substitutes.

5.3.5 Composites

Composite materials for bone tissue engineering have become the primary design space in the field of late. Novel research has focused on integrating the respective advantages of each material class while reducing its disadvantages. The breadth of specific composite formulations in the literature exceeds the scope of this chapter. Instead, the structural and functional characteristics of polymer—ceramic and metal—ceramic families of composites will be discussed.

Polymer—ceramic composites have been adopted with the intent to more closely mimic the natural nanocomposite structure of bone, leveraging the osteoconductivity imparted by ceramic materials while simultaneously improving construct toughness and resistance to brittle failure through the introduction of a ductile polymeric matrix. Additionally, scaffold degradation rates can be tuned by varying the relative amounts of polymer and ceramic [175]. Common polymer—ceramic formulations reported in the literature include ceramic phases of HA, β-TCP, bioglass, and calcium carbonate combined with PLA, PGA, PLGA, PCL, PPF, chitosan, silk, and collagen (see Table 5.1) [65]. A key challenge in the design of bone graft substitutes is the tradeoff between porosity and mechanical strength and stiffness [23]. Computational finite element analysis has been utilized to predict the mechanical behavior of 3-D printed (by SLS) PCL:HA composites with different relative compositions and porosities [176]. This technique allows for the direct design and manufacturing of a composite scaffold with mechanical properties specifically tailored for the application. Composite scaffolds consisting of bioglass and PLA with porosities of up to 77–80% have been reported to possess elastic moduli and strength close to that of trabecular bone [65]. Interestingly, some researchers have noted that the reported mechanical properties of numerous calcium phosphate–polymer composites fall below those of the mechanical properties reported for bulk and porous materials they are replacing (see Fig. 5.1) [150]. Additionally, toughness, fatigue, and fracture properties of polymer–ceramic composites are rarely reported. These properties are a key drawback to ceramic materials, and due to this deficiency in the literature, the relative mechanical benefits provided by many polymer–ceramic composite scaffolds are not well understood. Future work is needed to characterize the functional capabilities of polymer–ceramic composite bone graft substitutes for load-bearing applications.

Metal–ceramic composites predominantly consist of a ceramic surface coating deposited on a solid or porous metal implant to enhance osteoconductivity. HA, β-TCP, and bioglass surface coatings have been applied to numerous orthopedic metals including titanium, tantalum, magnesium, and their alloys through physical and chemical deposition techniques [79,177,178]. Bulk mechanical properties of the underlying metal scaffold are largely unchanged, although the literature is sparse of reports describing basic mechanical properties of metal–ceramic composites like both the elastic modulus and strength [66]. In vitro cell culture results have demonstrated significant improvements in bioactivity due to ceramic coatings. Titanium substrates coated with calcium phosphate increased the adherence, ALP activity, and BMP-2 production of osteoblasts compared to bare titanium [179,180]. However, conflicting results have been reported in vivo. Many studies have reported accelerated bone growth and biomechanical strength of composite scaffolds, but a systematic review of oral implants has called into question whether there is sufficient evidence of improved healing in ceramic coatings compared to metal surfaces that are simply roughened [177,181]. These inconsistent results indicate more research is needed to understand the importance of specific surface parameters including chemical composition, surface topography, crystallinity, and thickness [177]. Notably, calcium phosphate coatings have been utilized to slow the degradation rate of porous magnesium scaffolds and enhance surface bioactivity. In separate studies, the rates of scaffold corrosion and tensile strength reduction of HA-coated magnesium constructs implanted in vivo were drastically reduced compared to bare magnesium [182]. Thus, ceramic surface coatings have been identified as a promising approach to augment the bioactivity and tune the degradation of metal implants, although continued work is needed to better understand the influence of many surface characteristics.

Clearly, the ideal mechanical, architectural, and material properties of a bone graft substitute are still an active area of debate in the field. The vast range of bone regeneration strategies currently being explored highlights the creativity of new research. Rather than universal adoption of a singular bone graft substitution strategy, a wide range of application-specific designs tailored to specific indications of a given injury and patient is needed. As numerous material synthesis, processing, and characterization techniques are developed, it is critical that researchers and physicians are knowledgeable of device classifications, regulatory pathways, and testing considerations to accelerate translation of new technologies to the clinic. In the following section, a brief review of the United States Food and Drug Administration's medical device classification system and regulatory pathways for clinical translation of bone graft substitutes is provided.

5.3.6 FDA regulatory pathways and testing considerations

The Federal Food Drug and Cosmetic Act (FD&C Act or the Act) defines a medical device, in part, as an article intended to diagnose, cure, mitigate, treat, or prevent a disease or other condition, which does not achieve its primary intended purposes through chemical action or dependent upon being metabolized by the body. Medical devices are classified based on the risk of the device to the patient and/or user. This classification system provides the framework for the level of regulatory control needed to provide a reasonable assurance of safety and effectiveness of medical devices. Low- to moderate-risk devices are designated as Class I devices, moderate- to high-risk devices are designated as Class II devices, and high-risk devices are designated as Class III. Some Class I, most Class II, and all Class III devices require FDA clearance or approval before the device can be marketed and made available to the public.

Class I devices are the lowest-risk devices with the least regulatory controls. The regulatory controls for this class of devices are general controls that include, but are not limited to, device registration, listing, misbranding and adulteration provisions, notification and recall provisions, adverse event reporting, and good manufacturing practices as outlined in the Quality System Regulations. Many Class I devices are exempt and thus may be marketed without FDA clearance. Examples of orthopedic Class I exempt devices are crutches, casts for stabilizing fractures, and bone cement dispensers.

In the case of Class II devices, which are of moderate to high risk, general controls alone are insufficient to provide reasonable assurance of the safety and effectiveness and there is sufficient information to establish special controls to provide such assurance. Special controls are additional device-specific controls that are needed to provide reasonable assurance of the safety and effectiveness for a particular device type. Special controls include, but are not limited to, guidelines, premarket data requirements, compliance with specified performance standards (e.g., ASTM or ISO standards), postmarket surveillance, patient registries, and special labeling requirements. Examples of orthopedic Class II devices include resorbable calcium salt bone void fillers (BVFs), intervertebral body fusion devices (i.e., interbody cages), and PMMA bone cement. Although some Class II devices are exempt from FDA review, the vast majority of Class II devices require premarket notification submissions (referred to as a 510(k) submission in reference to the section of the FD&C Act that describes this process). In a 510(k) submission device manufacturers provide information in a marketing submission in order to establish that the device is substantially equivalent to a legally marketed device (known as a predicate device). To demonstrate equivalence, the new device must have the same intended use and either the same technological characteristics or, in cases where the technological characteristics are different, not raise any different types of safety and effectiveness questions when compared to the predicate device. The information necessary to establish substantial equivalence typically includes, among other items, a device description, proposed labeling, indications for use, and performance testing (i.e., bench and/or animal testing), and in some cases can also include clinical data.

Class III devices are associated with the highest risk. These devices are intended to be used in supporting or sustaining human life or preventing impairment of human health, or that may present a potential unreasonable risk of illness or injury for which general controls and special controls are insufficient to provide reasonable assurance of the safety and effectiveness of a device or for which there is insufficient information to make such a determination. For many Class III devices, clinical data are needed to establish that there is reasonable assurance that the device is safe and effective for the identified intended use and patient population. For these devices, a premarket approval (PMA) application is required which includes both preclinical and clinical data, as well as manufacturing, sterilization, packaging, labeling, and other information. Class III devices are also required to comply with the general controls listed previously. Examples of Class III orthopedic devices are spinal disc replacements, metal-on-metal hip replacement systems, and BVFs that include a recombinant protein or synthetic peptide (e.g., rhBMP-2). Clinical studies conducted in the United States that evaluate significant risk devices, such as implants, must receive approval from the FDA prior to initiation. This is accomplished through the investigational device exemptions (IDE) process. Among other things, an IDE application contains a risk analysis of the device, preclinical testing, and clinical trial design (including patient population, enrollment criteria, study endpoints, and statistical analysis plan). An IDE allows a device that has not received approval or clearance for the identified investigational use or patient population to be used in a clinical study to obtain safety and/or effectiveness data.

There are other device submissions and regulatory pathways for medical devices, but these are utilized less frequently under special conditions or if certain criteria are met. The de novo classification request provides a pathway to classify low- to moderate-risk devices for which general and special controls provide reasonable assurance of safety and effectiveness, but for which there is no legally marketed predicate device. The data and information in the de novo request must demonstrate that general controls or general and special controls are adequate to provide reasonable assurance of safety and effectiveness. Humanitarian device exemption (HDE) application is another pathway for devices intended to benefit patients by treating a disease or condition that affects fewer than 4000 patients in the United States per year. An HDE application is similar to the PMA process; however, the clinical data presented in the HDE do not need to demonstrate efficacy of the device. An HDE application, however, must contain sufficient information for FDA to determine that the device does not pose an unreasonable or significant risk of illness or injury and that the probable benefit to health outweighs these risks, taking into account the probable risks and benefits of alternative forms of treatment. Additionally, the submission should demonstrate that no comparable devices are available to treat or diagnose the disease or condition, and that they could not otherwise bring the device to market.

The regulatory pathway for BVFs can vary based on the approach taken to treat bone defects. The use of autografts as BVFs is not regulated as a device; however, allografts may be regulated as a HCT/P (human cells, tissues, and cellular and tissue-based product) if they meet criteria specified in 21 CFR §1270–1271. These criteria state that an HCT/P (1) is minimally manipulated, (2) is intended for homologous use, (3) does not involve the combination of cells or tissues (with some exceptions), and (4) does not have a systemic effect and is not dependent upon the metabolic activity of living cells for it primary function (with certain exceptions). If these criteria are met, tissue establishments do not need PMA prior to marketing their tissue-based product and are only required to maintain records and comply with the donor eligibility and screening requirements as described in the Good Tissue Practices regulations. The use of cellular approaches, recombinant protein, or synthetic peptide technologies in combination with synthetic or natural BVFs may be regulated as a combination product. A combination product is defined in 21 CFR 3.2(e) as a product comprised of two or more regulated components (i.e., drug/device, biologic/device, drug/biologic, drug/device/biologic) that are physically, chemically, or otherwise combined or mixed and produced as a single entity. A BVF device combined with another regulated component (e.g., recombinant protein, drug, or cells) would be considered a combination product and multiple centers within the FDA would be involved in the review.

Synthetic BVFs are regulated as medical devices in accordance with 21 CFR §888.3045. As described previously in this chapter, BVFs can be manufactured from various synthetic materials. Examples of BVFs that can fall under this regulation are those consisting of calcium sulfate, HA, β-TCP, calcium carbonate, Bioglass, and other calcium salt derivatives. BVFs consisting of demineralized bone matrix (DBM) combined with components that are not intended for sterilization, storage, or preservation (e.g., DBM combined with glycerin) also fall under this regulation. Resorbable synthetic BVFs are considered Class II devices if the intended use is to fill bony voids or gaps of the extremities, posterolateral spine, and pelvis that are caused by trauma or surgery and are not intrinsic to the stability of the bony structure. It is important to note that BVF devices that fall under this definition are not intended to be the main load-bearing component and other stabilization or fixation methods (e.g., cast, internal/external fixation) are required to prevent collapse.

As discussed previously, Class II devices are regulated by general and special controls. The special controls for BVFs are discussed in the FDA guidance document "Class II Special Controls Guidance Document: Resorbable Calcium Salt Bone Void Filler Device: Guidance for Industry and FDA." This guidance document recommends characterization of chemical composition and physical properties, biocompatibility testing, bench performance testing, and functional animal implantation testing. The chemical composition of the implant may include identification and purpose of all of the constituents, crystalline and noncrystalline phases, phase purity, and the weight percentage of phases. In addition, elemental analysis, identifying the cation to anion ratio (e.g., Ca/P, Ca/S) and all trace impurities are necessary. It is also important to identify the physical properties of the device such as the form of the device (e.g., granules, preformed block, or putty/paste), dimensions, device density, surface area and roughness, and device microstructure (e.g., porosity). A side-by-side comparison of these properties between a new device and a legally marketed predicate device aids in establishing substantial equivalence.

Establishing biocompatibility (e.g., assessing toxicity, sensitization, irritation, carcinogenicity, and pyrogenicity) of the BVF is critical since it is a permanent implant and contacts tissue (e.g., bone). These parameters are typically addressed by tests performed in accordance with ISO 10993-1 (Biological Evaluation of Medical Devices-Part 1: Evaluation and Testing). Because BVFs can be produced in a variety of forms and working conditions (e.g., preformed blocks vs liquid and powder components that must be combined intraoperatively to form a putty or paste), the types of recommended bench testing will vary depending on the specific device characteristics of the BVF. Devices that set in vivo have additional testing considerations, such as the evaluation of working and setting times, dimensional stability, setting reaction temperature, chemical analysis, curing in vivo, and migration potential during curing. For devices that are intended to be injected, assessing whether the device can be correctly applied to the surgical site or if phase separation may occur under the proposed injection pressures are important considerations. Handling (e.g., moldability, ability to be cut and/or be shaped) and viscosity testing (if applicable) are considerations for devices not injected directly into the surgical site. For BVFs that are to be hydrated prior to implantation it is important that the end-user be provided with adequate instructions for professional use and that the preclinical testing properly assesses the device's ability to cure in a simulated wet environment (e.g., blood, saline, bone marrow aspirate).

Animal models can provide an important functional assessment of BVF device performance. Animal testing can evaluate the potential impact of technological differences (e.g., surface charge, surface topography, porosity) on the in vivo behavior of BVF devices that may not be adequately assessed by bench testing. A rabbit or larger animal model is generally used for assessment of the device. For the posterolateral spine, validated animal models involve the use of rabbits or sheep. When evaluating the use of BVFs in the extremities, dogs and goats, in addition to rabbits and sheep, are often used for assessing the performance of BVF in critical size defects. Regardless of the animal model or indications for use, skeletal maturity of the animal should be documented through literature and/or confirmed by closure of the growth plate during radiography. For BVFs that require use with adjuncts (i.e., autograft or allograft, saline, blood, or bone marrow aspirate), the animal study is designed to evaluate the BVF with each adjunct in all proposed anatomical locations. Because BVFs resorb and remodel at different rates in vivo, a minimum of three evaluation time points (e.g., 4, 8, and 12 weeks postimplantation) are useful for an assessment of graft resorption and new bone formation, as well as inflammatory reaction, over time. Assessing the performance of a BVF and establishing substantial equivalence to a legally marketed device typically involves the use of comparative testing of a predicate with similar technological characteristics (e.g., composition, configuration), as well as an autograft. In addition, assessment of a BVF in the extremities often incorporates a concurrent negative control (empty defect site) in the study design. Radiographic, histological, and histomorphometric evaluations during the course of the animal study will allow for the assessment of implant resorption and new bone formation over time.

The preceding information is intended to serve as an overview of the regulatory aspects of BVF development. This is not intended to be a complete and exhaustive review since there may be specific characterizations and/or study design considerations depending on BVF material(s) and configuration. In order to identify specific requirements for a particular BVF under development, it would be necessary to contact the relevant FDA review division to understand what information is needed to include as part of a marketing submission or request to initiate a US-based clinical trial.

5.4 CELL-LEVEL MECHANOBIOLOGY OF BONE REGENERATION

Physical forces are transduced into biochemical signals governing essential processes in almost all cells. Unsurprisingly, MSCs possess a number of mechanosensory systems and their differentiation processes are exquisitely sensitive to their micromechanical environment. After surgical implantation, the bone graft substitute acts as the initial cell substrate and template upon which healing will take place. Thus, the mechanical environment conferred by a specific bone defect treatment strategy is an essential factor dictating the healing mechanism and eventual patient outcome. Some of these critical physical factors include substrate stiffness, substrate topography, cell shape, and cell deformation resulting from interactions with the tissue matrix and surrounding fluids [183–185]. Similarly, mechanical strain and flow-induced shear are known to regulate growth and maturation of neovascular networks formed by endothelial cells [19–21]. These cellular-level phenomena have been demonstrated to correspond to tissue-level healing outcomes, as shown by numerous in vivo studies in the large bone defect and fracture healing literature investigating the role of specific mechanical signals on bone healing and maturation [40,55,186]. One critical prerequisite to osteogenic differentiation and tissue mineralization is vascularization of the regenerating tissue with a functional blood vessel network [44,54]. In large bone defects, both intramembranous and endochondral healing mechanisms can take place simultaneously in different locations [186]. There is increasing evidence that the mechanism of healing, or lack thereof, is regulated significantly by the local mechanical environment and the level of neovascularization in the tissue. The growth of the neovascular network, in turn, is also highly sensitive to mechanical conditions, underscoring the complex and fundamental role of mechanics in the healing process. In the subsequent sections, we discuss mechanobiological processes known to regulate MSC and endothelial function at the microscale and their correspondence to macroscale tissue formation during bone regeneration.

5.4.1 Cell-level mechanosensors

Mechanotransduction is the process by which cells sense and respond to physical forces exerted by the ECM and surrounding cells. This process is generally classified to occur in four major steps: (1) sensing of the mechanical stimulus, (2) conversion of the mechanical stimulus into a biochemical signal, (3) transmission of the biochemical signal, and (4) response of the effector cell [187]. Nearly all cells possess multiple mechanotransduction mechanisms known to regulate cell proliferation, differentiation, factor secretion, and matrix synthesis. The intricacies of each step in these mechanotransduction processes are beyond the scope of this text. For the purposes of this chapter, we provide a basic outline of (1) how cells sense force and (2) the functional roles of specific biophysical cues and substrate properties on cells as it pertains to bone healing.

First, we discuss four common mechanosensitive transmembrane components expressed in numerous cell types, including MSCs, bone cells, and endothelial cells, which alter cell function in response to physical interactions with their environment:

integrins, cadherins, stretch-activated ion channels, and the primary cilia [188]. Transmembrane integrin cell adhesion receptors are the primary receptor linking type I collagen, fibronectin, and laminin fibers of the local ECM to actin filaments of the cytoskeleton [189,190]. The specialized sites in the cytoskeleton at which integrin receptors form clusters are known as focal adhesion complexes. When ECM proteins bind to the integrin dimer, a subunit of the integrin within the cytoplasm undergoes a conformational change [191]. Since integrins do not have inherent enzymatic activity, the conformational change in the cytoplasmic domain transduces extracellular signals to regulate intracellular biochemical activity via kinases docked at the focal adhesion complex [192]. Mechanical stresses and strains on the ECM are also transmitted directly to the actin cytoskeleton of adhered cells via integrin binding sites. Conversely, cells exert traction forces and remodel their respective substrate via integrins [193]. In this manner, integrin complexes are the primary mechanism by which deformation and force are transferred bidirectionally between a cell and its substrate.

Cadherin receptors are the primary transmembrane component cells utilize to transmit traction forces and deformation to neighboring cells. Cell–cell connections formed at cadherin receptors are also anchored to the intracellular cytoskeleton by protein complexes including vinculin, α-catenin, and β-catenin, which regulate important downstream cell functions including differentiation, proliferation, and apoptosis [194]. Observations of highly localized strain concentration at cadherin-linked adherens junctions between endothelial cells subjected to flow-induced shear have led researchers to hypothesize that their structure is designed to target and amplify mechanical signals on cellular interfaces, increasing communication of mechanical signals between neighboring cells [195,196].

Stretch-activated transmembrane cation channels (SA-CATs) are gated by tension generated within the cytoskeleton acting along the plane of the cell membrane [197]. These nonselective mechanosensitive channels have been found in numerous cell types including endothelial cells and osteoblasts [198–200]. They respond to the magnitude and frequency of membrane deformation induced by changes in hydrostatic pressure by increasing channel open probability in response to larger or more frequent mechanical stimuli [198,201]. SA-CATs are considered a primary mechanism of load-induced bone formation. In osteoblasts, depolarization of SA-CATs triggers the opening of neighboring voltage-sensitive cation channels, eventually resulting in increased production of bone matrix proteins [194,202].

Primary cilia are immotile organelles formed by microtubules running from the centrosome and protruding 4–6 μm above the apical cell membrane surface. The cilia of osteoblasts deflect due to fluid flow-induced shear stress, and mice with bone-specific primary cilia knockouts exhibit reduced load-induced bone formation [203,204]. In human MSCs subjected to oscillatory fluid flow (OFF), removing expression of primary cilia with small-interfering RNA inhibits flow-induced osteogenic gene expression, confirming their role in flow mechanotransduction [205]. However, the precise signaling mechanisms mediating this response are not well characterized. One hypothesis cites that integrin focal adhesion complexes are known to localize at the same locations as primary cilium in several cell types including chondrocytes [206]. Thus, the cilia might signal interdependently with integrin to alter cell function and phenotype in response to fluid-mediated shear independent of cell substrate deformation [205]. Interestingly, cilia on endothelial cells are only found in regions of low or disturbed flow and they disassemble in response to laminar flow, but their role in cell function remains unclear [207,208].

Cells utilize their intrinsic mechanosensitive components to regulate their function based on feedback from the local environment, and conversely they also remodel their surroundings through these same mechanisms. This two-way mechanical communication is a critical process underlying tissue-level growth and development during healing. Through in vitro studies, specific substrate properties and extrinsic mechanical stimuli acting at the micro- and nanoscale have been elucidated as controllers of cell migration, lineage, proliferation, and protein synthesis. Physical mechanisms known to direct cell behavior include substrate stiffness, substrate topography and shape, substrate deformation, fluid flow-induced shear, and hydrostatic pressure. These in vitro mechanobiological studies have begun to quantify relative and categorical ranges of stimuli that would be considered beneficial or detrimental to clinically pertinent processes such as bone regeneration. Thus, understanding basic mechanical stimuli that promote bone healing in the cellular microenvironment is critical to inform rational scaffold design and selection decisions at the organ level.

5.4.2 Intrinsic physical factors

Cells in vivo inhabit a vast array of tissues, each with different degrees of elasticity and stiffnesses. Cells that adhere to an underlying substrate form focal adhesion complexes and exert contractile forces, creating tension in the actin cytoskeleton and local deformation of the bound substrate [209]. The mechanical stiffness of this substrate is known to have a direct effect on cell behaviors including migration, proliferation, apoptosis, and differentiation [183]. Vincent et al. fabricated gels with stiffness gradients encompassing the majority of soft tissues (1−12 kPa) and observed that MSCs preferentially migrated to the region with the highest stiffness with a migration rate proportional to the gradient slope [210]. Increasing the stiffness of the underlying cell substrate has also been shown to promote cell proliferation and to decrease the rate of apoptosis in fibroblasts and endothelial cells [211−214].

The influence of substrate mechanical properties on stem cell differentiation is of particular importance for bone regeneration, where MSCs serve as the primary source for skeletal tissue growth and differentiation. One of the first studies to isolate the role of substrate stiffness on MSC lineage showed that cells cultured on polyacrylamide gels possessing a modulus similar to unmineralized osteoid matrix (25–40 kPa) adopted an osteogenic morphology and produced osteogenic gene and protein profiles, while cells seeded on more compliant substrates mimicking neurogenic and myogenic environments assumed neurogenic and myogenic phenotypes, respectively [185]. While the preceding experiment was conducted in a two-dimensional (2D) culture environment, osteogenic commitment has also been replicated by Huebsch and colleagues in three-dimensional (3D) culture with mouse MSCs encapsulated in gels of approximately 11–30 kPa [215]. However, MSCs in 3D did not exhibit the drastic change in morphology as observed in 2D monolayer conditions. Interestingly, cells encapsulated in an even stiffer gel of approximately 110 kPa showed a drop-off in the production of osteogenic markers compared to cells within the 11–30 kPa gel. They demonstrated that integrin binding and the formation of tension-generating traction forces within the actin cytoskeleton are directly proportional to the rigidity of the substrate and mediate this process of stiffness-dependent osteogenesis, as blocking cell contractility with (2,3)-butanedione-monoxime prevents lineage commitment [215]. It is important to note that the substrate elastic moduli utilized in all the preceding experiments did not come close to reaching that of native mineralized bone, yet consistent patterns of stiffness-dependent osteogenic differentiation were observed in the presence of identical culture media, challenging the idea that bone graft substitutes should possess mechanical properties mimicking intact bone to promote osteogenesis. These data indicate that implants possessing more compliant material properties in the range of unmineralized osteoid might hold regenerative potential if supplementary load-bearing fixation is used.

The surface topography of a cell's substrate controls the spatial distribution of internal cytoskeletal stresses by altering the cell shape as well as the density of integrin and cadherin-mediated traction forces formed with the surroundings. Consequently, intracellular mechanical signaling transmitted through the actin cytoskeleton is altered. Human endothelial cells cultured on microstructural features, such as square islands and asymmetric annuluses (on the order of hundreds of μm), created asymmetric stress distributions, and cells in regions of high local stress concentrations proliferated faster than neighboring cells in low-stress regions [216]. Dalby and colleagues observed that nano-textured surfaces with equally spaced pit features 120 nm in diameter and 100 nm deep inhibit formation of focal adhesions and prevent osteogenic differentiation in human MSCs [217]. Interestingly, when the identical pit feature was distributed in a random pattern more representative of nanoscale disorder seen in native tissue, cells adopted osteoblastic morphology and produced early markers of osteogenic differentiation measured at 14 and 21 days [217].

In 3D microenvironments seen in vivo, there is a complex interplay between substrate architecture, cell shape, and cytoskeletal stress distribution, making it difficult to elucidate their relative importance [218]. Khetan and colleagues attempted to decouple the role of cell shape and cell-mediated tractions by encapsulating human MSCs in degradable hyaluronic acid hydrogels that promoted cell spreading, formation of focal adhesions, and osteogenic differentiation [219]. Secondary crosslinkers were added after 1 week of culture, which effectively halted further degradation of the hydrogel and inhibited cell-substrate tractions while the cells were still in a spread morphology. In response, cells switched from osteogenic to adipogenic differentiation without significantly altering their shape, indicating that cell adhesion-mediated traction forces with the matrix are more potent regulators of stem cell fate than shape alone [219].

5.4.3 Extrinsic physical factors

In load-bearing organs like bones, the tissue is subjected to complex spatiotemporal patterns of force and deformation. Stress and strain of the tissue by external biomechanical loads are transferred to cells and microvasculature primarily in the form of compressive and tensile mechanical strains of the underlying matrix, interstitial fluid flow-induced shear stress, and hydrostatic pressure. The regulatory role of each of these physical stimuli in MSCs and endothelial cells has been studied in vitro. First, we discuss the effect of tensile and compressive substrate deformation on MSC and endothelial cell function.

Cytoskeletal tensile strain can be transmitted to a cell by stretch of the underlying ECM and is known to affect MSC phenotype. However, the role of strain in osteogenesis has not been fully elucidated, as independent studies have shown that tension can induce upregulation of bone [220–222], muscle [223], and fibrous [224,225] tissue markers in MSCs. Sumanasinghe et al. found that human MSCs cultured in 3D collagen matrices subjected to daily bouts of cyclic 10% uniaxial strain for 7 or 14 days upregulated BMP-2 mRNA expression, while unstrained cells did not [220]. Kearney and colleagues subjected rat MSCs cultured on a type I collagen-coated silicone substrate to 2.5% uniaxial cyclic tensile strain for 14 days and observed reduced MSC proliferation and increased expression of osteogenic genes including core-biding factor alpha 1 (Cbfa1/Runx2), type Col I, OC, and BMP-2 [221]. Using biochemical inhibitors, they identified that stretch-activated cation channels were required for increased Col I expression and that kinases ERK, p38 and PI-3K each contribute to the observed increase in BMP-2. These findings indicate that multiple parallel signaling mechanisms mediate cellular responses to tension [221]. Simmons et al. also found that ERK and p38 signaling pathways were activated in human MSCs exposed to a biaxial cyclic strain of 3%, but osteogenic media supplements were utilized [226].

Tensile strain can also enhance MSC differentiation down other tissue lineages. Subramony and colleagues cultured human MSCs on poly(lactide-*co*-glycolide) nanofiber scaffolds with either aligned or unaligned fiber matrices and applied 1% cyclic tensile strain [224]. Differing from the findings of the previous studies, cells seeded on aligned matrices and subjected to tensile loading increased production of fibroblastic or tendon-related markers including Col I, type Col III, and tenascin-C after 14 and 28 days with no significant increases in osteogenic markers [224]. Chen et al. found that tensile strain can induce fibrogenesis or osteogenesis in human MSCs cultured on Col I-coated substrates in a strain magnitude-dependent fashion [227]. Cells exposed to 3% cyclic tensile strain for a period of 8 hours increased expression of osteogenic genes. However, cells subjected to higher magnitude strains (10%) for 48 hours showed increased expression of tendon-related markers. This increase in connective tissue expression was sustained after 48 additional hours of nonloaded culture [227]. Jang and colleagues have also shown magnitude-dependence to tensile strain in rabbit MSCs on fibronectin-coated polydimethylsiloxane substrates [223]. Cells subjected to higher cyclic strains (10%) for 72 hours increased production of smooth-muscle markers while cells exposed to identical conditions but reduced (3%) strain expressed more osteogenic markers [223]. These findings support that relatively large-magnitude, sustained tensile strains tend to promote fibroblastic or myogenic differentiation of MSCs, whereas lower-magnitude or shorter-duration tension supports osteogenic differentiation. Several in vivo studies have also found evidence supporting that an upper threshold of mechanical strain may exist for osteogenesis. These findings are reviewed in Section 5.5.

Compressive deformation of a 3D ECM creates a complex micromechanical environment which can result in direct strain of cells, increased hydrostatic pressure, and extracellular fluid flow [228]. The individual contribution of each type of mechanical perturbation is difficult to uncouple experimentally in 3D cultures which better replicate the in vivo niche. Nonetheless, several studies have found evidence that direct, unconfined compression of 3D hydrogels enhances chondrogenic differentiation of MSCs [229]. Huang and colleagues suspended rabbit MSCs in 2% agarose, with or without administration of the chondrogenic cytokine transforming growth factor-β1 (TGF-β1), and subjected the gels to daily sessions of 10% compressive strain [230]. They observed increased expression of chondrogenic markers collagen type II (Col II) and aggrecan in mechanically stimulated MSCs with no significant differences due to the administration of exogenous TGF-β1, indicating compressive strain is a chondrogenic stimulus independent of biochemical supplements in vitro [230]. Other studies of encapsulated MSCs have supported that exposure to TGF-β1 or compressive loading are both chondrogenic, but instead have shown that TGF-β1 is a significantly more potent stimulus [231,232]. Notably, Thorpe and colleagues found that when MSCs were cultured within a fibrin hydrogel which typically guided encapsulated cells down a myogenic lineage, long-term (42 days) dynamic compression superseded the myogenic effect of the fibrin substrate and instead cells adopted a chondrogenic phenotype [233]. To better elucidate the intracellular mechanism facilitating compression-induced chondrogenesis, Pelaez et al. cultured human MSCs within a fibrin hydrogel with or without administration of an inhibitor of the extracellular signal-related kinase 1/2 (ERK 1/2) pathway, a widely conserved signaling pathway modulated by integrin adhesion with the ECM [234,235]. Dynamic compression was applied to the gels immediately followed by measurement of osteogenic and chondrogenic markers. They found that inhibition of the ERK 1/2 pathway abrogated the chondrogenic response observed in cells loaded without the inhibitor. Instead, blocking the ERK 1/2 pathway promoted osteogenic marker expression. Thus, it appears that dynamic compression-induced chondrogenesis or osteogenesis is primarily regulated by activation of the ERK 1/2 pathway, with ERK 1/2 activation promoting cartilage formation [235]. Likewise, Steward and colleagues showed that integrin adhesion of MSCs with the ECM at least in part mediates chondrogenic differentiation in response to dynamic compression [236]. Based on these studies, it is clear that compressive stimuli regulate the differentiation profile, and particularly chondrogenesis, of MSCs. Future work is needed to investigate the role of mechanical loads in endochondral ossification of newly formed cartilage, and if compressive loading can be tuned to promote early formation of a cartilage callus in large bone defects with poor vascular supplies.

Mechanical stretch due to hemodynamic forces has long been known to regulate vascular structure and function [237]. Increasing evidence has also elucidated that stretch mediated by the external matrix or substrate influences the collective behavior of endothelial cells, capillaries, and microvascular structures in vitro. Zheng et al. showed that rat and human endothelial cells seeded in 2D on Col I increased production of proangiogenic receptors in response to cyclic tensile strain (15%, 0.5 Hz) [238]. Thus, mechanical stretch can increase endothelial cell sensitivity to paracrine VEGF signaling to promote vascular growth. Wilkins and colleagues observed that tensile strain promotes angiogenesis but is dependent on the loading frequency [239]. Endothelial cells were seeded on top of 3D collagen gels and subjected to 10% or 20% strain at 1/12 or 1 Hz. Only the higher, 1 Hz strain frequency induced neovascular sprouting, which grew perpendicular to the direction of stretch [239]. Likewise, Joung and colleagues cultured vascular endothelial cells in a 3D collagen gel subjected to cyclic tensile stretch and observed that cord-like cellular structures formed perpendicular to the stretch direction [240]. Numerous other 2D studies of endothelial cells exposed to tensile strain have also shown that cells tend to minimize their deformation and orient perpendicular to the primary axis of the deformation field [241–243].

To better understand the effect of micromechanical stimuli on multicellular structures with a 3D vascular morphology, Krishnan and colleagues cultured microvessel fragments within 3D rectangular collagen gels and subjected the constructs to four different mechanical boundary conditions: 6% static stretch, 6% cyclic stretch

(1 Hz, 12 hours per day), unstretched but anchored, and free on both ends (shape control) [20]. Each of the three anchored or stretched construct groups had significantly more vessels per construct compared to the shape control, indicating tension formed by external stretch and contraction of the gel enhanced microvascular growth. Interestingly, they found that the microvessel fragments in these same three groups preferentially oriented themselves parallel to the direction of stretch [20]. This seemingly contradictory result to cellular-level studies may be due to enhanced contact guidance provided by the surrounding collagen matrix with the multicellular microvessel fragments, since the ECM tends to align in the primary direction of stress [244]. Thus, the role of mechanical cues like matrix deformation in more geometrically complex models recapitulating in vivo tissue architecture can be drastically different to reproducible results in simpler models. Nonetheless, in vitro models have established that tensile strains in the ECM can enhance neovascular growth. Strikingly little is known about the role of compressive strains on endothelial cells and the microvasculature, which is the primary stimulus induced by functional loading of bone defects. Future work to understand how compression or shear of the pericellular matrix influences neovascular growth, branching, and orientation is critical to inform novel approaches to improve vascularization in regenerative processes like bone repair.

As mentioned briefly, the application of cyclic external loads also induces oscillatory patterns of interstitial fluid flow away from regions of large compressive deformation, like a sponge releasing water when squeezed [191]. This fluid flow exerts shear stress on the apical surface of adhered cells within the tissue, activating membrane mechanosensors like the primary cilia which in turn transduce the cytoskeleton [205]. Additionally, perfusion of the cells increases convective transport of nutrients throughout the ECM. Fluid-induced shear force on the cell surface is related to the magnitude and the velocity of the external load application, and is widely accepted as a principal extracellular stimulus regulating the maintenance and adaptation of native bone to biomechanical loads [187,194]. Fluid-flow-induced shear is also a critical determinant of the function of MSCs, regulating their migration, proliferation, and differentiation. Meinel et al. showed that fluid flow increased calcium and ALP in human MSCs on collagen scaffolds, and that the degree of osteogenesis is dependent on the flow pattern (spinner flask or perfused reactor) and scaffold degradation rate [245]. Li and colleagues cultured human MSCs in 2D on glass and subjected them to 2 hours of laminar OFF [246]. After 24 hours, increased proliferation and expression of osteogenic genes was measured in cells subjected to OFF relative to cells in static culture. Conversely, ALP activity was actually reduced 3 days after OFF, although the expression of ALP is known to be highly transient during osteogenic differentiation of MSCs [246,247]. Datta and colleagues looked at the role of OFF in more complex 3D environments by culturing rat MSCs on a titanium mesh with or without a pregenerated ECM perfused with peristaltic flow and saw that the presence of a native

ECM increased mineral deposition, calcium content, and ALP compared to titanium alone [248]. Additionally, mineral content was fivefold higher in perfused Ti/ECM constructs compared to static constructs, indicating a synergistic effect of native ECM soluble factors and flow [248]. Hoey et al. demonstrated that OFF-induced osteogenesis in MSCs is partially facilitated by the primary cilia [205]. Notably, inhibiting primary cilia formation significantly increased proliferation in the presence of flow, indicating cilia regulate the extent of cell proliferation in the presence of mechanical stimuli [205].

Similarly, external fluid shear stress is also known to affect the proliferation and migration of endothelial cells, although most research has focused on steady rather than oscillatory flow patterns. Ando and colleagues were the first to show that endothelial cell proliferation is significantly enhanced in proportion with the intensity of the applied shear stress [249]. Li et al. demonstrated that endothelial cells subjected to flow migrate in the direction of the flow stimulus by successively forming focal adhesions at the front of the cell and disassembling focal adhesions at the rear [250]. These observations provide evidence that flow-induced shear stress within a graft substitute might enhance endothelial cell migration and proliferation. For bone tissue engineering, the benefits of fluid flow on osteogenic differentiation and endothelial proliferation is one advantage of highly interconnected porous architectures for graft substitutes [251]. OFF-induced osteogenesis has also been leveraged by in vitro scaffold preconditioning in perfusion bioreactor culture platforms [252].

Local changes in hydrostatic fluid pressure (HP) due to tissue deformation are also known to control MSC phenotype. Numerous in vitro studies of MSCs in aggregate, pellet, and hydrogel-encapsulated cultures have established that cyclic HP enhances expression of chondrogenic genes, proteoglycans, and collagen [253–255]. The mechanosensory mechanism mediating this response is unclear, though intracellular and extracellular ion transport is known to be responsive to changes in HP, supporting a role for stretch-activated ion channels [256–259]. Steward and colleagues have also elucidated that cell–matrix interactions and substrate stiffness play a complex role in MSC adaptation to cyclic HP [260]. They cultured porcine MSCs in agarose hydrogels of varying stiffness, with the stiffest gel supporting the formation of stress fibers and an osteogenic phenotype. When subjected to cyclic HP for 3 weeks only MSCs encapsulated in stiff gels increased chondrogenic marker expression, indicating that cell–matrix interactions also facilitate HP mechanotransduction [260].

In vitro models have established that all cells, including MSCs and endothelial cells, are extremely sensitive to physical interactions with their surroundings. These mechanobiological interactions regulate cellular processes critical to bone defect healing. The mechanical environment of a cell is primarily determined by intrinsic properties of the underlying substrate, the configuration of cell adhesions, and the external stresses and strains transmitted by the underlying substrate and interstitial fluids.

During bone regeneration, the graft substitute and fixation equipment govern all of these physical factors. Thus, observations gleaned from well-controlled in vitro studies of cell mechanobiology can be used to inform rational design improvements for bone tissue engineering. For example, repeatable osteogenic differentiation has been demonstrated in vitro within hydrogels possessing a much lower stiffness than native bone. This result would appear to contradict the widely held theory that an ideal bone graft substitute should replicate the mechanical properties of the tissue it is replacing. Additionally, mechanical strain has been demonstrated to promote bone, cartilage, and neovascular growth, depending on the magnitude, direction, timing, and frequency of the stimulus. Likewise, deformation-induced fluid flow and hydrostatic pressure changes can enhance osteogenesis and chondrogenesis. This motivates the long-held theory that controlled load transfer through the regenerating tissue within a predetermined threshold could be used to augment the healing process and direct the mechanism by which it occurs [261].

5.5 TISSUE-LEVEL MECHANOBIOLOGY OF BONE REGENERATION

While in vitro models have been critical to elucidate how distinct mechanical cues regulate cells responsible for bone regeneration, the environment of healing tissue in vivo is a spatiotemporally heterogeneous, complex combination of both mechanical and biochemical signals. In vivo models of bone regeneration are critical to establish the relative importance of mechanical stimuli on functional healing outcomes. Numerous studies have explored the effects of different types of loading on fracture and large bone defect healing. However, the ability to experimentally measure local mechanical stresses and strains in vivo is extremely challenging. Many researchers, particularly in the fracture healing literature, have leveraged computational models based on experimental data to back calculate tissue-level estimates of stress and strain. These numerical simulations have reinforced various mechanobiological regulation theories, which define quantities of mechanical stimuli as thresholds for tissue differentiation. In this section, we review key findings from in vivo and in silico studies that have helped to clarify the functional significance of the mechanical environment on bone healing.

5.5.1 In vivo mechanobiology of bone regeneration

The regenerative niche in vivo is subjected to combined modes of mechanical loading, including compression, tension, bending, shear, and torsion. These organ-level stimuli are largely determined by the type of fixation used as well as the structural and mechanical properties of the tissue and/or scaffold within the defect space. The experimental framework to study mechanical stimulation of bone healing is not standardized, making it difficult to compare findings across different studies. Generally, researchers transfer mechanical loads through a bone defect by three methods: (1)

using a defined loading protocol transmitted by an external loading device, (2) using fixation device designs that allow different ranges and modes of deformation, and (3) using fixation devices fabricated from different materials with distinct mechanical properties [262]. The latter two techniques do not allow active control of the stress or strain exerted on the defect region, but do permit the use of internal fixation devices.

The vast majority of experimental data investigating mechanical stimulation on bone healing is for fracture, whereas the literature on large defect regeneration is more limited. The fracture healing literature has established that certain levels of early interfragmentary movement promote the formation of an unmineralized callus and enhanced endochondral bone healing [56,263–265]. Increased callus formation can have a beneficial or detrimental effect on tissue growth and maturation, with a strong dependence on the magnitude, timing, and duration of the loading. Goodship and Kenwright were the first to show that controlled cyclic axial compression protocol initiated at day 0 (500 cycles/day, 33% maximum strain/360 N maximum load) in a sheep 3-mm tibial osteotomy model enhanced initial callus formation, increased tibia axial stiffness at 8–10 weeks in vivo, and increased tibia torsional stiffness at 12 weeks ex vivo [263].

The postoperative timing of load transfer is also critical to the healing outcome. Late load transfer has been shown to enhance the rate of bone remodeling and maturation after defect bridging has occurred. Gardner et al. observed that noninvasive cyclic compression (2 N peak load, 100 cycles per day) in a mouse tibial osteotomy from day 0 inhibited callus formation and ultimately prevented healing. Notably, a 4-day delay in compressive loading enhanced bone healing [266]. While these findings may appear contradictory to the prior reports of Goodship and Kenwright, an intramedullary nail with significantly reduced mechanical resistance to axial and torsional loads was used in the mouse model, highlighting the importance of fixation strategy. Multiple fracture and large bone defect models in the rat and mouse have also supported the functional healing benefit of increased load transfer at 3–4 weeks by utilizing a dynamic fixation system whose axial stiffness can be reduced at a given time point, permitting larger compressive loads through the tissue [40,58,186,267].

To elucidate the role of uniaxial compressive stimuli in a critically sized 6-mm rodent femoral defect model, Boerckel and colleagues showed that load transfer at 4 weeks after initial mineral bridging significantly enhances bone volume at 8 weeks and torsional stiffness at 12 weeks when treated with a graft substitute consisting of an alginate hydrogel delivering 5 μg BMP-2 and a dynamic internal fixator [186]. Qualitative histological observation demonstrated that loaded defects had increased cartilage formation at 5 weeks and an isotropic collagen microstructure characteristic of woven bone at 12 weeks, demonstrating that the chondral and remodeling phases of healing are prolonged in mechanically stimulated large bone defects in a manner analogous to fracture healing. In a separate study, Boerckel et al. studied the effect of delayed mechanical loading on neovascular growth in an 8-mm defect model and observed that compressive load transfer at 4 weeks increases the number of large-diameter blood vessels exceeding 300 μm in diameter and reduces the number of small vessels less than 100 μm in diameter within and around the defect region (Fig. 5.2F–K) [40]. From these data it was hypothesized that mechanical stimulation may rupture small vessels while concurrently enhancing arteriogenesis of larger vessels in and around the newly regenerated bone. Notably, immediate postsurgical load transfer in defects treated with 2.5 μg BMP-2, which produced axial strains of approximately 5–10%, significantly reduced bone formation by 75% and vascular volume by 50% in defects (Fig. 5.2A–E) [40]. Thus, it appears that an initial phase of tissue maturation and vascular infiltration must be achieved before relatively large-magnitude biomechanical loads can be transferred to the tissue.

Schwarz et al. showed that a controlled compressive loading protocol (six cycles, 10% strain) transmitted weekly by an external fixator from day 0 onward enhanced callus volume at 2, 4, and 6 weeks in a comparable rodent femoral defect model treated with a collagen sponge delivering a 10-fold larger dose of BMP-2 (50 μg) [268]. However no mechanical testing was completed to evaluate differences in functional load-bearing strength or stiffness of the newly regenerated bone. Glatt and colleagues treated a 5-mm rodent femoral defect with a collagen sponge delivering 11 μg BMP-2 and a dynamic external fixation system [269]. Interestingly, they found that initially affixing a relatively compliant fixator then increasing its stiffness at 2 weeks enhanced maximum torque to failure of the femur at 8 weeks. The bone and callus cross-sectional area of femurs secured with the dynamic fixation scheme was significantly lower than femurs secured with either high or low stiffness fixators throughout. Qualitative examination of micro-CT images indicated that dynamic fixation produced healed defects with thicker cortical bone and less trabecular bone compared to the other fixation systems. When comparing the experimental design of the three preceding rodent studies, it is important to note that Glatt and Schwarz utilized unilateral defects whereas bilateral defects were studied by Boerckel [40,186,268,269]. This may have affected the ambulatory load-share transferred through the operated limb. Additionally, the transition in the apparent axial stiffness of the "stiff" to "compliant" fixation configurations in the two studies utilizing dynamic fixation were dissimilar: approximately 25–30 N/mm for Glatt, and 8.4–349.5 N/mm for Boerckel [36,270]. Therefore, the relative change in the tissue mechanical environment introduced by actuation of the fixation system was drastically different between the two studies. Hou et al. studied a critically sized femoral defect in goats secured with either a stiff or spring-loaded intramedullary rod treated with DBM seeded with goat MSCs [271]. The uniaxially compliant fixation system exhibited increased callus formation and blood flow at early time points and improved torsional stiffness and strength at 8 and 16 weeks when compared to the static fixation system. These studies have

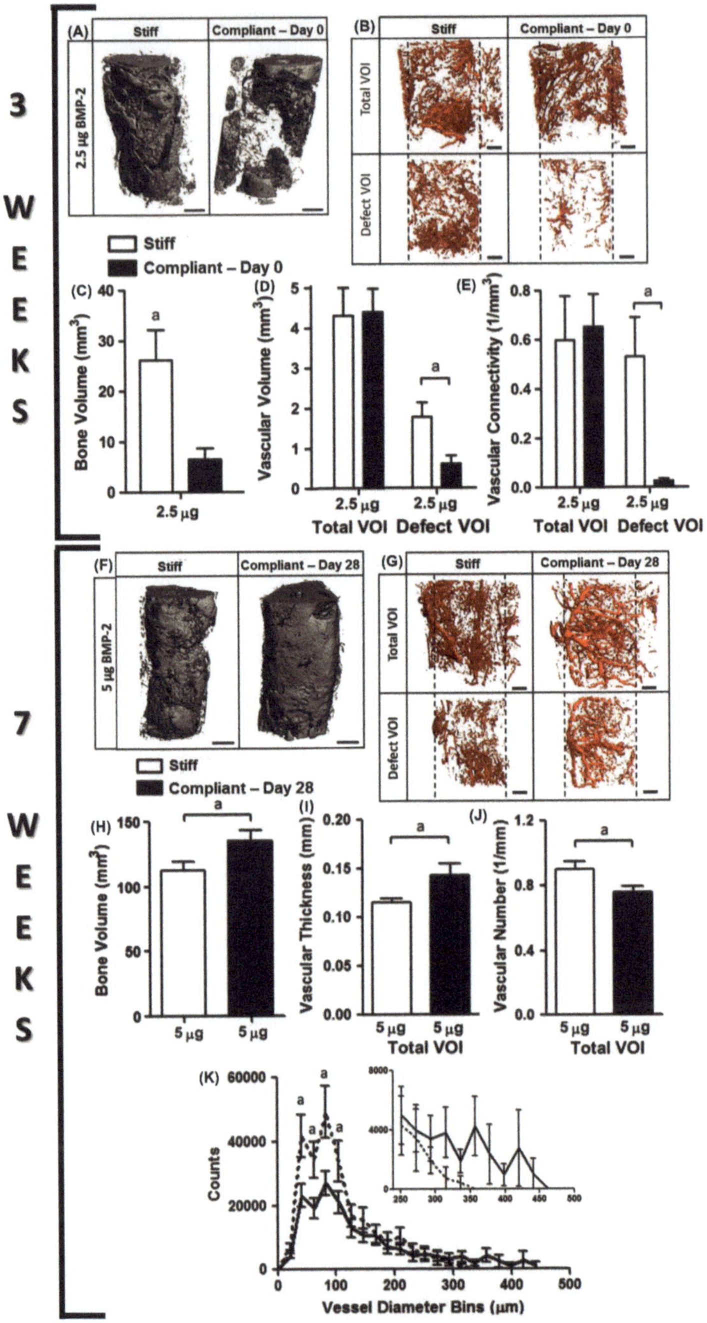

Figure 5.2 A rodent critically sized (8-mm) femoral defect model treated with BMP-2 and compliant fixation was used to investigate the effects of uniaxial load transfer through the defect due to physiological ambulatory loads. In defects treated with 2.5 μg BMP-2, load transfer immediately after surgery significantly attenuated bone formation, vascular volume, and vascular connectivity compared to load-shielded defects stabilized by stiff fixation (A—E). Delaying the onset of load transfer by 28 days significantly increased bone volume and vascular thickness, but reduced vascular number compared to stiff fixation in defects treated with 5 μg BMP-2 (F—K). Based on these observations, the authors hypothesized that large initial strains inhibited vascular invasion and bone formation. Smaller strains after initial stabilization of the defect were hypothesized to promote bone formation, vascular remodeling, and arteriogenesis of larger vessels, but reduce formation and growth of smaller vessels; (a) $P < 0.05$ [40].

demonstrated that a controlled compressive loading regimen can act as a potent anabolic stimulus to promote functional healing in bone defects treated with cells or biologics. Analysis of the mechanical boundary conditions imposed by the fixation system and scaffold over time is needed to elucidate the underlying mechanism modulating bone and vascular growth in disparate in vivo modeling approaches.

Although the research literature is not as well established, several studies have evaluated the effect of compressive load transfer on bone defects treated with a structural scaffold. Duty and colleagues developed a subcutaneous implant capable of exerting cyclic compressive loads on a cylindrical scaffold in vivo [272]. Porous PLDL scaffolds seeded with MSCs were subjected to six bouts of 13.3 N loads at 1 Hz over a 2-week period. Mineralization in loaded scaffolds increased significantly by nearly threefold versus the unloaded controls. Roshan-Ghias et al. implanted a composite PLA/β-TCP graft substitute into the distal femur of the rat and applied external cyclic loading to the entire limb [273]. The loading protocol was initiated 2 weeks postsurgery and consisted of five brief sessions of 10 N compressive loading. Bone formation was tracked longitudinally by micro-CT over 35 weeks, with loaded constructs exhibiting an 18% increase in bone volume compared to unloaded controls. Image registration of time-lapsed scans permitted quantification of local bone formation and resorption rates. Loaded scaffolds exhibited enhanced bone formation rates over 4–10 weeks postsurgery and decreased bone resorption rates throughout weeks 9–18. Interestingly, this would seem to indicate that mechanical conditioning not only enhances bone formation for an extended period of time but also inhibits bone resorption well after the stimulus has concluded [273]. Zhang and colleagues demonstrated that loading could potentially be leveraged to synchronize the rate of defect mineralization with the degradation of solid calcium sulfate cylindrical scaffolds implanted in the distal femur of the rat [157]. In this study, mechanical stimulation was introduced 1 week postoperation by a treadmill running regimen utilizing different belt speeds and lasting 30 consecutive days. The rate of bone formation at the defect site in animals completing an ascending speed running program matched closely with the rate of calcium sulfate degradation compared to constant speed or nonexercising animals [157]. These data suggest compressive load transfer can also enhance bone formation in defects treated with structural scaffolds with or without cells.

The regulation of bone healing by static tension is well established by the clinical practice of distraction osteogenesis, in which incremental tensile strains are introduced into an osteotomy gap by an external fixator to promote bone lengthening [274–276]. The distraction technique consists of a controlled surgical osteotomy, followed by up to a week of static rest. Then, the external fixator is actuated to gradually separate the osteotomy ends 1 mm per day in four 0.25-mm increments. Distraction proceeds for 1–2 weeks or until the desired length is achieved, followed by locking the fixator to permit consolidation of the gap over 8–12 weeks [277]. The application of a small tensile strain appears to promote robust intramembranous ossification and vascularization, while inhibiting cartilage formation [278,279]. Matsubara and colleagues demonstrated that distraction induces bone formation through cooperative secretion of angiogenic and osteogenic factors between mesenchymal cells in the defect region and vascular tissues in the surrounding muscle [279]. The healing response is highly sensitive to the mechanical environment produced by the distraction rate [280]. Increasing the distraction rate to 2 mm per day can result in fibrous nonunion, bone weakening, soft tissue contracture, and nerve lesions [281]. Conversely, decreasing the distraction rate can result in premature bridging of the gap [274,275]. Evidently, a relatively narrow range of small static tensile strains promotes intramembranous bone formation during distraction osteogenesis. The addition of short bouts of compression alternating with the standard distraction protocol, nicknamed the "accordion technique," has been investigated in an effort to simultaneously promote endochondral and intramembranous healing in defects with delayed callus formation [277,282]. Small clinical reports of the accordion maneuver have shown some anecdotal evidence of efficacy, but rigorous studies to elucidate any mechanistic changes in healing due to the addition of compression are lacking [283].

Bending, torsion, and shear deformations generate stress distributions with significantly higher spatial complexity, and their effect remains controversial. Boerckel and colleagues stimulated a critically sized rodent defect treated with a porous PLDL/TCP scaffold containing 2 μg BMP-2 by first installing a relatively stiff internal fixation plate, then replacing the stiff plate with a multiaxially compliant internal fixator possessing low stiffness to both bending and axial loads after 8 weeks of healing. Following the substitution, the defects failed structurally and nonunions formed, signifying the tissue had not matured to handle the full range of ambulatory loads [36]. Augat et al. compared pure shear versus compression up to 1.5 mm of a 3-mm tibial osteotomy in sheep. Shear significantly attenuated healing compared to axial motion, reducing defect bridging by 70%, callus area by 36%, and stiffness by over 60% [284]. Conversely, Bishop et al. reported improved intercortical mineralization in a 2.4-mm ovine osteotomy subjected to rotational shear compared to static or axially compressed specimens [285]. Thus, bone defects appear highly sensitive to shear stimuli, which can dramatically attenuate healing or result in tissue failure if excessive loads are applied.

While in vivo models have undeniably established the functional importance of mechanics in bone regeneration, experimental variability in species, injury model, loading regimen, and treatment intervention make it difficult to draw salient conclusions of how graft substitute treatments and mechanical stimuli can be implemented to augment bone healing in the clinic. Overall, the literature indicates that certain load levels can enhance bone or callus formation depending on the stage of healing. Relatively small early loads can promote initial callus formation, and larger magnitude loads can accelerate bone growth after initial defect bridging. However, excessive loads at any of these time points can promote fibrous tissue formation, inhibit vascularization, and result in nonunion or structural failure of the newly formed bone. The ability to predetermine these load thresholds and prescribe a controlled mechanical environment in the defect remains a complex challenge for future work. Changes in tissue volume, structure, and distribution over the time course of healing continuously alter the mechanical environment. Degradable scaffolds further increase the spatiotemporal complexity of mechanical signals in vivo. To clarify how healing is regulated across dissimilar treatment scenarios, the progression of the local stresses and strains within the healing tissue must be analyzed.

5.5.2 Computational modeling of bone regeneration

As described in Section 5.4, macroscopic mechanical boundary conditions ultimately correspond to cellular-level cues like deformation, interstitial fluid flow, and changes in hydrostatic pressure which regulate cell function. Due to the heterogeneity of healing tissue geometry and mechanical properties, the organ-level stress and strain tensor is not representative of the local stresses and strains encountered in the tissue microstructure. Since mechanotransduction is mediated at the cellular-level, quantifying the stress state within the microstructure provides deeper insight into how mechanical signals regulate healing outcomes. To address these gaps in experimental data, numerical finite element models of bone healing regulated by mechanical signals have been developed. The development of a governing "mechanoregulation" theory with mechanical thresholds able to predict local tissue differentiation and healing outcome a priori is an overarching goal of this analysis approach.

Numerous mechanoregulation theories of transverse fracture healing governed by specific mechanical stimuli have been proposed and reviewed in detail elsewhere [262,286]. To account for limitations in accurately computing individual components of stress and strain at the microstructural level, many researchers utilize a scalar parameter describing overall deformation (i.e., strain energy density) or a combination of parameters [262]. For example, Claes and colleagues developed a tissue differentiation model based on qualitative comparisons with histological tissue distributions of healing 1-, 2-, and 6-mm osteotomies subjected to different interfragmentary strains (7% or 31%) in sheep. They hypothesized that local tissue differentiation was governed by hydrostatic pressure and maximum strain. Based on an axisymmetric two-dimensional finite element model of a fracture callus at three time points, they determined that localized intramembranous ossification was promoted at hydrostatic pressures below ± 0.15 MPa and strains less than $\pm 5\%$. When compressive hydrostatic pressures exceeded -0.15 MPa but strains remained below $\pm 15\%$, endochondral ossification was predominant. Persistent fibrous connective tissue or cartilage was found in environments exceeding these bounds [56,287]. These findings help to quantify in vivo observations demonstrating increased fibrous tissue formation and delayed bridging or nonunion from premature or excessive magnitude mechanical stimulation [36,40,56,288,289].

To further recapitulate complexities of the healing environment, coupled algorithms considering other biological factors like neovascularization and diffusion of soluble factors have been developed [218,290–292]. Burke and Kelly investigated an innovative hypothesis that external mechanical signals act indirectly to influence the local oxygen environment [218]. In this finite element model of a 3-mm axisymmetric fracture callus, the regulatory variables determining stem cell differentiation were local oxygen tension and substrate stiffness. Angiogenesis and oxygen transport were both modeled as diffusive processes, where angiogenesis was inhibited by shear strains exceeding a threshold (4–8%). The simulation closely predicted experimental measurements of oxygen tension in a healing fracture callus and spatially averaged histological images of fracture healing, both taken from sheep [293,294]. Thus, there is increasing evidence of significant interplay between local mechanical cues and nutrient delivery in healing tissues. Future experimental and computational work exploring relationships between different biophysical stimuli in large bone defects and geometrically complex three-dimensional environments will continue to improve our understanding of their relative importance.

Computational studies have greatly enhanced our understanding of the spatial and temporal mechanical environment during bone regeneration, which is far too complex to be characterized solely by experimentation alone. A significant number of mechanoregulation models have been proposed to predict tissue differentiation within transverse fractures and bone graft substitutes. A number of these studies, however, lack quantitative validation against experimental data and their relevance to large bone defects is not well characterized at this point [262]. Studies that do reference experimental data primarily use qualitative comparisons to 2D histological cross sections at a single time point. Furthermore, the majority of computational models rely on simplifying assumptions including 2D axisymmetric callus geometries, uniform boundary conditions, and homogeneous tissue properties; yet, these factors are heterogeneous and dynamic in vivo [56,262]. Leong and Morgan demonstrated that the indentation moduli of tissues in the rodent fracture callus 35 days after fracture are highly heterogeneous, ranging from 0.61 to 1010 MPa, with woven bone spanning 26.92–1010 MPa [295]. In a separate study, Leong and Morgan showed that the average nanoindentation modulus within a sub-VOI of the callus correlates with the average tissue mineral density (TMD) as measured by micro-CT [55]. This relationship supports TMD as a promising metric to noninvasively account for tissue modulus heterogeneity in micro-CT-based finite element models of regenerating bone, although further investigation is needed to confirm its validity in large defects. Additionally, external loads on the defect are complex and continuously evolve over time as healing occurs and the regenerate tissue stiffens. Assumptions of tissue geometry, composition, and properties as well as boundary conditions, substantially alter the local mechanical environment predicted by computational models. Consequently, these assumptions could compromise the accuracy of conclusions obtained from the analysis. Therefore, a key challenge moving forward is longitudinally measuring and modeling external boundary conditions, tissue composition, and tissue geometry throughout healing to underpin models with improved accuracy and predictive capability.

To address the limitations of predicting local tissue deformation with a finite element model, Morgan and colleagues utilized digital image correlation to measure the 2D strain field in the midsagittal plane of a fracture callus during mechanical bending of the fracture callus over 35 degrees. Although the measurement technique only provided a 2D assessment of strain in a single plane at a single time point, it did not rely on any underlying assumptions of tissue mechanical properties or boundary conditions. Correlating the local strain with histomorphometry of multiple samples over time revealed that the probability of woven bone formation decreased and cartilage increased with increasing shear strain, and to a lesser extent, increasing maximum principal strain. These findings are in part agreement with mechanoregulation models of Prendergast et al. and Claes et al., which respectively consider shear strain and principal strain as governing stimuli [56,296].

Current computational analyses of bone defect healing mechanobiology rely on numerous simplifying assumptions, limiting their utility for direct quantitative comparison to experimental results. Nonetheless, models offer exciting potential to parametrically investigate the role of mechanical signals in physiologically relevant healing environments. Practically, computational simulations are a cost-effective and high-throughput approach to screen graft substitute design parameters before in vivo testing, reducing animal usage in the process. This approach could also be extended to simultaneously consider the pairing of a certain fixation configuration with a graft substitute to evaluate the osteogenic potential of the mechanical environment they confer. However, to improve our understanding of how local mechanical signals regulate tissue compositional changes in vivo, specimen-specific experimental measurements of external loads and tissue composition acquired at multiple time points (or continuous local measurements) are needed. Experimental measurements of these factors will help to validate the spatial and temporal accuracy of high-resolution finite element models describing the local stress and strain state throughout the entire process of bone regeneration.

5.6 CONCLUSIONS AND FUTURE DIRECTIONS

While a tremendous amount of progress has been made in the past decades, the field of bone tissue engineering remains a highly active field of research, and no consensus has been reached on what an "ideal" treatment approach looks like for many clinical procedures. Consequently, autografts remain the gold standard implant for bone defect treatment despite their inherent limitations. Increasing evidence has established the exquisite sensitivity of bone to mechanical cues. Therefore, a complete understanding of the role of the mechanical environment in osteogenesis is broadly applicable to the design of bone graft substitutes and treatment strategies for many clinical scenarios. In this chapter, we reviewed the process of bone defect healing, the mechanical properties of materials investigated for bone defect treatment, and the role of mechanical signals in bone repair. In addition, we reviewed relevant FDA device classifications and testing considerations for BVFs.

The optimal range of mechanical properties of a bone graft substitute remains a highly controversial topic. Inspection of Table 5.1 and Fig. 5.1 shows that the elastic modulus of bone graft substitutes reported in the literature spans seven orders of magnitude. While scaffold apparent elastic modulus is often reported, a wide range of factors ultimately determine the defect mechanical environment, including the scaffold material, scaffold architecture, fixation strategy, and anatomical site. Research analyzing the mechanical environment produced within the tissue by a particular treatment strategy over multiple length and timescales is needed to attain a more rigorous understanding of how scaffold properties can be leveraged to achieve successful bone defect healing. As an illustrative guide, Fig. 5.3 classifies key factors which play an important role in the design and selection of bone graft substitutes.

While many studies characterize the continuum-level properties of a bone graft substitute, both the continuum-level and micro-level mechanical and architectural properties are significant. During healing, the initial infiltrating cells flow into or migrate over the implanted graft substitute. The graft substitute serves as the initial substrate matrix upon which the cells interact. Consequently, the local elastic modulus, surface topography and local strain distribution of the implant regulate the mechanical signals transmitted to the cells. Notably, osteogenic differentiation of MSCs has been demonstrated to occur on substrates possessing much lower modulus than mineralized bone. These findings challenge a widely held paradigm in bone tissue engineering: that the mechanical properties of implanted scaffolds should match those of intact bone. Instead, a growing contingent of researchers has proposed that a more fitting approach to prompt endogenous bone repair is to deliver a scaffold with mechanical properties corresponding to unmineralized fracture callus, the precursor to healing, rather than the end product [297].

With a nonload-bearing graft substitute approach, supplementary fixation is required to ensure suitable mechanical stability is maintained prior to bridging. Fixation defines the mechanical boundary conditions and degree of load share transmitted to the defect throughout daily activity. Dynamic plate and screw systems have long been utilized to provide compressive mechanical stimuli to healing bone.

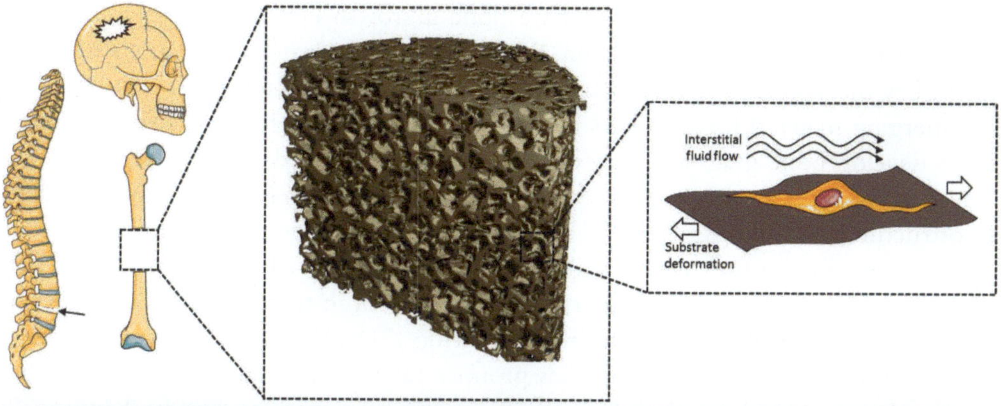

Design and selection criteria for bone graft substitutes		
Organ level cm → mm	*Scaffold/tissue level* mm → 100 μm	*Cell level* < 100 μm
• Physiological loads • Defect geometry • Supplementary fixation • Intended scaffold lifetime • Delivery method • Patient factors	• Apparent stiffness • Failure strength • Stress/strain distribution • Porosity and connectivity • Fracture toughness • Fatigue properties • Degradability	• Elastic modulus • Local stresses/strains • Interstitial fluid flow • Micro- and nanotopography

Figure 5.3 Structural considerations for the design and selection of bone graft substitutes is application-specific. The mechanical environment provided by the scaffold over multiple length scales should be taken into account when developing novel therapeutic strategies. Created using images from Servier Medical Art, CC-BY 3.0.

Distraction osteogenesis is another well-established fixation technique utilizing static tensile strain delivered by an external ring fixator, to promote bone formation over a small gap. For large bone defects, the fixation strategy and bone graft substitute work as a coupled system to provide a structurally stable, osteogenic mechanical environment. Once bridging occurs, controlled load transfer and mechanical stimulation are a promising approach to accelerate bone growth, but further investigations are needed to understand how the local mechanical environment progresses over the entire course of healing to improve the efficacy of bone regeneration strategies.

The intended lifetime of the implant is another important consideration. Procedures requiring a nondegrading, load-bearing implant demand strong and stiff materials to preserve the stability of the treated site. In this case, the fatigue life, fracture toughness, and apparent-level stiffness of the implant become critical design factors. Nano- and microscale mechanical properties are still critically important at the tissue interface where robust osseointegration is needed to provide a strong interlock between the tissue and implant. For long-term implants, load transfer to neighboring tissue is necessary to mitigate the risk of implant subsidence or loosening due to stress-shielding. In scaffold regions where bone ingrowth is desired, highly connected pore structures are crucial to permit functional vascularization and interstitial fluid flow, a key mechanical signal regulating bone formation and strength.

Emerging material formulations and fabrication technologies hold exciting potential to develop bone graft substitutes with tunable mechanical, architectural, and biological properties with spatiotemporal control. Novel approaches include nanostructured scaffolds designed to stimulate specific osteogenic mechanical and biological interactions at the cellular and molecular level, materials with controllable degradation rates, and scaffolds delivering osteogenic or osteoinductive biologics like BMPs or cells [298,299]. Additive manufacturing (3D printing) of polymers, metals, and even biological materials also holds promise for personalized approaches to fabricate implants tailored to the distinct challenges of a patient [300]. Additionally, advanced computational models and high-resolution in vivo imaging will continue to improve our understanding of how mechanical cues regulate bone regeneration at the local level [262]. While these technologies represent promising avenues for bone graft substitute development, ample consideration of the local mechanical environment over the implant lifetime is justified, given the importance of mechanical forces on bone healing. Continued research to clarify how mechanical signals regulate bone defect repair will inform rational improvements to the design and selection of mechanically tuned scaffolds and treatment strategies. Rapid translation of newly developed bone graft substitute platforms to the clinic is vital to increase the number of efficacious treatment options available to a large and growing number of patients worldwide.

REFERENCES

[1] Griffith LG, Naughton G. Tissue engineering—current challenges and expanding opportunities. Science 2002;295:1009–14. Available from: http://dx.doi.org/10.1126/science.1069210.

[2] Pollak A, Watkins-Castillo S. Fracture trends—the burden of musculoskeletal diseases in the United States; 2014. <http://www.boneandjointburden.org/2014-report/via23/fracture-trends>.

[3] Tzioupis C, Giannoudis PV. Prevalence of long-bone non-unions. Injury 2007;38:S3–9. Available from: http://dx.doi.org/10.1016/S0020-1383(07)80003-9.

[4] Loeffler BJ, Kellam JF, Sims SH, Bosse MJ. Prospective observational study of donor-site morbidity following anterior iliac crest bone-grafting in orthopaedic trauma reconstruction patients. J Bone Joint Surg Am 2012;94:1649–54. Available from: http://dx.doi.org/10.2106/JBJS.K.00961.

[5] Goulet JA, Senunas LE, DeSilva GL, Greenfield ML. Autogenous iliac crest bone graft. Complications and functional assessment. Clin Orthop Relat Res 1997;76–81. <http://www.ncbi.nlm.nih.gov/pubmed/9186204> (accessed December 15, 2015).

[6] Kim DH, Rhim R, Li L, Martha J, Swaim BH, Banco RJ, et al. Prospective study of iliac crest bone graft harvest site pain and morbidity. Spine J 2009;9:886–92. Available from: http://dx.doi.org/10.1016/j.spinee.2009.05.006.

[7] Stafford PR, Norris BL. Reamer-irrigator-aspirator bone graft and bi Masquelet technique for segmental bone defect nonunions: a review of 25 cases. Injury 2010;41:S72–7. Available from: http://www.dx.doi.org/10.1016/S0020-1383(10)70014-0.

[8] McCall TA, Brokaw DS, Jelen BA, Scheid DK, Scharfenberger AV, Maar DC, et al. Treatment of large segmental bone defects with reamer-irrigator-aspirator bone graft: technique and case series. Orthop Clin North Am 2010;41:63−73. Available from: http://dx.doi.org/10.1016/j.ocl.2009.08.002.

[9] Obremskey W, Molina C, Collinge C, Tornetta P, Sagi C, Schmidt A, et al. Current practice in the management of open fractures among orthopaedic trauma surgeons. Part B: management of segmental long bone defects. A survey of orthopaedic trauma association members. J Orthop Trauma 2014;28:e203−7. Available from: http://dx.doi.org/10.1097/BOT.0000000000000034.

[10] Brigman BE, Hornicek FJ, Gebhardt MC, Mankin HJ. Allografts about the knee in young patients with high-grade sarcoma. Clin Orthop Relat Res 2004;232−9. <http://www.ncbi.nlm.nih.gov/pubmed/15123953> (accessed May 9, 2015).

[11] Laurencin C, Khan Y, El-Amin SF. Bone graft substitutes. Expert Rev Med Devices 2006;3:49−57. Available from: http://dx.doi.org/10.1586/17434440.3.1.49.

[12] De Long WG, Einhorn TA, Koval K, McKee M, Smith W, Sanders R, et al. Bone grafts and bone graft substitutes in orthopaedic trauma surgery. A critical analysis. J Bone Joint Surg Am 2007;89:649−58. Available from: http://dx.doi.org/10.2106/JBJS.F.00465.

[13] Lewandrowski KU, Gresser JD, Wise DL, Trantol DJ. Bioresorbable bone graft substitutes of different osteoconductivities: a histologic evaluation of osteointegration of poly(propylene glycol-co-fumaric acid)-based cement implants in rats. Biomaterials 2000;21:757−64. <http://www.ncbi.nlm.nih.gov/pubmed/10721744> (accessed May 9, 2015).

[14] Muschler GF, Negami S, Hyodo A, Gaisser D, Easley K, Kambic H. Evaluation of collagen ceramic composite graft materials in a spinal fusion model. Clin Orthop RelatRes 1996;250−60. <http://www.ncbi.nlm.nih.gov/pubmed/8653966> (accessed May 9, 2015).

[15] Baroli B. From natural bone grafts to tissue engineering therapeutics: brainstorming on pharmaceutical formulative requirements and challenges. J Pharm Sci 2009;98:1317−75. Available from: http://dx.doi.org/10.1002/jps.21528.

[16] Rowlands AS, George PA, Cooper-White JJ. Directing osteogenic and myogenic differentiation of MSCs: interplay of stiffness and adhesive ligand presentation. Am J Physiol Cell Physiol 2008;295: C1037−44. Available from: http://dx.doi.org/10.1152/ajpcell.67.2008.

[17] Shih Y-R V, Tseng K-F, Lai H-Y, Lin C-H, Lee OK. Matrix stiffness regulation of integrin-mediated mechanotransduction during osteogenic differentiation of human mesenchymal stem cells. J Bone Miner Res 2011;26:730−8. Available from: http://dx.doi.org/10.1002/jbmr.278.

[18] Bear JE, Haugh JM. Directed migration of mesenchymal cells: where signaling and the cytoskeleton meet. Curr Opin Cell Biol 2014;30:74−82. Available from: http://dx.doi.org/10.1016/j.ceb.2014.06.005.

[19] Matsumoto T, Yung YC, Fischbach C, Kong HJ, Nakaoka R, Mooney DJ. Mechanical strain regulates endothelial cell patterning in vitro. Tissue Eng 2007;13:207−17. Available from: http://dx.doi.org/10.1089/ten.2006.0058.

[20] Krishnan L, Underwood CJ, Maas S, Ellis BJ, Kode TC, Hoying JB, et al. Effect of mechanical boundary conditions on orientation of angiogenic microvessels. Cardiovasc Res 2008;78:324−32. Available from: http://dx.doi.org/10.1093/cvr/cvn055.

[21] Yung YC, Chae J, Buehler MJ, Hunter CP, Mooney DJ. Cyclic tensile strain triggers a sequence of autocrine and paracrine signaling to regulate angiogenic sprouting in human vascular cells. Proc Natl Acad Sci USA 2009;106:15279−84. Available from: http://dx.doi.org/10.1073/pnas.0905891106.

[22] Kim J, Kim IS, Cho TH, Lee KB, Hwang SJ, Tae G, et al. Bone regeneration using hyaluronic acid-based hydrogel with bone morphogenic protein-2 and human mesenchymal stem cells. Biomaterials 2007;28:1830−7. Available from: http://dx.doi.org/10.1016/j.biomaterials.2006.11.050.

[23] Pilia M, Guda T, Appleford M. Development of composite scaffolds for load-bearing segmental bone defects. Biomed Res Int 2013;2013:458253. Available from: http://dx.doi.org/10.1155/2013/458253.

[24] McKibbin B. The biology of fracture healing in long bones. J Bone Joint Surg Br 1978;60-B:150−62. <http://www.ncbi.nlm.nih.gov/pubmed/350882> (accessed May 10, 2015).

[25] Claes L, Recknagel S, Ignatius A. Fracture healing under healthy and inflammatory conditions. Nat Rev Rheumatol 2012;8:133–43. Available from: http://dx.doi.org/10.1038/nrrheum.2012.1.

[26] Schmidt-Bleek K, Schell H, Schulz N, Hoff P, Perka C, Buttgereit F, et al. Inflammatory phase of bone healing initiates the regenerative healing cascade. Cell Tissue Res 2012;347:567–73. Available from: http://dx.doi.org/10.1007/s00441-011-1205-7.

[27] Kolar P, Gaber T, Perka C, Duda GN, Buttgereit F. Human early fracture hematoma is characterized by inflammation and hypoxia. Clin Orthop Relat Res 2011;469:3118–26. Available from: http://dx.doi.org/10.1007/s11999-011-1865-3.

[28] Taguchi K, Ogawa R, Migita M, Hanawa H, Ito H, Orimo H. The role of bone marrow-derived cells in bone fracture repair in a green fluorescent protein chimeric mouse model. Biochem Biophys Res Commun 2005;331:31–6. Available from: http://dx.doi.org/10.1016/j.bbrc.2005.03.119.

[29] Kon T, Cho TJ, Aizawa T, Yamazaki M, Nooh N, Graves D, et al. Expression of osteoprotegerin, receptor activator of NF-kappaB ligand (osteoprotegerin ligand) and related proinflammatory cytokines during fracture healing. J Bone Miner Res 2001;16:1004–14. Available from: http://dx.doi.org/10.1359/jbmr.2001.16.6.1004.

[30] Naik AA, Xie C, Zuscik MJ, Kingsley P, Schwarz EM, Awad H, et al. Reduced COX-2 expression in aged mice is associated with impaired fracture healing. J Bone Miner Res 2009;24:251–64. Available from: http://dx.doi.org/10.1359/jbmr.081002.

[31] Wang Y, Wan C, Deng L, Liu X, Cao X, Gilbert SR, et al. The hypoxia-inducible factor alpha pathway couples angiogenesis to osteogenesis during skeletal development. J Clin Invest 2007;117:1616–26. Available from: http://dx.doi.org/10.1172/JCI31581.

[32] Mizuno K, Mineo K, Tachibana T, Sumi M, Matsubara T, Hirohata K. The osteogenetic potential of fracture haematoma. Subperiosteal and intramuscular transplantation of the haematoma. J Bone Joint Surg Br 1990;72:822–9. <http://www.ncbi.nlm.nih.gov/pubmed/2211764> (accessed May 10, 2015).

[33] Park S-H, Silva M, Bahk W-J, McKellop H, Lieberman JR. Effect of repeated irrigation and debridement on fracture healing in an animal model. J Orthop Res 2002;20:1197–204. Available from: http://dx.doi.org/10.1016/S0736-0266(02)00072-4.

[34] Bhandari M, Tornetta P, Sprague S, Najibi S, Petrisor B, Griffith L, et al. Predictors of reoperation following operative management of fractures of the tibial shaft. J Orthop Trauma 2003;17:353–61 <http://www.ncbi.nlm.nih.gov/pubmed/12759640> (accessed May 10, 2015).

[35] Epari DR, Kassi J-P, Schell H, Duda GN. Timely fracture-healing requires optimization of axial fixation stability. J Bone Joint Surg Am 2007;89:1575–85. Available from: http://dx.doi.org/10.2106/JBJS.F.00247.

[36] Boerckel JD, Dupont KM, Kolambkar YM, Lin ASP, Guldberg RE. In vivo model for evaluating the effects of mechanical stimulation on tissue-engineered bone repair. J Biomech Eng 2009;131 084502–084502. doi:10.1115/1.3148472.

[37] Jain RK. Molecular regulation of vessel maturation. Nat Med 2003;9:685–93. Available from: http://dx.doi.org/10.1038/nm0603-685.

[38] van Royen N, Piek JJ, Buschmann I, Hoefer I, Voskuil M, Schaper W. Stimulation of arteriogenesis; a new concept for the treatment of arterial occlusive disease. Cardiovasc Res 2001;49:543–53. <http://www.ncbi.nlm.nih.gov/pubmed/11166267> (accessed February 2, 2015).

[39] Street J, Bao M, deGuzman L, Bunting S, Peale FV, Ferrara N, et al. Vascular endothelial growth factor stimulates bone repair by promoting angiogenesis and bone turnover. Proc Natl Acad Sci USA 2002;99:9656–61. Available from: http://dx.doi.org/10.1073/pnas.152324099.

[40] Boerckel JD, Uhrig BA, Willett NJ, Huebsch N, Guldberg RE. Mechanical regulation of vascular growth and tissue regeneration in vivo. Proc Natl Acad Sci 2011;108:E674–80. Available from: http://dx.doi.org/10.1073/pnas.1107019108.

[41] Hirao M, Tamai N, Tsumaki N, Yoshikawa H, Myoui A. Oxygen tension regulates chondrocyte differentiation and function during endochondral ossification. J Biol Chem 2006;281:31079–92. Available from: http://dx.doi.org/10.1074/jbc.M602296200.

[42] Wang Y, Wan C, Gilbert SR, Clemens TL. Oxygen sensing and osteogenesis. Ann N Y Acad Sci 2007;1117:1–11. Available from: http://dx.doi.org/10.1196/annals.1402.049.

[43] Sheehy EJ, Buckley CT, Kelly DJ. Oxygen tension regulates the osteogenic, chondrogenic and endochondral phenotype of bone marrow derived mesenchymal stem cells. Biochem Biophys Res Commun 2012;417:305–10. Available from: http://dx.doi.org/10.1016/j.bbrc.2011.11.105.

[44] Hankenson KD, Dishowitz M, Gray C, Schenker M. Angiogenesis in bone regeneration. Injury 2011;42:556–61. Available from: http://dx.doi.org/10.1016/j.injury.2011.03.035.

[45] Dennis SC, Berkland CJ, Bonewald LF, Detamore MS. Endochondral ossification for enhancing bone regeneration: converging native extracellular matrix biomaterials and developmental engineering in vivo. Tissue Eng Part B Rev 2014;. Available from: http://dx.doi.org/10.1089/ten.TEB.2014.0419.

[46] Fiedler J, Leucht F, Waltenberger J, Dehio C, Brenner RE. VEGF-A and PlGF-1 stimulate chemotactic migration of human mesenchymal progenitor cells. Biochem Biophys Res Commun 2005;334:561–8. Available from: http://dx.doi.org/10.1016/j.bbrc.2005.06.116.

[47] Yang Y-Q, Tan Y-Y, Wong R, Wenden A, Zhang L-K, Rabie ABM. The role of vascular endothelial growth factor in ossification., Int. J Oral Sci 2012;4:64–8. Available from: http://dx.doi.org/10.1038/ijos.2012.33.

[48] Deckers MML, van Bezooijen RL, van der Horst G, Hoogendam J, van Der Bent C, Papapoulos SE, et al. Bone morphogenetic proteins stimulate angiogenesis through osteoblast-derived vascular endothelial growth factor A. Endocrinology 2002;143:1545–53. Available from: http://dx.doi.org/10.1210/endo.143.4.8719.

[49] Zhang F, Qiu T, Wu X, Wan C, Shi W, Wang Y, et al. Sustained BMP signaling in osteoblasts stimulates bone formation by promoting angiogenesis and osteoblast differentiation. J Bone Miner Res 2009;24:1224–33. Available from: http://dx.doi.org/10.1359/jbmr.090204.

[50] Malladi P, Xu Y, Chiou M, Giaccia AJ, Longaker MT. Effect of reduced oxygen tension on chondrogenesis and osteogenesis in adipose-derived mesenchymal cells. Am J Physiol Cell Physiol 2006;290:C1139–46. Available from: http://dx.doi.org/10.1152/ajpcell.00415.2005.

[51] Tuncay OC, Ho D, Barker MK. Oxygen tension regulates osteoblast function. Am J Orthod Dentofacial Orthop 1994;105:457–63. Available from: http://dx.doi.org/10.1016/S0889-5406(94)70006-0.

[52] Utting JC, Robins SP, Brandao-Burch A, Orriss IR, Behar J, Arnett TR. Hypoxia inhibits the growth, differentiation and bone-forming capacity of rat osteoblasts. Exp Cell Res 2006;312:1693–702. Available from: http://dx.doi.org/10.1016/j.yexcr.2006.02.007.

[53] Hausman M, Schaffler M, Majeska R. Prevention of fracture healing in rats by an inhibitor of angiogenesis. Bone 2001;29:560–4. Available from: http://dx.doi.org/10.1016/S8756-3282(01)00608-1.

[54] Kanczler JM, Oreffo ROC. Osteogenesis and angiogenesis: the potential for engineering bone. Eur Cell Mater 2008;15:100–14. <http://www.ncbi.nlm.nih.gov/pubmed/18454418> (accessed February 2, 2015).

[55] Morgan EF, Salisbury Palomares KT, Gleason RE, Bellin DL, Chien KB, Unnikrishnan GU, et al. Correlations between local strains and tissue phenotypes in an experimental model of skeletal healing. J Biomech 2010;43:2418–24. Available from: http://dx.doi.org/10.1016/j.jbiomech.2010.04.019.

[56] Claes LE, Claes LE, Heigele C a, Heigele C a, Neidlinger-Wilke C, Neidlinger-Wilke C, et al. Effects of mechanical factors on the fracture healing process. Clin Orthop Relat Res 1998; S132–47. <http://www.ncbi.nlm.nih.gov/pubmed/9917634>.

[57] Shapiro F. Bone development and its relation to fracture repair. The role of mesenchymal osteoblasts and surface osteoblasts. Eur Cell Mater 2008;15:53–76. <http://www.ncbi.nlm.nih.gov/pubmed/18382990> (accessed April 7, 2015).

[58] Claes L, Blakytny R, Besse J, Bausewein C, Ignatius A, Willie B. Late dynamization by reduced fixation stiffness enhances fracture healing in a rat femoral osteotomy model. J Orthop Trauma 2011;25:169–74. Available from: http://dx.doi.org/10.1097/BOT.0b013e3181e3d994.

[59] Hou T, Li Q, Luo F, Xu J, Xie Z, Wu X, et al. Controlled dynamization to enhance reconstruction capacity of tissue-engineered bone in healing critically sized bone defects: an in vivo study in goats. Tissue Eng Part A 2010;16:201−12. Available from: http://dx.doi.org/10.1089/ten.TEA.2009.0291.

[60] Huiskes R, Weinans H, Grootenboer HJ, Dalstra M, Fudala B, Slooff TJ. Adaptive bone-remodeling theory applied to prosthetic-design analysis. J Biomech 1987;20:1135−50 <http://www.ncbi.nlm.nih.gov/pubmed/3429459> (accessed April 8, 2015).

[61] Chen Q, Thouas GA. Metallic implant biomaterials. Mater Sci Eng R Reports 2015;87:1−57. Available from: http://dx.doi.org/10.1016/j.mser.2014.10.001.

[62] Navarro M, Michiardi A, Castaño O, Planell JA. Biomaterials in orthopaedics. J R Soc Interface 2008;5:1137−58. Available from: http://dx.doi.org/10.1098/rsif.2008.0151.

[63] Velasco MA, Narváez-Tovar CA, Garzón-Alvarado DA. Design, materials, and mechanobiology of biodegradable scaffolds for bone tissue engineering. Biomed Res Int 2015;2015:1−21. Available from: http://dx.doi.org/10.1155/2015/729076.

[64] Van Lieshout EMM, Van Kralingen GH, El-Massoudi Y, Weinans H, Patka P. Microstructure and biomechanical characteristics of bone substitutes for trauma and orthopaedic surgery. BMC Musculoskelet Disord 2011;12:34. Available from: http://dx.doi.org/10.1186/1471-2474-12-34.

[65] Chen Q, Zhu C, Thouas GA. Progress and challenges in biomaterials used for bone tissue engineering: bioactive glasses and elastomeric composites. Prog Biomater 2012;1:2. Available from: http://dx.doi.org/10.1186/2194-0517-1-2.

[66] Amaral M, Lopes MA, Silva RF, Santos JD. Densification route and mechanical properties of Si3N4−bioglass biocomposites. Biomaterials 2002;23:857−62. Available from: http://dx.doi.org/10.1016/S0142-9612(01)00194-6.

[67] Hing KA, Best SM, Bonfield W. Characterization of porous hydroxyapatite. J Mater Sci Mater Med 1999;10:135−45. <http://www.ncbi.nlm.nih.gov/pubmed/15348161> (accessed May 18, 2015).

[68] Gomes ME, Ribeiro AS, Malafaya PB, Reis RL, Cunha AM. A new approach based on injection moulding to produce biodegradable starch-based polymeric scaffolds: morphology, mechanical and degradation behaviour. Biomaterials 2001;22:883−9. http://dx.doi.org/10.1016/S0142-9612(00)00211-8.

[69] Eosoly S, Brabazon D, Lohfeld S, Looney L. Selective laser sintering of hydroxyapatite/poly-epsilon-caprolactone scaffolds. Acta Biomater 2010;6:2511−17. Available from: http://dx.doi.org/10.1016/j.actbio.2009.07.018.

[70] Williams JM, Adewunmi A, Schek RM, Flanagan CL, Krebsbach PH, Feinberg SE, et al. Bone tissue engineering using polycaprolactone scaffolds fabricated via selective laser sintering. Biomaterials 2005;26:4817−27. Available from: http://dx.doi.org/10.1016/j.biomaterials.2004.11.057.

[71] Stakleff KS, Lin F, Smith Callahan LA, Wade MB, Esterle A, Miller J, et al. Resorbable, amino acid-based poly(ester urea)s crosslinked with osteogenic growth peptide with enhanced mechanical properties and bioactivity. Acta Biomater 2013;9:5132−42. Available from: http://dx.doi.org/10.1016/j.actbio.2012.08.035.

[72] Deng M, Kumbar SG, Nair LS, Weikel AL, Allcock HR, Laurencin CT. Biomimetic structures: biological implications of dipeptide-substituted polyphosphazene-polyester blend nanofiber matrices for load-bearing bone regeneration. Adv Funct Mater 2011;21:2641−51. Available from: http://dx.doi.org/10.1002/adfm.201100275.

[73] Tanner KE. Bioactive composites for bone tissue engineering. Proc Inst Mech Eng H 2010;224:1359−72. <http://www.ncbi.nlm.nih.gov/pubmed/21287825> (accessed September 17, 2015).

[74] Van der Stok J, Van Lieshout EMM, El-Massoudi Y, Van Kralingen GH, Patka P. Bone substitutes in the Netherlands—a systematic literature review. Acta Biomater 2011;7:739−50. Available from: http://dx.doi.org/10.1016/j.actbio.2010.07.035.

[75] Drosos GI, Babourda E, Magnissalis EA, Giatromanolaki A, Kazakos K, Verettas DA. Mechanical characterization of bone graft substitute ceramic cements. Injury 2012;43:266−71. Available from: http://dx.doi.org/10.1016/j.injury.2011.02.004.

[76] Albrektsson T, Johansson C. Osteoinduction, osteoconduction and osseointegration.. Eur Spine J 2001;10(Suppl. 2):S96–101. Available from: http://dx.doi.org/10.1007/s005860100282.

[77] Kienapfel H, Sprey C, Wilke A, Griss P. Implant fixation by bone ingrowth. J Arthroplasty 1999;14:355–68. Available from: http://dx.doi.org/10.1016/S0883-5403(99)90063-3.

[78] Ashman RB, Cowin SC, Van Buskirk WC, Rice JC. A continuous wave technique for the measurement of the elastic properties of cortical bone. J Biomech 1984;17:349–61. Available from: http://dx.doi.org/10.1016/0021-9290(84)90029-0.

[79] Rezwan K, Chen QZ, Blaker JJ, Boccaccini AR. Biodegradable and bioactive porous polymer/inorganic composite scaffolds for bone tissue engineering. Biomaterials 2006;27:3413–31. Available from: http://dx.doi.org/10.1016/j.biomaterials.2006.01.039.

[80] Zysset PK, Guo XE, Hoffler CE, Moore KE, Goldstein SA. Mechanical properties of human trabecular bone lamellae quantified by nanoindentation. Technol Health Care 1998;6:429–32. <http://www.ncbi.nlm.nih.gov/pubmed/10100945>. (accessed December 17, 2015).

[81] Turner CH, Rho J, Takano Y, Tsui TY, Pharr GM. The elastic properties of trabecular and cortical bone tissues are similar: results from two microscopic measurement techniques. J Biomech 1999;32:437–41. Available from: http://dx.doi.org/10.1016/S0021-9290(98)00177-8..

[82] Hernigou P, Homma Y. Tissue bioengineering in orthopedics. Clin Cases Miner Bone Metab 2012;9:21–3. <http://www.pubmedcentral.nih.gov/articlerender.fcgi?artid=3392675&tool=pmcentrez&rendertype=abstract> (accessed June 7, 2015).

[83] Albee FH. The various uses of the bone graft. Proc R Soc Med 1930;23:855–60. <http://www.pubmedcentral.nih.gov/articlerender.fcgi?artid = 2182036&tool=pmcentrez&rendertype=abstract>. (accessed June 7, 2015).

[84] Cypher TJ, Grossman JP. Biological principles of bone graft healing. J Foot Ankle Surg 1996;35:413–17. Available from: http://dx.doi.org/10.1016/S1067-2516(96)80061-5.

[85] Sandhu HS, Grewal HS, Parvataneni H. Bone grafting for spinal fusion. Orthop Clin North Am 1999;30:685–98. Available from: http://dx.doi.org/10.1016/S0030-5898(05)70120-6.

[86] Morgan HD, McCallister W, Cho MS, Casnellie MT, Leopold SS. Impaction allografting for femoral component revision: clinical update. Clin Orthop Relat Res 2004;160–8. <http://www.ncbi.nlm.nih.gov/pubmed/15057092> (accessed June 7, 2015).

[87] Dunlop DG, Brewster NT, Madabhushi SPG, Usmani AS, Pankaj P, Howie CR. Techniques to improve the shear strength of impacted bone graft: the effect of particle size and washing of the graft. J Bone Joint Surg Am 2003;85-A:639–46. <http://jbjs.org/content/85/4/639.abstract> (accessed June 7, 2015).

[88] Urist MR. Bone: formation by autoinduction. Science 1965;150:893–9. Available from: http://dx.doi.org/10.1126/science.150.3698.893.

[89] Einhorn TA, Lane JM, Burstein AH, Kopman CR, Vigorita VJ. The healing of segmental bone defects induced by demineralized bone matrix. A radiographic and biomechanical study. J Bone Joint Surg Am 1984;66:274–9. <http://jbjs.org/content/66/2/274.abstract> (accessed June 8, 2015).

[90] Catanese III J, Iverson EP, Ng RK, Keaveny TM. Heterogeneity of the mechanical properties of demineralized bone. J Biomech 1999;32:1365–9. Available from: http://dx.doi.org/10.1016/S0021-9290(99)00128-1.

[91] Pelker RR, Friedlaender GE, Markham TC, Panjabi MM, Moen CJ. Effects of freezing and freeze-drying on the biomechanical properties of rat bone. J Orthop Res 1984;1:405–11. Available from: http://dx.doi.org/10.1002/jor.1100010409.

[92] Shaw JM, Hunter SA, Gayton JC, Boivin GP, Prayson MJ. Repeated freeze-thaw cycles do not alter the biomechanical properties of fibular allograft bone. Clin Orthop Relat Res 2012;470:937–43. Available from: http://dx.doi.org/:10.1007/s11999-011-2033-5.

[93] Cornu O, Banse X, Docquier PL, Luyckx S, Delloye C. Effect of freeze-drying and gamma irradiation on the mechanical properties of human cancellous bone. J Orthop Res 2000;18:426–31. Available from: http://dx.doi.org/10.1002/jor.1100180314.

[94] Berrey BH, Lord CF, Gebhardt MC, Mankin HJ. Fractures of allografts. Frequency, treatment, and end-results. J Bone Joint Surg Am 1990;72:825–33. <http://www.ncbi.nlm.nih.gov/pubmed/2365716> (accessed June 7, 2015).

[95] Wheeler DL, Enneking WF. Allograft bone decreases in strength in vivo over time. Clin Orthop Relat Res 2005;36–42. <http://www.ncbi.nlm.nih.gov/pubmed/15930919> (accessed May 11, 2015).

[96] Gilardino MS, Chen E, Bartlett SP. Choice of internal rigid fixation materials in the treatment of facial fractures. Craniomaxillofac Trauma Reconstr 2009;2:49–60. Available from: http://dx.doi.org/10.1055/s-0029-1202591.

[97] Lane WA. Some remarks on the treatment of fractures. Br Med J 1895;1:861–3. <http://www.pubmedcentral.nih.gov/articlerender.fcgi?artid = 2509418&tool = pmcentrez&rendertype = abstract> (accessed June 27, 2015).

[98] Jones AR, Sir William. Arbuthnot Lane. J Bone Joint Surg Br 1952;34-B:478–82. <http://www.ncbi.nlm.nih.gov/pubmed/12999937> (accessed June 27, 2015).

[99] Byrne DP, Lacroix D, Planell JA, Kelly DJ, Prendergast PJ. Simulation of tissue differentiation in a scaffold as a function of porosity, Young's modulus and dissolution rate: application of mechanobiological models in tissue engineering. Biomaterials 2007;28:5544–54. Available from: http://dx.doi.org/10.1016/j.biomaterials.2007.09.003.

[100] Morra M. Biomolecular modification of implant surfaces. Expert Rev Med Devices 2007;4:361–72. Available from: http://dx.doi.org/10.1586/17434440.4.3.361.

[101] Puleo D. Understanding and controlling the bone–implant interface. Biomaterials 1999;20:2311–21. Available from: http://dx.doi.org/10.1016/S0142-9612(99)00160-X.

[102] Schwartz Z, Boyan BD. Underlying mechanisms at the bone-biomaterial interface. J Cell Biochem 1994;56:340–7. Available from: http://dx.doi.org/10.1002/jcb.240560310.

[103] Kieswetter K, Schwartz Z, Dean DD, Boyan BD. The role of implant surface characteristics in the healing of bone. Crit Rev Oral Biol Med 1996;7:329–45. <http://www.ncbi.nlm.nih.gov/pubmed/8986395> (accessed June 28, 2015).

[104] Gittens RA, Olivares-Navarrete R, Schwartz Z, Boyan BD. Implant osseointegration and the role of microroughness and nanostructures: lessons for spine implants. Acta Biomater 2014;10:3363–71. Available from: http://dx.doi.org/10.1016/j.actbio.2014.03.037.

[105] Wu S, Liu X, Yeung KWK, Liu C, Yang X. Biomimetic porous scaffolds for bone tissue engineering. Mater Sci Eng R Reports 2014;80:1–36. Available from: http://dx.doi.org/10.1016/j.mser.2014.04.001.

[106] Hirschhorn JS, McBeath AA, Dustoor MR. Porous titanium surgical implant materials. J Biomed Mater Res 1971;5:49–67. Available from: http://dx.doi.org/10.1002/jbm.820050608.

[107] Fantigrossi A, Galbusera F, Raimondi MT, Sassi M, Fornari M. Biomechanical analysis of cages for posterior lumbar interbody fusion. Med Eng Phys 2007;29:101–9. Available from: http://dx.doi.org/10.1016/j.medengphy.2006.02.007.

[108] Park HS, Kim YK, Yoon CH. Various applications of titanium mesh screen implant to orbital wall fractures. J Craniofac Surg 2001;12:555–60. <http://www.ncbi.nlm.nih.gov/pubmed/11711822> (accessed June 28, 2015).

[109] Schön R, Metzger MC, Zizelmann C, Weyer N, Schmelzeisen R. Individually preformed titanium mesh implants for a true-to-original repair of orbital fractures. Int J Oral Maxillofac Surg 2006;35:990–5. Available from: http://dx.doi.org/10.1016/j.ijom.2006.06.018.

[110] Niinomi M, Nakai M. Titanium-based biomaterials for preventing stress shielding between implant devices and bone. Int J Biomater 2011;2011 836587. Available from: http://dx.doi.org/10.1155/2011/836587.

[111] Vandendolder J, Farber E, Spauwen P, Jansen J. Bone tissue reconstruction using titanium fiber mesh combined with rat bone marrow stromal cells. Biomaterials 2003;24:1745–50. Available from: http://dx.doi.org/10.1016/S0142-9612(02)00537-9.

[112] St-Pierre J-P, Gauthier M, Lefebvre L-P, Tabrizian M. Three-dimensional growth of differentiating MC3T3-E1 pre-osteoblasts on porous titanium scaffolds. Biomaterials 2005;26:7319–28. Available from: http://dx.doi.org/10.1016/j.biomaterials.2005.05.046.

[113] Kanayama M, Hashimoto T, Shigenobu K, Oha F, Ishida T, Yamane S. Pitfalls of anterior cervical fusion using titanium mesh and local autograft. J Spinal Disord Tech 2003;16:513–18. <http://www.ncbi.nlm.nih.gov/pubmed/14657747> (accessed June 28, 2015).

[114] Proussaefs P, Lozada J. Use of titanium mesh for staged localized alveolar ridge augmentation: clinical and histologic-histomorphometric evaluation. J Oral Implantol 2006;32:237−47. Available from: http://dx.doi.org/10.1563/1548-1336(2006)32[237:UOTMFS]2.0.CO;2.

[115] Misch CM, Jensen OT, Pikos MA, Malmquist JP. Vertical bone augmentation using recombinant bone morphogenetic protein, mineralized bone allograft, and titanium mesh: a retrospective cone beam computed tomography study. Int J Oral Maxillofac Implants 2015;30:202−7. <http://www.ncbi.nlm.nih.gov/pubmed/25615925> (accessed June 28, 2015).

[116] Bauer TW, Schils J. The pathology of total joint arthroplasty. Skeletal Radiol 1999;28:483−97. Available from: http://dx.doi.org/10.1007/s002560050552.

[117] Körner C, Singer RF. Processing of metal foams—challenges and opportunities. Adv Eng Mater 2000;2:159−65. doi:10.1002/(SICI)1527-2648(200004)2:4 < 159::AID-ADEM159 > 3.0.CO;2-O.

[118] Ryan GE, Pandit AS, Apatsidis DP. Porous titanium scaffolds fabricated using a rapid prototyping and powder metallurgy technique. Biomaterials 2008;29:3625−35. Available from: http://dx.doi.org/10.1016/j.biomaterials.2008.05.032.

[119] Dunand DC. Processing of titanium foams. Adv Eng Mater 2004;6:369−76. Available from: http://dx.doi.org/10.1002/adem.200405576.

[120] Bobyn JD, Stackpool GJ, Hacking SA, Tanzer M, Krygier JJ. Characteristics of bone ingrowth and interface mechanics of a new porous tantalum biomaterial. J Bone Joint Surg Br 1999;81:907−14. <http://www.ncbi.nlm.nih.gov/pubmed/10530861> (accessed June 28, 2015).

[121] Sagomonyants KB, Hakim-Zargar M, Jhaveri A, Aronow MS, Gronowicz G. Porous tantalum stimulates the proliferation and osteogenesis of osteoblasts from elderly female patients. J Orthop Res 2011;29:609−16. Available from: http://dx.doi.org/10.1002/jor.21251.

[122] Blanco JF, Sánchez-Guijo FM, Carrancio S, Muntion S, García-Briñon J, del Cañizo M-C. Titanium and tantalum as mesenchymal stem cell scaffolds for spinal fusion: an in vitro comparative study., Eur. Spine J 2011;20(Suppl. 3):353−60. Available from: http://dx.doi.org/10.1007/s00586-011-1901-8.

[123] Zardiackas LD, Parsell DE, Dillon LD, Mitchell DW, Nunnery LA, Poggie R. Structure, metallurgy, and mechanical properties of a porous tantalum foam. J Biomed Mater Res 2001;58:180−7. <http://www.ncbi.nlm.nih.gov/pubmed/11241337> (accessed June 28, 2015).

[124] Levine BR, Sporer S, Poggie RA, Della Valle CJ, Jacobs JJ. Experimental and clinical performance of porous tantalum in orthopedic surgery. Biomaterials 2006;27:4671−81. Available from: http://dx.doi.org/10.1016/j.biomaterials.2006.04.041.

[125] Wauthle R, van der Stok J, Amin Yavari S, Van Humbeeck J, Kruth J-P, Zadpoor AA, et al. Additively manufactured porous tantalum implants. Acta Biomater 2015;14:217−25. Available from: http://dx.doi.org/10.1016/j.actbio.2014.12.003.

[126] Buehler WJ, Wang FE. A summary of recent research on the nitinol alloys and their potential application in ocean engineering. Ocean Eng 1968;1:105−20. Available from: http://dx.doi.org/10.1016/0029-8018(68)90019-X.

[127] Otsuka K, Ren X. Physical metallurgy of Ti−Ni-based shape memory alloys. Prog Mater Sci 2005;50:511−678. Available from: http://dx.doi.org/10.1016/j.pmatsci.2004.10.001.

[128] Itin VI, Gyunter VE, Shabalovskaya SA, Sachdeva RLC. Mechanical properties and shape memory of porous nitinol. Mater Charact 1994;32:179−87. Available from: http://dx.doi.org/10.1016/1044-5803(94)90087-6..

[129] Wu S, Liu X, Chan YL, Ho JPY, Chung CY, Chu PK, et al. Nickel release behavior, cytocompatibility, and superelasticity of oxidized porous single-phase NiTi., J. Biomed Mater Res A 2007;81:948−55. Available from: http://dx.doi.org/10.1002/jbm.a.31115.

[130] Wu SL, Chu PK, Liu XM, Chung CY, Ho JPY, Chu CL, et al. Surface characteristics, mechanical properties, and cytocompatibility of oxygen plasma-implanted porous nickel titanium shape memory alloy. J Biomed Mater Res A 2006;79:139−46. Available from: http://dx.doi.org/10.1002/jbm.a.30705.

[131] Shabalovskaya SA. On the nature of the biocompatibility and on medical applications of NiTi shape memory and superelastic alloys. Biomed Mater Eng 1996;6:267−89. <http://europepmc.org/abstract/med/8980835> (accessed June 29, 2015).

[132] Bansiddhi A, Sargeant TD, Stupp SI, Dunand DC. Porous NiTi for bone implants: a review. Acta Biomater 2008;4:773–82. Available from: http://dx.doi.org/10.1016/j.actbio.2008.02.009.

[133] Ritchie PK, McCarty EC. Metal and plastic suture anchors for rotator cuff repair. Oper Tech Sports Med 2004;12:215–20. Available from: http://dx.doi.org/10.1053/j.otsm.2004.07.004.

[134] Blum U, Voshage G, Lammer J, Beyersdorf F, Töllner D, Kretschmer G, et al. Endoluminal stent-grafts for infrarenal abdominal aortic aneurysms. N Engl J Med 1997;336:13–20. Available from: http://dx.doi.org/10.1056/NEJM199701023360103.

[135] Yakacki CM, Gall K, Dirschl DR, Pacaccio DJ. Pseudoelastic intramedullary nailing for tibio-talo-calcaneal arthrodesis. Expert Rev Med Devices 2011;8:159–66. Available from: http://dx.doi.org/10.1586/erd.10.93.

[136] Biesiekierski A, Wang J, Gepreel MA-H, Wen C. A new look at biomedical Ti-based shape memory alloys. Acta Biomater 2012;8:1661–9. Available from: http://dx.doi.org/10.1016/j.actbio.2012.01.018.

[137] Bertheville B. Porous single-phase NiTi processed under Ca reducing vapor for use as a bone graft substitute. Biomaterials 2006;27:1246–50. Available from: http://dx.doi.org/10.1016/j.biomaterials.2005.09.014.

[138] Saris NE, Mervaala E, Karppanen H, Khawaja JA, Lewenstam A. Magnesium. An update on physiological, clinical and analytical aspects. Clin Chim Acta 2000;294:1–26. <http://www.ncbi.nlm.nih.gov/pubmed/10727669> (accessed May 22, 2015).

[139] Staiger MP, Pietak AM, Huadmai J, Dias G. Magnesium and its alloys as orthopedic biomaterials: a review. Biomaterials 2006;27:1728–34. Available from: http://dx.doi.org/10.1016/j.biomaterials.2005.10.003.

[140] Witte F, Kaese V, Haferkamp H, Switzer E, Meyer-Lindenberg A, Wirth CJ, et al. In vivo corrosion of four magnesium alloys and the associated bone response. Biomaterials 2005;26:3557–63. Available from: http://dx.doi.org/10.1016/j.biomaterials.2004.09.049.

[141] Gu X, Zheng Y, Cheng Y, Zhong S, Xi T. In vitro corrosion and biocompatibility of binary magnesium alloys. Biomaterials 2009;30:484–98. Available from: http://dx.doi.org/10.1016/j.biomaterials.2008.10.021.

[142] Salahshoor M, Guo Y. Biodegradable orthopedic magnesium-calcium (MgCa) alloys, processing, and corrosion performance. Materials (Basel) 2012;5:135–55. Available from: http://dx.doi.org/10.3390/ma5010135.

[143] Li Z, Gu X, Lou S, Zheng Y. The development of binary Mg-Ca alloys for use as biodegradable materials within bone. Biomaterials 2008;29:1329–44. Available from: http://dx.doi.org/10.1016/j.biomaterials.2007.12.021.

[144] Dressman H, Knochenplombierung Ueber. Beitr Klin Chir 1892;9:804.

[145] Arinzeh TL, Tran T, Mcalary J, Daculsi G. A comparative study of biphasic calcium phosphate ceramics for human mesenchymal stem-cell-induced bone formation. Biomaterials 2005;26:3631–8. Available from: http://dx.doi.org/10.1016/j.biomaterials.2004.09.035.

[146] Kilpadi KL, Chang PL, Bellis SL. Hydroxylapatite binds more serum proteins, purified integrins, and osteoblast precursor cells than titanium or steel. J Biomed Mater Res 2001;57:258–67. <http://www.ncbi.nlm.nih.gov/pubmed/11484189> (accessed October 29, 2015).

[147] Banerjee SS, Bandyopadhyay A, Bose S. Biphasic resorbable calcium phosphate ceramic for bone implants and local alendronate delivery. Adv Eng Mater 2010;12:B148–55. Available from: http://dx.doi.org/10.1002/adem.200980072.

[148] Bose S, Tarafder S. Calcium phosphate ceramic systems in growth factor and drug delivery for bone tissue engineering: a review. Acta Biomater 2012;8:1401–21. Available from: http://dx.doi.org/10.1016/j.actbio.2011.11.017.

[149] Woodard JR, Hilldore AJ, Lan SK, Park CJ, Morgan AW, Eurell JAC, et al. The mechanical properties and osteoconductivity of hydroxyapatite bone scaffolds with multi-scale porosity. Biomaterials 2007;28:45–54. Available from: http://dx.doi.org/10.1016/j.biomaterials.2006.08.021.

[150] Wagoner Johnson AJ, Herschler BA. A review of the mechanical behavior of CaP and CaP/polymer composites for applications in bone replacement and repair. Acta Biomater 2011;7:16–30. Available from: http://dx.doi.org/10.1016/j.actbio.2010.07.012.

[151] Holmes RE. Bone regeneration within a coralline hydroxyapatite implant. Plast Reconstr Surg 1979;63:626–33. <http://www.ncbi.nlm.nih.gov/pubmed/432330> (accessed October 29, 2015).

[152] Guillemin G, Patat JL, Fournie J, Chetail M. The use of coral as a bone graft substitute. J Biomed Mater Res 1987;21:557–67. Available from: http://dx.doi.org/10.1002/jbm.820210503.

[153] Arnaud E, De Pollak C, Meunier A, Sedel L, Damien C, Petite H. Osteogenesis with coral is increased by BMP and BMC in a rat cranioplasty. Biomaterials 1999;20:1909–18. <http://www.ncbi.nlm.nih.gov/pubmed/10514067> (accessed October 29, 2015).

[154] Wu Y-C, Lee T-M, Chiu K-H, Shaw S-Y, Yang C-Y. A comparative study of the physical and mechanical properties of three natural corals based on the criteria for bone-tissue engineering scaffolds. J Mater Sci Mater Med 2009;20:1273–80. Available from: http://dx.doi.org/10.1007/s10856-009-3695-3.

[155] Beuerlein MJS, McKee MD. Calcium sulfates: what is the evidence? J Orthop Trauma 2010;24 (Suppl. 1):S46–51. Available from: http://dx.doi.org/10.1097/BOT.0b013e3181cec48e.

[156] Kelly CM, Wilkins RM, Gitelis S, Hartjen C, Watson JT, Kim PT. The use of a surgical grade calcium sulfate as a bone graft substitute: results of a multicenter trial. Clin Orthop Relat Res 2001;42–50. <http://www.ncbi.nlm.nih.gov/pubmed/11154003> (accessed October 29, 2015).

[157] Zhang J, Wang L, Zhang W, Zhang M, Luo Z-P. Synchronization of calcium sulphate cement degradation and new bone formation is improved by external mechanical regulation. J Orthop Res 2015;33:685–91. Available from: http://dx.doi.org/10.1002/jor.22839.

[158] Stevens MM. Biomaterials for bone tissue engineering. Mater Today 2008;11:18–25. Available from: http://dx.org.doi.org/10.1016/S1369-7021(08)70086-5.

[159] Xynos ID, Edgar AJ, Buttery LD, Hench LL, Polak JM. Ionic products of bioactive glass dissolution increase proliferation of human osteoblasts and induce insulin-like growth factor II mRNA expression and protein synthesis. Biochem Biophys Res Commun 2000;276:461–5. Available from: http://dx.doi.org/10.1006/bbrc.2000.3503.

[160] Bellantone M, Williams HD, Hench LL. Broad-spectrum bactericidal activity of Ag(2)O-doped bioactive glass. Antimicrob Agents Chemother 2002;46:1940–5. <http://www.pubmedcentral.nih.gov/articlerender.fcgi?artid=127232&tool=pmcentrez&rendertype=abstract> (accessed October 29, 2015).

[161] Jell G, Stevens MM. Gene activation by bioactive glasses. J Mater Sci Mater Med 2006;17:997–1002. Available from: http://dx.doi.org/10.1007/s10856-006-0435-9.

[162] Boutin P, Christel P, Dorlot JM, Meunier A, de Roquancourt A, Blanquaert D, et al. The use of dense alumina-alumina ceramic combination in total hip replacement. J Biomed Mater Res 1988;22:1203–32. Available from: http://dx.doi.org/10.1002/jbm.820221210.

[163] Affatato S, Traina F, De Fine M, Carmignato S, Toni A. Alumina-on-alumina hip implants: a wear study of retrieved components. J Bone Joint Surg Br 2012;94:37–42. Available from: http://dx.doi.org/10.1302/0301-620X.94B1.26956.

[164] Clarke IC, Manaka M, Green DD, Williams P, Pezzotti G, Kim Y-H, et al. Current status of zirconia used in total hip implants. J Bone Joint Surg Am 2003;85-A(Suppl.):73–84. <http://jbjs.org/content/85/suppl_4/73.abstract> (accessed September 17, 2015).

[165] Chen QZ, Boccaccini AR, Zhang HB, Wang DZ, Edirisinghe MJ. Improved mechanical reliability of bone tissue engineering (Zirconia) scaffolds by electrospraying. J Am Ceram Soc 2006;89:1534–9. Available from: http://dx.doi.org/10.1111/j.1551-2916.2006.00935.x.

[166] Soh E, Kolos E, Ruys AJ. Foamed high porosity alumina for use as a bone tissue scaffold. Ceram Int 2015;41:1031–47. Available from: http://dx.doi.org/10.1016/j.ceramint.2014.09.026.

[167] Kim H-W, Lee S-Y, Bae C-J, Noh Y-J, Kim H-E, Kim H-M, et al. Porous ZrO2 bone scaffold coated with hydroxyapatite with fluorapatite intermediate layer. Biomaterials 2003;24:3277–84. Available from: http://dx.doi.org/10.1016/S0142-9612(03)00162-5.

[168] Kolambkar YM, Dupont KM, Boerckel JD, Huebsch N, Mooney DJ, Hutmacher DW, et al. An alginate-based hybrid system for growth factor delivery in the functional repair of large bone defects. Biomaterials 2011;32:65–74. Available from: http://dx.doi.org/10.1016/j.biomaterials.2010.08.074.

[169] Diab T, Pritchard EM, Uhrig BA, Boerckel JD, Kaplan DL, Guldberg RE. A silk hydrogel-based delivery system of bone morphogenetic protein for the treatment of large bone defects. J Mech Behav Biomed Mater 2012;11:123–31. Available from: http://dx.doi.org/10.1016/j.jmbbm.2011.11.007.
[170] Berger J, Reist M, Mayer JM, Felt O, Peppas NA, Gurny R. Structure and interactions in covalently and ionically crosslinked chitosan hydrogels for biomedical applications. Eur J Pharm Biopharm 2004;57:19–34. Available from: http://dx.doi.org/10.1016/S0939-6411(03)00161-9.
[171] Drury JL, Mooney DJ. Hydrogels for tissue engineering: scaffold design variables and applications. Biomaterials 2003;24:4337–51. Available from: http://dx.doi.org/10.1016/S0142-9612(03)00340-5.
[172] Sun H, Mei L, Song C, Cui X, Wang P. The in vivo degradation, absorption and excretion of PCL-based implant. Biomaterials 2006;27:1735–40. Available from: http://dx.doi.org/10.1016/j.biomaterials.2005.09.019.
[173] Williams DF, McNamara A, Turner RM. Potential of polyetheretherketone (PEEK) and carbon-fibre-reinforced PEEK in medical applications. J Mater Sci Lett 1987;6:188–90. Available from: http://dx.doi.org/10.1007/BF01728981.
[174] Evans NT, Torstrick FB, Lee CSD, Dupont KM, Safranski DL, Chang WA, et al. High-strength, surface-porous polyether-ether-ketone for load-bearing orthopedic implants. Acta Biomater 2015;13:159–67. Available from: http://dx.doi.org/10.1016/j.actbio.2014.11.030.
[175] Chen QZ, Thompson ID, Boccaccini AR. 45S5 Bioglass-derived glass-ceramic scaffolds for bone tissue engineering. Biomaterials 2006;27:2414–25. Available from: http://dx.doi.org/10.1016/j.biomaterials.2005.11.025.
[176] Eshraghi S, Das S. Micromechanical finite-element modeling and experimental characterization of the compressive mechanical properties of polycaprolactone-hydroxyapatite composite scaffolds prepared by selective laser sintering for bone tissue engineering. Acta Biomater 2012;8:3138–43. Available from: http://dx.doi.org/10.1016/j.actbio.2012.04.022.
[177] Surmenev RA, Surmeneva MA, Ivanova AA. Significance of calcium phosphate coatings for the enhancement of new bone osteogenesis—a review. Acta Biomater 2014;10:557–79. Available from: http://dx.doi.org/10.1016/j.actbio.2013.10.036.
[178] Zhang Q, Leng Y, Xin R. A comparative study of electrochemical deposition and biomimetic deposition of calcium phosphate on porous titanium. Biomaterials 2005;26:2857–65. Available from: http://dx.doi.org/10.1016/j.biomaterials.2004.08.016.
[179] Feng B, Weng J, Yang BC, Qu SX, Zhang XD. Characterization of titanium surfaces with calcium and phosphate and osteoblast adhesion. Biomaterials 2004;25:3421–8. Available from: http://dx.doi.org/10.1016/j.biomaterials.2003.10.044.
[180] Gao Y, Hu J, Guan TH, Wu J, Zhang CB, Gao B. Physical properties and cellular responses to calcium phosphate coating produced by laser rapid forming on titanium. Lasers Med Sci 2014;29:9–17. Available from: http://dx.doi.org/10.1007/s10103-012-1226-9.
[181] Junker R, Dimakis A, Thoneick M, Jansen JA. Effects of implant surface coatings and composition on bone integration: a systematic review. Clin Oral Implants Res 2009;20(Suppl. 4):185–206. Available from: http://dx.doi.org/10.1111/j.1600-0501.2009.01777.x.
[182] Dorozhkin SV. Calcium orthophosphate coatings on magnesium and its biodegradable alloys. Acta Biomater 2014;10:2919–34. Available from: http://dx.doi.org/10.1016/j.actbio.2014.02.026.
[183] Guilak F, Cohen DM, Estes BT, Gimble JM, Liedtke W, Chen CS. Control of stem cell fate by physical interactions with the extracellular matrix. Cell Stem Cell 2009;5:17–26. Available from: http://dx.doi.org/10.1016/j.stem.2009.06.016.
[184] McBeath R, Pirone DM, Nelson CM, Bhadriraju K, Chen CS. Cell shape, cytoskeletal tension, and rhoa regulate stem cell lineage commitment. Dev Cell 2004;6:483–95. Available from: http://dx.doi.org/10.1016/S1534-5807(04)00075-9.
[185] Engler AJ, Sen S, Sweeney HL, Discher DE. Matrix elasticity directs stem cell lineage specification. Cell 2006;126:677–89. Available from: http://dx.doi.org/10.1016/j.cell.2006.06.044.
[186] Boerckel JD, Kolambkar YM, Stevens HY, Lin ASP, Dupont KM, Guldberg RE. Effects of in vivo mechanical loading on large bone defect regeneration. J Orthop Res 2012;30:1067–75. Available from: http://dx.doi.org/10.1002/jor.22042.

[187] Turner CH, Pavalko FM. Mechanotransduction and functional response of the skeleton to physical stress: the mechanisms and mechanics of bone adaptation. J Orthop Sci 1998;3:346–55. Available from: http://dx.doi.org/10.1007/s007760050064.

[188] Ingber DE. Cellular mechanotransduction: putting all the pieces together again. FASEB J 2006;20:811–27. Available from: http://dx.doi.org/10.1096/fj.05-5424rev.

[189] Giancotti FG. Integrin Signaling. Science 1999;285:1028–33. Available from: http://dx.doi.org/10.1126/science.285.5430.1028.

[190] Lee D-Y, Yeh C-R, Chang S-F, Lee P-L, Chien S, Cheng C-K, et al. Integrin-mediated expression of bone formation-related genes in osteoblast-like cells in response to fluid shear stress: roles of extracellular matrix, Shc, and mitogen-activated protein kinase. J Bone Miner Res 2008;23:1140–9. Available from: http://dx.doi.org/10.1359/jbmr.080302.

[191] Turner CH, Forwood MR, Otter MW. Mechanotransduction in bone: do bone cells act as sensors of fluid flow? FASEB J 1994;8:875–8. <http://www.ncbi.nlm.nih.gov/pubmed/8070637> (accessed August 15, 2015).

[192] Papachristou DJ, Papachroni KK, Basdra EK, Papavassiliou AG. Signaling networks and transcription factors regulating mechanotransduction in bone. Bioessays 2009;31:794–804. Available from: http://dx.doi.org/10.1002/bies.200800223.

[193] Hynes RO. Integrins: bidirectional, allosteric signaling machines. Cell 2002;110:673–87. <http://www.ncbi.nlm.nih.gov/pubmed/12297042> (accessed January 14, 2015).

[194] Thompson WR, Rubin CT, Rubin J. Mechanical regulation of signaling pathways in bone. Gene 2012;503:179–93. Available from: http://dx.doi.org/10.1016/j.gene.2012.04.076.

[195] Helmke BP, Rosen AB, Davies PF. Mapping mechanical strain of an endogenous cytoskeletal network in living endothelial cells. Biophys J 2003;84:2691–9. Available from: http://dx.doi.org/10.1016/S0006-3495(03)75074-7.

[196] Orr AW, Helmke BP, Blackman BR, Schwartz MA. Mechanisms of mechanotransduction. Dev Cell 2006;10:11–20. Available from: http://dx.doi.org/10.1016/j.devcel.2005.12.006.

[197] Sokabe M, Sachs F, Jing ZQ. Quantitative video microscopy of patch clamped membranes stress, strain, capacitance, and stretch channel activation. Biophys J 1991;59:722–8. Available from: http://dx.doi.org/10.1016/S0006-3495(91)82285-8.

[198] Duncan RL, Hruska KA. Chronic, intermittent loading alters mechanosensitive channel characteristics in osteoblast-like cells. Am J Physiol 1994;267:F909–16. <http://www.ncbi.nlm.nih.gov/pubmed/7528987> (accessed June 30, 2015).

[199] Duncan RL, Kizer N, Barry EL, Friedman PA, Hruska KA. Antisense oligodeoxynucleotide inhibition of a swelling-activated cation channel in osteoblast-like osteosarcoma cells. Proc Natl Acad Sci USA 1996;93:1864–9. <http://www.pubmedcentral.nih.gov/articlerender.fcgi?artid = 39873 &tool = pmcentrez&rendertype = abstract> (accessed August 16, 2015).

[200] Lansman JB, Hallam TJ, Rink TJ. Single stretch-activated ion channels in vascular endothelial cells as mechanotransducers?. Nature 2002;325:811–13. Available from: http://dx.doi.org/10.1038/325811a0.

[201] Kizer N, Guo XL, Hruska K. Reconstitution of stretch-activated cation channels by expression of the alpha-subunit of the epithelial sodium channel cloned from osteoblasts. Proc Natl Acad Sci USA 94 1997;1013–18. <http://www.pubmedcentral.nih.gov/articlerender.fcgi?artid = 19631 &tool = pmcentrez&rendertype = abstract> (accessed August 16, 2015).

[202] Rawlinson SCF, Pitsillides AA, Lanyon LE. Involvement of different ion channels in osteoblasts' and osteocytes' early responses to mechanical strain. Bone 1996;19:609–14. Available from: http://dx.doi.org/10.1016/S8756-3282(96)00260-8.

[203] Malone AMD, Anderson CT, Tummala P, Kwon RY, Johnston TR, Stearns T, et al. Primary cilia mediate mechanosensing in bone cells by a calcium-independent mechanism. Proc Natl Acad Sci USA 2007;104:13325–30. Available from: http://dx.doi.org/10.1073/pnas.0700636104.

[204] Temiyasathit S, Tang WJ, Leucht P, Anderson CT, Monica SD, Castillo AB, et al. Mechanosensing by the primary cilium: deletion of Kif3A reduces bone formation due to loading. PLoS One 2012;7:e33368. Available from: http://dx.doi.org/10.1371/journal.pone.0033368.

[205] Hoey DA, Tormey S, Ramcharan S, O'Brien FJ, Jacobs CR. Primary cilia-mediated mechanotransduction in human mesenchymal stem cells. Stem Cells 2012;30:2561–70. Available from: http://dx.doi.org/10.1002/stem.1235.
[206] McGlashan SR, Jensen CG, Poole CA. Localization of extracellular matrix receptors on the chondrocyte primary cilium. J Histochem Cytochem 2006;54:1005–14. Available from: http://dx.doi.org/10.1369/jhc.5A6866.2006.
[207] Iomini C, Tejada K, Mo W, Vaananen H, Piperno G. Primary cilia of human endothelial cells disassemble under laminar shear stress. J Cell Biol 2004;164:811–17. Available from: http://dx.doi.org/10.1083/jcb.200312133.
[208] Davies PF. Hemodynamic shear stress and the endothelium in cardiovascular pathophysiology. Nat Clin Pract Cardiovasc Med 2009;6:16–26. Available from: http://dx.doi.org/10.1038/ncpcardio1397.
[209] Ingber DE, Tensegrity I. Cell structure and hierarchical systems biology. J Cell Sci 2003;116:1157–73. Available from: http://dx.doi.org/10.1242/jcs.00359.
[210] Vincent LG, Choi YS, Alonso-Latorre B, del Álamo JC, Engler AJ. Mesenchymal stem cell durotaxis depends on substrate stiffness gradient strength. Biotechnol J 2013;8:472–84. Available from: http://dx.doi.org/10.1002/biot.201200205.
[211] Hadjipanayi E, Mudera V, Brown RA. Close dependence of fibroblast proliferation on collagen scaffold matrix stiffness. J Tissue Eng Regen Med 2009;3:77–84. Available from: http://dx.doi.org/10.1002/term.136.
[212] Yeh Y-T, Hur SS, Chang J, Wang K-C, Chiu J-J, Li Y-S, et al. Matrix stiffness regulates endothelial cell proliferation through septin 9. PLoS One 2012;7:e46889. Available from: http://dx.doi.org/10.1371/journal.pone.0046889.
[213] Wang H-B, Dembo M, Wang Y-L. Substrate flexibility regulates growth and apoptosis of normal but not transformed cells. Am J Physiol Cell Physiol 2000;279:C1345–50. <http://ajpcell.physiology.org/content/279/5/C1345.short> (accessed August 16, 2015).
[214] Leight JL, Wozniak MA, Chen S, Lynch ML, Chen CS. Matrix rigidity regulates a switch between TGF-β1-induced apoptosis and epithelial-mesenchymal transition. Mol Biol Cell 2012;23:781–91. Available from: http://dx.doi.org/10.1091/mbc.E11-06-0537.
[215] Huebsch N, Arany PR, Mao AS, Shvartsman D, Ali OA, Bencherif SA, et al. Harnessing traction-mediated manipulation of the cell/matrix interface to control stem-cell fate. Nat Mater 2010;9:518–26. Available from: http://dx.doi.org/10.1038/nmat2732.
[216] Nelson CM, Jean RP, Tan JL, Liu WF, Sniadecki NJ, Spector AA, et al. Emergent patterns of growth controlled by multicellular form and mechanics. Proc Natl Acad Sci USA 2005;102:11594–9. Available from: http://dx.doi.org/10.1073/pnas.0502575102.
[217] Dalby MJ, Gadegaard N, Tare R, Andar A, Riehle MO, Herzyk P, et al. The control of human mesenchymal cell differentiation using nanoscale symmetry and disorder. Nat Mater 2007;6:997–1003. Available from: http://dx.doi.org/10.1038/nmat2013.
[218] Burke DP, Kelly DJ. Substrate stiffness and oxygen as regulators of stem cell differentiation during skeletal tissue regeneration: a mechanobiological model. PLoS One 2012;7:e40737. Available from: http://dx.doi.org/10.1371/journal.pone.0040737.
[219] Khetan S, Guvendiren M, Legant WR, Cohen DM, Chen CS, Burdick JA. Degradation-mediated cellular traction directs stem cell fate in covalently crosslinked three-dimensional hydrogels. Nat Mater 2013;12:458–65. Available from: http://dx.doi.org/10.1038/nmat3586.
[220] Sumanasinghe RD, Bernacki SH, Loboa EG. Osteogenic differentiation of human mesenchymal stem cells in collagen matrices: effect of uniaxial cyclic tensile strain on bone morphogenetic protein (BMP-2) mRNA expression. Tissue Eng 2006;12:3459–65. Available from: http://dx.doi.org/10.1089/ten.2006.12.3459.
[221] Kearney EM, Farrell E, Prendergast PJ, Campbell VA. Tensile strain as a regulator of mesenchymal stem cell osteogenesis. Ann Biomed Eng 2010;38:1767–79. Available from: http://dx.doi.org/10.1007/s10439-010-9979-4.
[222] Simmons CA, Matlis S, Thornton AJ, Chen S, Wang CY, Mooney DJ. Cyclic strain enhances matrix mineralization by adult human mesenchymal stem cells via the extracellular signal-regulated

kinase (ERK1/2) signaling pathway. J Biomech 2003;36:1087–96. <http://www.ncbi.nlm.nih.gov/pubmed/12831733> (accessed August 23, 2015).
[223] Jang J-Y, Lee SW, Park SH, Shin JW, Mun C, Kim S-H, et al. Combined effects of surface morphology and mechanical straining magnitudes on the differentiation of mesenchymal stem cells without using biochemical reagents. J Biomed Biotechnol 2011;2011:860652. Available from: http://dx.doi.org/10.1155/2011/860652.
[224] Subramony SD, Dargis BR, Castillo M, Azeloglu EU, Tracey MS, Su A, et al. The guidance of stem cell differentiation by substrate alignment and mechanical stimulation. Biomaterials 2013;34:1942–53. Available from: http://dx.doi.org/10.1016/j.biomaterials.2012.11.012.
[225] Chen Y-J, Huang C-H, Lee I-C, Lee Y-T, Chen M-H, Young T-H. Effects of cyclic mechanical stretching on the mRNA expression of tendon/ligament-related and osteoblast-specific genes in human mesenchymal stem cells. Connect Tissue Res 2008;49:7–14. Available from: http://dx.doi.org/10.1080/03008200701818561.
[226] Simmons CA, Matlis S, Thornton AJ, Chen S, Wang C-Y, Mooney DJ. Cyclic strain enhances matrix mineralization by adult human mesenchymal stem cells via the extracellular signal-regulated kinase (ERK1/2) signaling pathway. J Biomech 2003;36:1087–96. Available from: http://dx.doi.org/10.1016/S0021-9290(03)00110-6.
[227] Chen Y-J, Huang C-H, Lee I-C, Lee Y-T, Chen M-H, Young T-H. Effects of cyclic mechanical stretching on the mRNA expression of tendon/ligament-related and osteoblast-specific genes in human mesenchymal stem cells. Connect Tissue Res 2015; <http://www.tandfonline.com/doi/abs/10.1080/03008200701818561?journalCode = icts20#.VdoPbflViko> (accessed August 23, 2015).
[228] Michalopoulos E, Knight RL, Korossis S, Kearney JN, Fisher J, Ingham E. Development of methods for studying the differentiation of human mesenchymal stem cells under cyclic compressive strain. Tissue Eng Part C Methods 2012;18:252–62. Available from: http://dx.doi.org/10.1089/ten.TEC.2011.0347.
[229] Steward AJ, Kelly DJ. Mechanical regulation of mesenchymal stem cell differentiation. J Anat 2014; n/a–n/a. Available from: http://dx.doi.org/10.1111/joa.12243.
[230] Huang C-YC, Hagar KL, Frost LE, Sun Y, Cheung HS. Effects of cyclic compressive loading on chondrogenesis of rabbit bone-marrow derived mesenchymal stem cells. Stem Cells 2004;22:313–23. Available from: http://dx.doi.org/10.1634/stemcells.22-3-313.
[231] Kisiday JD, Frisbie DD, McIlwraith CW, Grodzinsky AJ. Dynamic compression stimulates proteoglycan synthesis by mesenchymal stem cells in the absence of chondrogenic cytokines. Tissue Eng Part A 2009;15:2817–24. Available from: http://dx.doi.org/10.1089/ten.TEA.2008.0357.
[232] Mauck RL, Byers BA, Yuan X, Tuan RS. Regulation of cartilaginous ECM gene transcription by chondrocytes and MSCs in 3D culture in response to dynamic loading. Biomech Model Mechanobiol 2007;6:113–25. Available from: http://dx.doi.org/10.1007/s10237-006-0042-1.
[233] Thorpe SD, Buckley CT, Steward AJ, Kelly DJ. European society of biomechanics S.M. Perren Award 2012: the external mechanical environment can override the influence of local substrate in determining stem cell fate. J Biomech 2012;45:2483–92. Available from: http://dx.doi.org/10.1016/j.jbiomech.2012.07.024.
[234] Iqbal J, Zaidi M. Molecular regulation of mechanotransduction. Biochem Biophys Res Commun 2005;328:751–5. Available from: http://dx.doi.org/10.1016/j.bbrc.2004.12.087.
[235] Pelaez D, Arita N, Cheung HS. Extracellular signal-regulated kinase (ERK) dictates osteogenic and/or chondrogenic lineage commitment of mesenchymal stem cells under dynamic compression. Biochem Biophys Res Commun 2012;417:1286–91. Available from: http://dx.doi.org/10.1016/j.bbrc.2011.12.131.
[236] Steward AJ, Wagner DR, Kelly DJ. Exploring the roles of integrin binding and cytoskeletal reorganization during mesenchymal stem cell mechanotransduction in soft and stiff hydrogels subjected to dynamic compression. J Mech Behav Biomed Mater 2014;38:174–82. Available from: http://dx.doi.org/10.1016/j.jmbbm.2013.07.020.
[237] Nerem RM. Hemodynamics and the vascular endothelium. J Biomech Eng 1993;115:510–14. <http://www.ncbi.nlm.nih.gov/pubmed/8302033> (accessed August 24, 2015).

[238] Zheng W, Christensen LP, Tomanek RJ. Stretch induces upregulation of key tyrosine kinase receptors in microvascular endothelial cells. Am J Physiol Heart Circ Physiol 2004;287: H2739–45. Available from: http://dx.doi.org/10.1152/ajpheart.00410.2004.

[239] Wilkins JR, Pike DB, Gibson CC, Kubota A, Shiu Y-T. Differential effects of cyclic stretch on bFGF- and VEGF-induced sprouting angiogenesis. Biotechnol Prog 2014;30:879–88. Available from: http://dx.doi.org/10.1002/btpr.1883.

[240] Joung IS, Iwamoto MN, Shiu Y-T, Quam CT. Cyclic strain modulates tubulogenesis of endothelial cells in a 3D tissue culture model. Microvasc Res 2006;71:1–11. Available from: http://dx.doi.org/10.1016/j.mvr.2005.10.005.

[241] Ives CL, Eskin SG, McIntire LV. Mechanical effects on endothelial cell morphology: in vitro assessment. Vitr Cell Dev Biol 1986;22:500–7. Available from: http://dx.doi.org/10.1007/BF02621134.

[242] Wang JH-C, Goldschmidt-Clermont P, Wille J, Yin FC-P. Specificity of endothelial cell reorientation in response to cyclic mechanical stretching. J Biomech 2001;34:1563–72. Available from: http://dx.doi.org/10.1016/S0021-9290(01)00150-6.

[243] Moretti M, Prina-Mello A, Reid AJ, Barron V, Prendergast PJ. Endothelial cell alignment on cyclically-stretched silicone surfaces. J Mater Sci Mater Med 2004;15:1159–64. Available from: http://dx.doi.org/10.1023/B:JMSM.0000046400.18607.72.

[244] Wang JH, Grood ES. The strain magnitude and contact guidance determine orientation response of fibroblasts to cyclic substrate strains. Connect Tissue Res 2000;41:29–36. <http://www.ncbi.nlm.nih.gov/pubmed/10826706> (accessed August 24, 2015).

[245] Meinel L, Karageorgiou V, Fajardo R, Snyder B, Shinde-Patil V, Zichner L, et al. Bone tissue engineering using human mesenchymal stem cells: effects of scaffold material and medium flow. Ann Biomed Eng 2004;32:112–22. Available from: http://dx.doi.org/10.1023/B:ABME.0000007796.48329.b4.

[246] Li YJ, Batra NN, You L, Meier SC, Coe IA, Yellowley CE, et al. Oscillatory fluid flow affects human marrow stromal cell proliferation and differentiation. J Orthop Res 2004;22:1283–9. Available from: http://dx.doi.org/10.1016/j.orthres.2004.04.002.

[247] Jaiswal N, Haynesworth SE, Caplan AI, Bruder SP. Osteogenic differentiation of purified, culture-expanded human mesenchymal stem cells in vitro. J Cell Biochem 1997;64:295–312. <http://www.ncbi.nlm.nih.gov/pubmed/9027589> (accessed July 27, 2015).

[248] Datta N, Pham QP, Sharma U, Sikavitsas VI, Jansen JA, Mikos AG. In vitro generated extracellular matrix and fluid shear stress synergistically enhance 3D osteoblastic differentiation. Proc Natl Acad Sci USA 2006;103:2488–93. Available from: http://dx.doi.org/10.1073/pnas.0505661103.

[249] Ando J, Nomura H, Kamiya A. The effect of fluid shear stress on the migration and proliferation of cultured endothelial cells. Microvasc Res 1987;33:62–70. Available from: http://dx.doi.org/10.1016/0026-2862(87)90007-0.

[250] Li Y-SJ, Haga JH, Chien S. Molecular basis of the effects of shear stress on vascular endothelial cells. J Biomech 2005;38:1949–71. Available from: http://dx.doi.org/10.1016/j.jbiomech.2004.09.030.

[251] Gomes ME, Sikavitsas VI, Behravesh E, Reis RL, Mikos AG. Effect of flow perfusion on the osteogenic differentiation of bone marrow stromal cells cultured on starch-based three-dimensional scaffolds. J Biomed Mater Res A 2003;67:87–95. Available from: http://dx.doi.org/10.1002/jbm.a.10075.

[252] McCoy RJ, O'Brien FJ. Influence of shear stress in perfusion bioreactor cultures for the development of three-dimensional bone tissue constructs: a review. Tissue Eng Part B Rev 2010;16:587–601. Available from: http://dx.doi.org/10.1089/ten.TEB.2010.0370.

[253] Angele P, Yoo JU, Smith C, Mansour J, Jepsen KJ, Nerlich M, et al. Cyclic hydrostatic pressure enhances the chondrogenic phenotype of human mesenchymal progenitor cells differentiated in vitro. J Orthop Res 2003;21:451–7. Available from: http://dx.doi.org/10.1016/S0736-0266(02)00230-9.

[254] Miyanishi K, Trindade MCD, Lindsey DP, Beaupré GS, Carter DR, Goodman SB, et al. Effects of hydrostatic pressure and transforming growth factor-beta 3 on adult human mesenchymal stem cell chondrogenesis in vitro. Tissue Eng 2006;12:1419–28. Available from: http://dx.doi.org/10.1089/ten.2006.12.1419.

[255] Puetzer J, Williams J, Gillies A, Bernacki S, Loboa EG. The effects of cyclic hydrostatic pressure on chondrogenesis and viability of human adipose- and bone marrow-derived mesenchymal stem cells in three-dimensional agarose constructs. Tissue Eng Part A 2013;19:299–306. Available from: http://dx.doi.org/10.1089/ten.TEA.2012.0015.
[256] Wright MO, Stockwell RA, Nuki G. Response of plasma membrane to applied hydrostatic pressure in chondrocytes and fibroblasts. Connect Tissue Res 1992;28:49–70. <http://www.ncbi.nlm.nih.gov/pubmed/1628490> (accessed August 30, 2015).
[257] Browning JA, Saunders K, Urban JPG, Wilkins RJ. The influence and interactions of hydrostatic and osmotic pressures on the intracellular milieu of chondrocytes. Biorheology 2004;41:299–308. <http://www.ncbi.nlm.nih.gov/pubmed/15299262> (accessed August 30, 2015).
[258] Mizuno S. A novel method for assessing effects of hydrostatic fluid pressure on intracellular calcium: a study with bovine articular chondrocytes. Am J Physiol Cell Physiol 2005;288:C329–37. Available from: http://dx.doi.org/10.1152/ajpcell.00131.2004.
[259] Hui TH, Zhou ZL, Qian J, Lin Y, Ngan AHW, Gao H. Volumetric deformation of live cells induced by pressure-activated cross-membrane ion transport. Phys Rev Lett 2014;113. 118-101. <http://www.ncbi.nlm.nih.gov/pubmed/25260007> (accessed August 30, 2015).
[260] Steward AJ, Thorpe SD, Vinardell T, Buckley CT, Wagner DR, Kelly DJ. Cell-matrix interactions regulate mesenchymal stem cell response to hydrostatic pressure. Acta Biomater 2012;8:2153–9. Available from: http://dx.doi.org/10.1016/j.actbio.2012.03.016.
[261] Perren SM. Physical and biological aspects of fracture healing with special reference to internal fixation. Clin Orthop Relat Res 1979;175–96. <http://www.ncbi.nlm.nih.gov/pubmed/376198> (accessed September 5, 2015).
[262] Betts DC, Müller R. Mechanical regulation of bone regeneration: theories, models, and experiments. Front Endocrinol (Lausanne) 2014;5:211. Available from: http://dx.doi.org/10.3389/fendo.2014.00211.
[263] Goodship AE, Kenwright J. The influence of induced micromovement upon the healing of experimental tibial fractures. J Bone Joint Surg Br 1985;67:650–5. <http://www.ncbi.nlm.nih.gov/pubmed/4030869> (accessed September 7, 2015).
[264] Goodship AE, Cunningham JL, Kenwright J. Strain rate and timing of stimulation in mechanical modulation of fracture healing. Clin Orthop Relat Res 1998;S105–15. <http://www.ncbi.nlm.nih.gov/pubmed/9917631> (accessed February 17, 2015).
[265] Claes LE, Wilke H-J, Augat P, Rübenacker S, Margevicius KJ. Effect of dynamization on gap healing of diaphyseal fractures under external fixation. Clin Biomech (Bristol, Avon) 1995;10:227–34. <http://www.ncbi.nlm.nih.gov/pubmed/11415558> (accessed January 20, 2015).
[266] Gardner MJ, van der Meulen MCH, Demetrakopoulos D, Wright TM, Myers ER, Bostrom MP. In vivo cyclic axial compression affects bone healing in the mouse tibia. J Orthop Res 2006;24:1679–86. Available from: http://dx.doi.org/10.1002/jor.20230.
[267] Willie BM, Blakytny R, Glöckelmann M, Ignatius A, Claes L. Temporal variation in fixation stiffness affects healing by differential cartilage formation in a rat osteotomy model. Clin Orthop Relat Res 2011;469:3094–101. Available from: http://dx.doi.org/10.1007/s11999-011-1866-2.
[268] Schwarz C, Wulsten D, Ellinghaus A, Lienau J, Willie BM, Duda GN. Mechanical load modulates the stimulatory effect of BMP2 in a rat nonunion model. Tissue Eng Part A 2013;19:247–54. Available from: http://dx.doi.org/10.1089/ten.tea.2012.0265.
[269] Glatt V, Miller M, Ivkovic A, Liu F, Parry N, Griffin D, et al. Improved healing of large segmental defects in the rat femur by reverse dynamization in the presence of bone morphogenetic protein-2. J Bone Joint Surg Am 2012;94:2063–73. Available from: http://dx.doi.org/10.2106/JBJS.K.01604.
[270] Glatt V, Evans CH, Matthys R. Design, characterisation and in vivo testing of a new, adjustable stiffness, external fixator for the rat femur. Eur Cell Mater 2012;23:289–98. discussion 299. <http://www.ncbi.nlm.nih.gov/pubmed/22522283> (accessed January 20, 2015).
[271] Hou T, Li Q, Luo F, Xu J, Xie Z, Wu X, et al. Controlled dynamization to enhance reconstruction capacity of tissue-engineered bone in healing critically sized bone defects: an in vivo study in

goats. Tissue Eng Part A 2010;16:201–12. Available from: http://dx.doi.org/10.1089/ten.TEA.2009.0291.

[272] Duty AO, Oest ME, Guldberg RE. Cyclic mechanical compression increases mineralization of cell-seeded polymer scaffolds in vivo. J Biomech Eng 2007;129:531–9. Available from: http://dx.doi.org/10.1115/1.2746375.

[273] Roshan-Ghias A, Lambers FM, Gholam-Rezaee M, Müller R, Pioletti DP. In vivo loading increases mechanical properties of scaffold by affecting bone formation and bone resorption rates. Bone 2011;49:1357–64. Available from: http://dx.doi.org/10.1016/j.bone.2011.09.040.

[274] Ilizarov GA. The tension-stress effect on the genesis and growth of tissues. Part I. The influence of stability of fixation and soft-tissue preservation. Clin Orthop Relat Res 1989;249–81. <http://www.ncbi.nlm.nih.gov/pubmed/2910611> (accessed January 12, 2016).

[275] Ilizarov GA. The tension-stress effect on the genesis and growth of tissues: Part II. The influence of the rate and frequency of distraction. Clin Orthop Relat Res 1989;263–85. <http://www.ncbi.nlm.nih.gov/pubmed/2912628> (accessed January 12, 2016).

[276] Mofid MM, Manson PN, Robertson BC, Tufaro AP, Elias JJ, Vander Kolk CA. Craniofacial distraction osteogenesis: a review of 3278 cases. Plast Reconstr Surg 2001;108:1103–14. Available from: http://dx.doi.org/10.1097/00006534-200110000-00001.

[277] Alzahrani MM, Anam EA, Makhdom AM, Villemure I, Hamdy RC. The effect of altering the mechanical loading environment on the expression of bone regenerating molecules in cases of distraction osteogenesis. Front Endocrinol (Lausanne) 2014;5:214. Available from: http://dx.doi.org/10.3389/fendo.2014.00214.

[278] Morgan EF, Hussein AI, Al-Awadhi BA, Hogan DE, Matsubara H, Al-Alq Z, et al. Vascular development during distraction osteogenesis proceeds by sequential intramuscular arteriogenesis followed by intraosteal angiogenesis. Bone 2012;51:535–45. Available from: http://dx.doi.org/10.1016/j.bone.2012.05.008.

[279] Matsubara H, Hogan DE, Morgan EF, Mortlock DP, Einhorn TA, Gerstenfeld LC. Vascular tissues are a primary source of BMP2 expression during bone formation induced by distraction osteogenesis. Bone 2012;51:168–80. Available from: http://dx.doi.org/10.1016/j.bone.2012.02.017.

[280] Natu SS, Ali I, Alam S, Giri KY, Agarwal A, Kulkarni VA. The biology of distraction osteogenesis for correction of mandibular and craniomaxillofacial defects: a review. Dent Res J (Isfahan) 2014;11:16–26. <http://www.pubmedcentral.nih.gov/articlerender.fcgi?artid = 3955310&tool = pmcentrez&rendertype = abstract> (accessed November 25, 2015).

[281] Nogueira MP, Paley D, Bhave A, Herbert A, Nocente C, Herzenberg JE. Nerve lesions associated with limb-lengthening. J Bone Joint Surg Am 2003;85-A:1502–10. <http://www.ncbi.nlm.nih.gov/pubmed/12925630> (accessed January 12, 2016).

[282] Claes L, Augat P, Schorlemmer S, Konrads C, Ignatius A, Ehrnthaller C. Temporary distraction and compression of a diaphyseal osteotomy accelerates bone healing. J Orthop Res 2008;26:772–7. Available from: http://dx.doi.org/10.1002/jor.20588.

[283] Makhdom AM, Cartaleanu AS, Rendon JS, Villemure I, Hamdy RC. The accordion maneuver: a noninvasive strategy for absent or delayed callus formation in cases of limb lengthening. Adv Orthop 2015;2015:912790. Available from: http://dx.doi.org/10.1155/2015/912790.

[284] Augat P, Burger J, Schorlemmer S, Henke T, Peraus M, Claes L. Shear movement at the fracture site delays healing in a diaphyseal fracture model. J Orthop Res 2003;21:1011–17. Available from: http://dx.doi.org/10.1016/S0736-0266(03)00098-6.

[285] Bishop NE, van Rhijn M, Tami I, Corveleijn R, Schneider E, Ito K. Shear does not necessarily inhibit bone healing. Clin Orthop Relat Res 2006;443:307–14. Available from: http://dx.doi.org/10.1097/01.blo.0000191272.34786.09.

[286] Isaksson H, Wilson W, van Donkelaar CC, Huiskes R, Ito K. Comparison of biophysical stimuli for mechano-regulation of tissue differentiation during fracture healing. J Biomech 2006;39:1507–16. Available from: http://dx.doi.org/10.1016/j.jbiomech.2005.01.037.

[287] Claes L, Heigele C. Magnitudes of local stress and strain along bony surfaces predict the course and type of fracture healing. J Biomech 1999;32:255–66. Available from: http://dx.doi.org/10.1016/S0021-9290(98)00153-5.

[288] Wazen RM, Currey JA, Guo H, Brunski JB, Helms JA, Nanci A. Micromotion-induced strain fields influence early stages of repair at bone-implant interfaces. Acta Biomater 2013;9:6663–74. Available from: http://dx.doi.org/10.1016/j.actbio.2013.01.014.

[289] Cheal EJ, Mansmann KA, DiGioia AM, Hayes WC, Perren SM. Role of interfragmentary strain in fracture healing: ovine model of a healing osteotomy. J Orthop Res 1991;9:131–42. Available from: http://dx.doi.org/10.1002/jor.1100090116.

[290] Geris L, Vander Sloten J, Van Oosterwyck H. Connecting biology and mechanics in fracture healing: an integrated mathematical modeling framework for the study of nonunions. Biomech Model Mechanobiol 2010;9:713–24. Available from: http://dx.doi.org/10.1007/s10237-010-0208-8.

[291] Simon U, Augat P, Utz M, Claes L. A numerical model of the fracture healing process that describes tissue development and revascularisation. Comput Methods Biomech Biomed Engin 2011;14:79–93. Available from: http://dx.doi.org/10.1080/10255842.2010.499865.

[292] Moore SR, Saidel GM, Knothe U, Knothe Tate ML. Mechanistic, mathematical model to predict the dynamics of tissue genesis in bone defects via mechanical feedback and mediation of biochemical factors. PLoS Comput Biol 2014;10:e1003604. Available from: http://dx.doi.org/10.1371/journal.pcbi.1003604.

[293] Epari DR, Lienau J, Schell H, Witt F, Duda GN. Pressure, oxygen tension and temperature in the periosteal callus during bone healing—an in vivo study in sheep. Bone 2008;43:734–9. Available from: http://dx.doi.org/10.1016/j.bone.2008.06.007.

[294] Vetter A, Witt F, Sander O, Duda GN, Weinkamer R. The spatio-temporal arrangement of different tissues during bone healing as a result of simple mechanobiological rules. Biomech Model Mechanobiol 2012;11:147–60. Available from: http://dx.doi.org/10.1007/s10237-011-0299-x.

[295] Leong PL, Morgan EF. Measurement of fracture callus material properties via nanoindentation. Acta Biomater 2008;4:1569–75. Available from: http://dx.doi.org/10.1016/j.actbio.2008.02.030.

[296] Prendergast PJ, Huiskes R, Søballe K. Biophysical stimuli on cells during tissue differentiation at implant interfaces. J Biomech 1997;30:539–48. Available from: http://dx.doi.org/10.1016/S0021-9290(96)00140-6.

[297] Willie BM, Petersen A, Schmidt-Bleek K, Cipitria A, Mehta M, Strube P, et al. Designing biomimetic scaffolds for bone regeneration: why aim for a copy of mature tissue properties if nature uses a different approach? Soft Matter 2010;6:4976. Available from: http://dx.doi.org/10.1039/c0sm00262c.

[298] Li X, Wang L, Fan Y, Feng Q, Cui F-Z, Watari F. Nanostructured scaffolds for bone tissue engineering. J Biomed Mater Res A 2013;101:2424–35. Available from: http://dx.doi.org/10.1002/jbm.a.34539.

[299] García-Gareta E, Coathup MJ, Blunn GW. Osteoinduction of bone grafting materials for bone repair and regeneration. Bone 2015;81:112–21. Available from: http://dx.doi.org/10.1016/j.bone.2015.07.007.

[300] Hollister SJ, Flanagan CL, Zopf DA, Morrison RJ, Nasser H, Patel JJ, et al. Design control for clinical translation of 3D printed modular scaffolds. Ann Biomed Eng 2015;43:774–86. Available from: http://dx.doi.org/10.1007/s10439-015-1270-2.

[301] Xu C, Su P, Chen X, Meng Y, Yu W, Xiang AP, et al. Biocompatibility and osteogenesis of biomimetic Bioglass-Collagen-Phosphatidylserine composite scaffolds for bone tissue engineering. Biomaterials 2011;32:1051–8. Available from: http://dx.doi.org/10.1016/j.biomaterials.2010.09.068.

[302] El-Fiqi A, Lee JH, Lee E-J, Kim H-W. Collagen hydrogels incorporated with surface-aminated mesoporous nanobioactive glass: improvement of physicochemical stability and mechanical properties is effective for hard tissue engineering. Acta Biomater 2013;9:9508–21. Available from: http://dx.doi.org/10.1016/j.actbio.2013.07.036.

[303] Hussain A, Bessho K, Takahashi K, Tabata Y. Magnesium calcium phosphate as a novel component enhances mechanical/physical properties of gelatin scaffold and osteogenic differentiation of bone marrow mesenchymal stem cells. Tissue Eng Part A 2012;18:768–74. Available from: http://dx.doi.org/10.1089/ten.TEA.2011.0310.

[304] Bhumiratana S, Grayson WL, Castaneda A, Rockwood DN, Gil ES, Kaplan DL, et al. Nucleation and growth of mineralized bone matrix on silk-hydroxyapatite composite scaffolds. Biomaterials 2011;32:2812–20. Available from: http://dx.doi.org/10.1016/j.biomaterials.2010.12.058.
[305] Kong H-J, Lee KY, Mooney DJ. Decoupling the dependence of rheological/mechanical properties of hydrogels from solids concentration. Polymer (Guildf) 2002;43:6239–46. Available from: http://dx.doi.org/10.1016/S0032-3861(02)00559-1.
[306] Harley BA, Leung JH, Silva ECCM, Gibson LJ. Mechanical characterization of collagen-glycosaminoglycan scaffolds. Acta Biomater 2007;3:463–74. Available from: http://dx.doi.org/10.1016/j.actbio.2006.12.009.
[307] Kisiel M, Martino MM, Ventura M, Hubbell JA, Hilborn J, Ossipov DA. Improving the osteogenic potential of BMP-2 with hyaluronic acid hydrogel modified with integrin-specific fibronectin fragment. Biomaterials 2013;34:704–12. Available from: http://dx.doi.org/10.1016/j.biomaterials.2012.10.015.
[308] Shimko DA, Shimko VF, Sander EA, Dickson KF, Nauman EA. Effect of porosity on the fluid flow characteristics and mechanical properties of tantalum scaffolds. J Biomed Mater Res B Appl Biomater 2005;73:315–24. Available from: http://dx.doi.org/10.1002/jbm.b.30229.
[309] Marolt D, Augst A, Freed LE, Vepari C, Fajardo R, Patel N, et al. Bone and cartilage tissue constructs grown using human bone marrow stromal cells, silk scaffolds and rotating bioreactors. Biomaterials 2006;27:6138–49. Available from: http://dx.doi.org/10.1016/j.biomaterials.2006.07.015.
[310] Baker D, Hastings R, Pruitt L. Compression and tension fatigue resistance of medical grade ultra high molecular weight polyethylene: the effect of morphology, sterilization, aging and temperature. Polymer (Guildf) 2000;41:795–808. Available from: http://dx.doi.org/10.1016/S0032-3861(99)00199-8.

CHAPTER 6

Ceramics in Bone Grafts and Coated Implants

M. Roy[1], A. Bandyopadhyay[2] and S. Bose[2]
[1]Indian Institute of Technology (IIT), Kharagpur, India
[2]Washington State University, Pullman, WA, United States

Contents

6.1 INTRODUCTION

Ceramics that are used for musculoskeletal restoration are generally called bioceramics. These materials can be bioinert, such as alumina, bioresorbable, such as tricalcium phosphate, or bioactive, such as hydroxyapatite (HA) [1]. Bioceramics are used in orthopedics such as in articulation components in total hip prostheses or as bio-active coatings to enhance bone tissue integration in vivo, as bone cement or in maxillofacial reconstruction, just to name a few. Bioceramics are also used as drug delivery vehicles, and in dentistry toward dental restorations [2]. Table 6.1 and Fig. 6.1 show some of the applications of bioceramics in orthopedics and dentistry.

Bone is a living tissue that forms the skeletal system and provides shape and support to the body, as well as protection for many organs. Bone tissue remodels throughout life, and is a dynamic and coordinated biochemical process. Two primary cells that take part in this remodeling process are osteoclasts and osteoblasts. Osteoclasts resorb the old bone while osteoblasts synthesize new bone. Bone comprises nearly 70 wt% HA mineral, 20 wt% organic materials, and 10 wt% water. Collagen microfibers form the basic 3D matrix, where HA crystals deposit. Bone is

Table 6.1 Applications of bioceramics

	Application	Material
Orthopedics	Bone filler (Fig. 6.1F)	HA, α/β-TCP granules, bioglass
	Total knee arthoplasty (Fig. 6.1E)	Al_2O_3, ZrO_2, $Al_2O_3 + ZrO_2$ composite
	Femoral stem fixation (Fig. 6.1A)	Bone cement or HA coating
	Bone scaffold (Fig. 6.1D)	HA, α/β-TCP, bioglass
	Bone screw	Al_2O_3
	Femoral head (Fig. 6.1B)	Al_2O_3, ZrO_2, $Al_2O_3 + ZrO_2$ composite
	Acetabular cup fixation	Bone cement or HA coating
	Posterolateral spinal fusion	α/β-TCP
Dental	Fixed partial denture	Al_2O_3, ZrO_2, $Al_2O_3 + ZrO_2$ composite
	Periodontal pocket obliteration	Al_2O_3, HA
	Dental crown (Fig. 6.1C)	ZrO_2
	Coating on dental screw	HA
Cranio-maxilofacial	Facial reconstruction	HA, α/β-TCP, bone cement, bioglass
	Alveolar ridge (Fig. 6.1G)	Al_2O_3
	Reconstruction	Al_2O_3, HA
ENT	Middle ear ossicular replacements	Al_2O_3
Drug delivery	Osteomyelitis	Nano HA as drug carrier
	Bone tumor/cancer	Nano HA with cancer drugs, bone cement loaded with cancer drugs

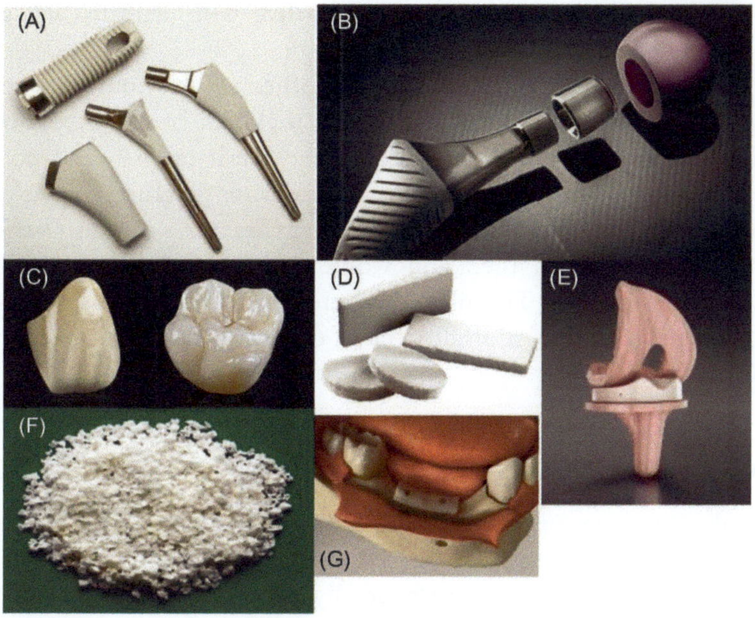

Figure 6.1 Examples of (A) HA-coated hip stem and dental implants (http://apsmaterials.com), (B) ceramic femoral head (https://www.ceramtec.com), (C) ZrO_2 dental crown (http://www.dentalart-slab.com), (D) HA/TCP resorbable ceramic scaffold (http://www.zimmer.com), (E) ceramic knee implants (https://www.ceramtec.com), (F) HA granules as bone filler (http://www.surgiwear.co.in), and (G) ceramic alveolar ridge (https://sigma-implants.com).

also a storage site for primary cations such as calcium and magnesium and maintains homeostasis. It also provides the marrow for the development and storage of blood cells. Because of numerous and complex functions of bone, there are many disorders that arise with time. In due course, these disorders turn so painful that clinical care by a physician or other healthcare professional becomes essential. Among these disorders, osteoarthritis, rheumatoid arthritis, osteoporosis, and bone cancer are predominant.

Osteoarthritis is a chronic disorder where the cartilage and surrounding tissues get seriously damaged. The typical symptoms of osteoarthritis are severe pain, stiffness, swelling, and loss of function. Damaged tissue and cartilage are one of the prime causes of osteoarthritis. The joints are normally of a low wear and tear region. However, obesity, excessive exercise, abnormal mobility, repeated injury, and metabolic disorders cause damage to cartilage and soft tissue. Cartilage protects the joint and absorbs shock when it is subjected to pressure. Cartilage also allows smooth movement of the joint. Without a protective cartilage layer, bones of the joint rub together, resulting in pain, swelling, and stiffness.

There are >100 different forms of arthritis, and chronic arthropathies are one of the most widespread and devastating health conditions in the United States and around the world. The number of people who live with arthritis will grow as life expectancy has increased in the last few decades.

Similar to osteoarthritis, osteoporosis is another severe kind of bone disorder, where bones become so porous and weak that they can break, even from a minor injury. It is referred to as the "silent disease" because it often shows no indications until a bone breaks. The most common osteoporosis fractures occur in the hip; however, vertebrae (bones in the spine) and wrist fractures are also very common. Osteoporosis can affect both men and women; however, typically women are at higher risk of bone fracture. The mortality rate associated with osteoporosis-related fractures is greater than the mortality rates of breast cancer and cervical cancer combined [3].

6.2 BIOINERT CERAMICS

A large number/volume of joint replacements are done worldwide, which are made of ceramics but do not have proven bioactivity, and are known as bioinert ceramics. These bioinert ceramics are generally oxides of aluminum (Al) and zirconium (Zr). The following properties make them suitable for load-bearing joint replacements.

6.2.1 Aluminum oxide

Application of alumina dates back to the 1960s as bone substitute and dental implants [4]. The primary reason for selecting alumina was low wear, chemical inertness, and resistance to corrosion, excellent hydrodynamic stability, and biocompatibility (bioinert). The standard specifications of alumina for medical applications are suggested by ASTM standard F603-12. Table 6.2 summarizes the characterization suggested by ASTM/ISO for alumina to be used in medical applications.

Although alumina was widely used in total hip and knee replacements during the 1980s, low fracture toughness was always a concern. Advancements in ceramic processing, along with better raw materials, resulted in higher densification of alumina at low temperature with finer grain size. Addition of magnesia (MgO) and calcia (CaO) allowed alumina to be sintered below 1600°C by enhancing solid-state diffusion mechanisms. The lower grain size improved the flexural strength and fracture toughness, making alumina suitable for load-bearing applications.

6.2.2 Zirconia

Zirconia ceramics was used as an alternative for alumina during the late 1980s due to improved fracture toughness. Zirconia found most promising use in dental implants

Table 6.2 Standard specification for high-purity dense aluminum oxide for medical application as suggestions made by ASTM/ISO

Chemical requirements	• Chemical compositions (measured by common analytical techniques) $Al_2O_3 \geq 99.5$ (wt%) $MgO \leq 0.5$ (wt%) Other oxides ≤ 0.1 (wt%)
Physical requirements	• Minimum density should be 3.94 ± 0.01 g/cm^3 • The median grain size should be 4.5 μm or less
Mechanical requirements	• Flexural strength $\geq$ 400 MPa (58 Kpsi) • Vicker's hardness $\geq$ 18 GPa (measured at 1 kg load) • The minimum Weibull modulus should be $\geq$ 8 (measured by four-point bend test and minimum of 30 samples)

and as femoral head in total hip replacements along with knee replacements. There are >1 million zirconia femoral heads in use worldwide [5]. The increased mechanical property of zirconia is the consequence of a phenomenon known as "transformation toughening." ZrO_2 can have three polymorphs depending on temperature: monoclinic at <1170°C, tetragonal between 1170°C and 2370°C, and cubic at >2370°C. Processing of zirconia requires it to be sintered at around 1600°C. During cooling, ZrO_2 goes through a phase transition at 1170°C from tetragonal to monoclinic phase, which is associated with 5% volume expansion. The stress associated with this transformation exceeds the fracture limits of ZrO_2 and leads to cracking. Therefore, successful sintering of ZrO_2 will require avoiding monoclinic phase transformation and stabilizing the tetragonal orcubic phase which is achieved by additives such as calcia (CaO), magnesia (MgO), and yttria (Y_2O_3). At times, a mixture of cubic, tetragonal, and small amounts of monoclinic phases is used for stress-induced phase transformation with concurrent toughening. These are known as partially stabilized zirconia (PSZ), whereas tetragonal zirconia polycrystals (TZP) consist of 100% tetragonal phase. Because of the transformation toughening, PSZ has almost twice the fracture toughness of alumina.

Although PSZ has been widely used as a femoral head, degradation of PSZ is a major concern among the orthopedic community and related industries. In 2001–02 a large amount of PSZ femoral heads failed, nearly 400 in number, which is quite a large number compared to almost no failures before that [5]. The failures were primarily corelated to degradation of PSZ in aqueous environments, which is also commonly known as aging. During aging, the metastable tetragonal phase in PSZ progressively transforms to monoclinic phase that follows with a reduction in strength, fracture toughness, and density [5,6]. The failures lead to a detailed understanding of the aging mechanism

Table 6.3 Standard specification for high-purity dense magnesia partially stabilized zirconia for surgical implant applications as suggested by ASTM/ISO

Chemical requirements	• Chemical compositions (measured by common analytical techniques) $ZrO_2 + HfO_2 + MgO \geq 99.8$ (wt%) MgO 3.1–3.4 (wt%) $HfO_2 \leq 2.0$ (wt%) Total other oxides <0.20 (wt%) Other oxides Fe_2O_3 <0.01 (wt%) SiO_2 <0.05 (wt%) CaO <0.02 (wt%) Al_2O_3 <0.05 (wt%)
Physical requirements	• Minimum density should be 5.800 g/cm^3 • Total porosity should be <1.0 vol% of which open porosity must be <0.1 vol% • The monoclinic phase in the PSZ should be <15% as determined by ASTM F2393-12
Mechanical requirements	• Flexural strength ≥600 MPa (87 Kpsi) • Vicker's hardness ≥ 1000 HV (measured at 1 kg load with dwell time of 15 s) • Room temperature elastic modulus should be ≥180 GPa

and pointed out that microstructure, distribution of sintering additives, flaw populations, and distribution are major contributors to aging [7].

Table 6.3 summarizes the characterization suggested by ASTM/ISO for PSZ to be used in medical applications.

Aging of zirconia bioceramics and some femoral head failures raised a few important points related to the use of inert bioceramics for orthopedic applications: (1) detailed specifications and testing procedures, (2) new processing techniques such as HIP (hot isostatic pressing/hot isostatic post-processing), and (3) development of new materials. Successful use of HIP made it possible to achieve the targeted specifications as laid out by ASTM/ISO. As mentioned by Metoxit, an orthopedic manufacturer, it would not be possible to market a nonhipped material for medical applications. Given the transformation toughening of PSZ, it is accepted that the future of load-bearing bioceramics has to come with zirconia. Therefore, a new development path was designed to reduce the aging effect of zirconia by making alumina–zirconia composite [8]. Table 6.4 summarizes some of the newly developed alumina–zirconia composites along with their physical properties.

Table 6.4 Different ceramic ball used as femoral head [8]

	Composition	Hardness (Hv)	Young's modulus (GPa)	Bending strength (MPa)	Density (g/cc)
TZP-A Bio-HIP	95% ZrO_2 + 0.25% Al_2O_3 + 5% Y_2O_3	1200	210	1200	6.05
BIOLOX delta	76.1% Al_2O_3 + 22.5% ZrO_2 + 1.4% Cr_2O_3 + Y_2O_3	1925	350	>950	4.37
Bioceram AZ209	79% Al_2O_3 + 19% ZrO_2 + 2% other additives				

Table 6.5 CaP family along with their physical properties

Symbol	Chemical formula	Chemical name	Ca/P	Solubility product
MCP	$Ca(H_2PO_4)_2\ H_2O$	Monocalcium phosphate	0.50	1.0×10^{-3}
DCPD	$CaHPO_4\ 2H_2O$	Dicalcium phosphate dihydrate	1.00	1.87×10^{-7}
DCP	$CaHPO_4$	Dicalcium phosphate	1.00	1.26×10^{-7}
OCP	$Ca_8H_2(PO_4)_6\ 5H_2O$	Octacalcium phosphate	1.33	5.01×10^{-15}
TCP	$Ca_3(PO_4)_2$	Tricalcium phosphate	1.5	2.83×10^{-30}
HA/HAP	$Ca_{10}(PO_4)_6(OH)_2$	Hydroxyapatite	1.67	2.35×10^{-59}
TTCP	$Ca_4O(PO_4)_2$	Tetracalcium phosphate	2.00	1×10^{-38}–1×10^{-44}

6.3 CALCIUM PHOSPHATES

The primary mineral component in bone is calcium phosphate (CaP) and specifically HA or calcium-deficient HA. In the last 50 years, major interest has been developed to use these materials as bone substitutes for obvious reasons. The CaPs are a class of materials having different solubility and bioactivity owing to their different Ca to P ratio. Table 6.5 shows different forms of calcium phosphates along with their physical properties [9].

Depending on the Ca/P ratio, the CaP can be bioactive, i.e., osteoconductive, or bioresorbable which is not only osteoconductive but also slowly resorbs in physiological media making a pathway for new bone formation [9]. Among different forms of CaPs, major interest has been developed for HA and tricalcium phosphate (TCP). Because of its lowest solubility, HA is primarily developed as a bioactive material. Over the years, a variety of methods have been explored to synthesize HA powder having different particle size and shape. Aqueous precipitation of HA is one of the simplest ways of synthesizing HA. A comprehensive review on different methods of HA powder synthesis has recently been published by Sadat-Shojai et al. [10]. Table 6.6 summarizes some of the processing routes and the properties of HA powders [10].

Processing of synthetic HA powder to applicable granules, beads, or preformed structures requires HA being heat treated at higher temperature or commonly known as sintering. Improper sintering of HA can easily lead to formation of α/β-TCP with higher solubility of the final product. It is found to be safe to sinter HA at 1250°C without significant α/β-TCP phase formation. As HA by itself is rarely used for load-bearing applications, the mechanical properties of sintered HA are not a major concern. However, for safety in application, sintered HA requires a compressive strength of >100 MPa (the majority of the values in the literature fall between 100 and 900 MPa). Excellent biocompatibility and bioactivity of HA have constantly been reported throughout the literature. Both in vitro and in vivo models have proven that HA can be successfully applied as bone substitutes and resulted in several commercial products of HA (Calcibon, Aperceram, Cortoss, Truebone, Osteograft, etc.).

Bioresorbable CaPs slowly degrade in physiological condition, both by physical and cell-mediated actions, and allow the new bone to grow [11]. Ideally, all of the CaPs are somewhat soluble in physiological condition, where solubility increases with decreasing Ca/P ratio. Moreover, solubility of a certain CaP can also be changed by addition of cations in the structure as dopants. For example, addition of Sr^{2+} and Mg^{2+} ions can lead to an increase in solubility of HA, whereas addition of Mg^{2+} in TCP decreases the solubility of TCP. Solubility can also be increased by decreasing crystallinity, grain size, and density. Given these choices to control solubility, a bioresorbable CaP can be tailormade to meet its application requirements.

Considering a balance between bioactivity and resorbability, TCP became a very popular bioresorbable bone replacement material. TCP has two commonly occurring polymorphs, α and β, where solubility of α-TCP (high-temperature phase) is higher than that of the β-polymorph (low-temperature phase). Phase transition generally occurs somewhere between 1120°C and 1300°C; however, stable β-TCP can be obtained by sintering at 1200°C with the addition of dopants. Several dopants have been tried to enhance the sinterability of β-TCP as shown in Table 6.7 [9]. Similar to HA, bioactivity and resorbability of TCP are beyond question as shown in recent and past literature [12].

Table 6.6 Different synthesis routes of HA powder [10]

Processing technique	Precursor	Powder property
Solid-state reactions	Calcium and phosphate containing compounds. Sintering ~1250°C	
Chemical precipitation	Slow mixing of $Ca(OH)_2 + H_3PO_4/(CH_3COO)_2Ca + KH_2PO_4/Ca(NO_3)_2 + (NH_4)_2HPO_4$ solutions using vigorous stirring, followed by aging	HA nanoparticles of 50–100 nm length HA nanorods of 50 nm diameter HA nanospheres of 200 nm size
Hydrothermal reactions	Hydrothermal treatment of an aqueous mixture of pH 4.5 comprising $Ca(NO_3)_2$, NaH_2PO_4, HNO_3, and urea at 160°C for about 3 h	HA whiskers of 10 μm width and 150 μm length
Sol-gel reactions	Aging an ethanol solution of pH 10 comprising $Ca(NO_3)_2$, $(NH_4)_2HPO_4$, NH_4OH, and PEG at 85°C for 4 h, followed by drying the resultant gel overnight at 40°C and subsequently calcination at 400°C for 2 h and then at 750 and 1100°C for 4 h	Sintered HA nanocrystals of 50–70 nm size
Citrate–nitrate method	Mixing $Ca(NO_3)_2$ and $(NH_4)_2HPO_4$ solutions with glycine (fuel), followed by evaporating the water at 100°C, burning and then calcination of the dried gel	HA nanocrystals
Emulsion method		
Sonochemical method	Ultrasonic irradiation (28–34 kHz, 100 W) of a pseudo-body solution containing NaCl, KCl, Na_2HPO_4, KH_2PO_4, $CaCl_2$, and $MgCl_2$ at 24°C, 37°C, and 55°C for 6–40 min	Spherical HA nanoparticles of 18 nm size with a specific surface area up to 107 m^2/g
From natural resources	Thermal treatment of a deproteinized bovine bone at 800°C for 3 h, then crushing and ball milling for 24 h, followed by vibro-milling using ethanol as a milling media for various milling times (1–8 h)	Needle-like HA nanopowder of ~100 nm size

Table 6.7 Effects of dopants on the properties of TCP [9]

Composition	Relative sintered density (%)	Average grain size (μm)
TCP	73.2	4.59 ± 0.4
TCP−1% SiO_2	75.6	3.85 ± 0.3
TCP−1% MgO	74.2	6.40 ± 0.5
TCP−0.25% ZnO	69.5	4.07 ± 0.4
TCP−1% SiO_2−0.25% ZnO	80.35	4.22 ± 0.4
TCP−1% SiO_2−1% MgO	81.7	4.99 ± 0.3
TCP−0.25% ZnO−1% MgO	81.1	4.30 ± 0.4
TCP−1% SiO_2−1% MgO−0.25% ZnO	83.1	3.89 ± 0.3
TCP−5 wt% SiO_2	76.4	5.43 ± 0.5

6.3.1 Bioceramics and bone remodeling

Bone remodeling is a dynamic and coordinated biochemical process of osteoclastic resorption and osteoblastic synthesis of new bone. The equilibrium of this bone remodeling can become unsettled by either increased osteoclastic activity (loss of bone density) or dysfunction of osteoblasts (increase in bone density), or both. Therefore, bone replacement materials should be able to support both osteoblast and osteoclast functions for bone remodeling. Osteoclasts, the bone-resorbing cells, are responsible for bone mineral degradation. Overactive osteoclasts result in rapid bone resorption, which is widely known as osteoporosis. In osteoporosis, the bone porosity increases at such a level that bone cannot carry the load according to its specific site and breaks from small accidents or injuries. Patients with osteoporotic bone are treated with drugs that prevent the osteoclasts from resorbing the bone cells by suppressing the recruitment and activity of osteoclasts. As a result, the dynamics of bone remodeling are disturbed and the bone disease is called osteoporosis (increase in bone mineral density), which increases the chance of bone fracture.

Bone replacement materials play important roles in determining the resorption activity of osteoclast cells, and the overall performance of bioactive and bioresorbable materials. As shown in Fig. 6.2, the attached osteoclast cells create a closed/isolated environment under it using integrins and other adhesive proteins. The pH in this closed environment is regulated by secretion of HCl, and can often go as low as 4.0. All of the CaPs used for bone replacement have considerable solubility at this pH, where solubility follows the same trend as shown in Table 6.5. The usual factors that control the solubility of CaPs, such as, crystallinity and grain size have a more profound effect at this pH condition. Osteoclastic degradation is one of the primary reasons for complete degradation of CaP materials. Therefore, to design and utilize the full potential of biodegradable CaPs it is essential to understand and regulate osteoclast formation and its resorption kinetics along with the chemical dissolution of

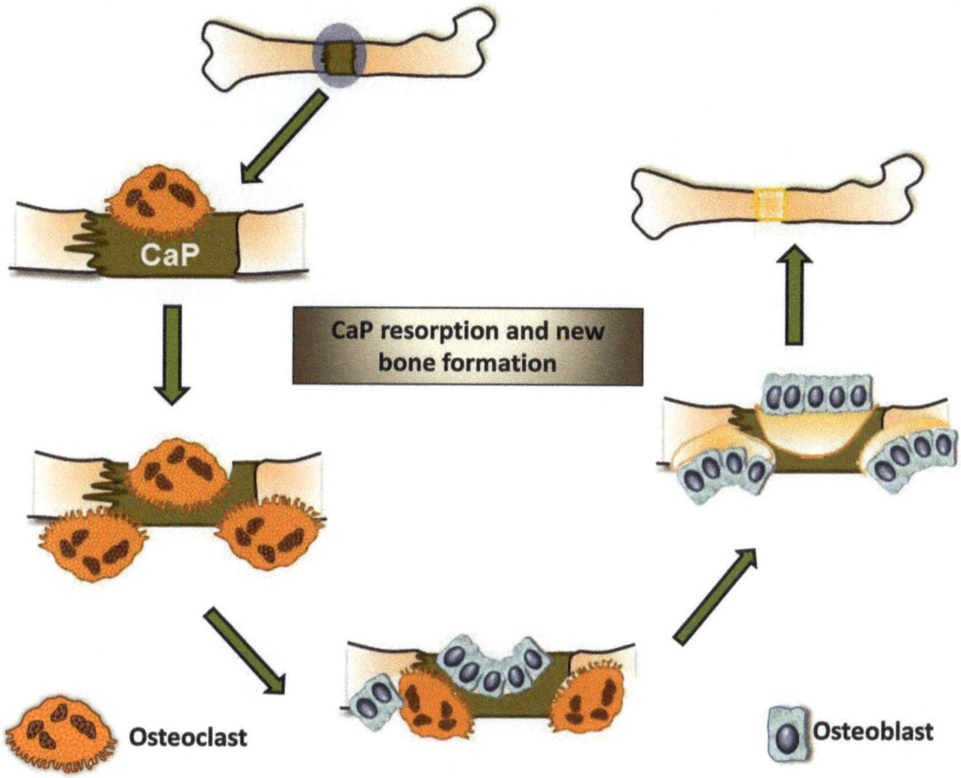

Figure 6.2 Schematics of osteoclastic resorption of bone.

the material. These new alternative approaches can modulate the osteoclast activity for a period of time to regain the bone mineral density, however resuming the bone remodeling at a later stage. Certain dopants are known to regulate osteoclastic activity on CaPs. Incorporation of Co^{2+} in the CaP increases osteoclast formation by 75% with a 2.3- to 2.7-fold increase in mineral resorption area, whereas addition of Mg^{2+} reduces osteoclast formation [13,14].

6.3.2 Role of trace elements on bioactivity of bioceramics

Inorganic compounds can effectively influence bone development or regeneration to influence the biological properties of these materials [15]. Among various dopants, strontium (Sr^{2+}) and silver (Ag^{1+}) gained significant interest as it shifts the bone remodeling equilibrium toward osteogenesis and infection control [16,17]. Five percent Sr-substituted biphasic CaP was shown to increase the expression of Type I collagen and mRNA with a reduction in matrix metalloproteinases (MMP-1 and MMP-2) production [16]. Sr—Hardystonite has been shown to enhance expression of alkaline phosphatase, Runx-2, osteopontin, osteocalcin (OC), and bone sialoprotein [18]. Nano Sr—HA has been shown to increase ALP activity and mineralization compared to nano-HA [19]. Overall it is predicted that the increased expression of these specific proteins not only increases the osteoconductive properties of Sr-doped CaPs, but also signifies osteoinductivity (Table 6.7).

Addition of zinc (Zn^{2+}) in CaP ceramics has been shown to significantly increase new bone formation in vivo when compared to the pure composition [20]. New bone formation in rabbit at 4 weeks was significantly promoted with 0.03 wt% Zn-doped α-TCP cement [20]. Recently, it has been shown that zinc suppresses significant repression of basal NF-κB activity in preosteoclast cells in vitro and also showed significant reduction in tumor necrosis factor alpha and stimulation of osteoblast mineralization [21]. Presence of Zn^{2+} in the culture media was also found to increase angiogenic growth factor, vascular endothelial growth factor (VEGF), secretion in osteoblast-like MC3T3-E1 cells [22].

Recently it has been shown that 0.6 at% Mg-doped octacalcium phosphate significantly promoted the synthesis of procollagen-Type I, transforming growth factor beta 1 (TGF-β1), ALP, and OC compared to pure octacalcium phosphate [23]. It has been shown that magnesium hydroxide temporarily (up to 4 weeks) reduced osteoclast formation in the surrounding area of a magnesium hydroxide implant [24]. The presence of Mg^{2+} can also locally restrict osteoclast proliferation and chemotaxis, which increases bone growth.

Silicon (Si) was also shown to have a significant effect on increased osteoblast proliferation, differentiation, and bone mineral density. α-TCP cement doped with 1% Si has been shown to have a 20% increase in bone contact area compared to undoped cement 3 weeks after surgery [25]. A composite scaffold of siloxane-doped poly(lactic acid) and vaterite composite coated with HA results in a 3—4-fold increase in osteoblast cells and a 1.5 times increase in ALP activity [26]. It has also been reported that the presence of Si also led to differentiation of human mesenchymal stem cells (MSCs) and a moderate increase in ALP activity after 14 and 21 days.

Recently it has been shown that silicon (Si) can be an effective element in inducing angiogenesis as well as improving the osteoinductivity of HA [27]. It has been shown that silicate substituted CaP results in a higher amount of bone formation (26 ± 7.8%) compared to stoichiometric CaP (2.2 ± 2.0%) in female sheep at 12 weeks [28]. Using micro-computed tomography (μCT) and nano-CT, Alt et al. have shown that a xerogel composed of 70 wt% sol-gel silica and 30 wt% collagen can induce 3.1 ± 1.2% volume vessel formation within the fracture zone of a rat femur in 6 weeks [29]. A higher endothelial specific cytokine release was noticed in biphasic CaP (60% HA and 40% β-TCP)—silica composite [30].

6.4 CERAMIC SCAFFOLDS

CaPs, being the major constituents of bone, have long been explored as scaffold material for bone tissue engineering. The structural and functional complexities of bone make it a real challenge to design and fabricate an ideal bone scaffold. The variation in mechanical properties from cortical to cancellous bone along with geometry complexity, make it difficult to design an ideal bone scaffold [31]. For successful bone tissue engineering, some essential factors are interconnected macro- (pore size $>100\ \mu m$) and microporosity (pore size $< 20\ \mu m$) and good mechanical strength with tailored degradation kinetics [11,32].

6.4.1 Ceramic scaffold fabrication techniques

Over the years, many different technologies have been developed to fabricate complex ceramic scaffolds. Some of the technologies along with their advantages and disadvantages are summarized in Table 6.8.

Solid freeform fabrication (SFF) is considered to be the most promising technology to fabricate ceramic scaffold with controlled properties (Table 6.9). SFF is also widely known as 3D printing or additive manufacturing, as the process is conceptually the same as a desktop computer printer [47–49]. During its early inception at MIT (Cambridge, MA, USA), Sachs et al. used a large ink-jet printer head to fabricate metallic and ceramic scaffolds from loose powder. Schematic of 3D printing is shown in Fig. 6.3A and B. The processes essentially fabricate/print 3D parts in a layer-by-layer approach based on a computer-aided design (CAD) file. A typical 3D printing system consists of a deposition bed, a feed bed, a binder holder and feeder, a powder spreader, a print head, and a drying unit. Initially the print head sprays the binder on the powder bed according to the specific instructions in the tool path created according to the computer model. The loose ceramic powder in the powder bed binds to the sprayed binder. Simultaneously, the deposition bed is lowered and the feeder bed is raised. A roller then evenly spreads the powder from feeder bed over the binder, after which the deposited layer goes to the dryer where the binder forces the ceramic particles to form a coherent 2D layer. The dryer is an important unit in the 3D printer as it allows the binder to dry out and prevent spreading between layers. The layer-by-layer printing process, when repeated in vertical direction, forms the 3D ceramic scaffold. The green ceramic scaffold is then heated to nearly 600–650°C to burn-out the binder. Finally, 3D printed parts are sintered at high temperature for densification (Fig. 6.3D).

Some of the critical aspects of 3D printing are essential to consider for preparing ceramic scaffold for bone-tissue engineering [31].

Table 6.8 Scaffold preparation techniques

	Characteristic properties	Advantages	Disadvantages
Solid freeform fabrication			
3D printing	In this process, a scaffold is printed directly from ceramic powder using a 3D printer. Process details are given below	Ability to form complex geometry with excellent dimensional accuracy, control over pore size, highly interconnected porosity, high compressive strength in its class	Expensive set up and running costs. Postprocessing complexity
Porogen-based techniques			
Thermally induced phase separation	Ultrafine HA powder is mixed with dioxane/water mixture to form a stable suspension. Often, polymer is added in the slurry. The mixture is then heated to 15–20°C above the measured cloud point temperature followed by quenching at predefined water bath temperature. After quenching, the sample is dipped in liquid nitrogen and freeze–dried to achieve the porous scaffold. The scaffold is sintered at higher sintering temperature to impart strength	Anisotropic pore structure with tubular morphology. Can have extremely high porosity (~95%)	Complex and expensive processing, poor mechanical properties
Solvent casting/particle leaching	Water-soluble element, such as NaCl, is mixed with ceramic powder to organic solvent or polymer solution to form a thick paste. The paste is then poured in a predefined mold and dried. The NaCl is then leached out from the scaffold by keeping them in water for a specific period of time. Eventually the compact is sintered at higher sintering temperature to impart strength. The initial particle size of NaCl determines the pore size of the final scaffold	Simple process, inexpensive, control over pore size	Weak in mechanical properties, possibility of residual porogen that can affect sintering and final scaffold performance

Polymer bead	In this process, polymer beads of specific size (porosifier) is mixed with HA/β-TCP powder and compacted. The compacts are heat-treated at nearly 550°C to burn off the polymer, leaving behind the porosity in the compact with the same size as the polymer beads. Eventually the compact is sintered at higher sintering temperature	Simple process, inexpensive	Weak in mechanical properties, poor control over distribution, unable to form complex geometry
Physical processes			
Freeze casting	In this process, ceramic slurries are prepared with appropriate dispersant and binder concentrations in aqueous medium. Once a stable slurry is prepared, unidirectional freezing technique is used to form a 3D solid component. The aqueous component is removed by freeze-drying technique to retain the shape and integrity of the scaffold. Once dried, the scaffold is sintered at higher sintering temperature to impart strength	High mechanical strength	Complex process, special and costly instrumentation. Poor control over pore geometry and distribution
Gas foaming	In this process, an in situ gas-forming agent is mixed with stable HA/β-TCP/Al_2O_3 slurry and cast to a predefined geometry. While setting, chemical reactions happen between the constituents and generally form CO_2 gas. The gas while escaping from the system leaves behind interconnected porosity.The CO_2 gas can also be formed by adding wood dust, naphthalene, in the slurry	Inexpensive process, good technique for preparing large samples	Complex process, weak in mechanical properties. Limited dimensional accuracy, poor control over pore size and its distribution
Sacrificial mold	In this process, polymer foam is coated with HA/β-TCP slurry. A suitable heat treatment is used to remove the polymer and sinter the scaffold	Simple process, inexpensive, good control over pore connectivity	Weak in compressive strength

Table 6.9 Physical and mechanical properties of ceramic scaffolds

Scaffold composition	Porosity (%)	Pore size (μm)	Compressive strength (MPa)	References
80 ± 3% HA + 20 ± 3% β-TCP	70	400	Not available	[33]
HA	41	250–350 and 2–8	34.4 ± 2.2	[34]
β-TCP	50	400	10.95 ± 1.28	[35]
β-TCP + 0.5% SiO_2 + 0.25% ZnO	46.44	343.74 ± 8.26	10.21 ± 0.11	[21]
β-TCP + 1.0%MgO + 1.0% SrO	42	3616 ± 9.1	9.38 ± 1.86	[36]
β-TCP + 1.0% ZnO + 0.5 wt% SiO_2	32.16	343 ± 8.3	11	[21]
β-TCP + 1.0%SrO + 0.5% SiO_2	42		22.40 ± 62.70	[37]
33% HA + 67% Si-β-TCP + BMSC	60			[38]
80 ± 5% HA + 20 ± 5% β-TCP + BMSC	70 ± 5	1–1000		[39]
Na_2O-K_2O-MgO-CaO-B_2O_3-P_2O_5–SiO_2	70	300–400		[40]
Bioactive glass (Ca/p/Si = 15/5/80 molar ratio)	0.30 cm^3/g	300–500 and 4–5 nm		[41]
6Na_2O, 8K_2O, 8MgO, 22CaO, 54B_2O_3, and 2P_2O_5	20	5–10		[42]
PGA: β-TCP = 1:3	88.4 ± 0.7	483.3 ± 113.6		[43]
HA: PU = 1:5	90 ± 2	200 ± 16		[44]
(40% HA + 60% β-TCP) coated with HA/PCL	90.8	550	2.1	[45]
TCP scaffold coated with 5% PCL	70	300–800	2.41	[46]

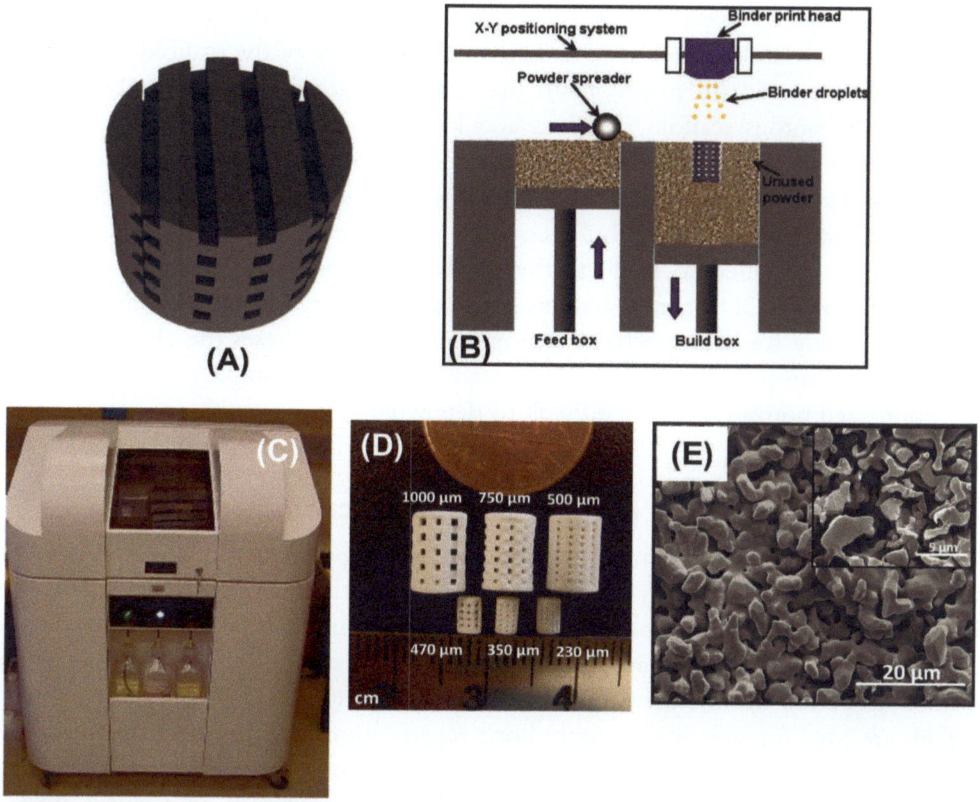

Figure 6.3 (A) CAD image of a porous scaffold. Square channels are oriented at 0/90 degrees for succeeding layers [21]. (B) Schematic drawing of the SFF 3D printing process. (C) The ExOne (Ex One Company, Irwin, PA) 3D printer. (D) Digital photograph showing 3D printed TCP scaffolds after sintering [35]. (E) Surface morphology of 3D printed TCP scaffolds after microwave sintering at 1250°C showing a porous scaffold strand. Inset scanning electron micrograph images show the presence of microporosity in the scaffold [35].

- Ceramic powder properties: The initial properties of ceramic powders play a significant role in fabricability and overall performance of 3D printed scaffolds [50]. Certain powder properties, such as particle size and shape, and its distribution play an important role in powder bed packing and sinterability of the 3D printed scaffold.
- Binder properties: Binder density and viscosity play an important role in determining the resolution of the 3D printed scaffolds. It also determines the green strength of the scaffold.
- Postprocessing complexities: The possibilities of making a 3D printed ceramic scaffold are limitless. If you can design it on a computer using suitable software, given an appropriate powder and binder combination, you can theoretically print

a 3D scaffold. However, certain postprocessing complexities pose major challenges for porous scaffolds and limit the design and usefulness of the scaffold. After a scaffold is fabricated (in green state), the loose powder is required to be removed from the porous scaffold which is also known as depowdering. If the designed porosities are very small, then it imposes a real challenge in the depowdering process as the ceramic powders have low flowability combined with the problem of agglomeration. Certain techniques, such as focused air blowing and ultrasonic vibrations, are used to facilitate the depowdering process. However, one has to remember that 3D printed ceramic scaffolds have very low green density and are subsequently weak in mechanical properties, which increases the chance of cracking the green part. Similarly, a 3D printed scaffold with complex network of interconnected porosities is very difficult to depowderize.

6.4.2 In vitro and in vivo properties of bone scaffolds

Being the major mineral content of bone, CaPs, especially HA, β-TCP, or their mixture, have been extensively studied as scaffold material for bone tissue engineering [51,52]. Depending on the application need, the composition of scaffold can be altered. For example, if the replacement scaffold is required to support the bone regeneration for a longer period of time then HA scaffolds are preferred. On the other hand, β-TCP scaffolds are used for sites with a faster bone regeneration rate. Irrespective of the scaffold material, bone tissue engineering scaffolds are proven to support active bone regeneration. Conventionally sintered β-TCP scaffold with 1 wt% of SrO and 1 wt% of MgO showed initial osteoid formation due to the presence of Sr and Mg elements as early as 4 weeks in a rat femur model (Fig. 6.4A). As time progressed, bone remodeling was found in both doped and undoped scaffolds with prominent osteon and haversian canal formation (Fig. 6.4B) [12]. In a similar study, naphthalene porogen-based β-TCP scaffold was prepared with SrO and SiO_2 doping. The doped scaffolds showed a significant increase in osteoid formation at 20 weeks compared to pure β-TCP scaffold [37]. More OC and haversian canal formation was found for SrO- and SiO_2-doped scaffolds, indicating faster bone regeneration and healing (Fig. 6.4D and E). A microwave sintered pure β-TCP scaffold with >60% porosity actively supported new bone formation within the pores when implanted in rat femur, as shown in Fig. 6.4F [35]. In one of the studies, both macroporosity (250–350 μm) and microporosity (2–8 μm) were designed in HA scaffold. When implanted in rabbit femur, the scaffold resulted in lamellar and woven bone formation, which was not seen in HA scaffolds without microporosity [34]. ABCP scaffold (80 ± 3% HA and 20 ± 3% β-TCP) with 70% interconnected porosity (68% pores are 400 μm, and ~3% are 0.7 μm in size), prepared by polymer replica method, successfully supported new bone formation in immune-deficient male mice [33].

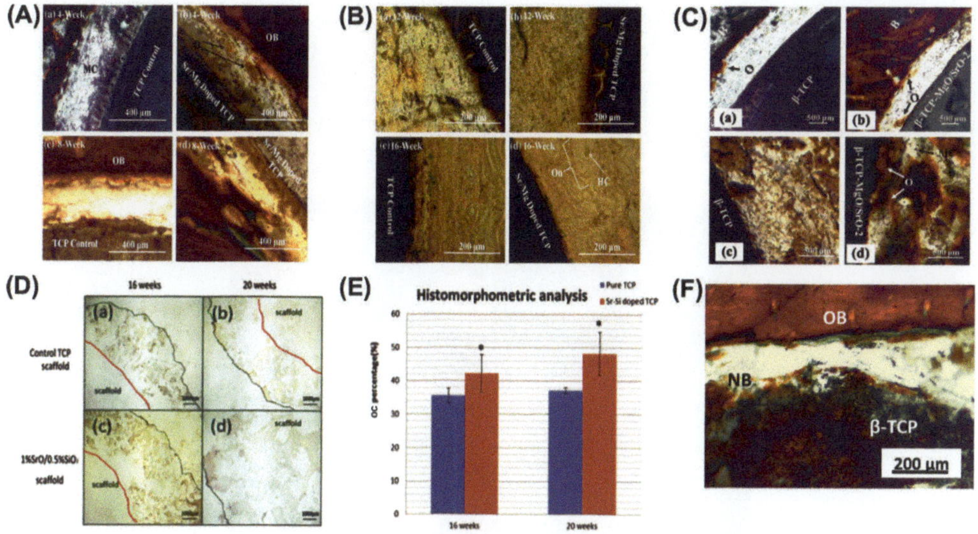

Figure 6.4 Photomicrographs showing the development of new bone formation and bone remodeling. (A and B) β-TCP implants (a and c), and β-TCP-MgO/SrO implants (b and d) at (A) 4 and 8 weeks and (B) 12 and 16 weeks [12], (C) β-TCP (a, low; c, high magnification) and β-TCP—MgO/SrO-2 (b, low; d, high magnification) implants at 4 weeks [53]. (D) Photomicrograph of 3DP pure TCP (a and c), and Sr-Mg-doped TCP scaffolds (b and d) showing osteon and haversian canal formation after 8 and 12 weeks [37]. (E) Histomorphometric analysis of haversian canal area (haversian canal area/total area, %) after 12 weeks [37]. (F) Photomicrograph of the 3D printed TCP scaffolds of 350 μm pore size showing development of new bone formation after 2 weeks implantation in rat femur [35].

Enhancement of biological performance of β-TCP scaffold in terms of better cell attachment, osteogenic differentiation, and osteoid formation leading to bone maturity has been achieved through addition of cationic dopants [12,21,36,37,53]. Addition of 0.5% SiO_2 and 0.25% ZnO in β-TCP scaffold resulted in a significant increase in compressive strength and up to 92% increase in cell viability when cultured with osteoblast cells [21]. The presence of micropores within the macroporous struts worked as anchor points for the cells and helped in rapid proliferation. Zn and Si addition in β-TCP increases type 1 collagen (COL1) gene expression and extracellular signal regulated kinases secretion. Both of these factors positively regulate osteoblast proliferation, differentiation, and morphogenesis along with angiogenesis, a key step in tissue bone tissue regeneration [54]. A 3D printed β-TCP scaffold, when doped with Sr and Mg ions, facilitated osteoid formation not only at the macropores but also within the micropores, indicating the true benefit of a 3D printed scaffold (Fig. 6.5A) [36]. No such behavior was observed in pure β-TCP scaffold or β-TCP scaffolds without micropores. The presence of dopants also increased the formation of osteon and haversian canal together, which is known as the "haversian system" (Fig. 6.5B and C). The results supported some key hypotheses behind the use of 3D printed bone ceramic scaffold such as (1) the presence of micropores in the scaffold strut

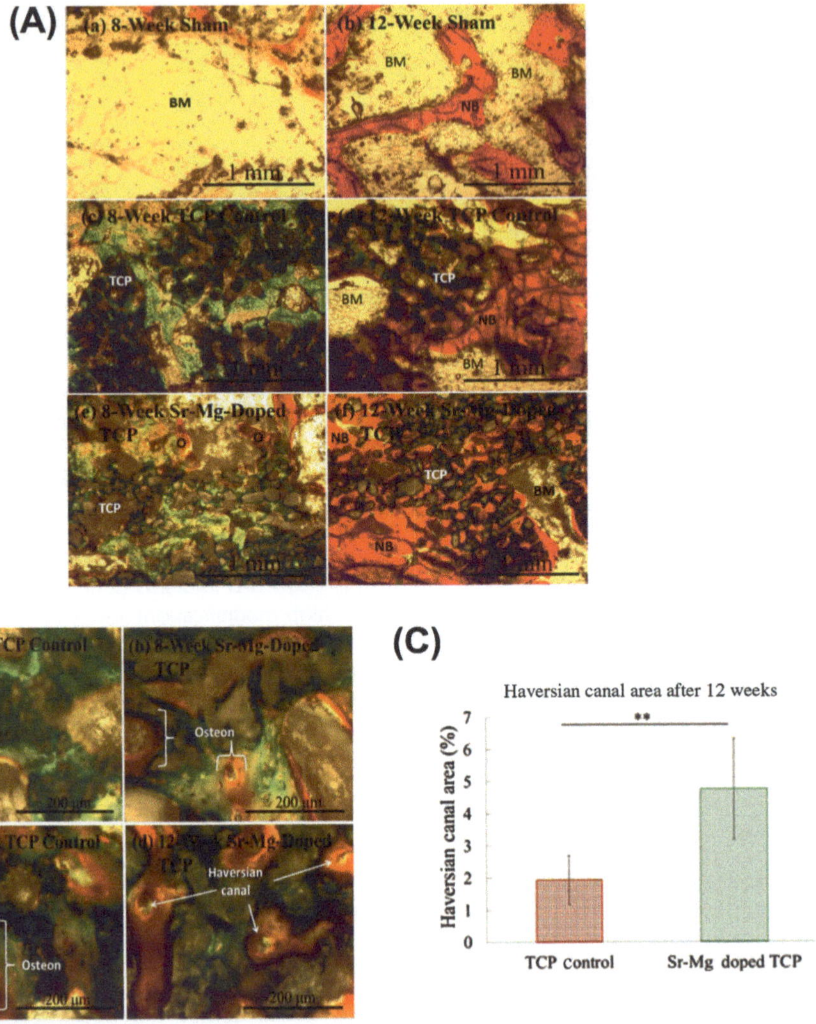

Figure 6.5 Photomicrographs of interconnected macro- and intrinsic micropores of the 3DP scaffolds after 8 and 12 weeks showing (A) mesenchymal cell and collagen infiltration during development of new bone formation in sham control (a and b), 3DP pure TCP (c and d), and Sr-Mg doped TCP scaffolds (e and f) and (B) osteon and haversian canal formation as part of the bone remodeling process in 3DP pure TCP (a and c), and Sr-Mg-doped TCP scaffolds (b and d). (C) Histomorphometric analysis of haversian canal area (haversian canal area/total area, %) after 12 weeks [36].

increases the overall exposed surface area to body fluid and thereby increases the dissolution rate of the scaffold, (2) rapid dissolution of scaffold releases the osteogenic factors (metal ion dopants) at a faster rate, which enhances osteoid formation, and (3) higher dissolution rate increases the Ca^{2+} in the vicinity of the implant site and increases bone mineralization with an overall effect of increased bone regeneration.

6.4.3 In vivo and in vitro performance of CaP–polymer composite scaffold

The concept of combining CaP and polymer to form an interconnected porous scaffold has been developed, where superior bioactivity and mechanical property of CaP can be combined with biodegradable polymer. These composite scaffolds have the potential to meet the stringent mechanical and physiological requirements of the host bone tissue. Two primary approaches have been widely used to prepare CaP–polymer porous scaffold: (1) mixing ceramic particles with molten polymer followed by scaffold preparation and (2) polymer infiltration in preformed porous ceramic scaffold.

Because of their excellent biocompatibility and biodegradability, polymers are an interesting choice for bioresorbable scaffolds. Flexibility in processing and ability to tailor the chemistry and mechanical properties of these materials are added advantages. Synthetic polyesters, such as poly(lactic acid) (PLA), poly(glycolic acid) (PGA), their copolymer poly(lactide-co-glycolide) (PLGA), and poly(ε-caprolactone) (PCL), have been clinically tried for various applications. These synthetic polymers can be processed relatively easily to control molecular weights, functional groups, configurations, and conformations, which give flexibility in manipulating the degradation rates. A high-molecular weight PCL can take up to 36 months to completely degrade in vivo. The degradation products of these polymers are monomers which are readily removed by the natural physiological pathway. Although PLA and PGA have been utilized to make 3D scaffolds, their bulk erosion often leads to a sudden decrease in mechanical properties and premature failure. In addition, degradation can also lead to an acute inflammatory response, a localized decrease in pH, and possible loss in bioactivity. In comparison, PCL, cleared by the US Food and Drug Administration (FDA) for craniofacial applications, has better mechanical stability in vivo and in vitro. Other polymers, such as polypropylene fumarate (PPF), also have a very high compressive strength, which is comparable to cortical bone and its degradation time can be controlled over a wide range. To address some of the challenges of PLA and PGA polymeric scaffolds, CaP reinforcement has been used. Incorporation of CaP in polymer scaffold is intended to improve the bioactivity of synthetic polymers and alter the degradation kinetics to better suit it with the bone tissue. In almost all studies, an improvement in osteoconductive properties of the HA and β-TCP incorporated polymeric scaffold has been reported. Incorporation of HA in PPF scaffold significantly increased the serum protein adsorption followed by enhanced cellular activity. Expression of osteogenic signals such as bone morphogenetic protein 2 (BMP-2), fibroblast growth factor 2, and TGF-β1 was also noticed for HA–PPF composite scaffold. Although, CaP-reinforced polymer scaffold is expected to improve strength, few literatures have reported actually that. It has generally been noted that addition of HA in polymer matrix does not increase the strength of composite [55]. Only a few studies have reported an increase in strength with HA or β-TCP addition.

In another approach, toughness and compressive strength of porous CaP scaffolds can be significantly increased by polymer infiltration. Being the major constituent of bone, CaPs have been extensively studied as scaffold for bone tissue engineering. Among the CaPs, research has been focused on HA, β-TCP, or biphasic calcium phosphate (BCP) due to their compositional similarity to apatite mineral. Numerous in vitro and in vivo studies have shown excellent biocompatibility as well as new bone formation. However, the real limitations for CaP scaffolds are low compressive and flexural strength, toughness, reliability, and complex manufacturing. Moreover, the relatively slow degradation rate of CaPs and difficulty in matching it with the regeneration rate of the replacing tissues is a challenge. To address these limitations, polymer can be introduced into the prefabricated porous CaP scaffold. A threefold increment in biodegradation of HA and β-TCP scaffolds has been reported due to PGA incorporation [43]. A solvent casting and particulate leaching method was used to prepare a PGA/β-TCP (1:3 weight ratios) porous 3D scaffold with $88.4 \pm 0.7\%$ open porosity with an average pore size of 483.3 ± 113.6 μm. It was found that the scaffold will degrade up to $96.2 \pm 3.3\%$ after 90 days of implantation in Sprague–Dawley male rats [43]. In another study, HA/poly(ester-urethane) (PU) composite scaffolds were prepared using a salt leaching phase inversion process with a total porosity of 90% and a pore size of 200 μm and strut wall thickness of 31 μm. The composite scaffold showed higher adsorbed amounts of bovine serum albumin (BSA), bovine fibrinogen, and fetal calf serum in vitro compared to PU scaffold [44]. Blood vessel growth in the border zones of 49 and 55 cm/cm^{-2} was found for HA/PU and PU scaffolds and between 0.4 and 3 cm/cm^{-2} in the center zones when implanted in mice dorsal skinfold chamber for 14 days. A twofold increase in compressive strength was found when a BCP porous scaffold surface was modified with HA/PCL [45]. A surface modification approach also encouraged differentiation of bone cells, with significant upregulation of alkaline phosphatase (ALP) activity and osteogenic gene expression (Runx2, collagen Type I, OC, and bone sialoprotein).

The compressive strength of these scaffolds was generally found to vary from 0.8 to 342 MPa with the majority <10 MPa. The major contributing factors are chemical composition, processing technique, porosity, and pore size range [56]. Although numerous literatures exist for compressive strength of these scaffolds, their toughness has rarely been characterized. Moreover, there is a universal lack of knowledge about the correlation of porosity and pore size range on the mechanical properties of the composite scaffolds.

6.5 CERAMICS IN DRUG DELIVERY

Localized deliveries of biomolecules, drugs, antibiotics, and growth factors through CaP cements, nanoparticles, and scaffold have drawn much attention for their ability

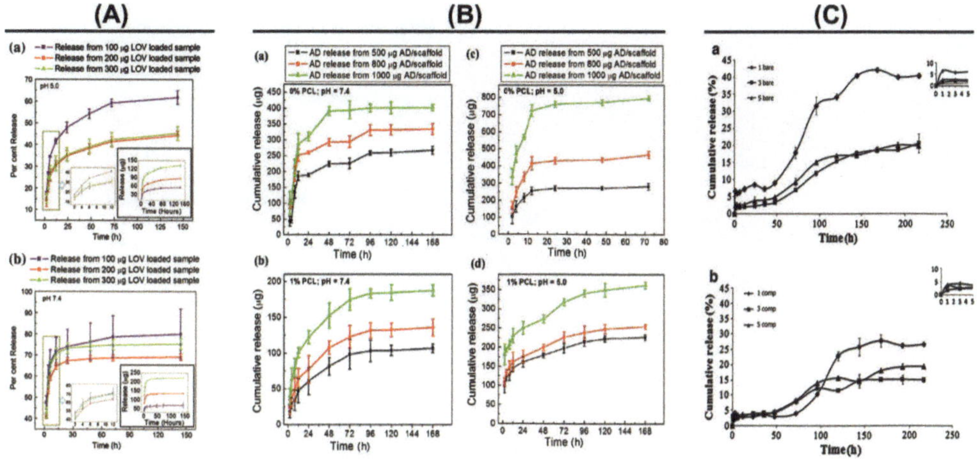

Figure 6.6 (A) Per cent and microgram (inset) release of lovastatin with increased lovastatin and fixed PCL concentration in the coating at pH 5.0 (a) and pH 7.4 (b) [62]. (B) Cumulative AD release at pH 7.4 phosphate buffer (a and b) and at pH 5.0 acetate buffer (c and d) from bare TCP (i.e., no PCL coating: indicated by 0% PCL) scaffolds (a and c), and PCL-coated (1% PCL in acetone [w/v] solution was used for coating) scaffolds (b and d) [60]. (C) BSA release profiles from 100 nm particles, (a) uncoated and (b) PCL-coated (error bars show the standard deviation) [61].

to stimulate bone remodeling on a functionalized surface and reducing healing time [57,58]. HA and β-TCP nanoparticles were studied as carriers for BSA protein [59]. Not only nanoparticles, but ceramic scaffolds can also be used for drug delivery [60]. The study suggests that controlled and sustained BSA release can be achieved by manipulating CaP particle size, crystallinity, dopants, and surface modifying agent. Vahabzadeh et al. have shown that BSA loading in β-TCP particles can be increased by decreasing the particle size and the release profile can be delayed with the addition of PCL on the particle surface (Fig. 6.6C) [61].

Other than BSA, drugs such as lovastatin (LOV) and alendronate can also be delivered using CaP nanoparticles [60,62,63]. Other than particles, TCP/PCL composite scaffolds can also be used for protein and drug delivery. Controlled and sustained release of BSA was achieved due to PCL coating for several weeks. The polymer toughened the ceramic scaffold by coating the struts or filling the surface flaws, such as cracks or both. Steady LOV release was observed from PCL coating compared to a burst release from bare TCP (Fig. 6.6A). Alendronate, an antiosteoporotic drug, was successfully load and delivered in vivo using β-TCP scaffold and modified further by coating with PCL (Fig. 6.6B). All scaffolds with AD showed higher bone formation and reduced tartrate-resistant acid phosphatase (TRAP)-positive cell activity than bare TCP and TCP coated with only PCL. TCP + PCL scaffolds did not show any adverse effects on in vitro osteoblast cells proliferation because of the presence of PCL (Fig. 6.6B). When implanted in vivo, these scaffolds showed new bone formation inside the macro- and micropores

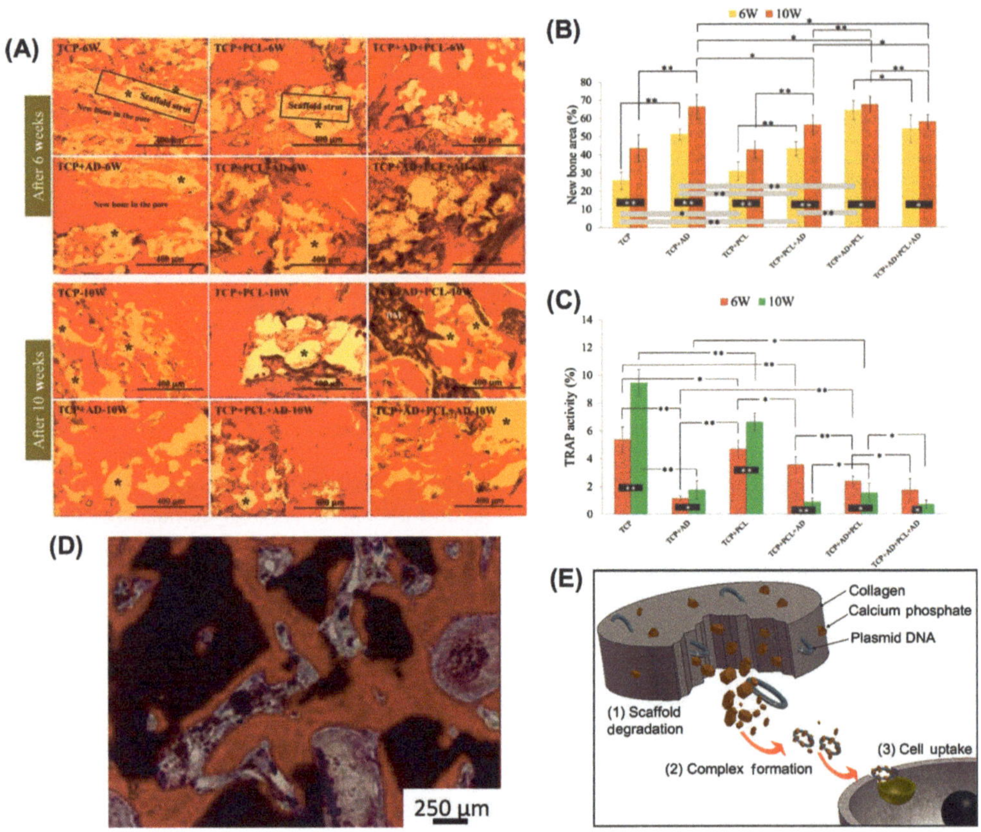

Figure 6.7 (A) Photomicrographs of representative histological sections after H&E staining of decalcified tissue sections showing the development of bone formation after 6 and 10 weeks. BM, bone marrow. Asterisk indicates acellular regions derived from scaffold [60]. (B, C) Histomorphometric analysis comparing (B) total new percent bone formation and (C) percent TRAP activity between the treatment and control groups [60]. (D) Micrographs showing bone formation and scaffold degradation of a TCP scaffold loaded with bone marrow-derived stem cells (BMSCs) [39]. (E) Schematic representation showing degradation behavior and delivery of VEGF from a CaP/collagen scaffold without a nonviral vector. The concept is that the degradation of scaffold will release the plasmid DNA along with CaP. Both CaP and DNA will form a complex that can be taken up by targeted cells and express VEGF and lead to angiogenesis [64].

of the scaffolds [60]. Fig. 6.7A shows the histological images of H&E-stained decalcified tissue sections of TCP scaffold coated with PCL and loaded with AD. The corresponding histomorphometric analysis is shown in Fig. 6.7B. The presence of AD significantly reduced in vivo osteoclast cell formation as indicated by TRAP activity in Fig. 6.7C.

The new generation of CaP biomaterials is designed not only to support bone growth but also to induce new bone deposition on their surfaces, whether in particular or scaffold form. Several growth factors, such as TGF-β, BMP, insulin-like growth factor (IGF), and VEGF, have been researched by various groups. These growth factors, along with other cytokines and hormones, control fracture repair by recruiting and differentiating the osteoprogenitor cells to specific lineages to form the extracellular matrix [31]. One example is BMP which not only stimulates the recruitment, proliferation, and differentiation of osteoprogenitor cells but also controls the activity of osteoclasts at an early stage. When used in vivo, the BMP-2 incorporated HA coatings showed significantly higher bone deposition on their surfaces [65]. Similarly, in nanoHA/collagen/poly (L-lactic acid) scaffolds, when loaded with BMP-2, the bone deposition rate increased compared to pure scaffolds (as shown in Fig. 6.8A and B) [67]. BCP scaffolds are also used to deliver VEGF for enhancement of blood vessel formation and bone regeneration. A dosage of 5 μg/ml VEGF increased the blood vessel density (counts/mm^3) of 83.8 ± 16.5 compared to 53.8 ± 10.9 pure BCP scaffold after 28 days of implantation in mice (Fig. 6.8C). The addition of VEGF not only resulted in enhanced vascularization but also resulted in a threefold increase in bone formed inside the macropores [68]. It is hypothesized that enhanced vascularization provided abundant

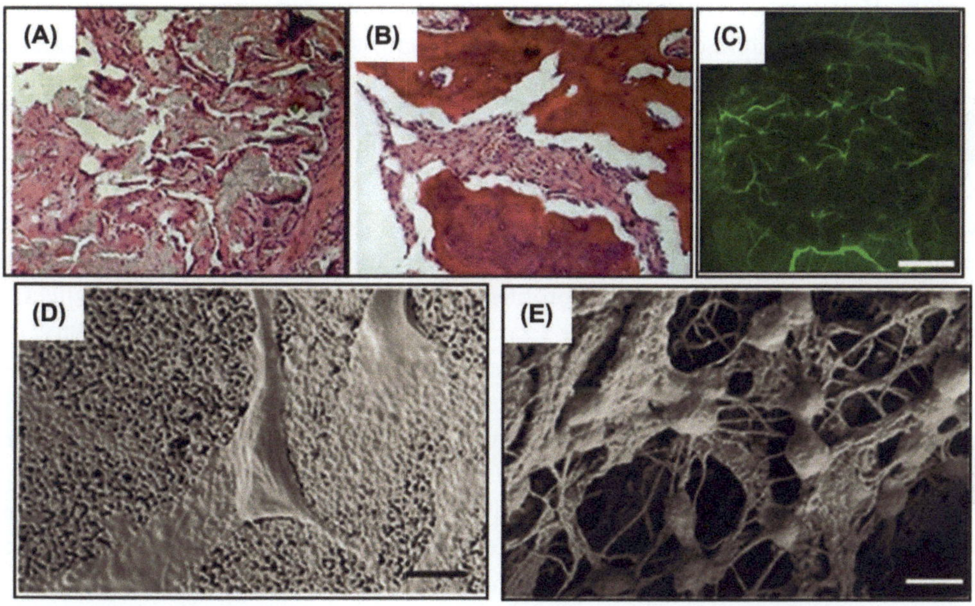

Figure 6.8 (A and B) Photomicrographs of 12 weeks postoperative histological samples of nanoHA/collagen/poly (L-lactic acid) and nanoHA/collagen/poly (L-lactic acid)/BMP-2, respectively. BMP-2 loading results in a larger area of new bone formation (dark red regions) [67]. (C) Visualization of blood vessel formation in effect of VEGF added BCP ceramics implanted into the cranial window for 2 days, using a vertical illumination fluorescence microscope. Plasma marker fluorescein-isothiocyanate (FITC)-labeled dextran was used to study the microcirculation [68]. Cellular interactions with (D) HA and (E) HA–collagen scaffolds indicate the differences between cellular adhesion behaviors [66].

osteoprogenitor cells to the defect site along with direct stimulating effects on osteoblast migration and differentiation, leading to higher bone deposition [68]. A combinational delivery of both BMP-2 and VEGF is also studied to understand any added advantage on overall bone regeneration rate. It was found that a ceramic scaffold coloaded with BMP-2 and VEGF resulted in both enhanced vascularization and new bone formation [69]. The results had encouraged a new research area where combinational and sequential biomolecule delivery is studied for controlled and efficient bone regeneration. Because of the ability of IGF to stimulate, proliferate, and chemotactic migration of different bone regeneration cells, significant interest has developed to deliver IGF through CaP scaffolds [70]. Addition of IGF-2 has the potential for osteogenic differentiation of embryonic stem cell (ESCs), which can potentially differentiate into all types of somatic cells [71]. The CaP scaffolds are also seeded with cells to enhance the acceptance of the scaffold as well as faster bone regeneration and are expected to be as good as autograft scaffold. A 70% porous BCP scaffold (80 wt% HA and 20 wt% β-TCP) and 100% β-TCP scaffold resulted in higher bone formation compared to natural bone grafts. Fig. 6.7D shows abundant bone formation for BMSC-loaded porous BCP scaffold [39]. Bone replacement scaffolds are also loaded with antibiotics to reduced bacterial infections. Commonly used drugs include gentamicin, vancomycin, alendronate, methotrexate, and ibuprofen [57,72]. To modulate the osteoinductive properties of growth and transcription factors, gene delivery through CaP nanoparticles has been explored [73]. In this process, genes encoding growth factor delivery to specific cells are used to express exogenous genes and proteins in the surrounding tissues [74]. A schematic presentation of CaP/polymer degradation, the release of incorporated VEGF and uptake by cell without a nonviral vector and a possible future angiogenesis, is shown in Fig. 6.7E [64].

Appropriate dosage and release profiles are the key to achieve the best effects of these drugs and growth factors. For example, BMP-2 induces osteoinductivity in a dose-dependent manner: differentiation stimulation for direct endochondral ossification and chondrogenesis of MSCs for microgram quantities and nanogram levels recruit stem cells through chemotaxis [75]. Likewise, controlled release of VEGF produces well-functioning blood vessels, whereas uncontrolled release of VEGF can lead to abnormal and nonfunctional blood vessels [76]. Controlling the release of biomolecules from CaP particles or a scaffold is one of the primary concerns in achieving the best out of the biomolecule. Further studies focusing on the adsorption and desorption kinetics of biomolecules can result in optimized drug delivery through CaPs.

6.6 BIOCERAMIC COATINGS

Load-bearing metallic implants suffer from poor osteoinductivity, which often results in aseptic loosening and leads to premature failure of the implant in vivo.

Therefore, to improve the bioactivity of metallic implants, an HA coating is used. The advantages of HA coating on metallic implants include rapid fixation and stronger bonding between the host bone and the implant. Since Furlong and Osborn first began clinical trials using the HA-coated implants in 1985, HA-coated implants have shown excellent results with $<2\%$ failure rate for follow-up study of 10 years [77].

6.6.1 Challenges of HA coatings

Although biocompatibility of HA is well documented, the application of HA-coated implants is not widespread. The long-term benefits of HA coatings are questioned by several researchers. Clinical studies contradict the need for HA-coating implants in hip replacement [78]. However, most clinical studies have shown early stages of bone formation shortly after the implantation and continued fixation for extended years. An analysis by Mäkelä et al. indicated that cementless total hip replacements had a reduced risk of revision compared with cemented hip replacements for aseptic loosening [79]. At younger age (patient age: 55–64 years), the 15-year survival rate was higher for coated groups compared to uncoated implants.

The schematic below (Fig. 6.9) represents possible reasons for questionable long-term performance of HA-coated metallic implants. Sustained bioactivity of HA coatings in the long term will not be evident if the coating disappears after a couple of years. In that case, bare metal will be exposed, leading to issues with it. It is even more evident as most of the clinical trials did not look at the coating condition after the retrieval surgery. Now, the HA coating can either delaminate or degrade (as shown in the schematic) in prolong use. HA, being a ceramic material, has a different thermal expansion coefficient than substrate metal (Ti or 316L stainless steel (SS)). Therefore, during coating preparation, thermal stresses generate at the metal–ceramic interface, making it the weakest section and delamination prone in physiological environment. On the other hand, the HA can just chemically degrade in physiological environment with its modest solubility product (2.35×10^{-59}). The dissolution kinetics of HA will increase even further with the presence of secondary phases such as α/β-TCP and amorphous HA. The only commercial coating technique is plasma spray that employs high temperature for HA-coating preparation. Often, plasma spray will result in a high amount of amorphous HA (owing to its faster cooling) and phase decomposition of HA to α/β-TCP or tetracalcium phosphate (TTCP) (owing to high-temperature treatment), leading to increased dissolution of HA coating in physiological environment. Therefore, newer coating techniques are constantly being developed to make phase pure and strongly adherent HA coating for better and longer in vivo performance (Fig. 6.9).

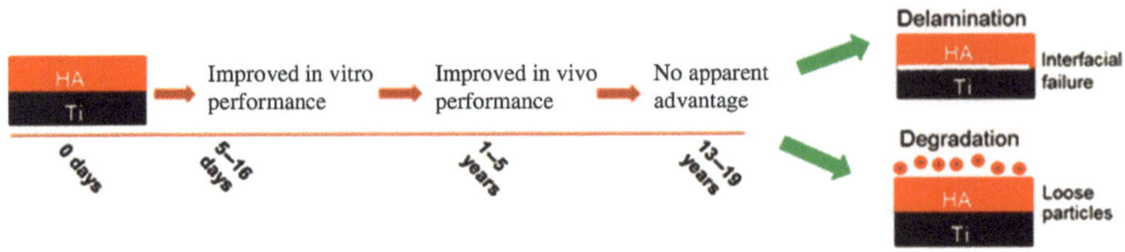

Figure 6.9 Schematic of HA coating failure.

6.6.2 Significance of HA coating in revision surgeries

For various reasons, such as, pain, polyethylene liner wear, dislocation, loosening, infection, and osteolysis, revision of the primary hip replacement may be necessary. Revision surgeries are much more complex and technically much more difficult than primary hip arthroplasty. Moreover, overall performances of revision prostheses have inferior results than primary prostheses. Therefore, much attention has been given to primary arthroplasty for its improved performance. In total hip replacements, the stem is generally cemented, HA-coated, porous-coated, or smooth. Although a variety of implant types and designs exist in the market, the replacement procedure is highly dictated by nation and surgeon. Clinical successes of HA-coated metallic implants are well documented. At an early stage of implantation (up to 5 years), HA coatings showed better performance than uncoated implants in terms of osseous ingrowth, fewer loosening followed by revisions [78]. Although, some long-term clinical follow-up studies (up to 13 years) indicated little to no advantage of HA-coated implants over uncoated or cemented implants, the majority of the studies indicated reliable and promising results for HA-coated metallic implants. Moreover, the performance of HA-coated implants is among the very best of cemented implants, where the implant design and surgical procedures have a significant impact on the performance of cemented implants. However, the most promising results of HA-coated metallic implants were found in revision hip surgeries. It has been claimed that, if needed, a revision is more straightforward for HA-coated implants than cemented implants [80]. The revision hip surgery is primarily done for the femoral component and/or acetabular cup. Femoral revision with extensively HA-coated femoral components showed excellent results in short-term revision [81]. Long-term clinical and radiological performance was excellent for fully HA-coated femoral components. The results are even promising for HA-coated acetabular cup revisions. A survival rate of 90.8% (mean follow-up of 7.6 years) for nonaseptic loosening and 98.1% for aseptic loosening is reported for HA-coated cups for acetabular revision [82]. The performance of acetabular revision with impacted allograft into localized defects and acetabular cavity with an HA-coated cup and supplementary screw showed a $>90\%$ survival rate. It has also been found that when host bone support is reduced to $<50\%$, the acetabular revision is reliable with an HA-coated cup.

Other than total hip arthopalsty (THA), HA coating was found to improve the performance of total knee arthroplasty. HA coating is primarily used in the lower part of the tibia and the upper region of the femoral component. At 12 years follow-up, 96.2% "Knee Score" and 87.1% "Function Score" have been reported [83]. Over time, the HA-coated components formed an intimate contact with bone and filled the interface gaps. A survivorship of 98.6% has been reported at 8 years for HA-coated Duracon (Stryker Corporation) total knee arthroplasties [84].

6.6.3 Coating properties and characterization standards

The applicability of CaP coatings is subjected to certain physical and mechanical properties that have been described by ASTM and ISO standards (ISO 13779-2). Table 6.10 summarizes the characterization suggested by ASTM/ISO for CaP coatings to be used in surgical applications. Some of the important characterizations are explained in detail below.

Table 6.11 provides the maximum allowable trace elements in the CaP (specifically HA) coatings (ASTM F1609-08).

6.6.3.1 Crystallographic Information

HA is the choice of coating materials for CaP-coated metallic implants for its proven bioactivity and long-term stability in physiological environments. However, often, the high temperature associated with coating preparation (primarily plasma spray-coating techniques), leads to the formation of amorphous calcium phosphate (ACP). On the other hand, HA also gets decomposed to α/β-TCP, TTCP, CaO with varying solubility factor. Therefore, it is not only essential to identify the secondary phases present in HA coating, but also to quantify them.

Crystallinity of HA phase in the coatings can be measured according to the following equation:

$$\text{Crystallinity}(\%) = A_c/(A_c + A_a) \times 100$$

where A_c is the integrated intensity of HA peaks in the range of 25 and 37 degrees. The value of A_c is calculated via multiplying the area of the most intense (211) peak of HA by 3.23, which is the ratio of the total intensity of all HA peaks within 25 and 37 degrees in JCPDS #9-432 file for HA to the intensity of the (211) peak. The value of A_a is the integrated intensity of the ACP phase, which can be calculated by the area of the amorphous hump between 25 and 37 degrees [85].

To determine the secondary phases in the crystalline part of plasma-sprayed HA coating, the following method (ASTM F2024-10) is generally used; however, it can be extended to other techniques as well. According to the standard, an external standard technique, also known as the relative intensity ratio method, is used to determine the weight fractions of individual phases. The process is time-consuming and also the mass absorption coefficients of the sample and standard must be known.

Table 6.10 Suggested HA coating properties

Nature of characterization	Suggestions made by ASTM/ISO
Chemical analysis	• Elemental analysis for major and trace elements • Ca/P ratio before and after coating
Crystallographic information	• Determine the relative amount of crystalline HA, α/β-TCP, TTCP, CaO • HA ≥ 50% by mass of which 45% (out of 100% HA) should be crystalline (ISO 13779-3) • α/β-TCP, TTCP, CaO should each be ≤ 5% by mass
Environmental stability	The dissolution characteristics of the coatings should be determined according to ASTM F1926M-14. Dissolution should be checked at pH of 5.5 (with 1M MES buffer) and pH 7.0 (with 1M TRIS buffer). The calcium ion concentration and media pH should be measured as a function of time [85]
Coverage of substrate	• Coating should be checked for uniformity in desired surface coverage of the substrate • Coating surface should be checked microscopically (10 × magnification) for pinholes, cracking, chipping, and unevenness in coating (ASTMF1609)
Thickness	• There is no ideal thickness of a coating; however, coating thicknesses between 50 and 100 μm are preferred. A thicker coating generally compromises the adhesive strength of the coating while a thinner coating is not sufficient for biological bonding • As HA coatings generally have relatively higher soluble phases, a thinner coating poses the challenge of physiological degradation in long-term implant performance
Porosity	The coatings should be microscopically checked for any residual porosity or designed porosity and reported accordingly. Porosity generally enhances the biological bonding of the coating with surrounding tissues; however, it degrades the mechanical properties of the coating. Therefore, porous metallic coatings are generally preferred over porous ceramic coatings
Color	To ensure a uniform and consistent coating for a specific process, geometry and thickness, color of the coating should be macroscopically observed
Surface topography	Surface roughness plays a vital role in the bioactivity of a coated implant. A surface profilometer can be used to accurately measure the surface roughness
Density	Density of both the starting powder and coating have to be determined with a suitable technique
Tensile bond strength	Should be 15 MPa or higher (ISO 13779-4). Lower value is only accepted with proper justification based on application [86,87]

Table 6.11 Maximum allowable trace elements in the CaP (ASTM F1609-08)

Elements	Concentrations (ppm)
Arsenic (As)	3
Cadmium (Cd)	5
Mercury(Hg)	5
Lead (Pb)	30
Total heavy metals (as lead)	50

6.6.3.2 *Environmental stability*

To accomplish long-term stability of a coating, it is important to understand the dissolution behavior of the CaP coatings. The two primary factors that control the dissolution characteristics are (1) material properties such as chemical composition (Ca/P ratio), presence of secondary phases (α/β-TCP, TTCP, CaO, etc.), crystallinity, particle size, surface morphology, and roughness and (2) environmental factors such as media composition and pH [85,88,89]. Poorly crystalline HA coatings have been shown to degrade faster than their crystalline counterpart, whereas the presence of relatively higher soluble secondary phases increases the dissolution rate [85]. The environmental stability is measured by the ASTM 1926M-14 standard. In brief, HA-coated samples should be immersed in sealed tubes containing appropriate proportions (based on surface area) of dissolution media (mentioned in Table 6.11) [85]. The experiment should be continued for 4–6 weeks at temperature of $36.5 \pm 0.5°C$ and subjected to a constant shaking at 150 rpm. A prefixed volume of media should be collected at regular intervals and the same volume of fresh media should be replenished. Coating surface morphology and weight change after dissolution should be monitored along with the Ca^{2+} concentration in the collected media.

6.6.3.3 *Tensile bond strength*

The applicability of CaP coating is primarily dictated by its adhesive bond strength. An uncoated implant is preferred over a weakly bonded coating, as the weak coating may delaminate in the body. The delamination or the wear-debris can lead to osteolysis, limiting the effectiveness of a coated implant. A strongly bonded coating ensures long-term success of the implant and also prevents osteolysis. During testing or practical applications, a CaP coating can fail at the coating substrate interface (adhesive mode of failure), within coating (cohesive mode of failure), or a combination of both. The failed surface morphology should be studied after adhesive testing and reported appropriately [90]. The adhesive bond strength is generally measured according to ASTM C633. The basic principle of this characterization is bonding the coating surface with another uncoated surface using a suitable bonding agent and application of a load normal to the coating surface to measure the failure load [90,91]. The adhesive bond strength can be calculated as: failure load/sample area (*F/A*).

$$S = F/A$$

where,

S = adhesion or cohesion strength,
F = maximum load to failure, and
A = cross-sectional area.

6.6.4 Coating preparation techniques

A variety of surface-coating technologies have been developed to deposit CaP on Ti-based alloys. Most of these techniques are intended to improve short- and long-term performance of implants by encouraging bone ingrowth and providing improved fixation [92]. Furthermore, coatings of these bioceramics on Ti-based alloys also provide the appropriate surface chemistry for tissue compatibility without altering the bulk mechanical properties of the material. The usefulness of a coated implant can only be realized if the coating is physically and mechanically stable in vivo. The physical stability of HA coatings is governed by its phase purity and crystallinity. Along with the physical properties of the coatings, the mechanical properties, such as adhesive bond strength, determine the applicability and in vivo lifetime of a coated implant. Although phase pure and crystalline HA coatings can be prepared with techniques, such as sol-gel coating, dip coating, electrophoretic deposition (EPD), and biomimetic coating, they lack the prerequisite of an HA-coated metallic implant for clinical applications and adequate adhesive bond strength. Among different coating techniques, plasma spraying is most widely used commercially for mass production of implants. However, phase decomposition is a very common problem in conventional plasma-sprayed HA coatings along ACP phase formation and cracking. A comparison of the different coating methods is summarized in Table 6.12.

6.6.4.1 Plasma-sprayed HA coating

Plasma spraying is regarded as the most efficient and economical technique to prepare CaP coatings for load-bearing orthopedic applications due to its simplicity in operation, high deposition rates, low substrate temperature, and economic viability. In plasma spray, the molten or heat-softened CaP bioceramics are sprayed onto a metallic substrate to form the coating. The typical plasma gases are He, Ar, N_2, H_2, and a mixture of these gases. Argon is usually chosen as the base gas as it ionizes easily. The plasma spraying involves a temperature of >10,000°C. The decomposition and phase transformation temperatures of HA are 1670°C and 1300°C, respectively. Therefore, phase transformation and decomposition of HA during plasma-sprayed coating preparation are very common. As the heat-treated HA particles cool down very rapidly during the coating preparation, the coating generally contains varying amounts of

Table 6.12 Different techniques to deposit HA coatings [92]

Technique	Thickness	Advantages	Disadvantages
Thermal spraying	30–200 μm	High deposition rates; low cost	Line-of-sight technique; high temperatures induce decomposition; rapid cooling produces amorphous coatings
Sputter coating	0.5–3 μm	Uniform coating thickness on flat substrates; dense coating	Line-of-sight technique; expensive, time-consuming; produces amorphous coatings
PLD	0.05–5 μm	Coating with crystalline and amorphous; coating dense and porous	Line-of-sight technique
Dynamic mixing method	0.05–1.3 μm	High adhesive strength	Line-of-sight technique; expensive; produces amorphous coatings
Dip coating	0.05–0.5 mm	Inexpensive; coatings applied quickly; can coat complex substrates	Requires high sintering temperatures; thermal expansion mismatch
Sol-gel	<1 μm	Can coat complex shapes; low processing temperatures; relatively cheap as coatings are very thin	Some processes require controlled atmosphere processing; expensive raw materials
EPD	0.1–2.0 mm	Uniform coating thickness; rapid deposition rates; can coat complex substrates	Difficult to produce crack-free coatings; requires high sintering temperatures
Biomimetic coating	<30 μm	Low processing temperatures; can form bone-like apatite; can coat complex shapes; can incorporate bone growth-stimulating factors	Time consuming; requires replenishment and a constant pH of simulated body fluid
HIP	0.2–2.0 mm	Produces dense coatings	Cannot coat complex substrates; high temperature required; elastic property differences; expensive; removal/interaction of encapsulation material

amorphous CaP phases. In vivo studies indicated that coating longevity is primarily dictated by the crystallinity of the HA phase in the coating.

Radio frequency (RF) and direct current (DC) are the two main types of plasma used in biomedical applications. Plasma is generally created by ionizing argon (Ar) gas with the help of an electric or electric/magnetic field. In DC plasma, the gaseous discharge is created between the cathode and the anode and the powder is fed at 90 degrees (perpendicular) to the plasma stream. Because of the feeding system, the precursor powder does not get an even treatment in the plasma and creates turbulence in the plasma. The lighter (finer) particles get carried away from the plasma stream, while heavy (bigger) particles fall close to the powder feeder and may not even enter the plasma stream. The various DC plasmas are (1) without magnetic confinement: discharge tubes, parallel plate, and hollow cathode or (2) with magnetic confinement: magnetron and cold cathode penning ionization gauge discharges. The two most commonly used RF plasmas are capacitively coupled and inductively coupled. In a capacitively coupled system, the electrodes are placed inside the reactor that may cause subsequent reactive chemical species. In comparison, electrodes stay completely outside the reaction chamber in inductively coupled RF plasma, which eliminates the risk of contamination from the electrodes, and is advantageous especially for preparing high-purity biomaterials. Axial feeding of precursor, which reduces turbulence in the plasma, is an important advantage of the RF plasma spray process. When using induction plasmas for feed stock preparation, the material is axially injected with a carrier gas into the center of the discharge. As the particles contact the plasma, they are heated in-flight and are deposited on the substrate.

Excellent in vivo bone tissue integration results are obtained when induction plasma-sprayed HA-coated Ti implants were inserted in rat femur. Significantly, higher bone formation was reported for HA coatings, which was further enhanced by Sr doping in the HA coating as shown in Fig. 6.10 [85]. Presence of dopants or trace elements in coated implants can not only help with osteogenesis and angiogenesis but also with infection control [85,86,87].

6.6.4.2 Laser-assisted coating

Laser-assisted techniques have been successfully used to prepare CaP coatings on metallic implants. Two main approaches of laser-assisted coating have been explored: direct laser melting and pulsed laser deposition (PLD). In direct laser melting, the CaP powders are premixed with an organic binder and then sprayed on the metallic substrate. The laser is then used to melt the substrate and form the coating with metallurgically strong interface. The focused and short energy input from the laser creates a molten metal pool on the substrate surface where HA is added concurrently. $X-Y$ axis movement of the stage solidifies the metal with the entrapped HA particles and creates the HA coating. PLD has been successfully used to prepare strongly adhering HA coatings. PLD creates thin ($<5\ \mu m$) and relatively phase-pure HA coatings.

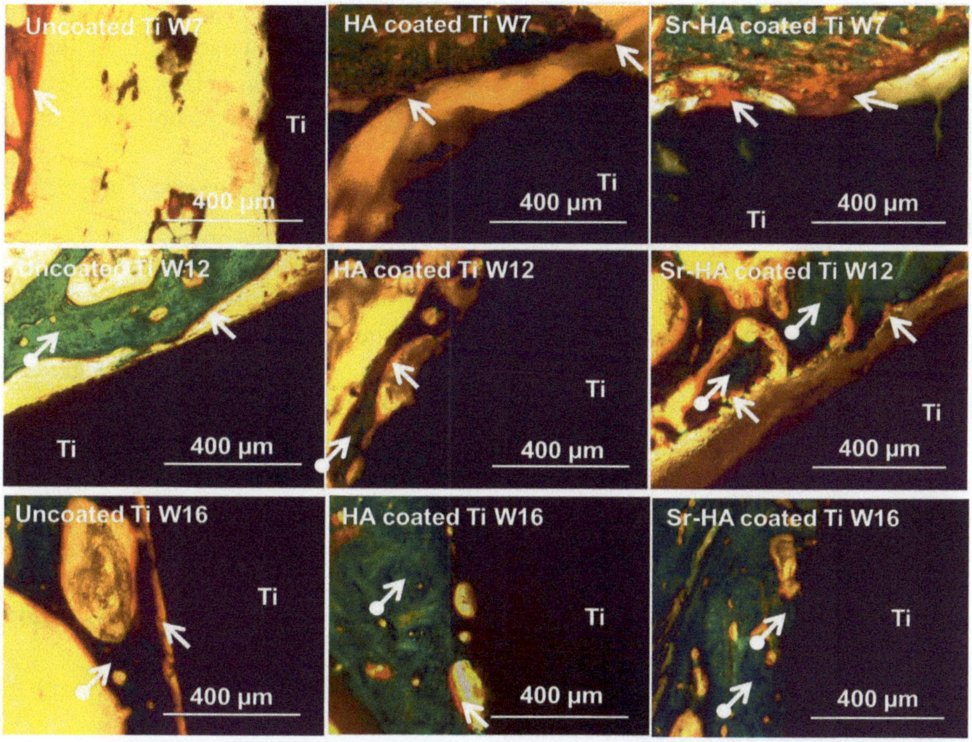

Figure 6.10 Optical photomicrograph of a longitudinal section of uncoated Ti, HA-coated Ti, and Sr-HA coated Ti implants showing the development of new bone formation on the surface of implants after 7, 12, and 16 weeks. Modified Masson–Goldner's trichrome staining of transverse section. Arrows indicate nonmineralized osteoid; circled arrows indicate mineralized bone [85].

6.6.4.3 Electrophoretic deposition

EPD is a solution-based deposition technique to achieve uniform CaP coatings on metallic substrates. In the EPD process, HA powder is suspended in organic media (ethanol/isopropanol) with polymer to create a stable suspension. Once a stable suspension is achieved, deposition is carried out with the application of high potential. The coating thickness can be varied by changing the electrical field strength, time of deposition, and suspension concentration. Some advantages associated with EPD can be listed as follows:[93]

- Non–line-of-sight process and therefore can coat complex shapes;
- Relatively inexpensive and quick process.

6.6.4.4 Sol-gel deposition

The solution sol-gel route is used to prepare CaP coatings with excellent chemical and microstructural homogeneity. In this method CaP coatings are prepared by using an HA sol and dipping the substrate in them for an appropriate time. The coatings are generally very thin (<1 μm). Poor adhesion is a major concern of sol-gel coating techniques. Therefore, to increase the adhesive strength, these coatings are sintered at high temperatures. Depending upon the sintering temperatures, HA can decompose to different CaP phases. Because of the complexities, sol-gel deposition has limited industrial applications.

6.6.4.5 Biomimetic deposition

Biomimetic is a solution-based HA-coating technique. In this process, metallic substrates are immersed in SBF for a specific period of time at 37°C. During immersion, HA crystals nucleate and grow from the supersaturated Ca solution on the substrate, resulting in HA coating. The thickness of this CaP coating is generally low (<30 μm). However, it can be increased substantially by increasing the deposition time. Most of the coatings have an amorphous oramorphous-crystalline structure, with a preferred crystallographic orientation. The biomimetic coating process can coat complex shapes and is also capable of incorporating bone growth-stimulating factors in the coating. Several orthopedic manufacturing industries are exploring the biomimetic deposition technique due to the fact that the coating is prepared at low temperature and therefore biologically active ingredients, such as drugs and growth factors, can be incorporated within the coating itself.

6.6.4.6 Compositionally graded coating

Compositionally graded coating comprises of a bioactive surface which slowly changes the composition to the base metal. The advantage of compositionally graded coating is the increased bond strength and higher environmental stability of the coating. A functionally graded α-TCP/HA coating on Ti-6Al-4V substrates can be prepared by plasma spraying, where HA was used as a bond coat to provide the necessary adhesive strength. The top layer can be designed to be made of highly bioresorbable α-TCP for accelerated bone formation.

6.7 BONE CEMENT

Calcium phosphate cements (CPCs) are a class of degradable ceramics that are primarily made with one or a mixture of CaP powders to an aqueous solution to form a paste. The cement paste hardens in a stipulated period of time directly at the application site. In this regard, CPCs are quite different from the traditional ceramics which are preformed to a specific shape and size. CPCs find wide application in treating cancellous bone defects, vertebral body fracture, craniomaxillofacial surgery, stabilizing hip implants, ligament anchor, reinforcement of osteosynthesis screws and as biosensors, and in drug delivery [94,95]. These cements are also used in reinforcing osteoporotic bone [96]. The wide acceptance of CPCs as bone graft material is due to their

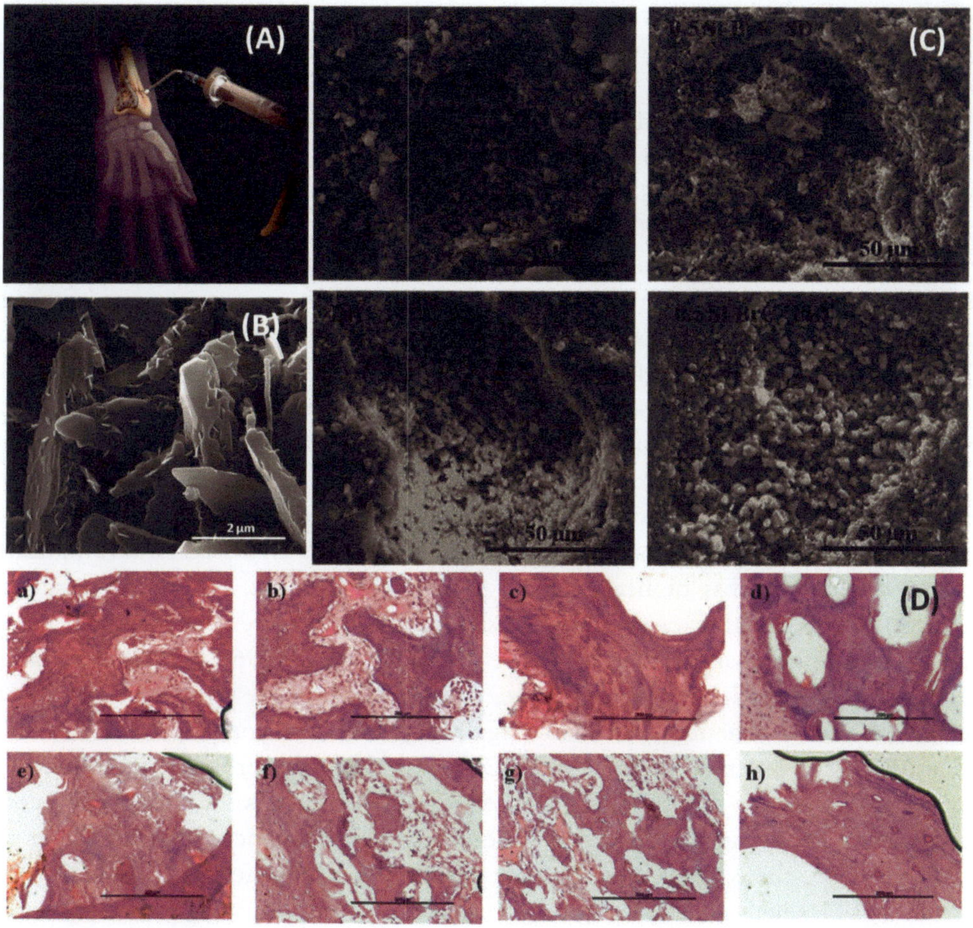

Figure 6.11 (A) Injection of CPC directly at the application site (https://www.arthrex.com). (B) Microstructure of brushite cement showing plate-like structures with anchor points for mechanical interlocking (Mangal Roy's Ph.D. thesis at Washington State University, 2010). (C) Osteoclast cell-mediated surface degradation of brushite cement [97]. (D) Histological images depicting bone formation at 2 and 4 months postimplantation in IGF-1-loaded samples. Subpanel descriptions: (a) BrC 2 months, (b) Si–BrC 2 months, (c) Zn–BrC 2 months, (d) Si/Zn–BrC 2 months, (e) BrC 4 months, (f) Si–BrC 4 months, (g) Zn–BrC 4 months, (h) Si/Zn–BrC 4 months [97].

chemical similarity to bone, injectability (Fig. 6.11A), and self-setting at the defect site, low setting temperature, and easy deformability to complex geometry [98,99]. Several in vivo studies have indicated that CPCs can have extensive resorption within the first few months of surgery that lead to new bone formation [94,100].

Years of research and commercial interest have resulted in many different forms of CPCs. Depending on the final set product CPCs are classified into two broad categories: (1) apatite cement and (2) brushite cement. Apatite cements are more widely studied as the final set product is a natural mineral content of the bone, HA. This kind of cement is prepared from either TTCP ($Ca_4(PO_4)_2O$) or α-tricalcium phosphate (α-TCP, $Ca_3(PO_4)_2$) [96,101]. The widespread acceptance of apatite cements is generally because of: (1) the set product is apatite which is the natural mineral phase found in bone, (2) minimal change in local pH due to the setting reactions, and (3) good mechanical strength [94,96]. However, limited solubility of apatite cements is a concern for orthopedic applications. Therefore, there is a growing interest in faster soluble brushite cements [94]. Brushite cements owing to their high solubility have a distinctive advantage from the application point of view. CaP cements are generally used for temporary support and should dissolve when the application purpose is fulfilled. In this regard, brushite cement is preferred over apatite cement. Moreover, faster degradation of brushite cement will increase the Ca^{2+} concentration and enhance bone mineralization. Brushite cement can be prepared by reacting β-TCP and monocalcium phosphate monohydrate (MCPM) or mixing β-TCP with phosphoric acid [96,102]; however, the reaction is often acidic and decreases the local pH while setting, which is considered as one of the major drawbacks of brushite cement. Several in vivo studies have indicated that brushite cement has higher solubility than apatite cement, leading to rapid new bone formation. Another concern of brushite cement is its relatively shorter setting time ($\geq$10s) which makes it difficult to be used by surgeons [96]. Setting time modifiers, such as sodium hydrogen phosphate, are often used with the liquid medium to increase the setting time to a workable range [103]. The commonly used CaPs, such as HA or TCP, are generally sintered to $>$1200°C to form the predefined geometry. In contrast, CPCs are set at body temperature (37°C) and still have a considerable compressive strength owing to its reaction mechanism. For instance, while forming the brushite cement, the MCPM phase readily dissolves in the aqueous phase, leading to a decrease in pH where the β-TCP phase is soluble. Once β-TCP dissolves in the liquid medium, the solution is supersaturated with Ca^{2+} ion and recrystallizes as dicalcium phosphate dihydrate. The interlocking mechanism during the crystal growth, as shown in Fig. 6.11B, is primarily responsible for the strength in the cement. Applications of bone cements are subjected to its degradability as the degrading cement surface provides the new surface for bone apposition. The bone cement with degradation rate matching with bone regeneration rate is the ideal situation. Bone cement degrades by both chemical dissolution and osteoclast cell-mediated resorption. Studies have shown that CaP cement can be successfully degraded by osteoclast-like cells (Fig. 6.11C) [104]. Table 6.13 describes the required properties and their usefulness for bone cements.

Biocompatibility of brushite cements has been extensively studied both in in vitro and in vivo models. It is reported that 90% of the brushite cement can be resorbed in vivo within 6 months, and is replaced by new bone [94]. Several researchers have successfully modified the brushite cement composition to achieve control over setting time, mechanical properties, degradation rate, and cellular activity. It has been

Table 6.13 Standard physical and mechanical characterizations for bone cements

Cement property	Usefulness	Characterization details
Setting time	Gives an idea about the cement formation reactions. It also allows the surgeons to know the exact time for wound closure where the cement has achieved an appropriate strength. Too short a setting time makes the cement unworkable before the surgeons can implant it	Time required for the cement to achieve sufficient strength to resist an applied force. Generally determined by gillmore needles or Vicat needle [105]. Two setting times are determined where the "initial setting time" indicates the end of workability of the cement paste, whereas the "final setting time" indicates sufficient mechanical strength
Cohesion time	Is an indication of time required to harden the cement in a stable environment without disintegrating or washing out. This property ensures that after setting the cement will not breakdown into pieces at the application site or washout by the flow of blood and body serum	There is no specific standard to determine the cohesion of cement paste. However, several approaches have been used to understand the cohesion property. Putting the cement paste in simulated physiological solution and measuring the Ca^{2+} ion concentration as a function of time. This approach poses a challenge as the cement is supposed to be somewhat soluble in physiological environment. Therefore, the obtained Ca^{2+} ion concentration will be from both cement washout and chemical dissolution. Another simpler approach is to measure the continuous mass loss of a suspended cement paste in physiological solution as a function of time
Injectability	The CPC cement has to be premixed in a plate using a spatula and then applied at the surgical site. A better and much more convenient option is to inject the cement paste directly at the surgical site with the help of a syringe and needle. Injectability is a property of the cement paste that determines whether the cement can be successfully injected at the surgical site without phase separation (known as filter press). Injectability enhances the surgeon's efficiency and allow for minimally invasive surgeries with complex-shaped defect sites	Currently there is no known standard to determine the injectability of cement paste. It depends on cement composition, polymer additives, syringe and needle diameter and length

(*Continued*)

Table 6.13 (Continued)

Cement property	Usefulness	Characterization details
Microstructure and porosity	As CPC cements are essentially formed by dissolution and reprecipitation process, porosity is an inherent characteristic of CPC. These internal and interconnected porosities not only contribute to the enhanced resorption of CPC but also contribute to excellent biomechanical locking through interporous cell migration. However, these porosities decrease the mechanical strength of CPC, which may or may not be of major concern depending on the application site	Standard microscopic studies are usually done to determine the porosity of the cement after setting along with its other features; such as needle-like microstructure with interlocking features
Mechanical strength	Although CPC is not used for direct load-bearing applications, a certain amount of mechanical strength is required for holding the load-bearing implants (hip or knee prosthesis) in place, proper biomechanical load transfer, and mechanically supporting the bone remodeling process. In the majority of the cases, the compressive strength of CPC is reported, which varies from 0.2 to 184 MPa depending on total porosity and pore size, composition, additives, aging time, and environment. Along with strength, fracture toughness and fatigue properties of cements are of primary interest. CPCs primarily used for bone defects are subjected to cyclic loading and therefore fatigue properties provide the suitable life cycle analysis of CPC	Standard testing for compressive strength is usually done and strength is correlated to its microstructure and variation in composition. Fracture toughness, K_{IC}, and fatigue properties are not commonly determined for CPCs; however, they should be tested according to standards

reported that Zn and Sr single or cosubstitution in brushite cement can reduce the setting time. Moreover, they have improved the compressive strength and preosteoblast proliferation and maturation [106]. Mg doping improved mechanical properties and setting time along with osteoblast cell proliferation and differentiation [107]. Zn and Si doping also enhance bone regeneration, as shown in Fig. 6.11D. The addition of Si has enhanced new bone formation as early as 4 weeks and enhanced vascularization by a factor of 3 (Fig. 6.12) [104]. A dose-dependent effect of silicon on new blood vessel formation was studied by implanting Si-doped brushite cement in rat femur. The von Willebrand factor (vWF) staining indicated significantly higher new blood vessel formation for 1.1 wt% Si-doped cement, as shown in Fig. 6.12A and B. Histomorphometric analysis also indicated enhanced tissue integration due to the presence of Si in the brushite cement. Effects of polyethylene glycol (PEG) addition in brushite cement are known to enhance injectability, a much needed quality for successful application of CPC. Addition of PEG is also known to enhance osteoblast differentiation [105].

The most widely used forms of bone cements are made of CaPs. However, for various clinical applications, faster-setting magnesium phosphate cements (MPCs) are preferred. MPCs are prepared from magnesium oxide (MgO) and ammonium dihydrogenphosphate. Faster-setting cements can provide certain distinct advantages where complete hemostasis in fracture repair cannot be achieved. Moreover, MPCs have higher initial strength, which helps in fracture stabilization [108]. Yu et al. have

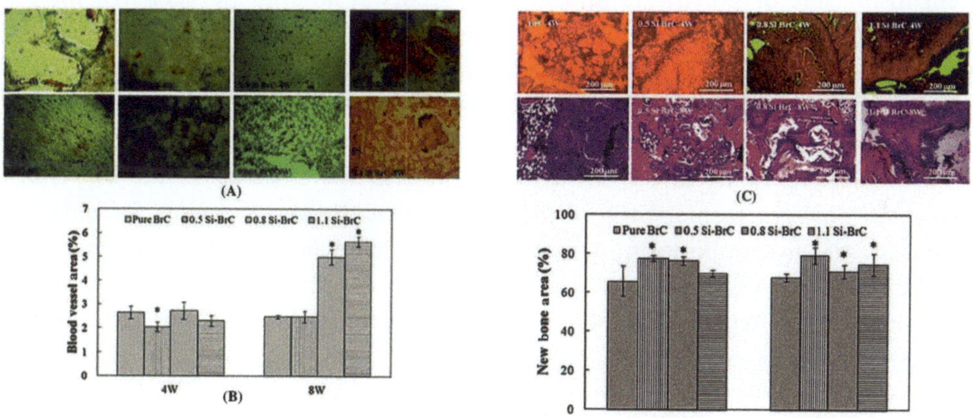

Figure 6.12 (A) Photomicrograph of vWF-stained tissue sections showing blood vessel formation after 4 and 8 weeks in BrCs. vWF-positive signals are brown/red with hematoxylin counterstaining [104]. (B) Histomorphometric analysis showing new blood vessel area comparisons between pure and Si-doped BrC (vWF positive area/total area, %) [104]. (C) Photomicrographs of H&E-stained histological sections of decalcified tissue sections showing the development of bone formation after 4 and 8 weeks [104]. (D) Histomorphometric analysis of bone area fraction (total newly formed bone area/total area, %) [104]. *indicates statistical significance.

studied the biocompatibility and genetic toxicity of MPC and reported apparent safety of these materials through in vitro study [108]. In another work, Mestres and Ginebra showed better mechanical properties of MPCs compared to conventionally used CaP cements. They even claimed the better applicability of MPC for its antimicrobial activity against *Streptococcus sanguinis* [109]. The chemical stability of MPCs has been studied by Tamimi et al. [110]. They have also shown that genetic expression of these materials is comparable to commonly used CaP bioceramics. However, no reported literatures exist for cell-mediated degradation of MPCs. Without the cell-mediated resorption mechanism, the true degradation potential of MPCs cannot be fully realized. Therefore, future research can focus on understanding the degradation of magnesium phosphate-based cement by osteoclast cells.

6.8 BIOGLASS FOR BONE REGENERATION

Bioglass is commonly referred to as a class of bioactive glasses specifically composed with silica (SiO_2), calcium oxide (CaO), sodium oxide (Na_2O), and phosphorous pentoxide (P_2O_5). Larry Hench pioneered the bioglass development in late 1960s with the development of widely known 45S5 Bioglass [111]. The concept of bioglass development was derived from the lack of tissue integration on metallic and polymeric bone implants. Being soluble at physiological environment, bioglass directly bonds with the surrounding tissue leading to biological fixation which is normally absent in metallic or polymeric implants. Bioglass was among the very first materials designed to be bioactive and resulted in several commercial products, like Novabone (Nova-Bone Products LLC), Biogran (BIOMET 3i, Palm Beach Gardens, FL), and BonAlive (BonAlive Biomaterials, Turku, Finland) [111].

Bioglass is in general more soluble than other bioactive materials such as HA and α/β-TCP. The solubility of bioglass comes from the hydrolization of the Si—O bond of the glass network former SiO_2. It is believed that the key elements for bioactivity of bioglass are its composition, which comprises of $<60\%$ SiO_2, moderately high network modifiers (CaO, Na_2O), and high CaO/P_2O_5 ratio. The popular 45S5 has a composition of 45 wt% SiO_2, 24.5 wt% CaO, 24.5 wt% Na_2O, and 6 wt% P_2O_5. This specific composition gives rise to a rapidly reacting bioglass surface when implanted at physiological environment where the SiO_2 reacts with H_2O to form Si—OH. When a complete unit of SiO_2 breaks down, it forms $Si(OH)_4$ and is released. After polycondensation, two $Si(OH)_4$ form a Si—O—Si bond and form a silica gel. In parallel, Ca, Na, and phosphate ions are also released due to breakdown of the silica network and are adsorbed on the glass surface. Together they form an amorphous hydroxy carbonate apatite (HCA) which crystallizes in due course. The bone bonding ability of bioglass or the shear strength of the interface is profoundly dependent on the HCA layer thickness. Typically, an interface thickness of nearly 20 μm provides good shear strength and interfacial bonding.

Since the inception of 45S5 Bioglass, many different compositions have been discovered over the years [112]. SiO_2 has been replaced with B_2O_3, CaO with CaF_2 or MgO, K_2O for Na_2O, and other minor compositional changes. All of the substitutions have increased the bioactivity to some extent, with effects on resorbability. Borate bioglass and borosilicate bioglass have higher solubility rates than silicate bioglass and completely convert to HCA mineral, making them a choice of material for ultrashort-period implant material. On the other hand, the addition of Al_2O_3 and TiO_2 has proven to be detrimental to the bone bonding ability of bioglass. The extensive research on compositional variance of bioglass resulted in exceptional control over bioglass dissolution with a common factor of increased bioactivity. Among the many different approaches, melt derived and sol-gel are the two most promising techniques for preparing bioglass [113]. The choice of route has a profound effect on the surface degradation, HCA layer formation, and effective bone bonding ability. While the melting process is relatively simple, inexpensive, and high-throughput, the sol-gel technique provides better chemical homogeneity and higher specific surface area for enhanced surface reactivity. Both of these techniques are used to prepare bioglass powder as well as 3D scaffolds. Almost all of the scaffold preparation techniques detailed in Table 6.8 can also be used to prepare bioglass scaffold.

Over the years, osteoconductivity and osteoinductivity of bioglass have been proven by several in vitro and in vivo models [113–115]. A 70% porous 3D bioglass scaffold with 300–400 μm pore size showed HCA layer formation in vitro that enhanced osteoblast activity [40]. HCA layer formation also enhances protein and growth factor absorption to facilitate new bone formation in vivo [40]. In more recent work, cobalt (Co)-incorporated bioglass has been studied in vitro. The results indicated that Co addition in mesoporous bioglass scaffold induced hypoxia (low oxygen pressure), which increased BMSC proliferation, differentiation, VEGF secretion, hypoxia-inducible factor 1-alpha expression, and bone-related gene expression [41]. The degradation product of bioglass in the form of Si^{4+} is shown to be angiogenic [27,116]. The ionic degradation of 45S5 bioglass has significantly upregulated specific genes, such as CD44 and integrin β1, metalloproteinases-2 and 4, and their inhibitors, TIMP-1 and TIMP-2 [114]. High degradability of bioglass particles and their tunable property have been explored for drug delivery [117,118]. Antibiotics such as gentamycin, functional cations such as Li, Sr, Zn, Cu, and biomolecules such as BMP, VEGF, and IGF have been delivered through mesoporous bioglass particles or scaffolds [118].

Bioglass found its wide application in the form of particles as filler for small-scale bone defects and not so much as a monolithic body or coating. The bioglass particles are mixed with blood in the surgery room and, while clotting, the blood and bioglass particles form a paste-like consistency that can easily be applied to the defect site, more like bone cement. In dentistry, bioglass has been used to improve the bone bed for anchoring metallic implants. The high solubility of bioglass results in faster bone regeneration at the implanted site, leading to increased bone density, which is often required to mechanically fix a dental fixture. Ultrafine bioglass is also used in toothpaste to reduce hypersensitivity around the gum line which happens due to the exposure of dentin (NovaMin; NovaMin Technology, FL; now owned by GlaxoSmithKline, UK) [111].

6.9 SUMMARY AND FUTURE DIRECTIONS

The concept of bioactive materials in orthopedic biomaterials was first introduced through ceramics in the form of bioglass in the late 1960s. Since then ceramic materials have revolutionized the field of orthopedic biomaterials through new material development along with break-through processing techniques. The application of alumina and zirconia as femoral heads had opened a new frontier of hip replacement surgery. These bioinert ceramics provided better articulating surfaces with lower friction and wear damage of femoral heads compared to their metallic counterparts, which resulted in lower metal ion release. The overall outcome was enhanced performance of total hip replacement and quality of patient's life. However, the use of alumina and zirconia was not beyond controversy. While alumina was questioned for low fracture toughness, the concern regarding zirconia was aging. Advancement in ceramic processing such as hot pressing made it possible to reduce the grain size of sintered alumina and thus increasing fracture toughness. A new material composition of alumina–zirconia had improved the strength loss behavior. More work is necessary to understand the long-term effect of sintering kinetics and composition of alumina–zirconia on the strength loss and associated failure mechanism. Advanced sintering techniques such as spark plasma sintering, microwave sintering, and flash sintering can make new stories in bioinert ceramics for improved or newer application in articulating surfaces.

The bioactive ceramics, which started in the form of bioglass, had moved into a new category of material named CaPs. CaP is a family of materials with varying Ca:P ratio that dictates its solubility as well as bioactivity. The early use of CaP was in the form of bone cement which had certain advantages, such as ease of application (injectability), setting at body temperature (minimal tissue necrosis), and excellent solubility. These cements were used to stabilize dental, hip, or knee metallic implants, and to treat small-scale bone defects. With time, newer CaP ceramics emerged in the form of HA and TCP. HA and TCP are probably the most studied bioceramics in the last two decades, focusing its acceptance in biological environment and mechanical properties. Among these two materials TCP emerged as a better bioactive material owing to its high solubility at physiological environment and ability for faster bone regeneration. TCP is used both as granules or scaffolds material for bone regeneration. On the other hand, HA, being less soluble, is used in places where sustained bioactivity is required for a longer period of time. One of the most successful commercial uses of HA is coating in femoral stems of hip replacement.

The new generations of bioactive ceramics are no longer designed only to provide a surface for bone growth (osteoconductive) but also to enhance the bone regeneration rate. The current perspective is to modulate the chemistry of HA/TCP/bioglass in such a way that these materials become osteoinductive. It is expected that the new class of materials will guide the progenitor cell recruitment and differentiation in order to achieve osteogenesis and angiogenesis. Only a synchronized performance of these two processes can lead to better bone regeneration. New frontiers of bioactive ceramics focused on modulating its chemistry through metal ion doping on improving its sinterability and overall biological performance. Elements such as Sr, Mg, Zn, and Si played a major role in improving the bone bonding ability of these materials. Research has also been directed to deliver drugs, proteins, and growth factors through bioglass, HA/TCP particles, and their respective scaffolds. The delivery of bisphosphonate through TCP particles and scaffolds reduced osteoclast formation, which can have a significant effect on osteoporosis. One of the primary challenges of biomolecule delivery is controlling its absorption and desorption kinetics. New drug immobilization techniques have to be developed for maximum drug incorporation on the ceramic particles or scaffolds, along with sustained and controlled release. Pore size and its distribution in ceramic scaffolds could show a new direction in biomolecule delivery. The future success of bioceramics will depend on new material development, better understanding of their in vivo performance, and ability to deliver biomolecules in a controlled manner that will require an interdisciplinary approach from chemists, material scientists, engineers, and biologists.

REFERENCES

[1] Hench LL. Bioceramics: from concept to clinic. J Am Ceram Soc 1991;74:1487–510.
[2] Vallet-Regí M, González-Calbet JM. Calcium phosphates as substitution of bone tissues. Prog Solid State Chem 2004;32:1–31.
[3] Dell RM, Greene D, Anderson D, Williams K. Osteoporosis disease management: what every orthopaedic surgeon should know. J Bone Jt Surg Am 2009;91:79–86.
[4] Smith L. CEramic-plastic material as a bone substitute. Arch Surg 1963;87:653–61.
[5] Chevalier J. What future for zirconia as a biomaterial? Biomaterials 2006;27:535–43.
[6] Piconi C, Maccauro G. Zirconia as a ceramic biomaterial. Biomaterials 1999;20:1–25.
[7] Lughi V, Sergo V. Low temperature degradation -aging- of zirconia: a critical review of the relevant aspects in dentistry. Dent Mater 2010;26:807–20.
[8] Kurtz SM, et al. Advances in zirconia toughened alumina biomaterials for total joint replacement. J Mech Behav Biomed Mater 2014;31:107–16.
[9] Bandyopadhyay A, Bernard S, Xue W, Bose S. Calcium phosphate-based resorbable ceramics: influence of MgO, ZnO, and SiO2 dopants. J Am Ceram Soc 2006;89:2675–88.
[10] Sadat-Shojai M, Khorasani M-T, Dinpanah-Khoshdargi E, Jamshidi A. Synthesis methods for nanosized hydroxyapatite with diverse structures. Acta Biomater 2013;9:7591–621.
[11] Olszta MJ, et al. Bone structure and formation: a new perspective. Mater Sci Eng R Rep 2007;58:77–116.
[12] Bose S, Tarafder S, Banerjee SS, Davies NM, Bandyopadhyay A. Understanding in vivo response and mechanical property variation in MgO, SrO and SiO2 doped β-TCP. Bone 2011;48:1282–90.

[13] Patntirapong S, Habibovic P, Hauschka PV. Effects of soluble cobalt and cobalt incorporated into calcium phosphate layers on osteoclast differentiation and activation. Biomaterials 2009;30: 548–55.
[14] Roy M, Bose S. Osteoclastogenesis and osteoclastic resorption of tricalcium phosphate: effect of strontium and magnesium doping. J Biomed Mater Res A 2012;100A:2450–61.
[15] Yang L, et al. The effects of inorganic additives to calcium phosphate on in vitro behavior of osteoblasts and osteoclasts. Biomaterials 2010;31:2976–89.
[16] Braux J, et al. A new insight into the dissociating effect of strontium on bone resorption and formation. Acta Biomater 2011;7:2593–603.
[17] Seeley Z, Bandyopadhyay A, Bose S. Influence of TiO_2 and Ag_2O addition on tricalcium phosphate ceramics. J Biomed Mater Res Part A 2007;82(1):113–21.
[18] Zreiqat H, et al. The incorporation of strontium and zinc into a calcium–silicon ceramic for bone tissue engineering. Biomaterials 2010;31:3175–84.
[19] Hao Y, et al. Evaluation of osteoinduction and proliferation on nano-Sr-HAP: a novel orthopedic biomaterial for bone tissue regeneration. J Nanosci Nanotechnol 2012;12:207–12.
[20] Li X, et al. The optimum zinc content in set calcium phosphate cement for promoting bone formation in vivo. Mater Sci Eng C Mater Biol Appl 2009;29:969–75.
[21] Fielding GA, Bandyopadhyay A, Bose S. Effects of silica and zinc oxide doping on mechanical and biological properties of 3D printed tricalcium phosphate tissue engineering scaffolds. Dent Mater 2012;28:113–22.
[22] Hanai Y, et al. Up-regulation by zinc of FGF-2-induced VEGF release through enhancing p44/p42 MAP kinase activation in osteoblasts. Life Sci 2006;80:230–4.
[23] Boanini E, et al. Magnesium and strontium doped octacalcium phosphate thin films by matrix assisted pulsed laser evaporation. J Inorg Biochem 2012;107:65–72.
[24] Janning C, et al. Magnesium hydroxide temporarily enhancing osteoblast activity and decreasing the osteoclast number in peri-implant bone remodelling. Acta Biomater 2010;6:1861–8.
[25] Camiré CL, et al. Material characterization and in vivo behavior of silicon substituted α-tricalcium phosphate cement. J Biomed Mater Res B Appl Biomater 2006;76B:424–31.
[26] Obata A, Kasuga T. Stimulation of human mesenchymal stem cells and osteoblasts activities in vitro on silicon-releasable scaffolds. J Biomed Mater Res 2008;A91A:11–17.
[27] Gorustovich AA, Roether JA, Boccaccini AR. Effect of bioactive glasses on angiogenesis: a review of in vitro and in vivo evidences. Tissue Eng Part B Rev 2010;16:199–207.
[28] Coathup MJ, et al. The osteoinductivity of silicate-substituted calcium phosphate. J Bone Jt Surg Am 2011;93:2219–26.
[29] Alt V, et al. Assessment of angiogenesis in osseointegration of a silica-collagen biomaterial using 3D-nano-CT. Acta Biomater 2011;7:3773–9.
[30] Thimm BW, Unger RE, Neumann H-G, Kirkpatrick CJ. Biocompatibility studies of endothelial cells on a novel calcium phosphate/SiO_2—xerogel composite for bone tissue engineering. Biomed Mater 2008;3:15007.
[31] Bose S, Roy M, Bandyopadhyay A. Recent advances in bone tissue engineering scaffolds. Trends Biotechnol 2012;30:546–54.
[32] Rouwkema J, Rivron NC, van Blitterswijk CA. Vascularization in tissue engineering. Trends Biotechnol 2008;26:434–41.
[33] Teixeira S, et al. In vivo evaluation of highly macroporous ceramic scaffolds for bone tissue engineering. J Biomed Mater Res A 2010;93A:567–75.
[34] Woodard JR, et al. The mechanical properties and osteoconductivity of hydroxyapatite bone scaffolds with multi-scale porosity. Biomaterials 2007;28:45–54.
[35] Tarafder S, Balla VK, Davies NM, Bandyopadhyay A, Bose S. Microwave-sintered 3D printed tricalcium phosphate scaffolds for bone tissue engineering. J Tissue Eng Regen Med 2013;7: 631–41.
[36] Tarafder S, Dernell WS, Bandyopadhyay A, Bose S. SrO- and MgO-doped microwave sintered 3D printed tricalcium phosphate scaffolds: mechanical properties and in vivo osteogenesis in a rabbit model. J Biomed Mater Res B Appl Biomater 2015;103:679–90.

[37] Ke D, Dernell W, Bandyopadhyay A, Bose S. Doped tricalcium phosphate scaffolds by thermal decomposition of naphthalene: Mechanical properties and in vivo osteogenesis in a rabbit femur model. J Biomed Mater Res B Appl Biomater 2015;103:1549–59.
[38] Papadimitropoulos A, et al. Kinetics of in vivo bone deposition by bone marrow stromal cells within a resorbable porous calcium phosphate scaffold: An X-ray computed microtomography study. Biotechnol Bioeng 2007;98:271–81.
[39] Eniwumide JO, Yuan H, Cartmell SH, Meijer GJ, de Bruijn JD. Ectopic bone formation in bone marrow stem cell seeded calcium phosphate scaffolds as compared to autograft and (cell seeded) allograft. Eur Cell Mater 2007;14:30–8. discussion 39.
[40] Miguel BS, et al. Enhanced osteoblastic activity and bone regeneration using surface-modified porous bioactive glass scaffolds. J Biomed Mater Res A 2010;94A:1023–33.
[41] Wu C, et al. Hypoxia-mimicking mesoporous bioactive glass scaffolds with controllable cobalt ion release for bone tissue engineering. Biomaterials 2012;33:2076–85.
[42] Fu Q, Huang W, Rahaman MN, Tomsia AP. Three-dimensional visualization of bioactive glass-bone integration in a rabbit tibia model using synchrotron x-ray microcomputed tomography. Tissue Eng Part A 2011;17:3077–84.
[43] Cao H, Kuboyama N. A biodegradable porous composite scaffold of PGA/β-TCP for bone tissue engineering. Bone 2010;46:386–95.
[44] Laschke MW, Strohe A, Menger MD, Alini M, Eglin D. In vitro and in vivo evaluation of a novel nanosize hydroxyapatite particles/poly(ester-urethane) composite scaffold for bone tissue engineering. Acta Biomater 2010;6:2020–7.
[45] Roohani-Esfahani S-I, Nouri-Khorasani S, Lu Z, Appleyard R, Zreiqat H. The influence hydroxyapatite nanoparticle shape and size on the properties of biphasic calcium phosphate scaffolds coated with hydroxyapatite–PCL composites. Biomaterials 2010;31:5498–509.
[46] Xue W, Bandyopadhyay A, Bose S. Polycaprolactone coated porous tricalcium phosphate scaffolds for controlled release of protein for tissue engineering. J Biomed Mater Res B Appl Biomater 2009;91B:831–8.
[47] Bandyopadhyay A, Vahabzadeh S, Shivaram A, Bose S. Three-dimensional printing of biomaterials and soft materials. MRS Bull 2015;40:1162–9.
[48] Darsell J, Bose S, Hosick HL, Bandyopadhyay A. From CT scan to ceramic bone graft. J Am Ceram Soc 2003;86:1076–80.
[49] Bose S, Vahabzadeh S, Bandyopadhyay A. Bone tissue engineering using 3D printing. Materials Today 2013;16:496–504.
[50] Suwanprateeb J, Sanngam R, Panyathanmaporn T. Influence of raw powder preparation routes on properties of hydroxyapatite fabricated by 3D printing technique. Mater Sci Eng C 2010;30:610–17.
[51] Karageorgiou V, Kaplan D. Porosity of 3D biomaterial scaffolds and osteogenesis. Biomaterials 2005;26:5474–91.
[52] Rezwan K, Chen QZ, Blaker JJ, Boccaccini AR. Biodegradable and bioactive porous polymer/inorganic composite scaffolds for bone tissue engineering. Biomaterials 2006;27:3413–31.
[53] Banerjee SS, Tarafder S, Davies NM, Bandyopadhyay A, Bose S. Understanding the influence of MgO and SrO binary doping on the mechanical and biological properties of β-TCP ceramics. Acta Biomater 2010;6:4167–74.
[54] Shie M-Y, Ding S-J, Chang H-C. The role of silicon in osteoblast-like cell proliferation and apoptosis. Acta Biomater 2011;7:2604–14.
[55] Lee K-W, Wang S, Yaszemski MJ, Lu L. Physical properties and cellular responses to crosslinkable poly(propylene fumarate)/hydroxyapatite nanocomposites. Biomaterials 2008;29:2839–48.
[56] Wagoner Johnson AJ, Herschler BA. A review of the mechanical behavior of CaP and CaP/polymer composites for applications in bone replacement and repair. Acta Biomater 2011;7:16–30.
[57] Bose S, Tarafder S. Calcium phosphate ceramic systems in growth factor and drug delivery for bone tissue engineering: a review. Acta Biomater 2012;8:1401–21.
[58] Bose S, Fielding G, Tarafder S, Bandyopadhyay A. Understanding of dopant-induced osteogenesis and angiogenesis in calcium phosphate ceramics. Trends Biotechnol 2013;31:594–605.

[59] Dasgupta S, Banerjee SS, Bandyopadhyay A, Bose S. Zn- and Mg-doped hydroxyapatite nanoparticles for controlled release of protein. Langmuir 2010;26:4958–64.
[60] Tarafder S, Bose S. Polycaprolactone-coated 3D printed tricalcium phosphate scaffolds for bone tissue engineering: in vitro alendronate release behavior and local delivery effect on in vivo osteogenesis. ACS Appl Mater Interfaces, 6. 2014. p. 9955–65.
[61] Vahabzadeh S, Edgington J, Bose S. Tricalcium phosphate and tricalcium phosphate/polycaprolactone particulate composite for controlled release of protein. Mater Sci Eng 2013;C33:3576–82.
[62] Tarafder S, Nansen K, Bose S. Lovastatin release from polycaprolactone coated β-tricalcium phosphate: Effects of pH, concentration and drug–polymer interactions. Mater Sci Eng 2013;C33: 3121–8.
[63] Banerjee SS, Roy M, Bose S. pH tunable fluorescent calcium phosphate nanocomposite for sensing and controlled drug delivery. Adv Eng Mater 2011;13:B10–17.
[64] Keeney M, van den Beucken JJJP, van der Kraan PM, Jansen JA, Pandit A. The ability of a collagen/calcium phosphate scaffold to act as its own vector for gene delivery and to promote bone formation via transfection with VEGF165. Biomaterials 2010;31:2893–902.
[65] Liu Y, de Groot K, Hunziker EB. BMP-2 liberated from biomimetic implant coatings induces and sustains direct ossification in an ectopic rat model. Bone 2005;36:745–57.
[66] Scaglione S, et al. Order versus disorder: in vivo bone formation within osteoconductive scaffolds. Sci Rep 2012;2.
[67] Li J, et al. Repair of rat cranial bone defects with nHAC/PLLA and BMP-2-related peptide or rhBMP-2. J Orthop Res 2011;29:1745–52.
[68] Wernike E, et al. VEGF incorporated into calcium phosphate ceramics promotes vascularisation and bone formation in vivo. Eur Cell Mater 2010;19:30–40.
[69] Young S, et al. Dose effect of dual delivery of vascular endothelial growth factor and bone morphogenetic protein-2 on bone regeneration in a rat critical-size defect model. Tissue Eng Part A 2009; 15:2347–62.
[70] Pollak M. The insulin and insulin-like growth factor receptor family in neoplasia: an update. Nat Rev Cancer 2012;12:159–69.
[71] Kang H, Sung J, Woo KM, Roh S. Insulin-like growth factor 2 promotes osteogenic cell differentiation in the parthenogenetic murine embryonic stem cells. Tissue Eng Part A 2012;18:331–41.
[72] Verron E, Khairoun I, Guicheux J, Bouler J-M. Calcium phosphate biomaterials as bone drug delivery systems: a review. Drug Discov Today 2010;15:547–52.
[73] Kimelman-Bleich N, et al. Targeted gene-and-host progenitor cell therapy for nonunion bone fracture repair. Mol Ther 2010;19:53–9.
[74] Fischer J, et al. Future of local bone regeneration—protein versus gene therapy. J Cranio-Maxillofac Surg 2011;39:54–64.
[75] Lan Levengood SK, et al. The effect of BMP-2 on micro- and macroscale osteointegration of biphasic calcium phosphate scaffolds with multiscale porosity. Acta Biomater 2010;6:3283–91.
[76] Kempen DHR, et al. Effect of local sequential VEGF and BMP-2 delivery on ectopic and orthotopic bone regeneration. Biomaterials 2009;30:2816–25.
[77] Furlong RJ, Osborn JF. Fixation of hip prostheses by hydroxyapatite ceramic coatings. J Bone Joint Surg Br 1991;73:741–5.
[78] Gandhi R, Davey JR, Mahomed NN. Hydroxyapatite coated femoral stems in primary total hip arthroplasty: a meta-analysis. J Arthroplasty 2009;24:38–42.
[79] Mäkelä KT, Eskelinen A, Pulkkinen P, Paavolainen P, Remes V. Total hip arthroplasty for primary osteoarthritis in patients fifty-five years of age or older. An analysis of the Finnish arthroplasty registry. J Bone Joint Surg Am 2008;90:2160–70.
[80] Moroni A, Vannini F, Mosca M, Giannini S. State of the art review: techniques to avoid pin loosening and infection in external fixation. J Orthop Trauma 2002;16:189–95.
[81] Crawford CH, et al. Femoral component revision using an extensively hydroxyapatite-coated stem. J Arthroplasty 2004;19:8–13.
[82] Geerdink CH, Schaafsma J, Meyers WGM, Grimm B, Tonino AJ. Cementless hemispheric hydroxyapatite-coated sockets for acetabular revision. J Arthroplasty 2007;22:369–76.

[83] Epinette J-A. Long lasting outcome of hydroxyapatite-coated implants in primary knee arthroplasty: a continuous series of two hundred and seventy total knee arthroplasties at fifteen to twenty two years of clinical follow-up. Int Orthop 2014;38:305–11.
[84] Chana R, et al. Five- to 8-year results of the uncemented Duracon total knee arthroplasty system. J Arthroplasty 2008;23:677–82.
[85] Vahabzadeh S, Roy M, Bandyopadhyay A, Bose S. Phase stability and biological property evaluation of plasma sprayed hydroxyapatite coatings for orthopedic and dental applications. Acta Biomater 2015;17:47–55.
[86] Fielding G, Roy M, Bandyopadhyay A, Bose S. Antibacterial and biological characteristics of plasma sprayed silver and strontium doped hydroxyapatite coatings. Acta Biomaterialia 2012;8:144–52.
[87] Roy M, Fielding G, Beyenal H, Bandyopadhyay A, Bose S. Mechanical and in Vitro Anti-Bacterial and Biological Properties of Plasma Sprayed Silver Doped Hydroxyapatite Coatings. ACS Applied Materials and Interfaces 2012;4:1341–9.
[88] Sun L, Berndt CC, Khor KA, Cheang HN, Gross KA. Surface characteristics and dissolution behavior of plasma-sprayed hydroxyapatite coating. J Biomed Mater Res 2002;62:228–36.
[89] Zhang Q, et al. Dissolution and mineralization behaviors of HA coatings. Biomaterials 2003;24:4741–8.
[90] Roy M, Bandyopadhyay A, Bose S. nduction plasma sprayed nano hydroxyapatite coatings on titanium for orthopaedic and dental implants. Surf Coat Technol 2011;205:2785–92.
[91] Roy M, Bandyopadhyay A, Bose S. Induction plasma sprayed Sr and Mg doped nano hydroxyapatite coatings on Ti for bone implant. J Biomed Mater Res B Appl Biomater 2011;99B:258–65.
[92] Yang Y, Kim K-H, Ong JL. A review on calcium phosphate coatings produced using a sputtering process—an alternative to plasma spraying. Biomaterials 2005;26:327–37.
[93] Besra L, Liu M. A review on fundamentals and applications of electrophoretic deposition (EPD). Progress in Materials Science 2007;5:21–61.
[94] Apelt D, et al. In vivo behavior of three different injectable hydraulic calcium phosphate cements. Biomaterials 2004;25:1439–51.
[95] Tamimi F, Sheikh Z, Barralet J. Dicalcium phosphate cements: brushite and monetite. Acta Biomater 2012;8:474–87.
[96] Bohner M. Reactivity of calcium phosphate cements. J Mater Chem 2007;17:3980.
[97] Vahabzadeh S, Bandyopadhyay A, Bose S, Mandal R, Nandi SK. IGF-loaded silicon and zinc doped brushite cement: physico-mechanical characterization and in vivo osteogenesis evaluation. Integr Biol 2015;7:1561–73.
[98] Pina S, et al. Biological responses of brushite-forming Zn- and ZnSr- substituted beta-tricalcium phosphate bone cements. Eur Cell Mater 2010;20:162–77.
[99] Ginebra MP, Traykova T, Planell JA. Calcium phosphate cements as bone drug delivery systems: A review. J Controlled Release 2006;113:102–10.
[100] Ohura K, et al. Resorption of, and bone formation from, new beta-tricalcium phosphate-monocalcium phosphate cements: an in vivo study. J Biomed Mater Res 1996;30:193–200.
[101] Han B, et al. β-TCP/MCPM-based premixed calcium phosphate cements. Acta Biomater 2009; 5:3165–77.
[102] Grover LM, Knowles JC, Fleming GJP, Barralet JE. In vitro ageing of brushite calcium phosphate cement. Biomaterials 2003;24:4133–41.
[103] Bohner M, Gbureck U, Barralet JE. Technological issues for the development of more efficient calcium phosphate bone cements: A critical assessment. Biomaterials 2005;26:6423–9.
[104] Vahabzadeh S, Roy M, Bose S. Effects of silicon on osteoclast cell mediated degradation, in vivo osteogenesis and vasculogenesis of brushite cement. J Mater Chem B 2015;3:8973–82.
[105] Roy M, DeVoe K, Bandyopadhyay A, Bose S. Mechanical property and in vitro biocompatibility of brushite cement modified by polyethylene glycol. Mater Sci Eng C 2012;32:2145–52.
[106] Pina S, et al. In vitro performance assessment of new brushite-forming Zn- and ZnSr-substituted β-TCP bone cements. J Biomed Mater Res B Appl Biomater 2010;94B:414–20.
[107] Klammert U, et al. Phase composition, mechanical performance and in vitro biocompatibility of hydraulic setting calcium magnesium phosphate cement. Acta Biomater 2010;6:1529–35.

[108] Yu Y, et al. Evaluation of inherent toxicology and biocompatibility of magnesium phosphate bone cement. Colloids Surf B Biointerfaces 2010;76:496–504.
[109] Mestres G, Ginebra M-P. Novel magnesium phosphate cements with high early strength and antibacterial properties. Acta Biomater 2011;7:1853–61.
[110] Tamimi F, et al. Biocompatibility of magnesium phosphate minerals and their stability under physiological conditions. Acta Biomater 2011;7:2678–85.
[111] Jones JR. Review of bioactive glass: From Hench to hybrids. Acta Biomater 2013;9:4457–86.
[112] Jones JR, Ehrenfried LM, Hench LL. Optimising bioactive glass scaffolds for bone tissue engineering. Biomaterials 2006;27:964–73.
[113] Rahaman MN, et al. Bioactive glass in tissue engineering. Acta Biomater 2011;7:2355–73.
[114] Xynos ID, Edgar AJ, Buttery LDK, Hench LL, Polak JM. Gene-expression profiling of human osteoblasts following treatment with the ionic products of Bioglass® 45S5 dissolution. J Biomed Mater Res 2001;55:151–7.
[115] Xynos ID, et al. Bioglass ®45S5 stimulates osteoblast turnover and enhances bone formation in vitro: implications and applications for bone tissue engineering. Calcif Tissue Int 2014;67: 321–9.
[116] Zhai W, et al. Silicate bioceramics induce angiogenesis during bone regeneration. Acta Biomater 2012;8:341–9.
[117] Wu C, Chang J. Multifunctional mesoporous bioactive glasses for effective delivery of therapeutic ions and drug/growth factors. J Control Release Off J Control Release Soc 2014;193:282–95.
[118] Li Y, et al. Mesoporous bioactive glass as a drug delivery system: fabrication, bactericidal properties and biocompatibility. J Mater Sci Mater Med 2013;24:1951–61.

CHAPTER 7

Ceramic Coatings in Load-Bearing Articulating Joint Implants

V. Thomas, S.A. Catledge, P. Baker, G.P. Siegal and Y.K. Vohra
University of Alabama at Birmingham, Birmingham, AL, United States

Contents

7.1 INTRODUCTION

More than 800,000 joint replacement procedures are done in the United States every year, according to the American Academy of Orthopaedic Surgeons. Among them, knee replacements are the most common, followed by hips and shoulders. As Baby Boomers age, the number of joint replacements is projected to increase substantially to improve mobility and enhance quality of life. The number of knee replacement surgeries is expected to reach 3.48 million annually by 2030 [1]. In the most commonly used knee replacement implant, cobalt−chromium−molybdenum (CoCrMo) alloy articulates against an ultrahigh-molecular-weight polyethylene (UHMWPE) acetabular liner component. Metallic and polyethylene wear-debris, as well as the release of potentially toxic metallic ions, is a major concern for these components. A long-term concern related to prosthetic bearings in the human body is the adverse host biological response to accumulated, nano- to microscopic wear-debris in the periprosthetic joint space, especially metallic and polyethylene (PE) wear particles. Polyethylene debris has been identified as a major factor inducing activation of macrophages which leads to the production of bone-resorbing cytokines with resultant loss of bone stock, especially in younger populations [1]. Strategies to reduce PE wear in the ball-and-socket joint of artificial hips, and the sliding–rolling articulation of artificial knees, have been pursued vigorously by orthopedic implant manufacturers and material scientists, with varied success. Bearings made of ceramics (e.g., alumina and zirconia) have been shown to possess extremely low wear properties that make them suitable for both hip and knee arthroplasties. When compared to the most commonly used bearing couple in joint arthroplasty, which consists of cobalt–chrome (CoCr) metal alloy articulating against UHMWPE, ceramic components such as alumina or zirconia offer significant reductions in bearing wear rates [2–4]. However, previous experience has shown that each new bearing technology applied to total joint arthroplasty can have unforeseen complications. For ceramics, such complications have ranged from relatively minor (squeaking noises during articulation) [5] to severe (catastrophic fracture) [6]. Ceramic technology continues to evolve, and new materials based on diamond ceramics, composites of existing ceramics, and surface modifications will offer more options to the arthroplasty surgeon.

Alumina (Al_2O_3) and zirconia (ZrO_2) ceramics were introduced in the 1970s and 1980s, respectively, to replace CoCr femoral components in hip and knee replacements. Al_2O_3 bearings are the only prosthetic hip bearings with over 30-year clinical survivorship, with no evidence of periprosthetic bone dissolution related to particulate debris [7,8]. Although alumina has excellent compression strength, its bending strength is limited and design options are often limited due to its mechanical properties. Al_2O_3, in composite form, is the most widely used ceramic in orthopedic surgery today, but despite its wear reduction and long-term durability, sporadic cases of catastrophic alumina bearing failure continue to be a clinical concern [6,9]. Improved materials, implantation techniques, manufacturing variables, and implant design are reducing the risk of catastrophic failure of this ceramic bearing. Nevertheless, potential for fracture of alumina and zirconia ceramic femoral heads has been, along with cost and restricted design options, a major limitation to their expanded use worldwide.

Pure zirconia is an unstable material showing three different crystalline phases: monoclinic, tetragonal, and cubic. The tetragonal-to-monoclinic phase transformation results in a large variation in volume and significantly decreases the mechanical properties of the material [10,11]. Despite attempts to stabilize the tetragonal and cubic phase with yttria, it can still undergo an undesirable transformation to the monoclinic phase in vivo [11], leading to catastrophic failure. This aging process is triggered by water molecules and leads to surface roughening and microcracking. Slow degradation during long-term implantation in the human body may occur and become pronounced after several years [12]. Mixed composites of ZrO_2 and Al_2O_3, named zirconia-toughened alumina (ZTA), have also been marketed and used in hip replacements, but a potential drawback is that ZTA is still an unstable, ZrO_2-based material and there is evidence that spontaneous hydrothermally induced phase transformation will occur with it as well. More recently, silicon nitride (Si_3N_4) ceramics have been actively investigated [13–15]. Silicon nitride has a distinctive combination of material properties such as high strength and fracture toughness, inherent phase stability, scratch resistance, low wear, biocompatibility, hydrophilic behavior, excellent radiographic imaging, and resistance to bacterial adhesion, all of which make it an attractive choice for orthopedic implants.

Surface modification can be a more economic and efficient way to adjust existing conventional biomaterials to meet current and ever-evolving clinical needs. Oxidized zirconium [16–18], titanium nitride [19,20], and diamond-like carbons (DLCs) [21,22] have been considered for orthopedic devices with a major aim to improve scratch and wear resistance. The most clinically successful of these is oxidized zirconium (Oxinium, Smith & Nephew, Memphis, TN, USA), which has about 15 years of clinical history and combines the improved wear performance and abrasion resistance of ceramics with the toughness of metals. The transformed surface oxide has high adhesion and cohesion properties, but is not considered as a discrete coating. This results in improvements in resistance to in vivo roughening, in reducing friction, and in improving biocompatibility without the risk of catastrophic fracture [23]. While it provides half the friction of CoCrMo, it is twice as hard and therefore expected to result in less wear-related device failure. However, some concerns about Oxinium surface damage and exposure of underlying substrate have been documented from retrieval studies [24–26]. As with any implant material system, long-term retrieval studies will be a primary indication of device success.

Clearly, the combination of high hardness, toughness, and low friction is important in the implant design, as is the mechanical integrity of the surface over many years of in vivo service. With increasing numbers of orthopedic devices being implanted, many ceramic coatings [27] are being investigated to reduce the friction and wear in mating total joint replacement components, in hopes of greatly improving implant function and increasing device life-span. Adhesion of the coating to the metallic implant surface is of paramount concern and so this must be closely tested and scrutinized. To this end, functionally graded materials [28] and nanostructured or nanocomposite materials [29–31] offer a promising direction to enhance mechanical strength and toughness, while also reducing the propensity for brittle fracture and/or coating delamination.

A potential coating system to address the issues associated with wear as well as metal ion release in orthopedic and dental implants is that of ultrasmooth nanostructured diamond (NSD) coatings. These have been developed for metal implant surfaces

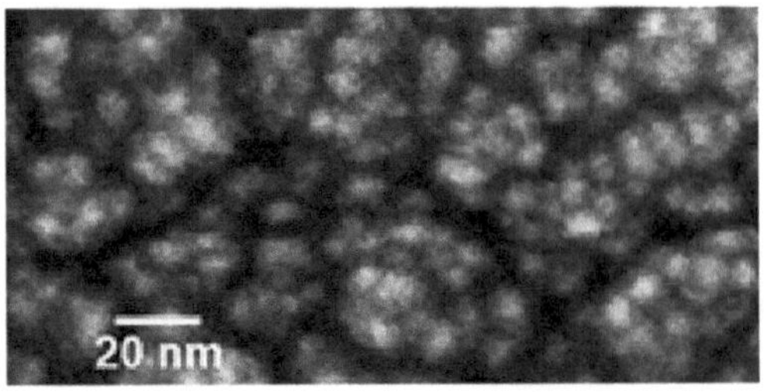

Figure 7.1 Representative scanning electron microscopy (SEM) image of NSD coatings using microwave plasma chemical vapor deposition (CVD) on a metal surface. *Reprinted from Baker PA, Thompson RG, Catledge SA. A wear simulation study of nanostructured CVD diamond-on-diamond articulation involving concave/convex mating surfaces. J Coat Technol Res 2016;13(2):385–93 [32], Copyright (2015), with permission from American Coatings Association.*

including titanium and cobalt-based alloys using microwave plasma chemical vapor deposition (CVD) [33–35]. The NSD coatings could prove to be more resistant to scratching by third-body wear particles, such as bone cement, due to the high hardness (56–80 GPa) and low surface roughness (rms value $<$ 10 nm) of the coatings [36–39]. Fig. 7.1 is a representative SEM image of NSD developed in our labs. They have been characterized as a mixture of sp^3 and sp^2 bonded carbon, with nanometer-sized diamond particles embedded in an amorphous carbon matrix. While adhesion and wear resistance of NSD to titanium is excellent [32,40–43], NSD coating of cobalt–chromium (CoCr) alloys that are so widely used as wear bearings in the orthopedic industry remains a challenge. The high cobalt content of this alloy acts as a catalyst for graphite that inevitably forms as an interfacial layer to limit NSD–metal adhesion strength [44]. The use of oxygen in the feed gas can promote early formation of chromium oxides that act as an effective diffusion barrier to cobalt and therefore minimize interfacial graphite. These chromium oxides combined with chromium carbides that form at elevated substrate temperature are believed to be important interfacial phases that have led to improved adhesion of NSD coatings on CoCr orthopedic alloys [33]. More recently, metal borides, also grown by CVD on CoCr as a graded interfacial layer for NSD deposition, have been reported [45]. The robust boride interlayer was effective in suppressing graphitic carbon during subsequent CVD of NSD, acting as a diffusion barrier against elemental cobalt. Migration of elemental cobalt to the surface of the interlayer is significantly reduced and undetectable on the surface of the subsequently grown NSD coating. A recent review on the process optimization and developmental characterizations, including bone-related cell interactions, has been published by the authors as a book chapter elsewhere [29]. This review focuses only on the diamond ceramic surfaces for the articulating joints based on an industry standard knee simulator (Fig. 7.2) and macrophage cell-interactions on nanodiamond wear-debris in vitro.

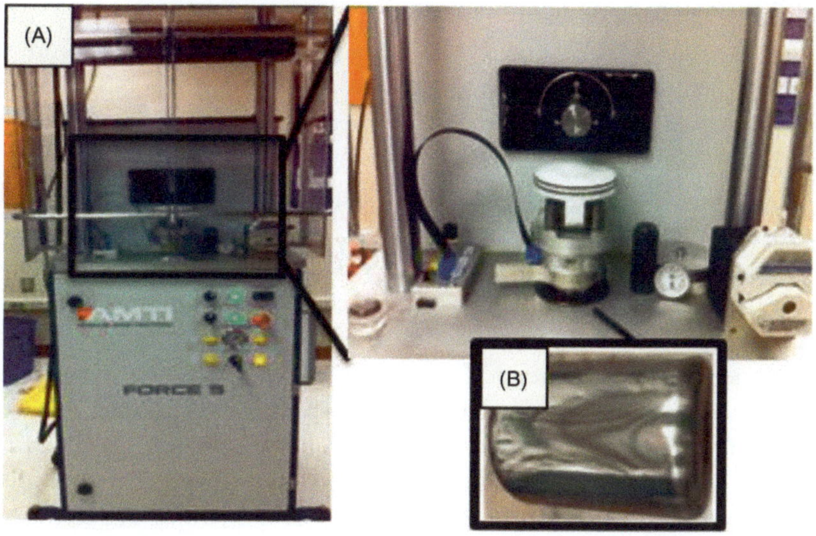

Figure 7.2 The AMTI Force 5 knee wear simulator (A) and NSD-coated hemisphere (B).

7.2 KNEE SIMULATOR STUDY INVOLVING NSD-COATED TITANIUM ARTICULATING AGAINST POLYETHYLENE

The wear of implants has been extensively studied, in vivo and in vitro [46–48]. Most wear studies can be classified into three categories: metal-on-UHMWPE, metal-on-metal, and ceramic-on-ceramic. As stated previously, cobalt–chrome alloys are often used for the metal in these load-bearing devices. Typically, wear of hard articulating surfaces reveals an initial wearing-in period of high surface material loss before establishing a significantly reduced linear wear rate [49]. This is due to the grinding away of surface asperities until the surfaces are mated such that the load is being applied uniformly. In a previous pin-on-disk study [50] using an OrthoPOD wear tester, we have shown that an NSD-coated Ti6Al4V disk surface resulted in reduced wear by a factor of two of the PE pin when compared to a noncoated CoCr disk. This study was not representative of the gait cycle experienced by the knee joint. In a recent study, we compared the effects of wear of an NSD-coated titanium alloy hemicylinder to a noncoated CoCr control using a multiaxis wear simulator, the AMTI Force 5 knee wear simulator, to more closely mimic the knee joint. The tests can be followed as per International Organization for Standardization (ISO) standard 14243-3: "Implants for surgery—Wear of total knee-joint prostheses—Part 3: Loading and displacement parameters for wear-testing machines with displacement control and corresponding environmental conditions." Flexion movement (rotation of flexion arm around a horizontal axis), anterior and posterior movement, and rotation of the stage were incorporated into the cyclic waveform representative of the knee gait cycle, according to the ISO standard.

Accordingly, for the comparison study [51] from the University of Alabama at Birmingham (UAB), the wear of UHMWPE against NSD-coated titanium alloy and uncoated CoCr hemicylinders was performed to determine if the NSD coating results in less volumetric wear of PE. A wear simulator was used with a gait cycle to mimic the knee joint, but with the axial force ranging from 30 to 700 N during the cycle. Both tests ran for 1.5 million cycles while immersed in bovine serum. Unfortunately, in the study the as-deposited surface roughness of the NSD coating was about 3–4 times higher than that of the starting polished CoCr surface, and so a direct comparison could not be made. The total PE volumetric wear when articulated against the NSD-coated alloy was greater than that of the noncoated control sample by a factor of five. No significant differences in the PE chemical structure or surface hardness were observed for either wear couple, as measured using Raman spectroscopy, X-ray diffraction, and nanoindentation [51]. The roughness of the PE (worn by the NSD-coated alloy) decreased faster than that of the control PE surface (worn by CoCr). It was suggested that a much higher abrasive wear occurred for the NSD-PE couple due to the high NSD surface roughness, ultimately leading to its inferior wear performance. This preliminary study [51] pointed out the importance of minimizing roughness of the hard bearing surface, and optimization of the NSD coating would be necessary to achieve a surface finish similar to the starting polish of CoCr in order to avoid accelerated abrasive wear.

An alternative bearing couple that could lead to more promising results involves articulation of NSD against NSD. Although minor surface "polishing" may occur as surface asperities are removed during initial stages of wear, the NSD coating is expected to experience very little wear over the long term while also acting as a barrier to prevent leaching of potentially toxic heavy metal ions from the substrate. The applications for this coating are more suitable for artificial hip joints (which also employ hard-on-hard bearings).

7.3 KNEE SIMULATOR STUDY INVOLVING ARTICULATION OF NSD ON NSD

To ensure that selected biomaterials meet the mechanical, tribological, and biological demands in vivo, agencies such as the ISO have established standards for biomaterials used for load-bearing applications [42]. For metallic articulating surfaces, a surface roughness below Ra = 50 nm is required, and minimum tensile strengths of 860–930 MPa and 725–1275 MPa are expected for titanium alloys and cobalt alloys, respectively. For ceramic surfaces, Ra better that 20 nm is required. For that, the Ti6Al4V alloy must be professionally polished to yield surface roughness within knee implant specifications (Ra = 50 nm). We have shown the surface roughness is reduced further to within Ra = 20 nm once the NSD coating is deposited with approximately 3–5 μm thickness [43].

Accordingly, a 3-μm-thick NSD layer was deposited by the CVD method onto polished, convex and concave components that were machined from Ti-6Al-4V alloy. These components had the same radius of curvature, 25.4 mm. Wear testing of the surfaces was performed by rotating articulation of the diamond-deposited surfaces (diamond-on-diamond) with a load of 225 N for a total of 5 million cycles in bovine serum resulting in polishing of the diamond surface and formation of very shallow, linear wear grooves of less than 50 nm depth [32]. The two diamond surfaces remained adhered to the components and polished each other to an average surface roughness that was reduced by as much as a factor of 80 for the most polished region located at the center of the condyle. Imaging of the surfaces showed that the initial wearing-in phase of the articulating surfaces by the end of the 5-million cycles. Fig. 7.3A shows the wear simulation setup in AMTI Force 5 wear simulator. Atomic force microscopy (AFM), scanning electron microscopy (SEM), Raman spectroscopy, and surface profilometry were used to characterize the surfaces and verify that the diamond remained intact and uniform over the surface, thereby protecting the underlying metal [32]. These wear simulation results show that diamond deposition on Ti alloy has potential application for joint replacement devices with improved longevity over existing devices made of cobalt chrome and UHMWPE [32].

The aim of the study was to create surfaces similar in size and function as those of the natural temporomandibular joint (TMJ) and simulate the articulation of the joint in a simple fashion to demonstrate their suitability in an implanted device [32]. Even after 5 million cycles only light polishing of the diamond surface occurred (Fig. 7.3B). It was expected that the full surface of the condyle component would slide across the surface of the fossa, but it can be seen that there was some mismatch in the radius of curvature of the two components, with the condyle having a slightly smaller radius. This change in shape is thought to be a result of the CVD deposition process, where the Ti alloy is expanded after heating and cooled by a small amount during the diamond growth process. The challenge was to produce clinically relevant conditions in terms of implant geometry and load/displacement for the articulating surfaces. Prior work using the NSD surface applied to titanium alloy substrates showed that when used in a pin-on-disk type configuration (under dry wear conditions) substantial wear and delamination of the diamond coating occurred [52]. However, this configuration placed the contact area under a large contact stress, approximately 2.8 GPa, leading to a deformation of the base metal and delamination of the film on the curved surface. The yield strength of the underlying metal was only 830 MPa, which was not enough to support the large contact stress without deformation. Thus the hard, brittle film could not be expected to survive this scenario in the long term. Another study using a condyle (convex) and fossa (concave) arrangement, where the surfaces were curved but still not matching in curvature, showed much improved performance of the diamond surfaces [53]. However, this setup was also conducted under dry wear conditions, and relatively short (2.25×10^5 cycles) simulations

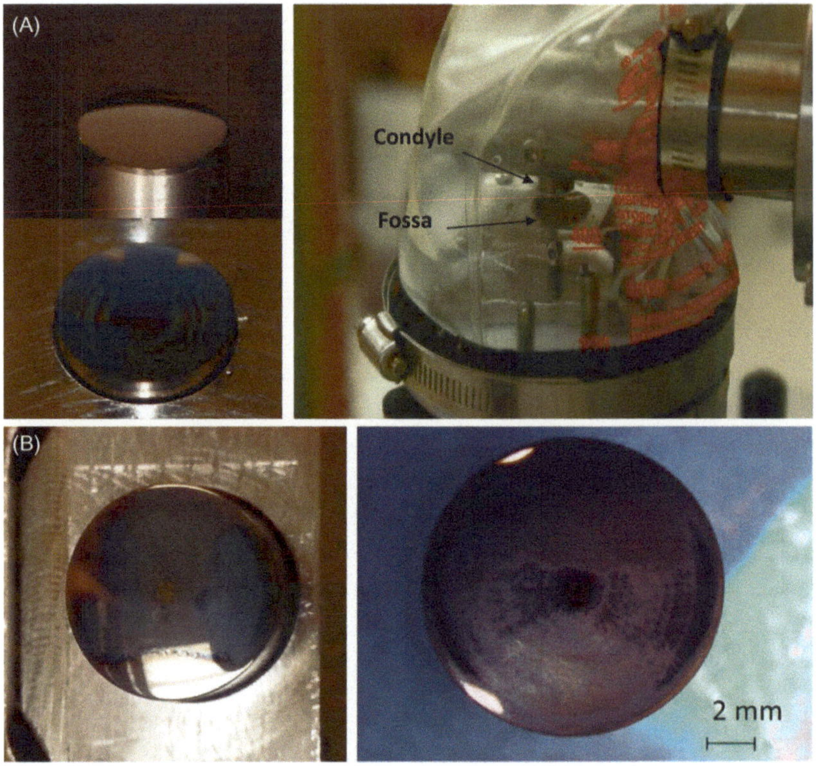

Figure 7.3 (A) NSD-coated wear couple; condyle (top-left) and fossa (bottom-left). Wear simulator set up with fluid housing and wear couple is also shown. (B) Optical imaging of the condyle contact area during and after 5 million cycles is shown. Even after 5 million cycles only light polishing of the diamond surface occurred. There was some mismatch in the radius of curvature of the two components, with the condyle having a slightly smaller radius. Currently experiments are being conducted to account for the mismatch by accurately measuring the amount of expansion of the material and then altering the initial curvature to account for the dimensional change. *Reprinted from Baker PA, Thompson RG, Catledge SA. A wear simulation study of nanostructured CVD diamond-on-diamond articulation involving concave/convex mating surfaces. J Coat Technol Res 2016;13 (2):385–93, Copyright (2015), with permission from American Coatings Association.*

were performed. Thus the next level of testing was to lubricate the surfaces with simulated body fluid and extend the simulation length, while making the surfaces more closely conforming to distribute the load (Fig. 7.3A).

The configuration used in a more current study was an attempt to lower the contact stress by matching the curvature of both surfaces so that the applied load was distributed evenly. In a perfect contact situation as in the current configuration, the stress would only be 3.46 MPa, well below the yield strength of the metal. In order to determine an appropriate load for the wear test, ASTM standard F732-00 (2011) was chosen, even though this standard is for wear testing polymeric materials used in total joint prosthesis. It was chosen due to the lack of existing wear simulation testing standards for ceramic on ceramic devices. In this standard, the average contact stress should be 3.54 MPa; this value is specified for a sliding wear test using polymer on metal. Another specification in the standard is for a "hip-type" wear test, with a designated contact stress of 2–10 MPa. The configuration chosen for the current test, with a calculated contact area of approximately 65 mm^2 and a load of 225 N provides a contact stress of 3.46 MPa. Therefore, the wear test performed in this study falls very close to the specification for linear wear and is well within the range for the "hip-type" test. At least for small mouth opening movements, the conventional "ball in cup" geometry of the hip joint is similar to that of the TMJ.

Another rationale for choosing the 225 N load for the TMJ in the wear simulator test follows from the work of Marks et al. [54], where they measured the strain on the condylar bones of miniature pigs and then used the surface area of the condyles to calculate the load on the condyle surface. They estimated the load at 135 N per condyle for mastication and 227 N for stimulation (single muscle contraction). Alternatively, a method of approximation is to use the value for the bite force reported by Hylander [55]which is 196 N. Multiplying this value by 80% (the condylar reaction force is approximately 75–80% of the bite force) [29] gives a value of 157 N for the load on the condyle during biting. The configuration used in our current study creates a simplified approximation to the type of articulation seen in the TMJ for small mouth opening movements. Thus the selection of 225 N load for the wear simulator test matches well or exceeds specified and published wear loads for similar tests and applications.

7.4 ROLE OF CERAMIC-BORIDING ON CoCr FOR SUBSEQUENT CVD DIAMOND DEPOSITION

Boriding results in a much higher hardness and higher resistance to wear, oxidation, and corrosion compared to other conventional thermochemical surface modification methods like carburizing and nitriding [56–59]. While boriding of steels (primarily using powder packing or molten salt methods) is widely reported, research on cobalt borides has become more active only in the past decade because of their catalytic and magnetic properties [60–62]. Previous reports show that boriding by high-temperature liquid baths and powder packing can improve CVD diamond compatibility with cobalt alloys. In a recent study by Johnston et al. [45], the microwave plasma-enhanced (PE) CVD process was used to deposit interlayers composed primarily of the borides of cobalt and chromium. The use of diborane (B_2H_6) in the plasma feedgas allows for the formation of a robust boride interlayer for suppressing graphitic carbon during subsequent CVD of NSD. This metal–boride interlayer is shown to be an effective diffusion barrier against elemental cobalt for improving nucleation and adhesion of NSD coatings on a CoCrMo alloy. Migration of elemental cobalt to the surface of the interlayer is significantly reduced and undetectable on the surface of the subsequently grown NSD coating. Boriding of CoCrMo resulted in improved adhesion of NSD coatings with low surface roughness.

The extent of boron diffusion was investigated using cross-sectional energy dispersive X-ray spectrum (EDS) and SEM (Fig. 7.4) [45]. The micrograph shows a dense surface layer (dark region) consisting primarily of body-centered tetragonal cobalt boride (Co_2B), with lesser concentrations of cobalt boride (CoB), chromium boride (CrB), and molybdenum boride (MoB). Furthermore, EDS confirmed graded boron diffusion into the bulk CoCrMo substrate. Diffusion of boron into the substrate is expected to form chemical compounds with cobalt, resulting in Co_2B and CoB structures. Up-diffusion of cobalt through a dense boride layer would occur predominately by a vacancy-assisted mechanism. The activation energy for vacancy exchange in the covalently bonded boride layer is expected to be sufficiently high compared to the alloy to limit cobalt up-diffusion to the growing NSD surface. Formation of these covalent boride compounds (and others) is expected to minimize access of elemental cobalt from the bulk to the surface where it could otherwise interact with carbon to form graphite during subsequent NSD deposition. The gradual variation in boron concentration across several microns near the interface is encouraging from the standpoint of boride adhesion and its potential to act as an effective barrier to elemental cobalt diffusion.

Modification by boriding has been known to increase the hardness of some metals, and it has been reported to form a robust and hard boride surface layer on CoCrMo [63–66]. Nanoindentation was used to evaluate the hardness and elastic versus plastic depth for both unborided (but polished) CoCrMo and borided CoCrMo (Fig. 7.5) [45]. The data with error bars represent average and standard deviation for 10 indents, each providing a single hardness at a specific depth. Tests on the unborided alloy to a 1500 nm depth showed an average hardness of 5.8 GPa. The large scatter in the data and higher average values closer to the surface may be due to localized regions of work-hardening from the grinding/polishing steps (Fig. 7.5A). The surface of the borided alloy showed significantly increased hardness, peaking to 25.2 GPa near the 400 nm depth, and dropping off with increasing depths into the bulk alloy (Fig. 7.5B). From glancing-angle XRD data (not shown), the surface hardness is expected to result from a mixture of the constituent metal-borides.

The reported hardness of CoB and Co_2B ranges significantly in the literature due to varied measurement techniques, surface conditions, and substrate material. CoB has reported microhardness values ranging from 18 to 21 GPa [62,67], and a Berkovich nanoindentation hardness of 30 GPa [62]. Co_2B has reported microhardness values ranging from 14 to 17 GPa [62,67], and a nanoindentation hardness of 18 GPa [62]. Additionally, combined CoB and Co_2B layers have been shown to have a

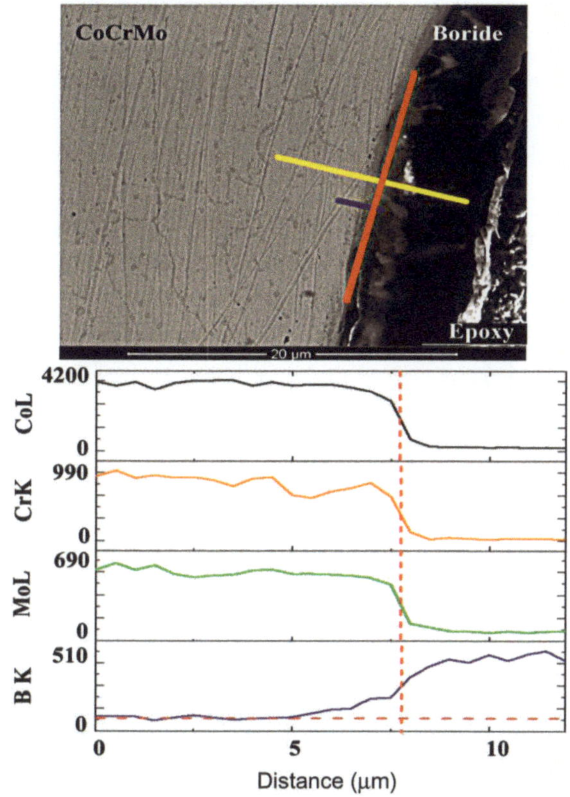

Figure 7.4 Cross-sectional SEM imaging and corresponding EDS. (Bottom) Line profile EDS of the cross-sectioned, borided CoCrMo disk. The vertical line is suggested as a midpoint between min/max elemental constituents. (Top) SEM of a cross-sectioned, borided CoCrMo disk. Yellow line represents line profile for EDS measurement. Blue line represents the approximate region of boron diffusion into the substrate. Red lines correspond to the estimated location of midpoint between min/max elemental constituents. The contrast-enhanced boride region show distinct areas near the surface and near the substrate that likely correspond to CoB and Co_2B borides, respectively. *Reprinted from Johnston JM, Jubinsky M, Catledge SA. Plasma boriding of a cobalt–chromium alloy as an interlayer for nanostructured diamond growth. Appl Surface Sci 2015;328:133–9, Copyright (2015), with permission from Elsevier.*

microhardness of only 9–12 GPa [68,69]. The measured peak nanoindentation hardness value of 25.2 GPa by Johnston et al. [45] falls within the range of other reported values for cobalt borides, but is much higher than microhardness of the combined CoB-Co_2B layer. We expect that there are two primary sources of variation in our hardness values. First the use of nanoindentation rather than microhardness testing reduces the influence of structural defects such as porosity. Second, the boride layer in this study [45] consists of a complex mixture of borides including not only CoB and Co_2B but also MoB (18 GPa [70]) and CrB (21 GPa [71]). Chromium in particular is known for forming very hard boride layers; mixed CrB and Cr_2B has a reported hardness of 28 GPa [72]. Fig. 7.5C and D shows average load-displacement data comparing unborided and borided alloy. The relative elastic versus plastic components of indentation depth are evident. For the unborided alloy, the elastic contribution is approximately 8% while that for the borided alloy is approximately 27%.

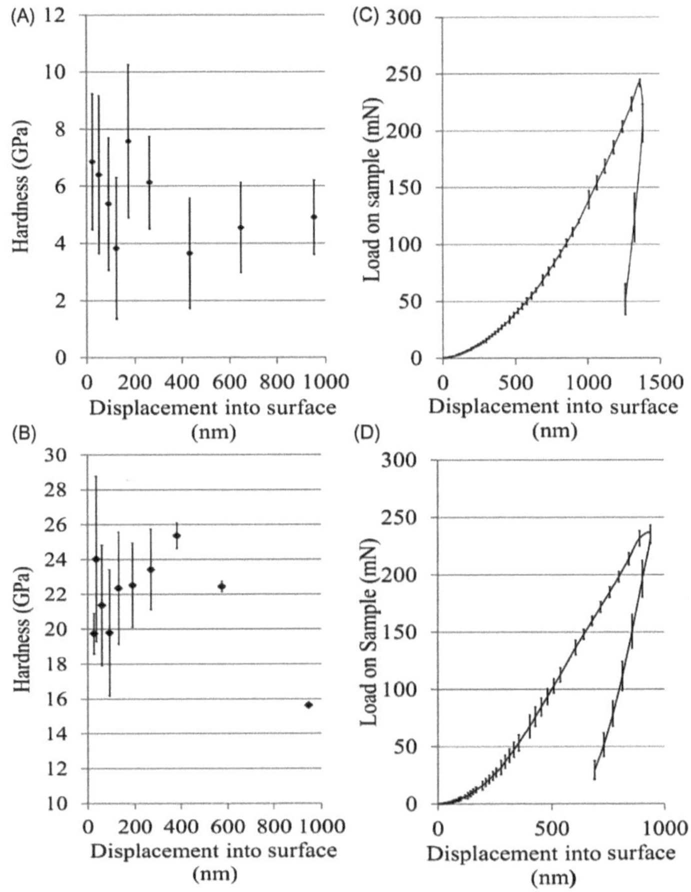

Figure 7.5 Nanoindentation test of unborided CoCrMo and borided CoCrMo. (A) Nanoindentation hardness testing on the raw CoCrMo alloy showed an average bulk hardness of 5.8 GPa. (B) The average hardness measured at 400 nm for CoCrMo-boride was 25.2 GPa. Hardness converged to bulk CoCrMo at an increasing depth (not shown). (C) Load vs displacement graph for CoCrMo up to 250 mN load shows a displacement of up to 1380 nm. (D) Load vs displacement graph for CoCrMo-boride up to 250 mN load shows a displacement of up to 938 nm. In all cases vertical error bars have been calculated using the standard of deviation ($n = 10$). *Reprinted from Johnston JM, Jubinsky M, Catledge SA. Plasma boriding of a cobalt–chromium alloy as an interlayer for nanostructured diamond growth. Appl Surface Sci 2015;328:133–9, Copyright (2015), with permission from Elsevier.*

One large area of interest in the investigation of CVD boriding is the effect that temperature and time play on the formation of surface borides and masking of elemental cobalt from the surface. While there are reported processes for producing boride layers for diamond deposition by way of powder packing or liquid bath boriding [56,60], an investigation of the microwave plasma CVD process for boriding and subsequent diamond growth remains relatively unexplored. Furthermore, the highly controllable CVD process allows a study of very specific surface temperatures and very precise deposition times as opposed to a thermal range and a more gradual cooling timeframe [73]. The effects of CVD surface temperature and deposition time on the presence of FCC Co and metal-borides was recently investigated [45]. A comparison of XRD peak intensity across a range of temperatures (Fig. 7.6A) and times

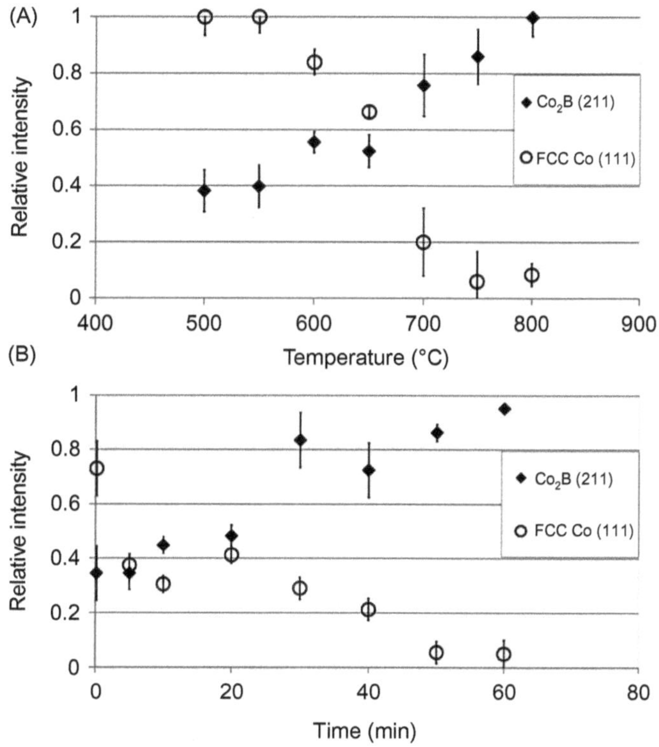

Figure 7.6 XRD peak intensity comparison of Co_2B and FCC Co after boriding at varied times and temperatures. (A) A comparison of XRD peak intensity for CoCrMo boriding at various temperatures, for a set time of 1 h, shows an increase in surface Co_2B and a decrease in FCC Co with increased temperature. (B) A comparison of peak intensity for various times, at a constant 750°C surface temperature, shows an increase in surface Co_2B and a decrease in FCC Co with increased time. Vertical error bars have been calculated using the standard of deviation ($n = 3$) at each temperature and time. *Reprinted from Johnston JM, Jubinsky M, Catledge SA. Plasma boriding of a cobalt–chromium alloy as an interlayer for nanostructured diamond growth. Appl Surface Sci 2015;328:133–9, Copyright (2015), with permission from Elsevier.*

(Fig. 7.6B) shows that as temperature or time increase the relative peak intensity caused by surface concentration of elemental cobalt is reduced. Additionally, the presence of Co_2B increased. The presence of FCC cobalt was effectively masked at 60 minutes and 750°C. Likewise, the presence of Co_2B was maximized at 60 minutes and 800°C. Temperatures over 750°C often resulted in inhomogeneous surface deposition and surface layer delamination. Data taken at 120 minutes revealed no significant change from 60 minutes.

Overall, the results indicate that boriding masks the presence of elemental cobalt and provides a sufficient layer of Co_2B that may be useful for subsequent NSD film growth. Ideal temperature conditions for CoCrMo borided were found to occur at a 750°C. Although no maximum could be identified for boride deposition time, the minimum time required to form a boride layer with full masking of FCC cobalt was found to be 50 minutes. NSD deposition was performed on CoCrMo disks that were borided at 750°C substrate temperature for 1 hour [45]. Depositing NSD over the boride layer (using a $H_2/CH_4/N_2$ feedgas mixture) resulted in a well-adhered coating with Raman spectra (Fig. 7.7) and surface morphology characteristic of NSD. The Raman feature at 1332 cm^{-1} (shown with dashed line) is attributed to ordered

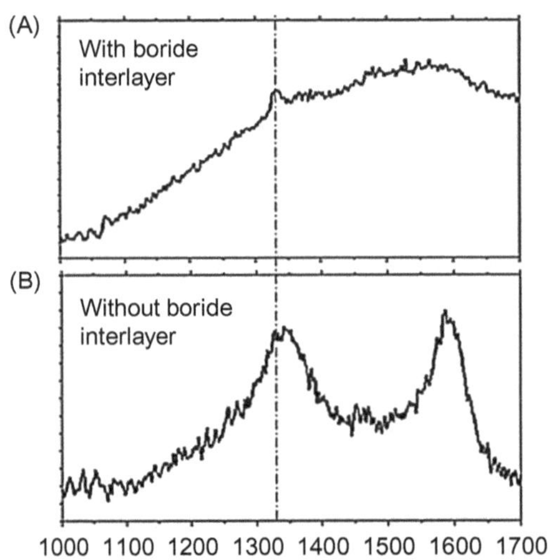

Figure 7.7 Raman spectra of diamond deposition on CoCrMo with and without boriding. (A) The Raman feature at 1332 cm^{-1} (shown with dashed line) is attributed to ordered sp^3-bonded carbon and the broad band c. 1550 cm^{-1} is associated with disordered carbon. (B) Without use of a boride, microcrystalline graphite is formed with characteristic "D" and "G" bands c. 1350 cm^{-1} and 1580 cm^{-1}. *Reprinted from Johnston JM, Jubinsky M, Catledge SA. Plasma boriding of a cobalt–chromium alloy as an interlayer for nanostructured diamond growth. Appl Surface Sci 2015;328:133–9, Copyright (2015), with permission from Elsevier.*

sp^3-bonded carbon and the broad band ca. 1550 cm^{-1} is associated with disordered carbon (Fig. 7.7A). Without the use of a boride interfacial layer, microcrystalline graphite is formed with characteristic "D" and "G" bands c. 1350 and 1580 cm^{-1}, respectively (Fig. 7.7B).

7.5 BIOCOMPATIBILITY AND OSTEO-INTEGRATION OF NANODIAMOND COATED IMPLANT

It is well understood that nanostructured materials respond to in vitro cells and in vivo differently compared to classic materials surfaces. NSD-coated implants interacted with most of the cells including human mesenchymal stem cells (hMSCs) favorably toward a better mineralization and biointegration. Data on the detailed cell–NSD interactions with various cells and surfaces with varying topology and roughness, terminal functional groups and wettability, surfaces with varying substrate chemistry were reported earlier [29,74] and the interactions of NSD with osteogenic and other cells in vitro is beyond the scope of this chapter. However, *p*-type electrical conductivity on nanodiamond films can be obtained by boron doping [75]. Only a couple of studies reported the influence of boron-doped nanodiamond films on the adhesion, growth, differentiation, and functions of osteoblasts [75,76]. This demands that more studies are required to evaluate the effect of boron-doped NSD and boride intermetallics and ceramics on biocompatibility and osteo-integration. We have studied the in vivo biocompatibility of NSD-coated diamond surfaces for TMJ devices in animal models for evidence of osteo-integration and biocompatibility. The initial in vivo biocompatibility profiles showed evidence that bone integration with NSD may be comparable with Ti6Al4V, observed from staining of bone on the diamond surface [77]. Recently, we have implanted NSD-based TMJ device in pigs for the long term (1 year) and the histological analyses of the periprostatic tissue confirmed the in vivo biocompatibility (unpublished data). Seven animals have undergone implantation of both left and right TMJ devices. After 1 year, the devices were explanted and four areas of soft tissue from around each joint were examined histologically for morphologic changes as previously described [78]. By semiquantitative methods [78] an ordinal score (0–3) was assigned to each soft tissue specimen based on three factors: the presence and extent of necrosis, amount of tissue area containing inflammatory cells, and presence and extent of lymphocytic vascular cuffing. There was a maximal score of nine. Histologic examination (Fig. 7.8) revealed only minimal alterations of the periprosthetic tissue with median scores for all devices of four or less. The tissue was characterized by neovascularization and an inflammatory composition of predominantly macrophages and lymphocytes. PMNs and plasma cells were only seen rarely and in a patchy distribution. Scattered isolated areas of

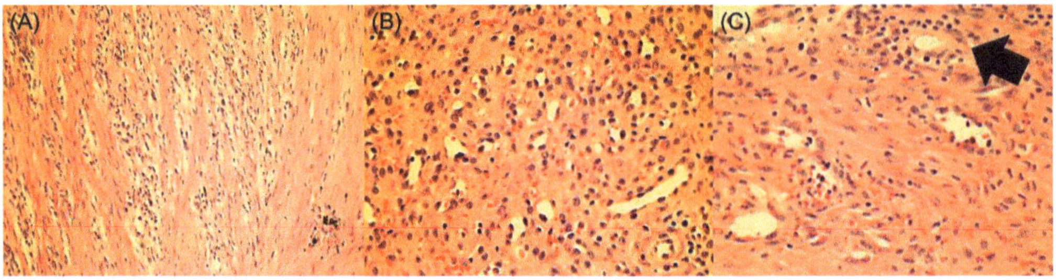

Figure 7.8 Periprostatic TMJ soft tissue consistent with low-grade inflammation and granulation tissue. (A) Specimens demonstrate primarily low-grade mononuclear cell infiltrates with rare neutrophils present. (B) Areas of prominent neovascularization. (C) Low-grade lymphocytic cuffing (arrow). Seven animals underwent implantation of both left and right TMJ devices. After 1 year, the devices were explanted and four areas of soft tissue from around each joint were examined histologically for morphologic changes.

necrosis were identified comprising <5% of the tissue. These features are consistent with granulation tissue related to device implantation [79].

7.6 NANODIAMOND (ND) WEAR-DEBRIS AND INFLUENCE OF SIZE AND CONCENTRATION OF WEAR-DEBRIS ON INFLAMMATION

An ongoing concern in conventional total joint replacement prostheses is osteolysis and aseptic loosening induced by wear-debris originating from the interfaces of articulating components [80–83]. Macrophages and multinuclear giant cells (MNGCs, formed by the fusion of macrophages) are the primary scavengers of wear particles and their response appears to depend on the nature, size, and concentration of particles accumulated [84,85]. Polyethylene debris surrounded by macrophages and phagocytosis of debris by macrophages has been frequently observed at the interface of tissues [81]. Phagocytic cells engulf wear-debris and become activated, releasing proinflammatory cytokines, degradative enzymes, and other factors that stimulate osteoclasts [80–83,86]. It is also known that particles of high-density polyethylene, bone cement, and chromium–cobalt cause inflammatory reactions and a marked decrease in the amount of ingrown bone [80]. Wearing and the generation of resultant wear-debris particles can lead to mechanical instability, decreased joint mobility, increased pain, deleterious biological responses, osteolysis, and ultimately component loosening and implant failure [84,85,87]. Large debris pieces are normally sequestered by fibrous tissue, while small debris pieces are phagocytosed by macrophages and multinucleated giant cells, which may release cytokines that result in inflammation. The inflammation cascade also leads to the recruitment of activated osteoclasts at the bone–implant interface and to bone resorption around the implant.

Studies have shown that less wear occurs with metal-on-metal hip prostheses, up to 100 times less than that of polyethylene-on-metal and CoCrMo metal articulation results in smaller debris particles than the metal-on-polyethylene articulation [87–89]. The CoCrMo debris from a metal-on-metal articulation was shown to be in the range of 6–744 nm, with an average size of 42 nm [89], but, polyethylene particles ranged from 0.1 to 5 μm (100–5000 nm) [90]. As the metal wear-particles are relatively smaller than polyethylene particles, they may be less prone to inflammation and osteolytic reaction. A study investigating bone and tissue reactions to metal debris using several metal-on-metal components revealed that there were fewer macrophages and giant cells than typically seen in tissues around metal-on-polyethylene joints [87]. Unfortunately, there are concerns and debate associated with metal sensitivity and metallosis, the release of alloy constituents into the surrounding tissue. The term "metallosis" has also been used to describe the intraoperative findings of gross metallic debris and blackening of periprosthetic tissue [91]. Metal sensitivity, which affects approximately 10–15% of the general population, is much higher among patients with failed implants [92–94].

The reduced wear volume and particle size expected for diamond articulation are a major advantage over conventional orthopedic bearings. However, a low wear volume in itself is not the only important factor governing the long-term clinical outcome of a total joint replacement. The number, morphology, and biological response to any wear particles released are also important. The majority of previous studies on the biological effects of metallic particles have been conducted using CoCr alloy particles, mainly in nanoscale [95–99]. CoCr prostheses are reported to produce up to 2.5×10^{14} particles/year of articulation and wear debris in the nanoscale range (with a diameter range of 50–115 nm) [86,89], which is 13–500 times more particles than the 5×10^{11} polyethylene particles produced per year in a typical metal-on-polyethylene prosthesis. For wear volumes even as low as 1 mm^3 per year, a very large number of nanoscale particles can exist. In addition to their biological effects on cells and tissues, the smaller metal particles may markedly increase the metal ion levels locally and in the bloodstream due to their large surface area per unit volume. Metal particles have been shown to be disseminated throughout the body including lymph nodes, liver, spleen, and bone marrow [100,101]. Fig. 7.9 shows the wear debris (size and number) for metal–polyethylene and metal–metal couples compared to that projected for NSD–polyethylene wear. Clinically relevant alumina ceramic wear particles have been shown to be less biologically active than polyethylene particles, and this coupled with dramatically reduced wear volumes means that the osteolytic potential of ceramic-on-ceramic hip prostheses is much lower than ceramic-on-polyethylene or metal hip prostheses. However, the use of zirconia as a bearing surface against polyethylene has not proven as successful clinically as alumina-on-polyethylene bearings. In comparing alumina-, zirconia-, and metal-on-conventional

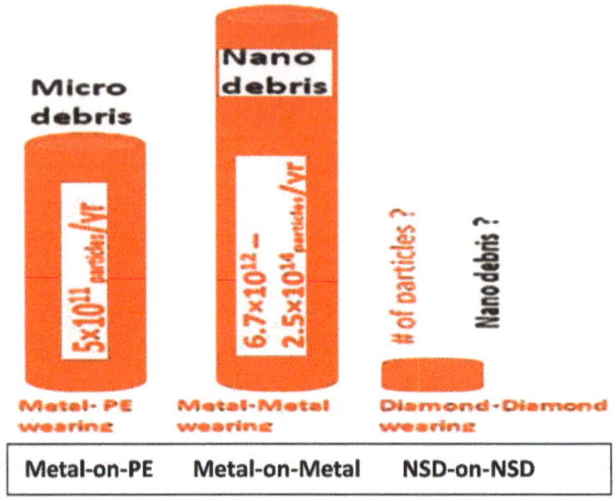

Figure 7.9 Potential number and size of wear debris produced per year from various wearing couples.

polyethylene bearings in total hip patients, the highest wear rate occurs in the zirconia group. Zirconia, which is as wear-resistant as alumina, tends to change its crystalline structure to a form that is less tough and more prone to wear. In general, alumina-on-alumina joints have shown very low wear rates clinically, though the results are design-dependent. Recent reports also show excellent wear resistance in young patients, with no measurable wear and no evidence of osteolysis even beyond a decade of follow-up [102]. Furthermore, very few implant fractures have been observed, even in this high-demand patient population, providing support for the improved mechanical properties of alumina. Oxidized zirconium is used for femoral heads in hip replacement and the femoral component in knee replacement, and initial results look promising. However, longer-term studies will be needed to prove that the improved bearing properties of oxidized zirconium lead to longer-lasting implants.

For a diamond-on-polyethylene couple, polyethylene has much lower hardness compared to diamond and would account for essentially all of the wear-particles generated. However, for a diamond-on-diamond couple, diamond wear-particles are expected to be produced. The reduced wear volume expected for NSD articulation is a major advantage over conventional orthopedic bearings. However, low wear in and of itself is not the only important factor governing the long-term clinical outcome of a total joint replacement. The number, morphology, and biological response to a given population of wear particles is also important. Although our preliminary pin/disk data [50] have demonstrated a factor of two reduction in wear for NSD—polyethylene compared to NSD—CoCr, this wear couple requires further study to evaluate wear-debris and biological response under simulated joint conditions. A limitation is that the amount of nanodiamond-debris generated from a wear couple in a simulator is expected to be negligible due to its superior hardness, smoothness, and wear-resistant properties as stated previously. Moreover, the particles produced in simulators or by other means do not consistently resemble wear-debris particles from joint-implants in vivo. Therefore, in one of our studies, synthetic nanodiamond particles of different sizes (ranging from 6 to 500 nm) and varying concentrations (10–200 μg/mL) were utilized to interact with macrophage cells in vitro [103]. Macrophage response to titanium dioxide (anatase) particles (~8 nm average size), a well-known nanoparticle, was evaluated for purpose of comparison. In order to quantify the inflammatory response of the macrophages to nanoparticles, cytokines such as TNF-α (tumor necrosis factor-α), IL-1β (interleukin-1β), chemokines such as Cxcl2 and MIP-1α (macrophage inhibitory protein), Ccl2 or MCP-1 (monocyte chemotactic protein), and growth factors such as VEGF (vascular endothelial growth factor) and PDGF (platelet-derived growth factor) synthesized by the macrophage cells were measured using quantitative reverse transcription (Fig. 7.10). The NSD wear particles have been shown to be less biologically active than titanium particles, as shown in apoptosis studies (Fig. 7.10). Wear-particle-induced inflammation is largely dependent on the debris characteristics such as size, dose (i.e., the number of particles per cell or tissue volume), and morphology (relative abundance of various shapes, including fibrillar) and surface chemistry of particulate debris [104–114], which in turn is dependent on the nature and properties of wearing surfaces. There is no consensus as to which size, shape, and dose ratio of nanoscopic particles within this osteolytic range (<1 μm), are maximally inflammatory. Our in vitro studies to evaluate the effect of nanodiamond particle size on macrophage proliferation, viability, and cytokine gene expression [103] suggest that exposure to nanodiamond wear debris may inhibit rather than increase inflammation. The qPCR results given in Fig. 7.10 show that most of the cytokines were reduced in the presence of nanodiamonds. This may possibly be due to decrease in cell viability as shown by an apoptosis assay (Fig. 7.11).

TNF-α and IL-1β are known bone-resorbing or osteolytic factors expressed by many cells such as macrophages, monocytes, and osteoclasts and their concentrations are low in cells in the absence of exogenous stimuli but become synthesized de novo when the cell is activated [115]. Studies have shown that TNF-α stimulates the production of proinflammatory adhesion molecules and increases the differentiation and maturation of osteoclasts, resulting in bone resorption both in vitro and in vivo [105,116–118]. IL-1β is a proinflammatory and prowound-healing cytokine that activates lymphocytes, chemokines such as MCP-1, and osteolytic cytokines such as TNF-α and IL-6. TNF-α production has been implicated in inducing apoptosis of adherent macrophage on biomaterials [117]. Of relevance to the present work was the absence of increased gene expression of both bone-resorbing proinflammatory factors when exposed to nanodiamond wear particles of varying sizes at a concentration of 50 μg/mL. Huang et al. [119] have also reported no significant variation in the mRNA levels for three genes (TNFα, IL-6, and iNOS) on exposure to very small-sized detonation nanodiamond (2–8 nm) at a relatively low concentration of

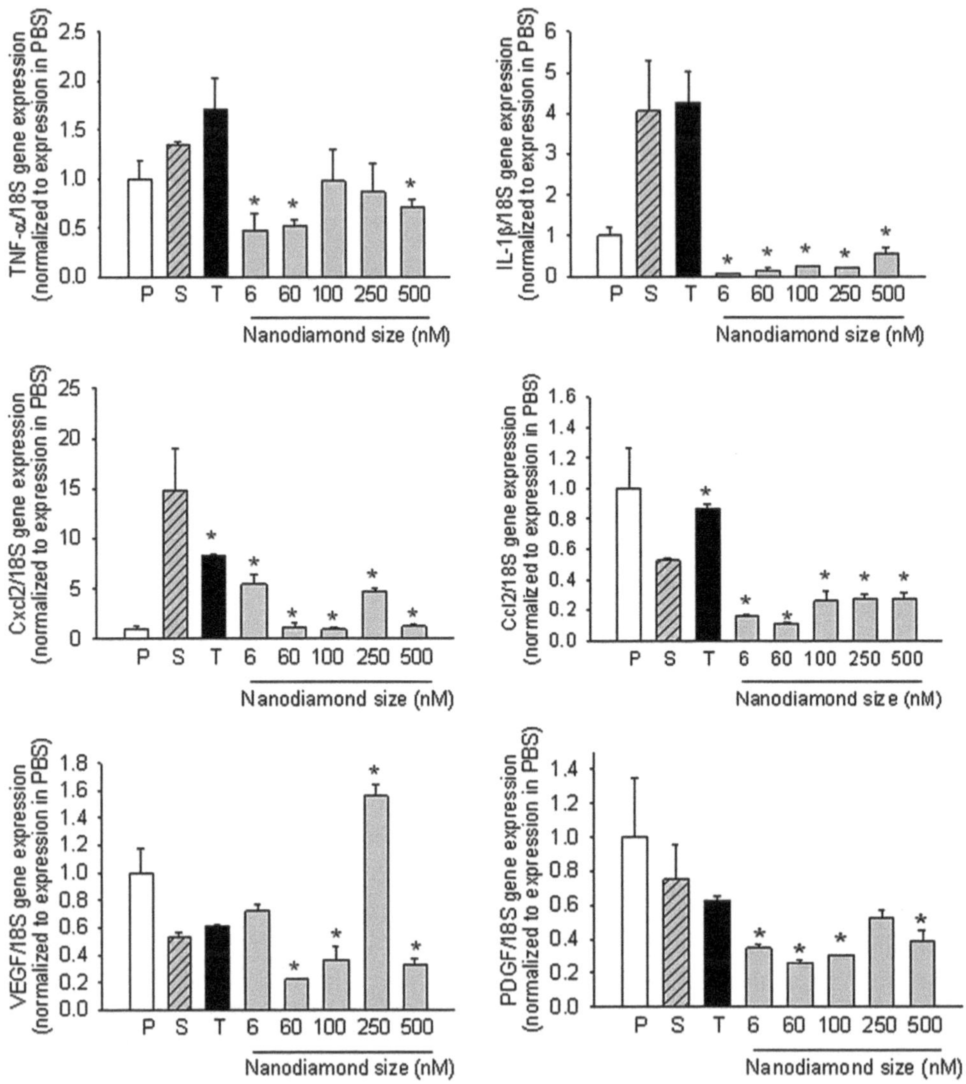

Figure 7.10 Gene expression of selected cytokines and growth factors. P, PBS; S, serum; T, TiO2 NP; $*P < 0.05$ vs serum control. *Reprinted from Thomas V, Halloran B, Ambalavanan N, Catledge SA, Vohra YK. In vitro studies on the effect of particle size on macrophage responses to nanodiamond wear debris. Acta Biomaterialia 2012;8(5):1939–47, Copyright (2012), with permission from Elsevier.*

30 μg/mL. The reduction noticed in our studies could be due to concentration-dependent effects. A comparable in vitro study of culturing RAW 264.7 cell line with metal particles (stainless steel) for 24 hours showed upregulation of both TNF-α and IL-1β with a significant number of late apoptotic cells [120].

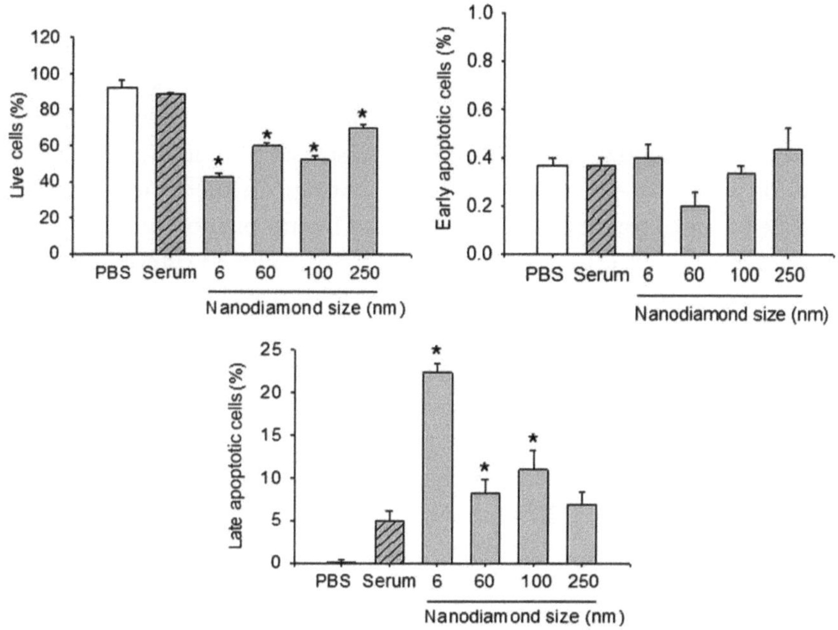

Figure 7.11 Cell viability and apoptosis as estimated by flow cytometry after culturing. A total of 200,000 cells/well with 50 μg/mL nanodiamonds in MEM containing 10% FCS in a 24-well plate for 24 h. Cells were washed with 250 μL PBS and labeled with propidium iodide and Annexin V-FITC (1:100). Unlabeled (nonnecrotic and nonapoptotic) cells were plotted for cell viability. $^{*}P < 0.05$ vs serum-only or PBS control. *Reprinted from Thomas V, Halloran B, Ambalavanan N, Catledge SA, Vohra YK. In vitro studies on the effect of particle size on macrophage responses to nanodiamond wear debris. Acta Biomaterialia 2012;8(5):1939–47, Copyright (2012), with permission from Elsevier*

Chemokine MIP-1α is involved in chemotaxis and recruitment of monocytes and leukocytes during inflammation, while chemokine MCP-1 recruits macrophages and stimulates murine FBGC fusion in vivo [105]. MCP-1 also stimulates interleukin-1 (IL-1) and IL-6 release from monocyte/macrophages. VEGF, a proangiogenic cytokine, and PDGF, a connective tissue mitogen, have been implicated in periprosthetic osteolysis and subsequent aseptic loosening of implants following total hip arthroplasty [121–123]. VEGF promotes blood vessel dilation and angiogenesis in the event of inflammation to promote wound healing in damaged tissue. Therefore, reduction or lack of upregulated expression of proinflammatory chemokines and prowound healing (VEGF) cytokine levels in the presence of nanodiamond particles suggests no severe signs of inflammation-related processes (compared to serum-only the control). However, the situation could be different in vivo as cells may release cytokines from preformed stores and then die, and these released cytokines might attract fresh macrophages from nearby tissue or the blood circulation. PCR and the gene expression experiments may be considered complementary to the measures of apoptosis/necrosis

(Fig. 7.11). However, in vitro studies may have results different from in vivo studies, as in vitro studies do not have recruitment of inflammatory cells from the circulation, and there is no translocation of the nanoparticles to other locations. This coupled with dramatically reduced wear and a resulting lower level of debris release indicates that the osteolytic potential of NSD-coated prostheses should be much lower than those involving metal-on-polyethylene. NSD coatings on metal are also expected to act as a barrier to metal ion release. Although the failure or loosening of joint replacement components is often multifactorial, wear-debris-induced osteolysis is a key factor among them. Macrophages activated by the phagocytosis of particulate wear debris are the key cells in this process, which can potentially occur in any implant system regardless of implant design or fixation mode. Our study [103] on the effect of nanodiamond particle size on macrophage responses was assessed by measuring the proliferation, viability, cellular morphology, apoptosis (Fig. 7.11), phagocytosis (Fig. 7.12), and genetic expression of proinflammatory cytokines and chemokines (Fig. 7.10) suggested there was no potential inflammation due to size effect at low concentrations (50–100 μg/mL) of diamond wear particles. However, the results mandate more studies to evaluate chemotaxis with nanodiamond particles and to evaluate in vivo responses in animal models.

7.7 SUMMARY AND FUTURE PERSPECTIVES

The clinical consequences of wear of articulating joints and wear debris formation cover a broad spectrum from radiolucencies to massive osteolysis and implant failure. For this reason, the reduction of wear-debris should be a primary goal of new-generation orthopedic joint implants. We have developed ultrasmooth nanodiamond coatings by CVD on orthopedic-implant metals (on titanium alloy for TMJ and on cobalt–chrome alloy for hip and knee joints). The measured hardness of our NSD coatings was shown to be significantly harder (40–90 GPa, depending on processing conditions) than other forms of carbon widely reported in the literature, including the several amorphous variations of DLC (15–35 GPa). The NSD coatings could be more resistant to scratching by third-body wear particles, such as bone cement, due to the high hardness and low surface roughness (rms value $<$ 8 nm) of the coatings. These NSD coatings are comprised of nanoscale diamond grains (less than 5 nm) within an amorphous carbon matrix and have also shown excellent biocompatibility and corrosion resistance in physiological fluids. However, the translational potential of these nanostructured coatings is in a large way determined by their bio-performance (wear-resistance of articulating surfaces and osteo-integration of the rest and bacterial infection resistance).

From a clinical perspective, the superior wear characteristics of NSD on metal prostheses may allow for a hard-on-hard approach of implant design providing a less invasive surgical procedure. In the current market, the industry standard for

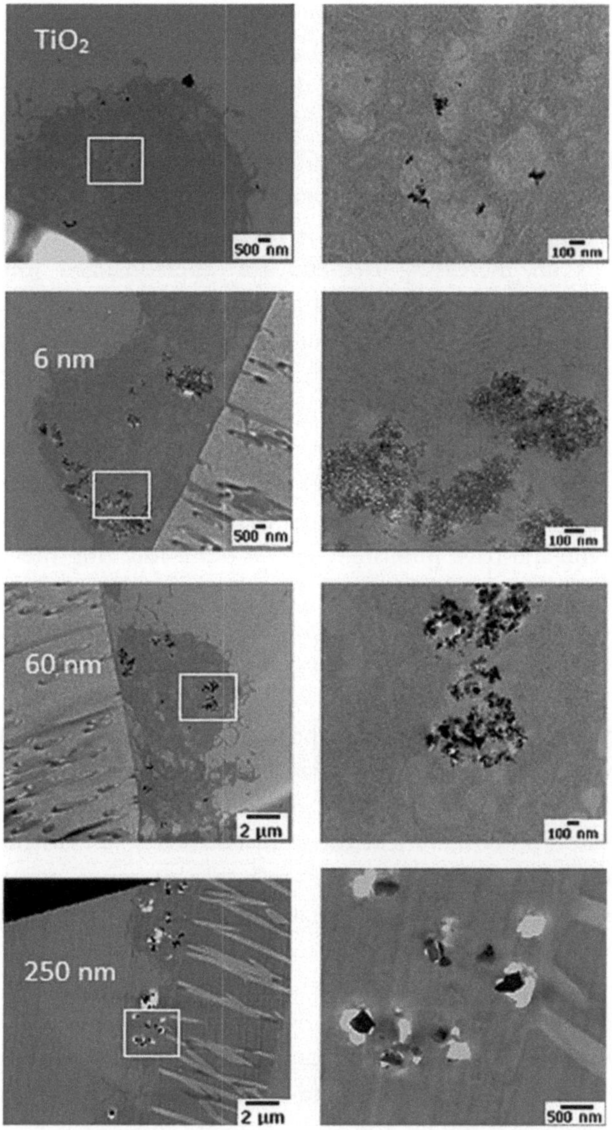

Figure 7.12 Transmission electron microscopic images showing the internalization of TiO_2 nanoparticles (~8 nm) and nanodiamond particles (6, 60, and 250 nm). Higher-magnification images of the corresponding marked area are given on the right side. *Reprinted from Thomas V, Halloran B, Ambalavanan N, Catledge SA, Vohra YK. In vitro studies on the effect of particle size on macrophage responses to nanodiamond wear debris. Acta Biomaterialia 2012;8(5):1939–47, Copyright (2012), with permission from Elsevier.*

orthopedic and dental total joint replacement involves articulation of UHMWPE against a cobalt–chromium alloy. The UHMWPE component requires considerable thickness to stand up to the articular loads. In the case of the hip and knee joints, e.g., a hard-on-hard device (metal-on-metal device with NSD coatings on articular surfaces) engineered to be of sufficient rigidity and smoothness with a suitable design of the articulating components for improving the life-span of the device. With the advancements in 3D printing and CAD/CAM technologies with additive manufacturing (AM), there is an increasing demand for "personalized joint devices" with improved wear properties for load-bearing articulating orthopedic and dental applications. The current market for total knee replacements (TKRs) includes many types of designs from various manufacturers. Two main categories of commonly available designs are those that are cruciate-retaining and posterior-stabilized designs. Another main differentiator of TKRs is whether or not they include a mobile or a fixed bearing. Owing to the extra costs and complexities involved in the design and fabrication of a mobile bearing design, the fixed simpler designs which have been in use for a longer period of time and have published studies demonstrating their wear characteristics, could be a better option.

AM and various 3D printing technologies have been gaining much attention recently in both orthopedic and dental medicine. An advantage of parts produced by AM methods is the ability to create a highly porous surface for greater bone ingrowth [124]. However, the materials properties of parts made via AM methods have not been fully investigated. The layer-by-layer melting technique can sometimes create a part that has different yield strength in the vertical direction as compared to the horizontal direction. This could affect the performance of a load-bearing device such as the knee prosthesis. Another known issue is the presence of small voids formed during the process. These voids could create a problem if they happen to be on the surface of the device. Furthermore, NSD-coated direct metal laser sintering (DMLS) parts have not been investigated. To our knowledge, no diamond-coating process has ever been reported for deposition onto DMLS-created components. This presents a great opportunity for discovery. Many grades of titanium alloy have been used including commercially pure Ti, Ti-6Al-4V, and Ti-10-2-3. Various forms of these alloys have been tested, such as wrought rod, rolled sheet, and cast bar, including forms of the material with different thermomechanical processing treatments. The closest type of manufacturing method that we have tested is a powder metallurgy sample, produced by hot isostatic pressing the Ti alloy powder. But even this does not relate very well to the conditions produced during the laser melting of the powder by DMLS. This provides a unique opportunity to investigate NSD-coated DMLS parts for its viability as a method of making medical devices.

There exists a strong interdependence of DMLS processing parameters such as laser energy density, scan speed, particle size, and powder bed temperature on the part's porosity and other structural features [125,126]. Each material (in starting powder form) responds differently to the DMLS process. For example, the use of aluminum (Al) alloys is still quite limited due to difficulties in processing that result in parts with high degrees of porosity [127]. Factors such as powder flowability, reflectivity, thermal conductivity, and oxidative tendency all impact the degree of porosity. Finally, due to the layer-wise part building nature of DMLS, orientation of the surface can lead to "stair-step" effect and impact surface structure. Mechanical anisotropy is common as a result of the directional scanning, and typically requires postprocessing heat treatment to minimize this effect [26–28]. Fig. 7.13 shows one of the designs of a knee implant by DMLS technology. Fig. 7.14 is the representative SEM images of a DMLS printed titanium disc before and after polishing as professional polishing is required for subsequent NSD coating.

Another, usual concern in joint implants in the medical device industry is infection-associated device failures. According to the Centers for Disease Control and Prevention (CDC), 65% of human bacterial infections involve biofilms [128]. Compared to planktonic cells, biofilms are up to 10–500 times more resistant to antimicrobial agents and disinfectants. The formation of biofilms is mediated by quorum sensing (QS). QS is a mechanism by which both Gram-negative and Gram-positive bacteria can assess their population density through the secretion and sensing of autoinducers (AIs) that regulate the expression of certain genes in a cell-density-dependent manner. Attenuating QS via sequestration of AIs represents a promising strategy to control biofilm development. However, conventional sequestration agents (i.e., antibodies) are unstable and their large-scale production is difficult to achieve.

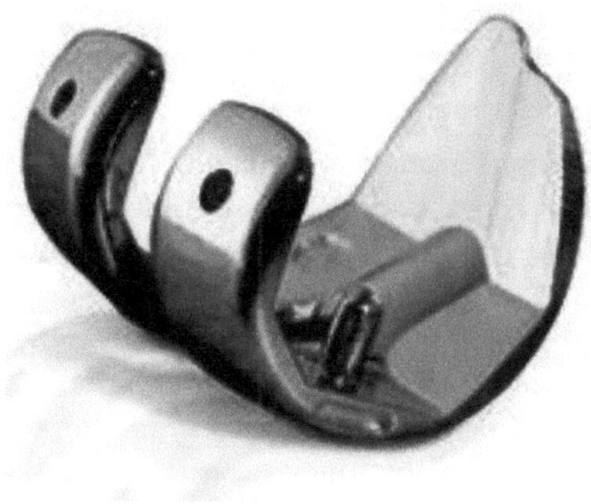

Figure 7.13 The above-knee implant was built by Direct Metal Laser-Sintering (DMLS) using a biocompatible cobalt–chrome alloy. Several such parts can be built fully automatically overnight, even if patient-specific, by Stryker Orthopaedics. *EOS Imaging. http://3dprinting.com/metal/3d-printing-metal/.*

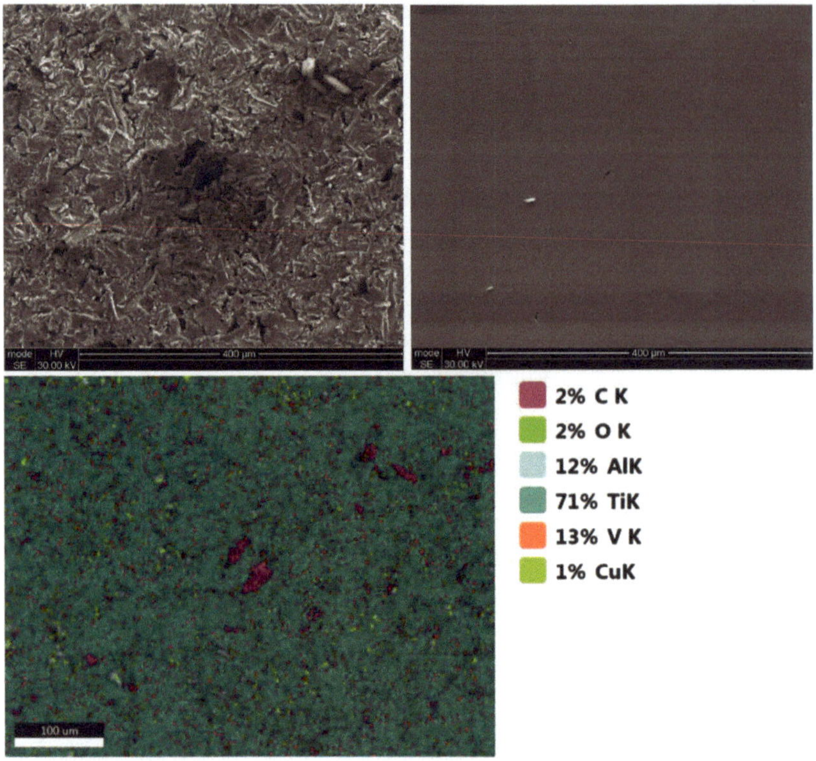

Figure 7.14 Representative SEM images of a neat 3D printed titanium alloy as received (top-left) and polished surface for NSD coating (top-right). The dark particle-like objects seen in SEM of unpolished surfaces are carbon after EDS elemental analyses. The elemental mapping and corresponding composition of the alloy surface are also given (at the bottom). Polishing is required to get a smooth surface for subsequent NSD coating.

Most pathogens delay their production of virulence factors until a critical population density is reached, which then allows a successful infection process against the host. Therefore, QS control may be an effective approach to mediate biofilm formation, and in this way prevent the adherence of pathogenic microorganisms. To address these disadvantages, molecularly imprinted polymers (MIPs), known as "artificial antibodies," offer a relatively new and promising route to specifically capture AIs [129].

MIPs are crosslinked polymers that are formed in the presence of a template molecule. Removal of the template creates binding cavities with affinity and selectivity for the template molecule [130]. Like other synthetic polymers, MIPs can be rapidly prepared and possess excellent chemical, thermal, and mechanical stability. Adsorption of some molecules to native implant surfaces exposed in vivo to a variety of pathogens can lead to an undesirable cascade effect resulting in infection and disease. If the

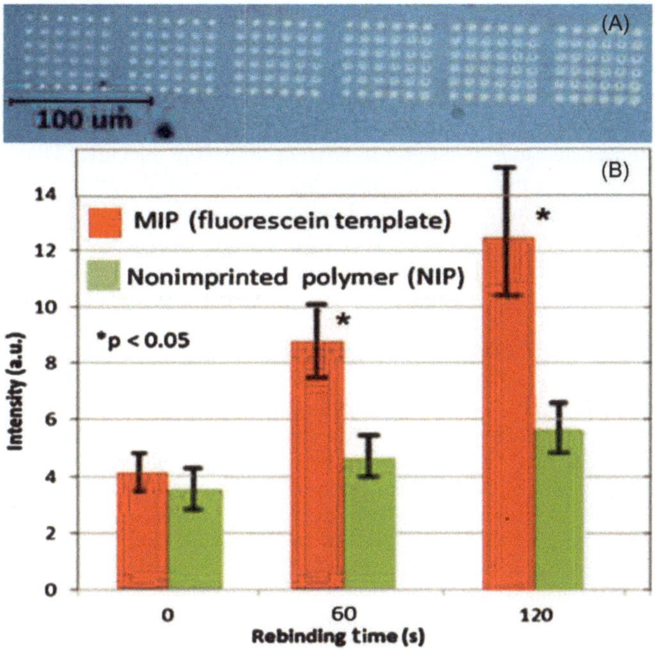

Figure 7.15 (A) Dip-pen lithographically printed MIP array consisting of polymer MIP dots imprinted with fluorescein. (B) Comparison of imprinted and nonimprinted (control) fluorescence after washing and then rebinding with 450 nM fluorescein for varying rebinding times up to 2 min.

implant surface could be modified to include MIPs designed to sequester the signaling molecules responsible for the cascade effect, then the potential for infection could be significantly reduced. Topographically patterned features can also influence the arrangement and the resulting behavior of cells on surfaces and, therefore, may also affect biofilm formation [131]. We have printed MIP using Dip-pen lithography as a promising method to pattern the stem of the joint implants and prevent the bacterial infection by inhibiting the QS and biofilm formation (Fig. 7.15). The interstitial spacing between surface features can be a critical parameter controlling assembly that drives long-range bacterial adhesion patterns and biofilm growth behavior. This passive, nonpharmaceutical approach to biofilm prevention has the added benefit that the sequestration of signaling molecules does not kill bacteria, and therefore the selection pressure to develop resistance is reduced. The use of nonadherent coatings on medical devices, such as catheters, is one strategy that can be used; however, the effect is confined to the device and offers no protection to adjacent tissues and surfaces [132]. The MIP approach disrupts the regulatory system responsible for initiating biofilm formation, thereby preventing biofilm formation in the first place.

ACKNOWLEDGMENTS

The material described in this chapter is partially based upon the work supported by the National Science Foundation Partnership for Innovation (NSF: PFI) program under Grant number IIP-1317210. We would like to thank all our collaborators including Dr. Patrick Louis and Dr. Raymond Thompson who contributed in our research publications referenced in this chapter. Thanks are also due to Mr. William Monroe for his assistance in obtaining SEM images of 3D printed Ti from SEM imaging facility at the Department of Materials Science & Engineering, UAB.

REFERENCES

[1] Goldring SR, Clark CR, Wright TM. The problem in total joint arthroplasty: aseptic loosening. J Bone Joint Surg Am 1993;75(6):799–801.
[2] Bascarevic Z, et al. Alumina-on-alumina ceramic versus metal-on-highly cross-linked polyethylene bearings in total hip arthroplasty: a comparative study. Int Orthop 2010;34(8):1129–35.
[3] Kim YH, Choi Y, Kim JS. Cementless total hip arthroplasty with alumina-on-highly cross-linked polyethylene bearing in young patients with femoral head osteonecrosis. J Arthroplasty 2011;26(2):218–23.
[4] Oonishi H, et al. Change in UHMWPE properties of retrieved ceramic total knee prosthesis in clinical use for 23 years. J Biomed Mater Res B Appl Biomater 2005;74(2):754–9.
[5] Tai SM, et al. Squeaking in large diameter ceramic-on-ceramic bearings in total hip arthroplasty. J Arthroplasty 2015;30(2):282–5.
[6] Rhoads DP, et al. Fracture of an alumina femoral head used in ceramic-on-ceramic total hip arthroplasty. J Arthroplasty 2008;23(8):1239 e25-30.
[7] Hannouche D, et al. Thirty years of experience with alumina-on-alumina bearings in total hip arthroplasty. Int Orthop 2011;35(2):207–13.
[8] Nizard R, et al. Alumina pairing in total hip replacement. J Bone Joint Surg Br 2005;87(6):755–8.
[9] Iwakiri K, et al. Alumina inlay failure in cemented polyethylene-backed total hip arthroplasty. Clin Orthop Relat Res 2008;466(5):1186–92.
[10] Catledge SA, et al. Surface crystalline phases and nanoindentation hardness of explanted zirconia femoral heads. J Mater Sci Mate Med 2003;14(10):863–7.
[11] Santos EM, et al. Examination of surface and material properties of explanted zirconia femoral heads. J Arthroplasty 2004;19(7 Suppl. 2):30–4.
[12] Chevalier J, Cales B, Drouin JM. Low-temperature aging of Y-TZP ceramics. J Amn Ceram Soc 1999;82(8):2150–4.
[13] Bock RM, et al. Surface modulation of silicon nitride ceramics for orthopaedic applications. Acta Biomaterialia 2015;26:318–30.
[14] Bal BS, Rahaman MN. Orthopedic applications of silicon nitride ceramics. Acta Biomaterialia 2012;8(8):2889–98.
[15] Özmen Y. Si3N4 as a biomaterial and its tribo-characterization under water lubrication. Lubr Sci 2016;28(4):243–54.
[16] Innocenti M, et al. The 5-year results of an oxidized zirconium femoral component for TKA. Clin Orthop Relat Res 2010;468(5):1258–63.
[17] Hui C, et al. Five-year comparison of oxidized zirconium and cobalt-chromium femoral components in total knee arthroplasty: a randomized controlled trial. J Bone Joint Surg Am 2011;93(7):624–30.
[18] Ahmed I, et al. Total knee arthroplasty with an oxidised zirconium femoral component: ten-year survivorship analysis. Bone Joint J 2016;98-B(1):58–64.
[19] Van Hove RP, et al. Titanium-nitride coating of orthopaedic implants: a review of the literature. BioMed Res Int 2015;2015:9.
[20] Gotman I, Gutmanas EY. Titanium nitride-based coatings on implantable medical devices. Adv Biomater Devices Med 2014;1(1):53–73.
[21] Oliveira LYS, Kuromoto NK, Siqueira CJM. Treating orthopedic prosthesis with diamond-like carbon: minimizing debris in Ti6Al4V. J Mater Sci Mater Med 2014;25(10):2347–55.

[22] Love CA, et al. Diamond like carbon coatings for potential application in biological implants—a review. Tribol Int 2013;63:141−50.
[23] Spector BM, et al. Wear performance of ultra-high molecular weight polyethylene on oxidized zirconium total knee femoral components. J Bone Joint Surg Am 2001;83-A(Suppl. 2 Pt 2):80−6.
[24] McCalden RW, et al. Damage of an Oxinium femoral head and polyethylene liner following 'routine' total hip replacement. J Bone Joint Surg Br 2011;93(3):409−13.
[25] Jaffe WL, et al. Surface oxidized zirconium total hip arthroplasty head damage due to closed reduction effects on polyethylene wear. J Arthroplasty 2009;24(6):898−902.
[26] Tribe H, et al. Advanced wear of an Oxinium(™) femoral head implant following polyethylene liner dislocation. Ann R Coll Surg Engl 2013;95(8):e133−5.
[27] Hee Ay, C, et al. Effects of surface coating on reducing friction and wear of orthopaedic implants. Sci Technol Adv Mater 2014;15(1):014402.
[28] Sola A, Bellucci D, Cannillo V. Functionally graded materials for orthopedic applications—an update on design and manufacturing. Biotechnol Adv 2016;34(5):504−31.
[29] Catledge SA, Thomas V, Vohra YK. Nanostructured diamond coatings for orthopaedic applications. Woodhead Publ Ser Biomater 2013;2013:105−50.
[30] Keshri AK, Agarwal A. Plasma processing of nanomaterials for functional applications: a review. Nanosci Nanotechnol Lett 2012;4(3):228−50.
[31] Leyland A, Matthews A. On the significance of the H/E ratio in wear control: a nanocomposite coating approach to optimised tribological behaviour. Wear 2000;246(1−2):1−11.
[32] Baker PA, Thompson RG, Catledge SA. A wear simulation study of nanostructured CVD diamond-on-diamond articulation involving concave/convex mating surfaces. J Coat Technol Res 2016;13(2):385−93.
[33] Catledge SA, et al. Improved adhesion of ultra-hard carbon films on cobalt-chromium orthopaedic implant alloy. J Mater Sci Mater Med 2011;22(2):307−16.
[34] Catledge S, Vohra Y. Effect of nitrogen addition on the microstructure and mechanical properties of diamond films grown using high-methane concentrations. J Appl Phys 1999;86:698.
[35] Chowdhury S, et al. Synthesis and mechanical wear studies of ultra smooth nanostructured diamond (USND) coatings deposited by microwave plasma chemical vapor deposition with He/H(2)/CH(4)/N(2) mixtures. Diam Relat Mater 2008;17(4-5):419−27.
[36] Papo MJ, et al. Mechanical wear behavior of nanocrystalline and multilayer diamond coatings on temporomandibular joint implants. J Mater Sci Mater Med 2004;15(7):773−7.
[37] Konovalov VV, et al. Ultra-smooth nanostructured diamond films deposited from He/H2/CH4/N2 microwave plasmas. J Nanosci Nanotechnol 2006;6(1):258−61.
[38] Chowdhury S, Hillman DA, Catledge SA, Konovalov VV, Vohra YK. Synthesis of ultrasmooth nanostructured diamond films by microwave plasma chemical vapor deposition using a He/H2/CH4/N2 gas mixture. J Mater Res 2006;21(10):2675−82.
[39] Catledge SA, et al. Nanostructured ceramics for biomedical implants. J Nanosci Nanotechnol 2002;2(3-4):293−312.
[40] Hill MR, et al. Preliminary tribological evaluation of nanostructured diamond coatings against ultra-high molecular weight polyethylene. J Biomed Mater Res B Appl Biomater 2008;85(1):140−8.
[41] Catledge SAFM, Vohra YK. Nanostructured surface modifications for biomedical implants. In: Nalwa HS, editor. Encyclopedia of nanoscience and nanotechnology, Vol. 7. American Scientific Publishers; 2004. p. 741−62.
[42] Catledge SA, Vohra YK. High density plasma processing of diamond films on titanium: residual stress and adhesion measurements. J Appl Phys 1995;78:7053.
[43] Booth L, et al. Synthesis and characterization of multilayered diamond coatings for biomedical implants. Materials (Basel) 2011;4(5):857−67.
[44] Lawson TR, Catledge SA, Vohra YK. Nanostructured diamond coated CoCrMo alloys for use in biomedical implants. Key Eng Mater 2005;284-286:1015.
[45] Johnston JM, Jubinsky M, Catledge SA. Plasma boriding of a cobalt−chromium alloy as an interlayer for nanostructured diamond growth. Appl Surface Sci 2015;328:133−9.

[46] Buford A, Goswami T. Review of wear mechanisms in hip implants: paper I-General. Mater Des 2005;25(5):385−93.
[47] Mattei L, et al. Lubrication and wear modelling of artificial hip joints: a review. Tribol Int 2011;44 (5):532−49.
[48] McGee MA, et al. Implant retrieval studies of the wear and loosening of prosthetic joints: a review. Wear 2000;241(2):158−65.
[49] Clarke I, et al. Ultra-low wear rates for rigid-on-rigid bearings in total hip replacements. Proc Instn Mech Engrs, Part H J Eng Med 2000;214(4):331−47.
[50] Hill MR, Catledge SA, Konovalov V, Clem WC, Chowdhury SA, Etheidge BS, et al. Preliminary tribological evaluation of nanostructured diamond coatings against ultra-high molecular weight polyethylene. J Biomed Mater Res B Appl Biomater 2008;85(1):140−8.
[51] Yamaleyeva D, Baker P, Sa C, A wear evaluation of ultra high molecualr weight polyethylene (UHMWPE) aganist nanostructured diamond coated Ti-6Al-4V alloy. Journal of Young Inverstigators, 2016.
[52] Fries M. Nanocrystalline diamond thin films on titanium-6 aluminum-4 vanadium alloy temporomandibular joint prosthesis simulants by microwave plasma chemical vapor deposition. ProQuest Dissertations And Theses; Thesis (Ph.D.)−The University of Alabama at Birmingham, Publication Number: AAI3078527; ISBN: 9780493990569; Source. Dissertation Abstracts International,. 2002. Volume: 64-01(Section: B): p. 139.
[53] Malesela J, et al. Mechanical wear behavior of nanocrystalline and multilayer diamond coatings on temporomandibular joint implants. J Mat Sci Mat Med 2004;15(7):773−7.
[54] Marks L, et al. Reaction strains on the condylar neck during mastication and maximum muscle stimulation in different condylar positions: an experimental study in the miniature pig. J Dent Res 1997;76(7):1412−20.
[55] Smith R. Mandibular biomechanics and temporomandibular joint function in primates.. Am J Anthropol 1978;49(3):341−9.
[56] Ulutan M, et al. Tribological properties of borided AISI 4140 steel with the powder pack-boriding method. Tribol Lett 2010;38(3):231−9.
[57] Davis JR, editor. Surface hardening of steels: understanding the basics; CH. 8 Boriding. Materials Park, OH: ASM International; 2002.
[58] Knotek O, Lugscheider E, Leuschen K. Surface layers on cobalt base alloys by boron diffusion. Thin Solid Films 1977;45(2):331−9.
[59] Mu D, et al. Oxidation resistance of borided pure cobalt. J Alloys Comp 2009;479 (1â€"2):629−33.
[60] Walter JC, Revankar S. Study of metal borides for sodium borohydride hydrolysis. Electrochem Soc Trans 2008;6(17):55−63.
[61] Legrand J, et al. Synthesis and XPS characterization of nickel boride nanoparticles. Langmuir 2002;18(10):4131−7.
[62] Campos-Silva I, et al. Growth kinetics and mechanical properties of boride layers formed at the surface of the ASTM F-75 biomedical alloy. Surface Coatings Technol 2013;237:402−14.
[63] Motojima S, Ihama Y. Preparation and some properties of CoB layers and crystals prepared by diffusion and CVD processes. J Crystal Growth 1986;76(2):373−8.
[64] Schmidt H, et al. Diffusion in transition metal diborides—an overview. Defect Diffusion Forum 2007;263:219.
[65] Sen U, Sen S. The fracture toughness of borides formed on boronized cold work tool steels. Mater Character 2003;50(4â€"5):261−7.
[66] Sue JA, Tucker RC, Nemeth JP. Chromium boride coatings, 1999, Google Patents.
[67] Chandler H. Heat Treater's Guide: Practices and Procedures for Irons and Steels. ASM International; 1994.
[68] CALIK A, et al. Boriding kinetics of pure cobalt.
[69] Zhunkovskii G, Navrotskii B, Kolosvetov YP. Boronizing of cobalt and some cobalt base alloys. Powder Metallurgy Metal Ceramics 1972;11(11):888−90.

[70] Yu L, Khor KA, Sundararajan G. Boride layer growth kinetics during boriding of molybdenum by the Spark Plasma Sintering (SPS) technology. Surface Coatings Technol 2006;201(6):2849–53.
[71] Zhou M, et al. Annealing effects on the structure and mechanical properties of r.f.-sputtered Cr-B hard thin films. Thin Solid Films 2000;359(2):165–70.
[72] Kulka M, et al. A study of nanoindentation for mechanical characterization of chromium and nickel borides' mixtures formed by laser boriding. Ceramics Int 2014;40(4):6083–94.
[73] Kaptay G, Kuznetsov S. Electrochemical synthesis of refractory borides from molten salts. Plasmas Ions 1999;2(2):45–56.
[74] Clem WC, Chowdhury S, Catledge SA, Weimer JJ, Shaikh FM, Hennessy KM, et al. Mesenchymal stem cell interaction with ultra-smooth nanostructured diamond for wear-resistant orthopaedic implants. Biomaterials 2008;29:3461–8.
[75] Grausova L, et al. Enhanced growth and osteoblastic differentiation of human osteoblast-like cells on boron doped nanocrystalline diamond thin films. PLoS One 2011;6:e20943. Available from: http://dx.doi.org/10.1371/journal.pone.0020943.
[76] Kopecek M, et al. Improved adhesion, growth and maturation of human bone-derived cells on nanocrystalline diamond films. Phys Stat Sol 2008;205:2146–53.
[77] Lemons J, et al. Biocompatibility of Nanostructured Diamond Surfaces for TMJ Articulation. 32nd Annual Meeting and Exhibition of the AADR. San Antonio, TX, 2003.
[78] Phillips EA, et al. Histological characterization of periprosthetic tissue responses for metal-on-metal hip replacement. J Long Term Eff Med Implants 2014;24(1):13–23.
[79] Thomas V, Jayabalan M. A new generation of high flex life polyurethane urea for polymer heart valve—studies on in vivo biocompatibility and biodurability. J Biomed Mater Res A 2009;89 (1):192–205.
[80] Purdue PE, et al. The cellular and molecular biology of periprosthetic osteolysis. Clin Orthop Relat Res 2007;454:251–61.
[81] Wang ML, Sharkey PF, Tuan RS. Particle bioreactivity and wear-mediated osteolysis. J Arthroplasty 2004;19(8):1028–38.
[82] Maloney WJ, Smith RL. Periprosthetic osteolysis in total hip arthroplasty: the role of particulate wear debris. Instr Course Lect 1996;45:171–82.
[83] Bauer TW. Particles and periimplant bone resorption. Clin Orthop Relat Res 2002;405:138–43.
[84] Mercuri L. The TMJ concepts patient fitted total temporomandibular joint reconstruction prosthesis in total temporomandibular joint reconstruction. Oral Maxillofac Surg Clin North Am 2000;12:73–91.
[85] Goldring S, et al. The synovial-like membrane at the bone-cement interface in loose total hip replacements and its proposed role in bone lysis. J Bone Joint Surg Am 1983;65(5):575–84.
[86] Ingham E, Fisher J. Biological reactions to wear debris in total joint replacement. Proc Inst Mech Eng 2000;H 214:21–37.
[87] Amstutz HC, et al. Mechanism and clinical significance of wear debris-induced osteolysis. Clin Orthop Relat Res 1992;276:7–18.
[88] Medley JB, et al. Comparison of alloys and designs in a hip simulator study of metal on metal implants. Clin Orthop Relat Res 1996;(Suppl. 329):S148–59.
[89] McKellop H, Park SH, Chiesa R, Doorn P, Lu B, Normand P, et al. In vivo wear of three types of metal on metal hip prostheses during two decades of use. Clin Orthop Relat Res 1996;(Suppl. 329):S128–40.
[90] Tipper JL, et al. Quantitative analysis of polyethylene wear debris, wear rate and head damage in retrieved Charnley hip prostheses. J Mater Sci Mater Med 2000;11(2):117–24.
[91] McGovern TF, Moskal JT. Radiographic evaluation of periprosthetic metallosis after total knee arthroplasty. J South Orthop Assoc 2002;11(1):18–24.
[92] Hallab NJ, Jacobs JJ. Biologic effects of implant debris. Bull NYU Hospital Joint Dis 2009;67 (2):182–8.
[93] Moran CG, Tourret LJ. Recent advances: orthopaedics. BMJ 2001;322(7291):902–5.
[94] Wagner M, Wagner H. Medium-term results of a modern metal-on-metal system in total hip replacement. Clin Orthop Relat Res 2000;379:123–33.

[95] Brown C, Fisher J, Ingham E. Biological effects of clinically relevant wear particles from metal-on-metal hip prostheses. Proc Inst Mech Eng H 2006;220:355–69.
[96] Kanaji A, Caicedo MS, Virdi AS, Sumner DR, Hallab NJ, Sena K. Co-Cr-Mo alloy particles induce tumor necrosis factor alpha production in MLO-Y4 osteocytes: a role for osteocytes in particle-induced inflammation. Bone 2009;45:528–33.
[97] Mostardi RA, Kovacik MW, Ramsier RD, Bender ET, Finefrock JM, Bear TF, et al. Comparison of the effects of prosthetic and commercially pure metals on retrieved human fibroblasts: the role of surface elemental composition. Acta Biomater 2010;6:702–7.
[98] Trindade MC, Lind M, Sun D, Schurman DJ, Goodman SB, Smith RL. In vitro reaction to orthopaedic biomaterials by macrophages and lymphocytes isolated from patients undergoing revision surgery. Biomaterials 2001;22:253–9.
[99] Wooley PH, Petersen S, Song Z, Nasser S. Cellular immune responses to orthopaedic implant materials following cemented total joint replacement. J Orthop Res 1997;15:874–80.
[100] Case CP, Langkamer VG, James C, Palmer MR, Kemp AJ, Heap PF, et al. Widespread dissemination of metal debris from implants. J Bone Joint Surg Br 1994;76(5):701–12.
[101] Langkamer VG, Case CP, Heap P, Taylor A, Collins C, Pearse M, et al. Systemic distribution of wear debris after hip replacement. A cause for concern? J Bone Joint Surg Br 1992;74(6):831–9.
[102] Wright T, et al. Joint replacement: implant bearing surface materials. New York; 2009.
[103] Thomas V, Halloran B, Ambalavanan N, Catledge SA, Vohra YK. In vitro studies on the effect of particle size on macrophage responses to nanodiamond wear debris. Acta Biomaterialia 2012;8(5):1939–47.
[104] Baumann B, Seufert J, Jakob F, Noth U, Rolf O, Eulert J, et al. Activation of NF-kappaB signaling and TNFalpha-expression in THP-1 macrophages by TiAlV- and polyethylene-wear particles. J Orthop Res 2005;23(6):1241–8.
[105] Epstein NJ, Bragg WE, Ma T, Spanogle J, Smith RL, Goodman SB. UHMWPE wear debris upregulates mononuclear cell proinflammatory gene expression in a novel murine model of intramedullary particle. Disease Acta Orthop 2005;76(3):412–20.
[106] Haynes DR, Crotti TN, Potter AE, Loric M, Atkins GJ, Howie DW, et al. The osteoclastogenic molecules RANKL and RANK are associated with periprosthetic osteolysis. J Bone Joint Surg Br 2001;83(6):902–11.
[107] Jacobs JJ, Roebuck KA, Archibeck M, Hallab NJ, Glant TT. Osteolysis: basic science. Clin Orthop Relat Res 2001;393:71–7.
[108] Kaufman AM, Alabre CI, Rubash HE, et al. Human macrophage response to UHMWPE, TiAlV, CoCr, and alumina particles: analysis of multiple cytokines using protein arrays. J Biomed Mater Res A 2008;84:464–74.
[109] Matthews JB, Green TR, Stone MH, Wroblewski BM, Fisher J, Ingham E. Comparison of the response of primary murine peritoneal macrophages and the U937 human histiocytic cell line to challenge with in vitro generated clinically relevant UHMWPE particles. Biomed Mater Eng 2000;10(3-4):229–40.
[110] Nakashima Y, Sun DH, Trindade MC, Maloney WJ, Goodman SB, Schurman DJ, et al. Signalingpathways for tumor necrosis factor-alpha and interleukin-6 expression in human macrophages exposed to titanium-alloy particulate debris in vitro. J Bone Joint Surg Am 1999;81(5):603–15.
[111] Purdue PE, Koulouvaris P, Potter HG, Nestor BJ, Sculco TP. The cellular and molecular biology of periprosthetic osteolysis. Clin Orthop Relat Res 2007;454:251–61.
[112] Ren W, Yang SY, Fang HW, Hsu S, Wooley PH. Distinct gene expression of receptor activator of nuclear factor-kappaB and rank ligand in the inflammatory response to variant morphologies of UHMWPE particles. Biomaterials 2003;24(26):4819–26.
[113] Shanbhag AS, Jacobs J, Black J, et al. Macrophage/ particle interactions: effect of size, composition and surface area. J Biomed Mater Res A 1994;28:81–90.
[114] Tuan RS, Lee FY, Konttinen Y, Wilkinson JM, Smith RL. What are the local and systemic biologic reactions and mediators to wear debris, and what host factors determine or modulate the biologic response to wear particles? J Am Acad Orthop Surg 2008;16(Suppl. 1):S33–8.

[115] Xia Z, Triffitt JT. A review on macrophage responses to biomaterials. Biomed Mater 2006;1(1): R1−9.
[116] Schwarz EM, et al. Tumor necrosis factor-alpha/nuclear transcription factor-kappaB signaling in periprosthetic osteolysis. J Orthop Res 2000;18(3):472−80.
[117] Huang Z, et al. Effects of orthopedic polymer particles on chemotaxis of macrophages and mesenchymal stem cells. J Biomed Mater Res A 2010;94(4):1264−9.
[118] Algan SM, Purdon M, Horowitz SM. Role of tumor necrosis factor alpha in particulate-induced bone resorption. J Orthop Res 1996;14(1):30−5.
[119] Huang H, et al. Protein-mediated assembly of nanodiamond hydrogels into a biocompatible and biofunctional multilayer nanofilm. ACS Nano 2008;2:203−12.
[120] Yuan Y, et al. Biodistribution and fate of nanodiamonds in vivo. Diamond Relat Mater 2009;18 (1):95−100.
[121] Xu JW, et al. Production of platelet-derived growth factor in aseptic loosening of total hip replacement. Rheumatol Int 1998;17(6):215−21.
[122] Kyriakides TR, et al. The CC chemokine ligand, CCL2/MCP1, participates in macrophage fusion and foreign body giant cell formation. Am J Pathol 2004;165(6):2157−66.
[123] Brodbeck WG, et al. Interleukin-4 inhibits tumor necrosis factor-alpha-induced and spontaneous apoptosis of biomaterial-adherent macrophages. J Lab Clin Med 2002;139(2):90−100.
[124] Matassi F, et al. Porous metal for orthopedics implants. Clin Cases Miner Bone Metab 2013;10 (2):111−15.
[125] Song B, et al. Process parameter selection for selective laser melting of Ti6Al4V based on temperature distribution simulation and experimental sintering. Int J Adv Manufact Technol 2012;61(9-12):967−74.
[126] Cherry JA, et al. Investigation into the effect of process parameters on microstructural and physical properties of 316L stainless steel parts by selective laser melting. Int J Adv Manufact Technol 2015;76(5-8):869−79.
[127] Aboulkhair NT, et al. Reducing porosity in AlSi10Mg parts processed by selective laser melting. Addit Manuf 2014;1-4:77−86.
[128] Costerton JW, Stewart PS, Greenberg EP. Bacterial biofilms: a common cause of persistent infections. Science 1999;284(5418):1318−22.
[129] Piletska EV, et al. Passive control of quorum sensing: prevention of Pseudomonas aeruginosa biofilm formation by imprinted polymers. Biomacromolecules 2011;12(4):1067−71.
[130] May A, Wang TJ. Biomarkers for cardiovascular disease: challenges and future directions. Trends Mol Med 2008;14(6):261−7.
[131] Kappell GM, Grover JP, Chrzanowski TH. Micro-scale surface-patterning influences biofilm formation. 2009.
[132] Caro A, et al. Grafting of lysozyme and/or poly(ethylene glycol) to prevent biofilm growth on stainless steel surfaces. J Phys Chem B 2009;113:2101−9.

CHAPTER 8

Polymers and Composites for Orthopedic Applications

S.V. Gohil[1], S. Suhail[2], J. Rose[2], T. Vella[3] and L.S. Nair[1,2]
[1]University of Connecticut Health Center, Farmington, CT, United States
[2]University of Connecticut, Storrs, CT, United States
[3]Simsbury High School, Simsbury, CT, United States

Contents

8.1 INTRODUCTION

The need to develop effective and reliable bone regeneration strategies is evident from the fact that, by 2020, half of all Americans over 50 will have bone-related medical conditions. An estimated 1.5 million individuals suffer from fracture every year and the orthopedic trauma device market is expected to exceed $9 billion by 2020 [1,2]. The increasing aging population and complications arising from osteoporosis-related fractures, trauma, congenital bone malformations, skeletal diseases, and tumor resection surgeries necessitates the development of novel bone graft substitutes. Consequently, the current annual growth rate of the bone graft substitutes market is in double digits [3].

Bone tissue engineering is a potential alternative to conventional strategies such as autografts (bone that is taken from an individual's body and transplanted into another part of the same individual) and allografts (bone from one individual is transplanted to another individual) [4]. Significant research is currently undergoing to identify effective biomaterials and graft substitutes with optimum regeneration capability, for both load-bearing and nonload-bearing orthopedic applications [5]. As per a consensus definition provided by the National Institute of Health, "a biomaterial is any substance (other than a drug) or combination of substances, synthetic or natural in origin, which can be used for any period of time, as a whole or as a part of a system which treats, augments, or replaces any tissue, organ, or function of the body" [6]. Ideally, a biomaterial should possess appropriate and preferably tunable mechanical, degradation, biological, and immunological properties as well as ease of processability [7]. Keeping the wide range of biomedical applications in mind, researchers have worked toward the development of novel biomaterials with varying physical, chemical, biological, and degradation characteristics, from both synthetic and natural sources. Unfortunately, no single biomaterial possesses all the desired characteristics for specific applications; hence "composite materials" have received significant attention in recent years. Inorganic–organic composites are particularly of interest for bone-related applications to mimic the composite nature of natural bone. They are prepared by combining the polymer phase with an inorganic phase (such as ceramics) to generate bioactive materials with improved mechanical properties and degradation profiles. Based on the earlier successes in single tissue regeneration, recent research efforts are being focused on regenerating complex tissues and organ systems to create translational technologies that are capable of addressing grand clinical challenges such as regenerating a functional knee or whole limb. The field of regenerative engineering has emerged to converge the cutting edge technologies in biology, material sciences, physical, chemical, and engineering sciences along with the potential to harness the body's innate healing capacity to support regeneration of complex tissues and organ systems [8–11]. The development of advanced biologically relevant biomaterials with good biological functionality is essential for developing strategies to support regeneration rather than repair or replace.

Currently, the use of polymeric biomaterials for bone-related applications include those for developing prosthetic devices such as nondegradable polymers and composites, and a wide range of three-dimensional (3D) scaffolds to support tissue regeneration, which are mostly based on biodegradable polymers, ceramics, and their composites. In addition to providing mechanical support, these biomaterials are also used for drug/cell/growth factor delivery. This chapter focuses on various polymeric biomaterials currently used for orthopedic applications, either alone or as composites, and highlights the recent advances in the field.

8.2 NONDEGRADABLE POLYMERS AND COMPOSITES FOR ORTHOPEDIC APPLICATIONS

The early 1960s saw the development and use of various "bioinert" biomaterials, which aimed to match the properties of the replaced tissue while exhibiting minimal toxic or immunological response. These materials belonged to the following major classes: metals, synthetic nondegradable polymers, and ceramics [9]. Nondegradable polymers such as poly(methyl methacrylate) (PMMA), polyaryletherketones (PAEK), and ultrahigh-molecular-weight polyethylene (UHMWPE) are some of the most extensively investigated polymers for orthopedic applications.

8.2.1 Poly(methyl methacrylate)

PMMA is a synthetic resin, created by the polymerization of methyl methacrylate (MMA) ($C_5H_8O_2$). Due to its good processability, handling properties, and biocompatibility, PMMA is considered to be a preferred material for a variety of biomedical applications [12]. PMMA can be prepared from MMA using a number of polymerization processes, including, but not limited to, anionic polymerization [13], bulk polymerization [14], emulsion polymerization [12], solution polymerization [15], and radical polymerization [12].

PMMA is a thermoplastic polymer with good mechanical strength and a good Young's modulus. The polymer exhibits low water absorptivity and thermal stability up to 65°C; however, heat-stabilized forms with an ability to withstand up to 100°C are now available. Even though PMMA was originally used to create plexiglass, it has since taken on many clinical applications, specifically in the field of orthopedics [16]. In 1936, Kulzer discovered that a "dough" or "cement" can be formed upon mixing PMMA powder with liquid MMA monomer, in the presence of benzoyl peroxide (BP) at 100°C. This discovery later led to the widespread use of PMMA as a bone cement [16]. Even though PMMA was initially used for dental fixtures, Dr. John Charnley is credited with the first use of PMMA bone cement for orthopedic applications [16]. In 1958, Dr. Charnley used cured PMMA to attach an acrylic cup of the hip to the femoral head. However, PMMA bone cement has some shortcomings including volumetric shrinkage, aseptic loosening of the graft, weak bone–cement interface, and toxicity; therefore more improved formulations are currently under development [17,18]. A number of PMMA composites incorporating radio-opacifying additives, drugs such as antibiotics and vitamin E, as well as metallic and ceramic nanoparticles have been investigated [16]. In a study, methacrylic monomer functionalized with vitamin E (MVE) was prepared and incorporated into acrylic bone cements to provide antioxidant properties. The addition of MVE led to a reduction in peak polymerization temperature values and an increase in setting time of the cement. The MVE-modified cements supported the attachment and proliferation of human osteoblasts, with the cements containing around 15% MVE showing the best cellular performance [19]. Additionally, copolymers of PMMA with other polymers have also been studied. A study showed the ability of the copolymer [poly(methyl methacrylate-acrylic acidallyl methacrylate) or poly(MMA-AA-AMA)] to reduce bone cement shrinkage associated with traditional PMMA compositions. This was attributed to the ability of the poly(MMA-AA-AMA) polymer to absorb body fluids and swell which could then compensate for PMMA shrinkage. The use of MMA:AA:AMA ratio of 80:20:10 was found to enhance the mechanical strength and improve fracture toughness of the bone cement, when compared to the PMMA control [20]. Another study evaluated the effect of adding multiwalled carbon nanotubes (MWCNTs) to PMMA, as a way to modulate the mechanical properties of Simplex P bone cement [21]. The study revealed that the addition of MWCNT to PMMA bone cement can significantly improve the mechanical properties and reduce the exothermic polymerization reaction of the bone cement [21]. A related study reported the feasibility of developing a porous, surface-modified bioactive PMMA-based bone cement, which could allow bone ingrowth and also maintain the desired mechanical properties [22]. The composite was prepared by incorporating bioactive glass as filler and chitosan particles as porogen within the PMMA matrix. The resultant porous structure led to enhanced bone ingrowth and improved interfacial bonding strength. Furthermore, the presence of bioactive glass led to improved handling characteristics, adequate mechanical properties, and osseointegration. The composite showed a setting time of 12.7 minutes and improved cellular attachment, proliferation, and osteogenic differentiation in vitro. In vivo evaluation in a rabbit femoral condyle defect model revealed higher interfacial bonding strength with the modified cement, which was attributed to the formation of an apatite layer and improved osseointegration upon implantation.

PMMA is also used as a delivery vehicle for antibiotics such as gentamicin, for the treatment of osteomyelitis and periprosthetic infections after arthroplasty [23]. A recent study investigated the feasibility of using quaternized chitosan derivative hydroxypropyl trimethyl ammonium chloride chitosan (HACC) with a 26% degree of substitution (26% HACC) as a biocompatible antibacterial for encapsulation in PMMA cements [24]. The 26% HACC-loaded PMMA was found to strongly inhibit biofilm formation, especially antibiotic-resistant staphylococci, when compared to PMMA, gentamicin-loaded PMMA, and chitosan-loaded PMMA. Similarly, incorporation of organic propylparaben nanoparticles in PMMA-based bone cements also showed antimicrobial activity, without evidence of adverse effects [25].

8.2.2 Polyaryletherketones

PAEK are high-performance semicrystalline thermoplastics composed of phenylene rings linked together through either carboxyl or ether groups. PAEK can be produced using nucleophilic or electrophilic polycondensation methods. The nucleophilic method creates rings connected by ether groups while the electrophilic method links the rings using carboxyl groups [26]. Generally, PAEK polymers possess high mechanical strength, very good impact strength, low moisture absorption and tendency to creep, good chemical resistance, sliding and wear properties, and radiation resistance [27]. The properties of PAEK can be further modulated by the addition of various reinforcing agents. For example, glass fiber-reinforced PAEK, carbon fiber-reinforced PAEK, as well as lubricated, nonlubricated, and load-bearing grades of PAEK are commercially available. Poly(etheretherketone) (PEEK) and poly(etherketoneketone) (PEKK) are two of the extensively investigated members of this family. The properties of these polymers can be further modulated by changing the sequence and ratio of ether–ketone linkage, the ratio of meta and para phenyl substitution, introduction of pendent alkyl or phenyl groups to PEKK, as well as incorporation of $-CR_2$- and $-SO_2$- in the backbone of PEEK.

Unlike PAEK, PEEK does not contain any aryl functional groups or substituents. The most widely used version of PEEK is PEEK-Optima from Invibio. According to the manufacturer, PEEK-Optima has a bone-like modulus of elasticity which could promote healing by reducing stress shielding, and is extremely strong and durable, with a high resistance to creeping and fatigue. PEEK has also been shown to be resistant to temperature, organic and aqueous solvents, has a density of 1.32 g/cm^3, melting temperature of 343°C and glass transition at 143°C. It also has a low coefficient of friction and outstanding abrasion/wear resistance. These desirable properties and customizable nature have made PEEK a polymer of choice for many biomedical applications. Due to its wide use as a substitute for traditional metal implants, PEEK has seen a recent upturn for applications like spinal fusions, disc arthroplasty, and as interspinal spacers.

Another common polymer in this class is poly(etherketoneetherketoneketone) or PEKEKK, which has similar structure and properties as PAEK. PEKEKK has low moisture absorption and has been modified by incorporating glass and carbon fiber reinforcements, carbon nanotubes, solid lubricants, and ceramics. These modifications help to improve its mechanical properties, provide outstanding chemical resistance, good electrical insulation, and thermal stability, depending on the components added [28].

8.2.3 Ultrahigh-molecular-weight polyethylene

Among the variety of nondegradable polymers and composites used for orthopedic applications, UHMWPE is one of the commonly used materials with excellent adaptability. The molecular weight of commercially available UHMWPE may range from 3 million g/mol (low) to 5 million g/mol (medium) and may reach up to 7–10 million g/mol (high). The high molecular weight and chemical properties of UHMWPE allow it to have good sliding wear resistance and impact toughness.

Karl Ziegler first synthesized UHMWPE in the early 1950s using Ziegler–Natta catalysts, although it was not introduced in the market until 1955 [29]. Reactive organo-titanate catalysts composed of titanium and aluminum alkyls are used to polymerize the feedstock composed of ethylene gas [30]. Initially, the aluminum alkyls form a titanium alkyl bond and subsequently UHWPE ethylene molecules get inserted into this titanium carbon bond to grow the UHMWPE chain. Molecular hydrogen is commonly used as a chain transfer agent, which terminates the growing chain without poisoning the catalyst, thereby allowing the chain to be terminated at the desired length [30].

The chemistry of the catalyst influences polymer attributes such as the average molecular weight and distribution, bulk density, degree of crystallinity, and particle size [30]. It is often difficult to measure the molecular weight of UHMWPE molecular chains as they are often too long and too entangled to permit measurable shear flow. Instead, the polymer's viscous behavior is commonly used to determine the molecular weight. UHMWPE powder is processed into a usable form by a sintering process which uses heat and high pressure to compact and fuse the powder [29,31]. Sintering processes include ram extrusion and compression molding. Compression molding involves cold compacting the powder to form a "green" preform followed by heating under pressure to fuse the compacted powder [31,32]. Ram extrusion is a continuous compression process wherein a reciprocating ram is used to compact the powder followed by transferring the compacted powder through a heated dye. Many additives may be utilized during the molding process to impart desirable properties [33]. For instance, surface lubricity may be enhanced with silicone oil, molybdenum disulfide, carbon black, graphite, mineral oils, and vegetable oils. Similarly, heat resistance may be enhanced with metal flakes, phosphite-based stabilizers, and electrical conductivity may be enhanced with carbon black and graphite. UHMWPE-based products have been used for fabrication of arthroscopic tools/implants due to the low elasticity, high modulus and lubricity, and good tactile feedback of the polymer. UHMWPE is also used in hip implants wherein the metal-on-metal interfaces are increasingly being replaced with metal-on-UHMWPE interfaces (commonly known as metal-on-poly), as UHMWPE can conform to the shape of the bone and help increase the contact surface area and lower contact pressure, thereby reducing the chances of failure [34].

Oxidative degradation is one of the main reasons for loss of mechanical strength of UHMWPE implants resulting in a reduced life span of joint arthroplasty. Recently, a study was done in which UHMWPE was stabilized with vitamin E to improve its longevity [35]. Vitamin E-stabilized UHMWPE was found to have superior oxidation resistance and mechanical strength, when compared to irradiated UHMWPEs. After in vitro trials, it was found that vitamin E-stabilized UHMWPEs offered good mechanical wear resistance and oxidation properties and thus their clinical use in joint arthroplasties is justified and beneficial [27].

8.2.4 Polypropylene

Polypropylene is another nondegradable polymer used in multiple orthopedic applications. Some of its characteristic properties include: low density, relatively high thermal stability, easy processing, and resistance to corrosion. It is the most commonly used thermoplastic polymer for injection molding applications [36]. In addition to injection molding, it is compatible with a number of processing techniques and is thus used in many commercial applications. Polypropylene is one of the lightest of all thermoplastics with a density of 0.9 g/cm^3 and thus may serve as a potential candidate for developing lightweight orthopedic implants [36]. In addition, the high melting temperature (160−170°C) makes it heat-resistant and provides it with an ability to withstand various molding techniques and environments [37]. Furthermore, it has excellent fatigue resistance and strong chemical resistance toward most organic solvents, except very strong oxidizing agents [36]. Polypropylene can be processed via injection molding, blow molding, extrusion, film casting, and thermoforming [37].

Polypropylene is prepared by polymerizing propylene, usually obtained from the gaseous by-products of petroleum refining (such as gas oil, naphtha, ethane, and propane) in the presence of catalysts, under controlled temperature and pressure [36]. A long, linear polymer chain of carbon atoms is formed with methyl (CH_3) groups attached to every other carbon atom of the chain and the crystallinity and molecular weight of the polypropylene can be controlled during the synthesis process [38]. Some of the most well-known suppliers of polypropylene in the world include Albis Plastics GmbH (Germany) and Arco Chemical Company (Pennsylvania). The major use of polypropylene is for the fabrication of bone fixation devices, specifically, ultrahigh-strength rods for bone fixation [39]. Researchers have also investigated the effect of addition of MWCNTs and nanohydroxyapatite (*n*HA) on the properties of a polypropylene-based biocomposite, for bone replacement. The MWCNTs of 0.1 and 0.3 wt% and *n*HA of 8−20 wt% were incorporated into the polypropylene rod using melt-compounding and injection molding techniques. Tensile and impact tests showed the enhanced stiffness, tensile strength, and impact toughness of the composite. Additionally, the biocomposite rods were effective in improving dimensional and thermal stability of polypropylene [40]. Similarly, incorporation of boron nitride and *n*HA in polypropylene via melt mixing and injection molding techniques has shown to improve its biocompatibility and mechanical strength [41]. The 20% *n*HA-enhanced polypropylene with boron nitride also showed greater elastic modulus when compared to standard polypropylene [41].

8.2.5 Polysulfone

Polysulfones (PS) are sulfur-containing nondegradable thermoplastic high-performance polymers used in orthopedic applications [42]. Polysulfones including poly(ether sulfone) and poly(phenyl sulfones) have been shown to have high thermal and chemical stability, high glass transition temperature, and excellent strength and flexibility. Polysulfone is formed of para-linked aromatic groups connected by ether, sulfone, as well as alkyl groups. Polysulfones are prepared by a polysulfonylation reaction by reacting aromatic sulfonyl halides with phenyl ethers or by the more commercially successful approach of polyestherification process. A typical reaction involves reaction of a diphenol with bis (4-chlorophenyl)sulfone forming a polyether by elimination of sodium chloride. Polysulfones are processed via extrusions, injection molding, and blow molding.

Wang et al. [44] investigated hydroxyapatite (HA)-reinforced polysulfone composites for tissue replacement. The composites were prepared by a standard procedure including drying, blending, and compounding followed by either injection molding (to obtain rectangular bars, discs, and dumbbell specimens) or compression molding process (to obtain thick plates). The study showed significant enhancement of mechanical properties (storage modulus) of the composites with increasing concentrations of HA. However, the storage modulus of the composite was found to decrease compared to polysulfone alone, after 7 days in distilled water. This was attributed to the enhanced water uptake by the composites containing HA.

Another study evaluated polyethersulfone and sulfonated polyether sulfone (SPES) nanofibers for bone regeneration applications [43]. Here, calcium ions were incorporated into the SPES nanofibers postfabrication, by immersion in calcium hydroxide solution. The calcium-ion-exchanged SPES (Ca-SPES) showed significant bioactivity and led to formation of an apatite layer after 7 days of immersion in simulated body fluid. The Ca-SPES scaffolds were able to enhance the in vitro osteogenic differentiation of stem cells, when compared to the polyether sulfone (PES) and SPES nanofibers. Furthermore, Ca-SPES scaffolds were found to induce "ectopic bone formation in the absence of exogenous cells" (Fig. 8.1), as shown by histological analysis of the isolated nanofiber and surrounding tissue explants, after 12 weeks of subcutaneous implantation in mice [37]. These studies indicate the potential of improving the suitability of polysulfone as a biomaterial for orthopedic applications, through hybrids and enhancements.

8.2.6 Polydimethylsiloxane

Polydimethylsiloxane (PDMS), commonly known as polysiloxane, or silicone, possesses good flexibility, flow properties, and film-forming capability. Due to the high bond energy of siloxane backbone (445 kJ/mol) and the presence of methyl CH_3 groups, PDMS is a chemically stable material [45]. It is able to resist extreme temperatures, aging, oxidation, moisture, and ultraviolet radiation and is generally nonirritating. PDMS has low surface tension (20.4 mN/m) and thus has good wettability. It is thermally stable and does not show significant changes in viscosity upon temperature changes, which makes it a suitable material for use in a wide temperature range

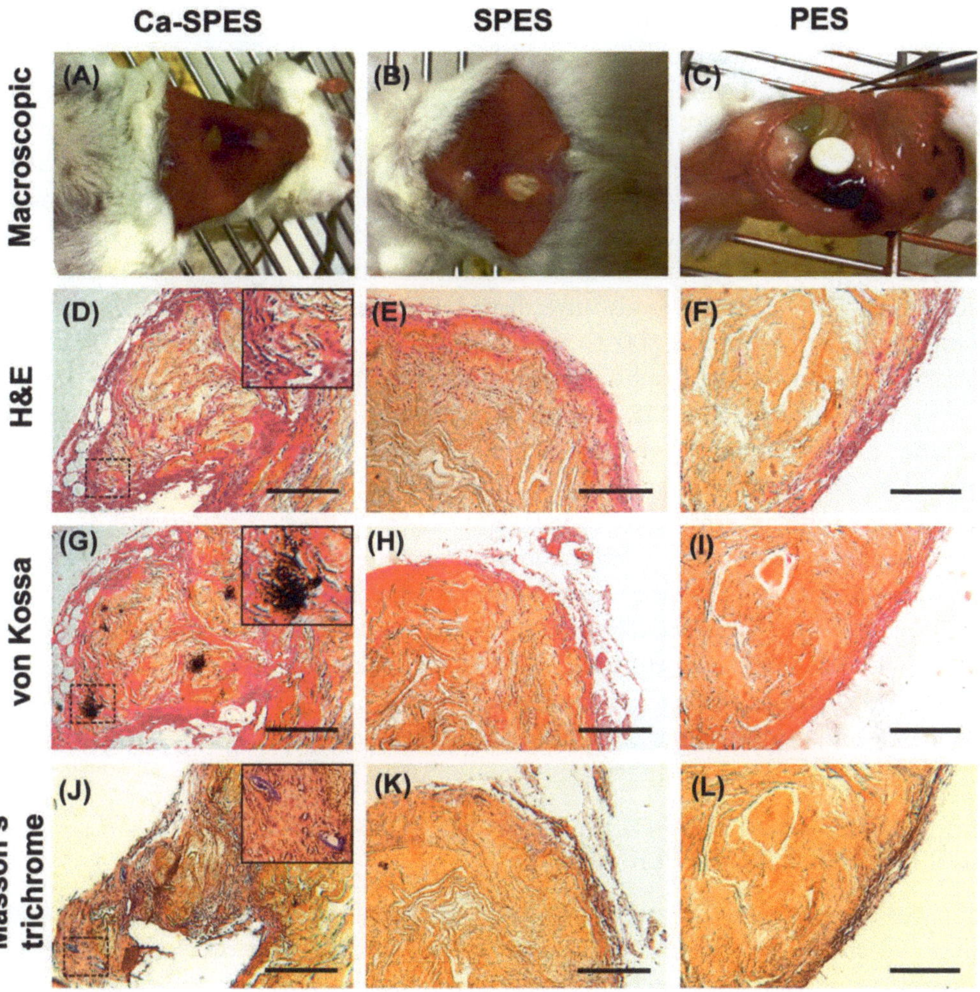

Figure 8.1 Macroscopic (A–C) and histological findings of ectopic bone formation, H&E staining (D–F), von Kossa staining (G–I), and Masson's trichrome (J–L) of calcium-enhanced sulfonated polyether sulfone (SPES) (A–J), sulfonated polyether sulfone (SPES) (B–K), and polyether sulfone (PES) (C–L). *Reprinted with permission from Shabani I, Haddadi-Asl V, Soleimani M, Seyedjafari E, Hashemi SM. Ion-exchange polymer nanofibers for enhanced osteogenic differentiation of stem cells and ectopic bone formation. ACS Appl Mater Interfaces 2014;6:72–82 [43] Copyright (2016) American Chemical Society.*

from $-40°C$ to $>150°C$. The open molecular structure of the polymer allows for high breathability, making it highly permeable to oxygen, nitrogen, and water vapor. Moreover, the high flexibility of PDMS allows it to be compressed, stretched, and bent repeatedly, making it ideal for coating applications. The physicochemical properties of PDMS make it a potential candidate for many medical applications.

Specific to orthopedics, the most common applications of PDMS include its use in hand and foot joint implants. Some of the following silicone-based joint implants have been developed: double-stemmed finger joint, metacarpophalangeal joints, and the single-stemmed silastic ulnar head implant [46]. A recent study investigated the effects of zirconia (a transition metal oxide known for its biointegration and injury repair properties) and PDMS hybrid coatings on proliferation and viability of human primary osteoblast and fibroblast cells. It was found that as zirconia concentration on the coating increased, so did cell proliferation, showing its potential as an orthopedic biomaterial [47]. Another study investigated the effect of PDMS coating, prepared using thermal treatment at 800°C and 1100°C, for surface modification of titanium surface. The surface topography analysis of the modified surface showed an increased surface roughness after PDMS coating. In addition, the surface tension between the polymer and the titanium sample, as well as the shear adhesion, was found to be affected by the PDMS coating temperature with the highest adhesion obtained with the PDMS coating thermally treated at 1100°C [48].

Overall, various nondegradable polymers and their composites have been widely used for a multitude of orthopedic applications, especially for the fabrication of medical devices aiming to replace damaged tissues. However, with the advent of novel biodegradable polymeric biomaterials, the orthopedic field has observed a significant use of these degradable alternatives which could not only replace but also repair and regenerate and can be ultimately replaced by healthy neotissue.

8.3 BIODEGRADABLE POLYMERS AND COMPOSITES FOR ORTHOPEDIC APPLICATIONS

The past two decades have seen a significant increase in the use of biodegradable polymers and composites for biomedical applications, as these materials not only exhibit appropriate physical and mechanical properties but also have the ability to get eliminated from the body. Consequently, biodegradable polymers and composites are ideal biomaterials to support tissue regeneration as they facilitate host tissue infiltration upon degradation. Biodegradable polymers and composites are currently used as surgical aids, controlled and local drug delivery systems as well as tissue engineering scaffolds. The following section discusses the commonly used synthetic and natural biodegradable polymers and composites for orthopedic applications.

8.3.1 Synthetic polymers

8.3.1.1 Poly(α-esters)

Poly(α-esters) are the most widely studied, diverse class of biodegradable thermoplastic polymers with aliphatic ester linkages. Commonly used polymers in this class include poly(α-hydroxy acids) such as poly(glycolic acid); the four chiral forms of poly(lactic acid): poly(L-lactic acid) (PLLA), poly (D-lactic acid) (PDLA), poly(D,L-lactic acid) (PDLLA), and meso-poly(lactic acid); polycaprolactone (PCL); polydioxanone; and copolymers thereof Refs. [49,50]. Table 8.1 shows the properties of some of the widely used poly(α-esters). Polyesters can be synthesized using ring-opening polymerization and polycondensation reactions. Self-condensation of difunctional monomers such as hydroxyl acids, condensation of diols with diacid chlorides or diacids and ester interchange reaction of diesters and diols, have been used to synthesize polyesters. However, it is difficult to achieve high-molecular-weight polymers using the condensation method. Ring-opening polymerization is therefore considered the preferred route of synthesis wherein one pot polymerization of cyclic lactones or cyclic anhydrides in the presence of catalysts such as stannous octoate and 2-ethylhexanoic acid leads to high-molecular-weight polyesters [7,51].

Most polyesters undergo degradation via bulk erosion due to nonspecific scission of the ester backbone and the rate of degradation depends on the molecular weight, copolymer ratio, crystallinity, and porosity of the matrix. The by-product of polylactic acid (PLA), i.e., lactic acid, is a normal human metabolic by-product and is broken down into water and carbon dioxide via the citric acid cycle. Polyglycolide (PGA) degrades to form glycolic acid which can be excreted in the urine or metabolized via the citric acid cycle [7]. Polyesters PGA, PLA, poly-lactic glycolic acid (PLGA), and PCL have been investigated for a plethora of clinical and biomedical applications such as drug delivery devices and as sutures, meshes, orthopedic pins and screws, and other medical devices [32].

Rahman et al. [52] developed novel PLGA/PEG-based scaffolds for the sustained delivery of recombinant human bone morphogenetic protein-2 (rhBMP-2). The scaffolds were prepared using PLGA/PEG particles (size range 100–200 μm), which could undergo temperature-induced PEG-leaching at 37°C and hence could be sintered at this temperature to form porous scaffolds. The scaffolds showed a burst rhBMP-2 release of 13% after 12 hours, followed by a sustained release (0.01–8% per day), with around 70% release in 23 days. In vivo implantation of the rhBMP-2-loaded scaffolds (1 μg per scaffold), in athymic nude-Foxn1^{nu} mice calvarial defect model led to a 55% increase in the bone volume when compared to empty defect controls. Another study utilized polydopamine-mediated surface modification to immobilize bone morphogenetic protein-2 (BMP-2) on to 3D PLGA scaffolds, via catechol chemistry [53]. The BMP-2-modified scaffolds led to in vitro osteogenic differentiation and mineralization of human adipose-derived stem cells (hADSCs) and also enhanced in vivo bone formation when transplanted with hADSCs.

In an attempt to fabricate an osteoconductive scaffold mimicking extracellular matrix, Kim et al. [54] developed PLGA/PLA-based meshes coated with human lung fibroblast-derived extracellular matrix. The cell derived matrix was then used to conjugate heparin to immobilize BMP-2. Human placenta-derived mesenchymal stem

Table 8.1 Properties of some widely used poly(α-esters)

Polymer	Thermal characteristics (°C)		Crystallinity	Degradation time (months)	Mechanical properties	
	T_g	T_m			Modulus (GPa)	Tensile strength (MPa)
Polyglycolide (PGA)	35–40	225–230	Highly crystalline 45–55%	6–12	5–7	60–80
Poly(L-lactic acid) (PLLA)	55–65	173–178	Semicrystalline 37%	>24	2.7–3	60–70
Poly(D,L)lactic acid (PDLLA)	50–60		Amorphous	12–16	1.9–2	2
Poly(L-lactide-*co*-glycolide) (PLGA)						
85/15	50–55	NA	Amorphous	5–6	2	
75/25	50–55			4–5	2	
65/35	40–50			3–4	2	
50/50	40–50			1–2	2	
Polycaprolactone (PCL)	−65 to −60	55–60	Semicrystalline	24–36	0.4	20–25
Poly(3-hydroxy butyrate) (PHB)	5	160–180	Crystalline		4	40
Poly(3-hydroxy butyrate-*co*-3-hydroxyvalerate) (PHBV)	−5 to 20	80–160				
Polydioxanone (PDS)	−10 to 0		NA	6–12	1.5	30
Poly(lactide-*co*-caprolactone) (PLCL)						

cells cultured on the modified scaffold showed significant upregulation of osteogenic markers compared to cells cultured on control and fibronectin-coated scaffolds. The modified scaffold was also able to induce significant new bone formation in a mouse ectopic and rat calvarial bone defect model.

Cylindrical, porous PLGA scaffolds were recently used for the combination delivery of anabolic rhBMP-2 with antiresorptive agents: bisphosphonates and IkappaB kinase (IKK) inhibitors. The PLGA scaffolds prepared by thermally induced phase separation were loaded with either zoledronic acid (ZA) alone, or ZA preadsorbed onto HA microparticles, or IKK inhibitor PS-1145 [55]. The PLGA scaffolds were found to provide better spatial control over the rhBMP-2-induced bone formation, when compared to collagen as a delivery system, in a 6-mm critical-sized femoral defect model. Moreover, the addition of antiresorptive agents further helped in augmenting new bone formation. The study thus showed the potential of local delivery of synergistic anabolic and antiresorptive agents using a polymeric delivery system to reduce rhBMP-2 dose and associated adverse side effects.

In another interesting study, high- and low-molecular-weight forms of three polyesters namely P(DL)LA, P(DL)LGA, and PCL were investigated for impaction bone grafting applications as potential allograft substitutes [56]. The polymers were milled, impacted into discs and, subsequently, the mechanical properties and skeletal stem cell (SSC) viability were evaluated in vitro. Both high- and low-molecular-weight P(DL)LA and P(DL)LGA discs fared better than the allograft in terms of shear strengths. The shear strength of PCL discs was, however, lower than the allograft. In addition, the high-molecular-weight P(DL)LA, and P(DL)LGA showed enhanced stem cell biocompatibility and cell viability demonstrating their efficacy as potential impaction bone grafting materials.

In addition to the use of polyester-based scaffolds as structural support and as drug delivery devices, many composite systems have been investigated for orthopedic applications. Composites can be designed to improve the bioactivity and mechanical properties or to incorporate other desirable functional characteristics to the system. Ceramics such as calcium phosphates and HA are most commonly used for this purpose. A study evaluated the effect of *n*HA content on bone regenerative capability, using *n*-HA PCL spiral scaffolds with different *n*-HA and PCL weight ratios. The in vitro biological activity was tested using human fetal osteoblasts [57]. A dose-dependent increase in bone phenotypic markers (bone sialoprotein, osteonectin, osteocalcin, and type-I collagen (Col-1)), alkaline phosphatase (ALP) activity, and mineralized matrix synthesis was observed in the composite matrix. Among these, the scaffold with 1:4 weight ratio of *n*-HA and PCL showed the optimal cellular performance demonstrating the unique biological activity of the composite matrix over the polymeric matrix. Tayton et al. [58] observed similar results, wherein addition of HA to porous PLA and PLGA scaffolds, significantly increased osteogenic activity and collagen-1 deposition by SSCs. In vivo analysis demonstrated increased bone formation in PLA–HA scaffolds. The study confirmed the better in vivo performance of the composite scaffold for impaction bone grafting compared to the polymer scaffold. Minton et al. [59] used melt molding and porogen leaching as a solvent-free approach to fabricate PCL–HA-based porous composites for bone tissue engineering. The study also showed improvement in cell adhesion with the addition of HA to PCL. In another study, supercritical carbon dioxide ($scCO_2$) processing was used to disperse organically modified montmorillonite clay in PDLA so as to fabricate nanocomposite bone grafts with improved structural and mechanical properties matching corticocancellous bone [60]. These nanocomposites were found to support osteogenesis in an ectopic bone formation model, in the presence of loaded BMP-2, demonstrating its ability to also serve as a protein delivery system.

Igwe et al. [61] developed a novel polymer/*n*-HA-hydrogel hybrid scaffold system composed of a self-assembling peptide gel solution (arginine-alanine-aspartic acid-alanine)$_4$ (RADA-16), infused into PLGA/*n*-HA macroporous sintered microsphere matrices. Biotinylated rhBMP-2 was tethered to the gel using biotin–streptavidin complexation. The hybrid scaffolds combined the load-bearing capability of the polymer/*n*-HA matrix with the osteoinductivity of the gel. The osteoinductive potential of the hybrid scaffold was demonstrated using rat bone marrow stromal cells and mouse preosteoblast cell line MC3T3-E1 cells, by following osteogenic gene expression.

The advantages of flexible composite matrices were shown in a study by Fujikura et al. [62], wherein composite membranes were prepared by electrospinning siloxane-containing vaterite and PLGA for guided bone regeneration. The composite showed good mechanical and cell adhesion properties. Similarly, Kutikov and Song [63] used amphiphilic poly(D,L-lactic acid)-*co*-poly-(ethylene glycol)-*co*-poly(D,L-lactic acid) (PELA) and HA to develop composite nanofiber matrices using the process of electrospinning. The PELA–HA composite fibers showed about an eightfold increase in storage modulus unlike HA–PLA composite fibers due to the unique interactions of HA with PEG demonstrating the role of polymers in modulating composite properties. The composite also promoted osteogenic differentiation of bone marrow-derived stromal cells (MSCs) in unstimulated culture. Based on the encouraging data, an in vivo study was subsequently performed using a rat femoral defect model [64]. The fibrous scaffolds were spiral-wrapped, and preseeded with MSCs or loaded with a low dose of rhBMP-2 (500 ng) before implantation (Fig. 8.2). These MSC-seeded spiral-wrapped scaffolds led to laminated endochondral ossification across the longitudinal span of the defect, which was templated by the scaffold. Hence, the defect showed formation of laminated new bone sandwiched in between adjacent electrospun scaffold layers. Addition of rhBMP-2, on the other hand, resulted in more robust but less templated bone formation. Another study investigated the efficacy of similar copolymer to serve as a rhBMP-2 delivery system to promote spinal fusion [65].

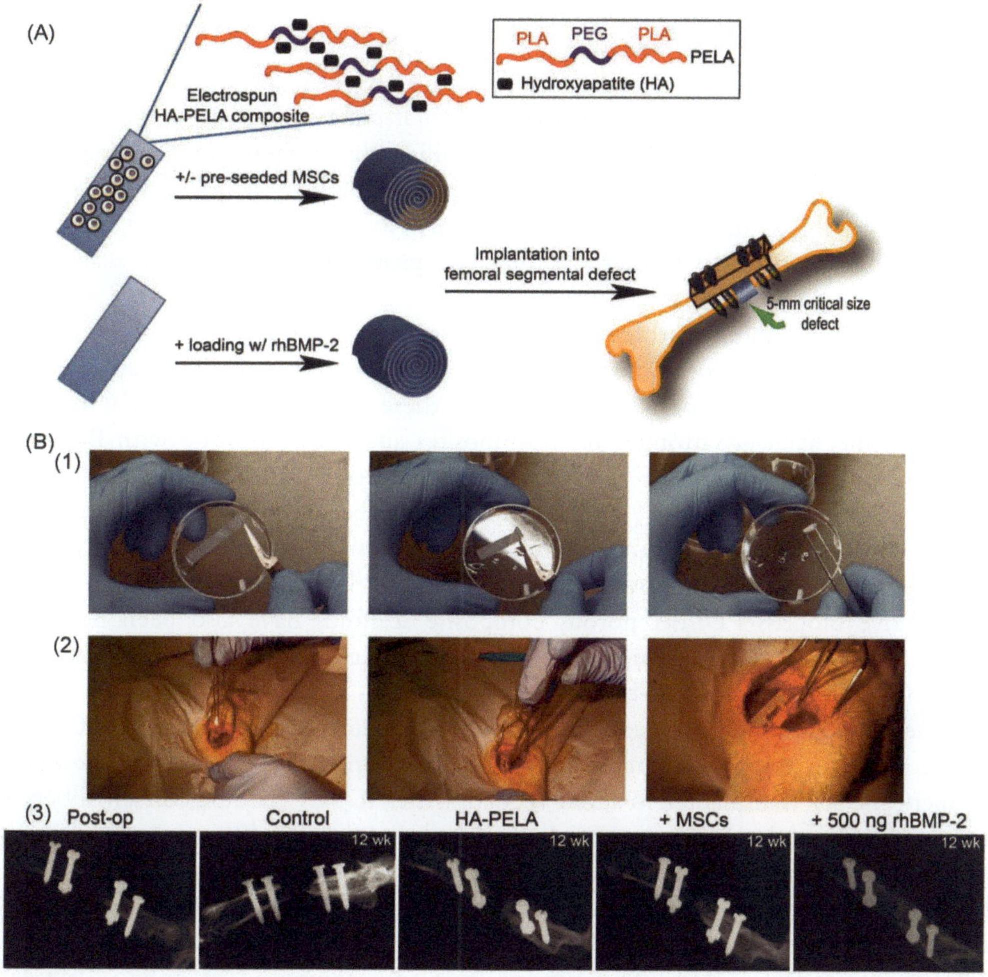

Figure 8.2 (A) Schematic of the spiral wrapping of HA—PELA scaffolds with or without preseeded cells or absorbed rhBMP-2 for implantation into a rat femoral defect stabilized by a PEEK fixation plate; (B) spiral wrapping and surgical implantation of HA—PELA scaffolds and postop radiographical follow-ups of the site of implantation. (1) Wrapping HA—PELA scaffolds into cylindrical spirals prior to surgery. (2) Implantation of spiral-wrapped HA—PELA scaffolds into rat femoral defects. (3) Radiographs of the scaffold-filled defect immediately postop, untreated control defect after 12 weeks, and scaffold-filled defects after 12 weeks. *Adapted with permission from Kutikov AB, Skelly JD, Ayers DC, Song J. Templated repair of long bone defects in rats with bioactive spiral-wrapped electrospun amphiphilic polymer/hydroxyapatite scaffolds. ACS Appl Mater Interfaces 2015;7:4890—4901 Copyright (2016) American Chemical Society.*

Composite graft made from poly-D,L-lactic acid/polyethylene glycol block copolymer (PLA—PEG) gel and β-tricalcium phosphate (TCP) was used as the delivery vehicle. In vivo evaluation confirmed the efficacy of this injectable composite for spinal repair as solid interspinous fusion was achieved in a rabbit lumbar fusion model.

The inherent osteogenic activity of many of the composite scaffolds raises significant interest to develop cost-effective bone graft substitutes. Tayton et al. [66] evaluated the in vivo osteogenic activity of a porous PLA–HA composite matrix in the presence and absence of SSCs in an ovine femoral condyle critical-size bone defect model. The study interestingly showed significantly higher bone formation in the unseeded composite scaffolds, when compared to those implanted with SSCs. The study highlights the potential osteogenic activity of these composite bone graft materials and the need to further optimize the protocol for cell-seeded scaffolds in order to develop translational technologies.

Another study evaluated three different perovskite ceramic nanoparticles, namely, calcium titanate (CT), strontium titanate (ST), and barium titanate (BT), as nanofillers for orthopedic applications [67]. Addition of these nanoparticles to PCL matrices resulted in mechanically stronger nanocomposites and the composite with BT particles showed piezoelectric properties. Moreover, the composite matrices also released small quantities of Ca^{2+}, Sr^{2+}, and Ba^{2+} ions. The biological activity of the nanocomposites was found to be enhanced and the composites induced cellular expression of osteogenic genes in the following order: PCL/CT > PCL/ST > PCL/BT > PCL.

Bioactive bioglass/PDLLA porous composite scaffolds have also been developed and evaluated as an osteogenic, cell delivery vehicle for bone regeneration [68]. The biological activity of the bioglass composites was demonstrated in vitro as they supported the growth and differentiation of adipose-derived stem cells (ADSCs), and the increase in biological activity was proportional to the bioglass content. Intraperitoneally transplanted scaffold seeded with ADSCs in diffusion chambers in nude mice, showed significant new bone formation in the 40 and 5 wt% bioglass composites compared to the PDLLA-only group, after 8 weeks. Another study investigated a layered scaffold formulation composed of highly porous 45S5 Bioglass coated with two polymer layers as a mechanically stable, osteoconductive, antibiotic-loaded multifunctional device [69]. The interior layer was composed of poly(D,L-lactide)/Pluronic P123, for improved mechanical stability, whereas the exterior coating composed of natural polymer (alginate or gelatin), served as an antibiotic drug carrier. The bilayered design improved the mechanical properties of the scaffold and also showed potential for drug delivery as well as enhanced bone regeneration applications.

One of the major issues subsequent to orthopedic surgeries is infection and therefore polymeric devices that can serve as antibiotic delivery systems raise significant interest. Brooks et al. reported an antibiotic-eluting bone void filler (ABVF) composed of calcium carbonate, HA, PCL, and PEG [70]. A solvent-free, molten-cast process was used to develop the filler and the fillers showed extended release of tobramycin sulfate and inhibited *Staphylococcus aureus* growth over 48 hours, at inoculums as high as 10^9 CFU/mL. In vivo efficacy was tested using a *S. aureus*-challenged rabbit radial defect window model [71]. The ABVF were able to eliminate the periprosthetic bacterial change during the tested time period of 8 weeks, whereas the controls without antibiotic required euthanasia 3 weeks postoperatively, due to infection.

Recently, shape memory polymers (SMPs), which are capable of reverting back to the original shape when exposed to certain stimuli after temporary deformation, have been investigated for various biomedical applications including orthopedics [72–75]. Xie et al. [73] reported electroactive SMP networks based on star-shaped (six-armed) polylactide and aniline trimer. These polymers showed excellent shape memory, high mechanical strength, tunable degradation properties, as well as enhanced osteogenic differentiation of C2C12 cells, indicating their potential for bone regeneration applications. Zhang et al. [74] developed a porous SMP scaffold via photocrosslinking PCL diacrylate using solvent casting/particulate leaching method. The porous scaffold showed the ability to conformally "self-fit" into irregular defects and the self-fitting property originated from the PCL crystalline domains. The biological activity of the scaffold was further improved by coating with "polydopamine." The polydopamine coating provided sites to nucleate HA on the surface for better bone bonding. The coating also improved the adhesion, proliferation, osteogenic gene expression, and extracellular matrix deposition by osteoblasts seeded on the scaffold. Another study reported the development of multifunctional fibrous electrospun scaffolds based on biodegradable poly(D,L-lactide-*co*-trimethylene carbonate) (denoted as PDLLA-*co*-TMC, or PLMC) with tissue architecture and shape memory effect, for minimally invasive applications [75]. The study demonstrated the feasibility to modulate fiber diameter, glass transition temperature, and mechanical properties by varying the ratios of building blocks (DLLA and TMC). The fibrous matrices showed excellent shape memory properties with shape recovery ratios of $R_r > 94\%$ and shape fixity ratios of $R_f > 98\%$. The scaffolds were also found to be cytocompatible and rat calvarial osteoblasts cultured on the scaffold showed increased ALP expression and mineral deposition, indicating the potential of the scaffold for bone tissue engineering.

Polydioxanone (PDS or PDO) is a colorless, crystalline, hydrophobic, biodegradable poly(ether–ester) polymer with a molecular structure of $(-O-CH_2-CH_2-O-CH_2-C=O)_n$. PDS was used to develop monofilament sutures in the 1980s [76]. PDS is commonly synthesized by ring-opening polymerization of *p*-dioxanone in the presence of an organometallic catalyst such as zirconium acetylacetone, diethylzinc, or zinc L-lactate (ZnLac2) and exhibits low glass transition temperature ranging from $-10°C$ to $0°C$ [77]. PDS is known to undergo hydrolytic degradation and is nonantigenic, nonpyrogenic, and elicits only minimal tissue reactivity upon absorption in the body. The degradation by-product of PDS is glyoxylate, which can be excreted in the urine or may be metabolized via citric acid cycle to form carbon dioxide and water. The PDS sutures are prepared using an extrusion process at the lowest possible temperature to prevent spontaneous depolymerization and the sutures possess high flexibility owing to the presence of an ether oxygen group within the polymer backbone. The PDS sutures typically lose half of their mechanical strength in about 3 weeks and undergo complete degradation by around 6 months, in humans. Antibacterial-loaded PDS sutures (PDS Plus) are now available for suturing wounds that exhibit a risk of dehiscence and infection. In addition to sutures, PDS has also been used to develop fixation screws for orthopedic applications. A recent study evaluated the efficacy of biodegradable PDS cages for reconstruction of large bone defects in rib cages of mongrel dogs [78]. Briefly, PDS sutures were used to weave cylindrical cages of 6 cm length and 1 cm diameter and used for enclosing two demineralized bone matrix scaffolds (molded into cuboids) preseeded with bone marrow-derived mesenchymal stem cells (BMSCs) differentiated toward osteogenic lineage. The PDS cage possessed appropriate degradation characteristics (complete degradation in 24 weeks), was radiolucent and flexible, and also presented optimum porosity for allowing exchange of nutrients and waste. The PDO cage/DBMs/BMSCs combination was able to retain their original shape on being subjected to external force and also showed bony union at all the construct interfaces, indicating its potential for repair of reconstructing large, nonload-bearing, bone defects.

Polycarbonates are linear, elastomeric, aliphatic polyester polymers with repeating carbonate (−O−C(O)−O−) linkages. They can be synthesized by the polycondensation between an aliphatic polyol with dialkyl carbonate, copolymerization of carbon dioxide with epoxides, and ring-opening polymerization of cyclic carbonate monomers [79]. Poly(trimethylene carbonate) (PTMC) is the most extensively investigated polycarbonate prepared using ring-opening polymerization of trimethylene carbonate. The polymer undergoes surface degradation to form biocompatible by-products, 1,3-propanediol, and carbonic acid. To overcome the slow degradation of aliphatic polycarbonates, several methods, including introduction of pendent hydroxyl groups, end group functionalization, and copolymerization with polyesters, have been attempted [80,81]. Polycarbonates and their block copolymers with glycolides (also termed polyglyconates) have been used as orthopedic tacks and screws and as sutures. The suitability of resorbable PTMC barrier membranes for guided bone regeneration of 5.0 mm circular mandibular defect in a rat model, has been recently demonstrated [82]. Histological analysis of the surrounding tissues showed only a mild tissue reaction corresponding to a normal foreign body reaction with minimal cellular capsule formation. Although the bone formation with the use of PTMC membranes was similar to that of control (collagen membrane), the space-maintaining properties of the PTMC membranes were found to be superior [83]. Polycarbonate-based scaffolds have also been used as a delivery vehicle for orthopedic applications. A study reported the use of $PTMC_{11}$-F127-$PTMC_{11}$ hydrogels for the controlled delivery of P24 peptide, an osteogenic peptide derived from the "knuckle" epitope of BMP-2 [84]. Increasing the polymer concentration resulted in reduced burst release, along with sustained release of the loaded peptide for up to 35 days. The P24 loaded matrices enhanced the in vitro osteogenic differentiation of BMSCs and also induced ectopic bone formation in rats. Another study utilized PTMC for the local delivery of gentamicin to inhibit biofilm formation due to osteomyelitis. Standard gentamycin-loaded nondegradable PMMA beads were used as control [85]. In an in vitro study using an in vivo mimicking solution (containing the enzyme lipase), surface-eroding gentamicin-loaded PTMC discs released 60% of loaded drug in 14 days, similar to that from the PMMA beads. Similar to PMMA beads, PTMC discs inhibited *S. aureus*-mediated biofilm formation by approximately 80% for at least 14 days. The study showed the potential of PTMC discs as a biodegradable alternative to PMMA delivery systems. Wang et al. [86] developed a peptide conjugated diblock copolymer using PEG and PTMC (PEG-*b*-PTMC), as a drug carrier capable of charge reversal in response to bone metastatic environments, for targeted drug delivery to the lesion sites. The stimuli-responsive carrier was developed by tethering a chimeric peptide CKGHPGGPQAsp8 consisting of an osteotropic anionic Asp8, a cathepsin K (CTSK)-cleavable substrate (HPGGPQ), and a cationic residue to PEG-*b*-PTMC chain (Pep-*b*-PEG-*b*-PTMC). The (Pep-*b*-PEG-*b*-PTMC) showed the ability to spontaneously self-assemble into negatively charged nanomicelles encapsulating anticancer drug doxorubicin ($30.0 \pm 1\%$ loading content and $90.1 \pm 2\%$ loading efficiency). The nanomicelles also showed enhanced binding to bone HA and exhibited charge conversion from -18.5 ± 1.9 to 15.2 ± 1.8 mV upon exposure to CTSK, an enzyme overexpressed in bone metastatic microenvironments. This unique charge conversion facilitated targeted and enhanced cellular uptake in the bone metastatic cancer lesion sites, making the system an excellent candidate for the treatment of metastatic osteosarcomas.

8.3.1.2 Polyfumarates

Polyfumarates are a class of injectable, biodegradable polymers which can undergo crosslinking in the presence of suitable initiators, owing to the presence of unsaturated double bonds within the polymer backbone. Polypropylene fumarate (PPF) is one of the most widely investigated polyfumarates as an injectable system for drug delivery and tissue engineering applications [87–89]. PPF undergoes bulk degradation via hydrolysis to form fumaric acid and propylene glycol. The rate of degradation depends on polymer molecular weight, the type of crosslinker used, and the crosslinking density of the polymer network.

Lewandrowski et al. [87] developed a nanocomposite bone graft substitute composed of PPF and nano/microHA and evaluated its biocompatibility and osseointegration using a rat tibial defect model. The study showed improved bioactivity of the graft upon addition of *n*-HA leading to superior biocompatibility and osseointegration, when compared to composites prepared using micron-sized HA.

The same group later developed a bone repair material using injectable PPF cross-linked in the presence of HA filler and effervescent agents as a biodegradable adjunct to relieve the disadvantages of wire fixation [90]. To evaluate the efficacy, rat osteotomies were fixed with threaded Kirschner wire or with Kirschner wire augmented with the injectable PPF composite. The study demonstrated enhanced osteotomy with PPF material demonstrating its suitability as an adjunct to wire fixation. Another study investigated the craniofacial bone repair applications of a two-phase biodegradable bone cement, which was fabricated analogous to conventional PMMA cement [91]. The system consisted of crosslinked PPF microparticles, BP as initiator; and a liquid phase of PPF macromer, *N*-vinyl pyrrolidone as the crosslinking agent, and dimethyl toluidine as the accelerator. Formulation parameters including particle weight percentage, particle size, and accelerator concentration were found to significantly influence the properties of crosslinked composites. Addition of PPF microparticles led to a significant increase in the compressive modulus and compressive strength of the cement and also increased its setting time, while reducing the temperature rise during crosslinking (from around $102.7 \pm 49.3°C$ for formulations without microparticles to around $28.0 \pm 2.0°C$ for two-phase composites containing 50% PPF microparticles).

A recent study reported the use of poly(ethylene glycol fumarate) (OPF) as a carrier for autologous or hADSCs for the treatment of critical-sized osteochondral defects in mini pigs [92]. Six months postimplantation, the defects implanted with autologous or hADSC-loaded OPF scaffold showed better neocartilage tissue formation with improved biomechanical properties and higher collagen II expression. The treatment group also showed more mature bone formation with higher expression of collagen I. Another study reported the potential of rehydrated freeze-dried OPF hydrogels for in vivo delivery of BMSCs, in an osteochondral defect model in Prestige World Genetics micropigs [93]. The extent of healing was evaluated 4 months postimplantation and the BMSC-loaded scaffold group showed significantly higher (~99%) defect filling, with 84% hyaline-like cartilage compared to the scaffold-alone group. Another fumarate-based polymer investigated for orthopedic applications is poly(ε-caprolactone fumarate) (PCLF). 3D porous PCLF scaffolds have also been evaluated as a rhBMP-2 delivery system to promote bone regeneration [94]. Incorporation of HA and PVA in the matrix significantly increased the release of rhBMP-2 in a bioactive manner and rhBMP-2-loaded scaffolds were found to induce significant bone formation in a rabbit critical-sized calvarial defect model. Fernandez et al. [95] investigated the feasibility of developing blends of PCL and poly(diisopropyl fumarate), using ultrasound. The blends showed mechanical properties similar to trabecular bone. Moreover, UMR106 and MC3T3E1 osteoblasts showed higher adhesion and also expressed more collagen I and mineral on the compatabilized blends compared to either homopolymers. Bodakhe et al. [96] developed an in situ hardening nanocomposite based on fumarate derivative of poly(glycerol sebacate) and *n*-HA.

The injectable nanocomposite was prepared by photocrosslinking the polymer in the presence of *n*-HA. Incorporation of *n*-HA significantly increased the mechanical properties and the composite showed good attachment, proliferation, and osteogenic differentiation of rat BMSCs. The results were corroborated by the in vivo studies, which showed the potential of the composite to support bone regeneration.

8.3.1.3 Polyurethanes

Polyurethanes are biologically stable polymers generally synthesized using polycondensation reaction of diisocyanates with alcohols and amines, and possess good biocompatibility and mechanical properties. To extend their applications to the field of drug delivery and tissue engineering, many degradable polyurethanes are now being developed. Giannitelli et al. [97] developed polyurethane foam-based graded porous scaffolds with a dense shell and a porous core for potential applications in guided bone regeneration of oromaxillary bone defects. The foam was synthesized via a one-pot reaction of PCL diol and polymethylene polyphenyl isocyanate. Water served as a foaming agent in the process as it could support CO_2 formation upon reaction with residual isocyanate groups. The degradable foam showed good cytocompatibility toward rat BMSCs. Another study investigated the feasibility to enhance the mechanical properties of polyurethane-based porous scaffolds by molecular modification of the polymer soft segments with glyceride of castor oil (GCO) and by the incorporation of HA [98]. The three-phase composite (*n*-HA/GCO − PU) showed significantly improved compressive strength (4.34 MPa) and elastic modulus (165.36 MPa), when compared to pure PU, *n*-HA/CO − PU, and μ-HA/polyurethane (HA/PU) scaffolds. The incorporation of *n*-HA in the scaffold improved the interface bonding with the GCO − PU matrix and bone as well as increased the biological activity of the scaffold. Dumas et al. [99] investigated the effect of the rates of new bone formation, matrix resorption, and polymer degradation on healing of settable weight-bearing polyurethane/allograft composites in a rabbit femoral condyle defect model. The degradable polyurethane was prepared by reacting lysine triisocyanate (LTI) modified PEG prepolymer with poly(ε-caprolactone-*co*-D,L-lactide-*co*-glycolide) triol. However, the unbalanced rates of polymer degradation and zero-order new bone formation resulted in incomplete healing in the interior of the composite, addition of rhBMP-2 to the composite balanced the rate of new bone formation and polymer degradation resulting in extensive healing in all regions of the graft.

Prieto et al. [100] developed and tested injectable composites made from lysine-derived polyurethanes and particulate allograft bone which could set to form bone void fillers, with mechanical strength similar to trabecular bone. In vivo evaluation in a rabbit femoral condyle plug defect model showed that composites containing large (105−500 μm) allograft particles could heal by the end of 12 weeks, whereas those prepared using smaller (<105 μm) particles showed only partial healing. Hence, particle size and surface connectivity could play a major role in overall regeneration capability of these injectable bone void fillers. Studies also investigated the efficacy of nanostructured biodegradable polyurethane scaffolds for bone tissue engineering. Composite, porous, electrospun scaffolds were developed from thermoplastic polyurethane (TPU) and HA [101]. Soft (lower Young's modulus and higher strain-at-break) and hard TPU as well as μ and *n*-HA were investigated. Although higher cellular proliferation and migration was observed in the hard scaffolds, the soft scaffolds showed better osteogenesis of human MSCs. The addition of *n*-HA to soft TPU scaffolds further enhanced the osteogenesis of hMSCs, when compared to those without *n*-HA. Das et al. [102] developed a nanocomposite composed of rapeseed protein functionalized MWCNTs and vegetable-oil-based hyperbranched polyurethane for bone repair. Protein functionalization resulted in significant improvement in the biocompatibility of the MWCNTs. In vivo implantation of the scaffold in a critical-sized fracture gap model led to rapid new bone formation within 30–45 days, with 90–93% filling of the defect area, without any immunogenic or toxic effects.

Studies have also investigated the efficacy of biodegradable polyurethane and its composites as delivery vehicles for bioactive small molecules. For instance, an anabolic agent, lovastatin-loaded porous biodegradable polyurethane scaffolds were evaluated to enhance bone regeneration [103]. The polyurethanes were prepared by reacting trifunctional polyester polyols derived from ε-caprolactone, glycolide, and D,L-lactide monomers with LTI. Lovastatin was incorporated in the scaffold by combining it with the hardener component before scaffold synthesis. Sustained release of biologically active lovastatin is evidenced from the significant enhancement of the in vitro osteogenic differentiation of osteoblastic cells. The in vivo biological activity was demonstrated using a rat plug defect model, wherein the local delivery of lovastatin enhanced new bone formation at 4 weeks postimplantation. Another study investigated the efficacy of biodegradable HA/PU composite scaffolds to locally release an antibiotic (ceftazidime) [104]. The antibiotic was first encapsulated in ethyl cellulose microspheres and incorporated in the composite scaffolds, leading to a sustained release of up to 60 days and good antibacterial properties. Another study utilized porous scaffolds composed of aliphatic polyurethanes made with a different ratio of hydrophilic poly(ethylene oxide) diol and hydrophobic PCL diol components. The scaffolds were loaded with calcium complexing moiety, a sucrose-based polyol Multranol 4035 (polysaccharide), or vitamin D3, so as to improve their biological performance [105]. Implantation of these scaffolds in bicortical defects generated in ovariectomized Warhill ewes, supported defect healing. The scaffolds incorporating calcium-complexing additive were found to be the most effective promoter of bone healing, followed by scaffolds containing vitamin D3 and polysaccharide-containing polymer.

8.3.1.4 Polyanhydrides

Polyanhydrides are hydrolytically unstable, surface eroding homo- or copolymers synthesized via melt condensation, ring-opening polymerization, and dehydrochlorination, as well as condensation reactions. Various aliphatic and aromatic monomers, such as diacid monomers (chlorides and esters), linear and nonlinear fatty acid dimers, and diacid chlorides, have been utilized for polyanhydride synthesis. They are biocompatible and nontoxic in nature [106,107]. Due to their surface erosion characteristics, polyanhydrides have the ability to provide zero-order drug release kinetics and have been widely investigated and in fact approved by Food and Drug Administration (FDA), as a drug delivery vehicle. Lucas et al. [108] investigated the ability of polyanhydride matrix to serve as a controlled-release vehicle for delivering water-soluble osteogenic proteins derived from demineralized bone matrix. The biological activity of the protein was preserved in polyanhydride matrix and the released protein was able to support cartilage and bone formation. Salicylic acid-based poly (anhydride ester) has been developed as an interesting biodegradable and biologically active polyanhydride. An in vitro drug release study demonstrated a lag period of 2 days and day 3 onwards a zero-order release of salicylic acid was observed due to its characteristic surface-eroding properties. In vivo study using critical-sized mandibular angle defects in diabetic rats demonstrated the ability of the polymer to resolve the local inflammatory response and enhance bone regeneration [109].

A study investigated nanocomposites prepared by homogeneously distributing HA nanoneedles in polyanhydrides by in situ photopolymerization [110]. The polyanhydrides were synthesized using methacrylated anhydride monomers of citric acid, sebacic acid (SA), and 1,4-bis(carboxyphenoxy) butane. HA addition was found to significantly improve the mechanical properties and mechanical integrity of the composites during degradation. A related study investigated a composite of polyanhydride copolymers, synthesized using SA and 1,6-bis(*p*-carboxyphenoxy)hexane (CPH), with PCL-grafted HA as a bone graft substitute [111]. The study found a CPH/SA ratio of 7:3 in combination with 10 wt% HA to be optimal for use as a bone substitute, as it could lead to increased cell attachment as well as good mechanical properties. The unique surface-eroding properties and controllable degradation profile of polyanhydrides make them a promising candidate for drug and protein delivery.

8.3.1.5 Poly(amino acids) and pseudo poly(amino acids)

Poly(amino acids), such as poly-γ-(glutamic acid) (γ-PGA), poly(aspartic acid) (PAA), poly(arginine), and poly(lysine), are naturally occurring biodegradable polymers. Poly(amino acids), as the name indicates, are composed of amino acids linked through amide bonds and are known to present some limitations such as immunogenicity, poor mechanical characteristics, and low/pH-dependent solubility. Pseudo(amino acids), on the other hand, are linked by nonamide bonds, such as esters, imino carbonates, and carbonates. Tyrosine-derived poly(amino acids) are one of the most commonly investigated pseudo poly(amino acids) and use desaminotyrosyl-tyrosine alkyl esters as the building blocks. Various functional group modifications have been reported for these polymers, including but not limited to aminolysis, ester exchange, condensation reactions, ring-opening polymerization, and introduction of block, branch, hyperbranched, or dendron-like architecture [51]. Most of the recent studies investigating the use of poly(amino acids) for orthopedic applications have focused on developing composite scaffolds so as to incorporate bioactivity and improved mechanical properties in the resulting constructs.

A study investigated the effect of poly(amino acids) (PAA and γ-PGA) incorporation on the properties of injectable calcium phosphate cements (CPCs) [112]. The addition of these polymers was found to significantly affect the dynamic viscosity (directly proportional to γ-PGA and inversely proportional to PAA) and increase the injectability of the CPCs. γ-PGA incorporation also decreased the initial setting time of the cements. Furthermore, Saos-2 cell spreading was enhanced on CPCs with poly (amino acids), when compared to CPC alone. Another study showed that the surface erosion of poly(amino acid) polymer could help in maintaining the mechanical strength during degradation of the TCP-poly(amino acid) composite [113]. The composite was prepared by in situ polymerization of TCP powder with a poly(amino acid) composed of alanine, phenylalanine, glycine, 6-aminocaproic acid, proline, and lysine, in the presence of water. In vivo implantation of the composites in dog femoral defects showed the formation of osteoid, 12 weeks postimplantation. The composites were biocompatible and did not show any inflammatory response or fibrous encapsulation. The degradability and bioactivity of poly(amino acid)/β-Ca_2SiO_4 composite fabricated using in situ melting polymerization, has also been investigated [114]. Here, a tyrosine-based poly(amino acid) polymer was used. The composite showed good bioactivity and degradation in vitro, when placed in simulated body fluid, indicating its potential for bone regeneration. Another study recently reported the successful regeneration of surgically created cancellous bone defects in rabbits with calcium sulfate/poly(amino acid) composite grafts [115]. The poly(amino acid) used in this study was composed of alanine, benzene alanine, glycine, 6-aminocaproic acid, proline, and lysine amino acids. Furthermore, the biocompatibility and ability of HA-poly(amino acid) composites to induce osteogenesis and reconstruct rabbit long bone defect, has also been demonstrated [116,117].

Lee et al. [118] reported a novel method to increase the osteogenic activity to titanium implants, by surface functionalizing them using adhesive poly(amino acid) diblock copolymer-based nanoparticles. The BMP-2-loaded nanoparticles were prepared by the self-assembly of catechol-poly(L-aspartic acid)-*b*-poly(L-phenylalanine) (Cat-PAsp-PPhe). The nanoparticle shell was composed of anionic PAsp, the inner core was PPhe and the peripheral catechol groups provided titanium immobilization properties. Nanoparticles immobilized on titanium surface showed the ability to release BMP-2 for up to 40 days and also enhanced surface osteogenicity as evidenced by the improved attachment, proliferation, and ALP activity of hADSCs.

8.3.1.6 Polyphosphazenes

Polyphosphazenes are hybrid polymers composed of a backbone of alternating phosphorus and nitrogen atoms containing two organic or organometallic side chains attached to each phosphorus atom. Polyphosphazenes can be synthesized using ring-opening polymerization and living cationic polymerization [119]. Many methods like esterification, etherification, and amidification have been used to incorporate a variety of side chains to the polymer backbone. The side chains invariably affect the degradation, physical, thermal, and mechanical properties of the polymer. The formation of nontoxic and neutral by-products upon degradation of polyphosphazenes has led to their use as drug carriers and tissue engineering scaffolds [120]. Biodegradable polyphosphazene polymers containing imidazolyl (I-PPHOS) or ethyl glycinato (EG-PPHOS) side chain substituents have been used for intraarticular delivery of the antiinflammatory agent, colchicine [121]. I-PPHOS released 20% of the loaded colchicine in 21 days, whereas EG-PPHOS released 60% of the loaded drug within the same time period. This could be attributed to the differences in the degradation rate of these polymers. Krogman et al., first reported the synthesis of block copolymers of polyphosphazenes linked to polyesters or polycarbonates, via ring-opening polymerization techniques [122]. Deng et al. [123] prepared blends of polyphosphazene (poly[(glycine ethyl glycinato)$_1$(phenyl phenoxy)$_1$phosphazene], PPHOS) and polyesters (PLGA) for bone tissue engineering applications. The blends showed higher tensile modulus and improved in vivo biocompatibility compared to the polyester. The degradation rate of the blends was found to be slower than the polyester. This was attributed to the neutralization of polyphosphazene degradation products with the acidic degradation products of PLGA. The blend was also used for the fabrication of electrospun nanofiber matrices as bone tissue regeneration scaffolds. The electrospun fiber matrix was concentrically folded to replicate the bone marrow cavity, as well as the lamellar structure of bone [124]. The scaffolds showed a compressive modulus in the mid-range for that of human trabecular bone and also supported in vitro osteoblast adhesion, infiltration, and extracellular matrix secretion. 3D porous scaffolds based on a degradable amino acid containing polymer, poly[(methylphenoxy)(ethyl glycinato) phosphazene] have also been fabricated by salt-leaching technique [125]. These 3D scaffolds showed good osteoblast attachment and growth, when compared to a 2D matrix. Nukavarapu et al. [126] synthesized three biodegradable polyphosphazenes substituted with leucine, valine, and phenylalanine ethyl ester side groups, for orthopedic applications. Furthermore, the phenylalanine ethyl ester substituted polyphosphazene (glass transition temperature 41.6°C) was used to fabricate composite microspheres with *n*-HA and sintered into porous scaffolds (pore size 86–145 μm), using a dynamic solvent sintering approach. Good cell adhesion, proliferation, and ALP expression of primary rat osteoblasts seeded on these 3D scaffolds indicated their potential for bone tissue engineering applications.

8.3.2 Natural polymers

8.3.2.1 Protein-based polymers

Collagen is the most abundant protein in the human body and is responsible for providing strength and flexibility to connective tissues and skin. It has excellent biocompatibility and cell adhesion properties, and has been extensively investigated for various tissue engineering and orthopedic applications [127]. Around 28 different collagens are currently known with types I–IV being the most common and widely studied. It is composed of three parallel polypeptide strands in a left-handed, polyproline II-type helical conformation which coil around each other with a one-residue stagger to form a right-handed triple helix, also known as tropocollagen. The strands have a repeating Xaa–Yaa–Gly sequence, where Xaa and Yaa can be any amino acid but are, most often than not, (2*S*)-proline (Pro, 28%) and (2*S*,4*R*)-4-hydroxyproline (Hyp, 38%), respectively. ProHypGly is thus the most common triplet (10.5%) in collagen [128]. The assembly of tropocollagen in a complex, hierarchical manner leads to the formation of macroscopic fibrous structures and networks which then form the extracellular matrix of various tissues, bone, and basement membranes [129]. Collagen can be dissolved in acidic aqueous solutions and degraded using enzymes like collagenase and metalloproteinases. It is mainly obtained from bovine or porcine skin and tendons and can also undergo crosslinking via thermal, chemical, and irradiation methods. Various collagen-based scaffolds such as fibers, foams, and sponges have been fabricated using techniques like freeze-drying, electrospinning, critical point drying, and rapid prototyping [127]. Collagenous scaffolds have also been a scaffold of choice for delivery of growth factors, with products such as Infuse, currently available in the market for the local delivery of rhBMP-2. Many modified forms of collagen scaffolds are currently under investigation to increase its biological activity. In one study, 3-glycidoxypropyl trimethoxysilane was used as a crosslinker for Col-1 to fabricate nanofibrous, porous, BMP-2-loaded silicate-collagen hybrid fibril sheets [130]. The hybrid sheets showed a loading efficiency of 64% with around 40% release of encapsulated BMP-2 in 2 weeks. The sheets also allowed for attachment, growth, and differentiation of MC3T3-E1 cells in vitro. Another study attempted to mimic the natural extracellular microenvironment by using sulfated polysaccharides, which are known to bind and regulate the bioactivity of BMP-2 through a heparin-binding domain [131]. Supramolecular nanofibrous networks were developed using peptide amphiphiles, which integrate the biological role of syndecan and fibronectin. The hybrid biomaterial was composed of collagen scaffold infiltrated with peptide nanofibers, heparan sulfate, and BMP-2. The presence of peptide nanofibers and heparin sulfate enhanced the biological activity of incorporated BMP-2 and was found to be more effective in bridging a rat critical-size femoral defect compared to BMP-2 delivered using conventional collagen.

Moreau et al. [132] developed a composite scaffold based on collagen and CPC for improving the fracture resistance, mechanical properties, and cellular response of the cement. The composite was injectable, self-setting, and showed a 10-fold increase in toughness and a twofold increase in MC3T3-E1 attachment, indicating its potential for regenerating bone in moderate stress-bearing applications. In an attempt to fabricate a matrix capable of regenerating bone in defects associated with bacterial infections, a study reported the development of silver nanoparticle-loaded, fibrillar collagen—HA matrices [133]. To this end, spherical silver nanoparticles (average diameter 25 nm) were attached to collagen molecules in solution followed by collagen self-assembly in modified SBF to form fibrils with native periodicity. The matrix could further undergo biomineralization upon incubation in SBF. The composites showed significant antibacterial activity against *S. aureus* and *Escherichia coli*, proportional to the concentration of silver nanoparticles. In addition, the composites were found to be hemocompatible and showed acceptable biocompatibility toward MG-63 osteoblasts.

Fibrin is another protein-based polymer, derived from fibrinogen and is involved in blood clotting wherein thrombin initiates the cleavage of soluble fibrinogen to form insoluble fibrin clot. Owing to its source and biological availability, fibrin shows excellent biocompatibility. It is also injectable, biodegradable, and contains several extracellular matrix proteins that can favorably affect cell adhesion and proliferation. The ability of fibrin to serve as a delivery vehicle for growth factors, including BMP-2, has been widely investigated [134]. The heparin-binding domain II of fibrinogen can act as a promiscuous high-affinity growth factor-binding domain [135]. Several growth factors from the platelet derived growth factor/vascular endothelial growth factor and FGF families and some growth factors from the transforming factor beta and neurotrophin families have been shown to possess high affinity toward fibrin matrix and could be retained via binding interactions. Incorporation of the heparin-binding domain of fibrin into synthetic fibrin-mimetic matrices was found to improve bone formation and wound healing in vivo, indicating the potential of such matrices for growth factor delivery and tissue regeneration [136].

Yang et al. [137] developed an injectable, heparin-conjugated fibrin (HCF) gel by mixing heparin-conjugated fibrinogen with thrombin, as a long-term BMP-2 delivery vehicle. Later, the group compared the bone-forming capability of the HCF gel with clinically used collagen sponge [138]. In vitro BMP-2 release studies showed a more sustained release from HCF when compared to collagen. HCF released around 80% of encapsulated BMP-2 in 20 days, whereas collagen released the same amount within 6 days. Interestingly, less than half of the BMP-2 dose delivered using collagen sponge could lead to similar bone formation and higher bone density in mouse calvarial defects, when delivered using HCF. The results indicate that long-term delivery vehicle "HCF" may be a better alternative to short-term delivery vehicle "collagen," for achieving good bone formation using BMP-2. A related study also confirmed the superiority of fibrin matrix over absorbable collagen sponge, as a carrier for BMP-2 [139]. The study showed equivalent in vivo bone formation in a critical-sized rat osteotomy model, with sevenfold lower dose of BMP-2 (dose: 10 μg) delivered using fibrin matrix, when compared with absorbable collagen sponge (dose: 72 μg). Another study investigated a hybrid construct composed of BMP-2 loaded poly (L-lysine) nanoparticles dispersed in fibrin gel, for inducing in vitro differentiation of encapsulated hMSCs [140]. The in vitro evaluation of the 3D hybrid constructs via reverse transcription polymerase chain reaction, Western blotting, histological, and immunohistochemical analysis showed improved potency of BMP-2-loaded nanoparticles to induce osteogenic differentiation of encapsulated hMSC, when compared to the control or BMP-2-loaded fibrin constructs without nanoparticles. BMP-2-loaded fibrin hydrogels implanted within porous titanium implants have also been shown to completely regenerate load-bearing segmental bone defects in rat femora within 4 weeks, with full restoration of the original bone functionality and anatomical shape, although the empty defects and fibrin gel alone controls did not show the same effects [141]. These studies demonstrate the improved efficacy of fibrin-based matrices for protein delivery for orthopedic applications.

Albumin is another water-soluble protein, and is a prominent blood plasma protein (50%) with a molecular weight of around 66.5 kDa. Albumin has been widely investigated as a drug delivery carrier as well as a scaffold for tissue regeneration. Albumin is of great significance for bone regeneration as its expression has been found to increase during healing of fractures and it has shown to possess anabolic effects during bone formation [142]. Recent studies have shown faster in vivo bone formation in critical-sized calvarial defects using serum albumin-coated demineralized bone matrices and similarly serum albumin-coated bone graft has been shown to successfully regenerate nonunion femoral defects [143,144]. Gallego et al. [145] have shown the feasibility of using porous, crosslinked albumin sponges as a scaffold for delivering human alveolar osteoblasts to treat critical-sized, rat mandibular defects. Unlike blank controls, cell-seeded albumin scaffolds supported complete healing of the mandibular defects. Another study reported the feasibility of fabricating highly porous scaffolds from human, porcine, and bovine albumin [146]. Here, instead of using the usual chemical methodology for crosslinking, microbial transglutaminase enzyme was used to polymerize albumin followed by freeze-drying to fabricate porous scaffolds with moderate mechanical strength. The approach is expected to reduce the compatibility issues associated with aldehyde-based crosslinkers and improve the biocompatibility of the scaffolds. In addition to scaffolds, albumin nanoparticles coated with positively charged polyethyleneimine, have also been used as a delivery vehicle for BMP-2 [147]. The nanoparticles showed a BMP-2 encapsulation efficiency of >90%. Uncoated nanoparticles, however, released >70% of loaded BMP-2 within the first day. Coating with PEI significantly reduced the burst release (<15% in 1 day) and extended the release for over 10 days, in a concentration-dependent manner. However, higher concentration of PEI also led to an increase in in vitro toxicity. The BSA nanoparticles coated with 0.1 mg/mL PEI showed tolerable toxicity with slow BMP-2 release, while maintaining the bioactivity of encapsulated BMP-2. These studies show the efficacy of albumin-based carriers for drug and cellular delivery to support regeneration.

8.3.2.2 Polysaccharide-based polymers

Chitosan is a linear polysaccharide composed of randomly located β(1−4)-linked D-glucosamine and *N*-acetyl glucosamine units. It is obtained by the deacetylation of chitin (fully acetylated form, i.e., degree of acetylation (DA) = 100%), found in the exoskeletons of crustaceans. Chitosan is known to be biocompatible, nontoxic, and even approved for oral administration as a food additive by FDA. It has inherent hemostatic and antibacterial properties, and is mucoadhesive in nature [148]. It has been widely explored as a hemostatic, permeation enhancer, scaffold for tissue regeneration and wound dressing, and as a carrier for drugs, genes, and other biomolecules. The physicochemical properties of chitosan depend on its molecular weight, DA, and crystal structure. The viscosity, solubility, permeability, hemostatic activity, mucoadhesivity, and biocompatibility of chitosan have an inverse relationship with DA [149]. However, the crystallinity and biodegradability increase with increasing DA [150]. The in vivo degradation of chitosan has been known to occur enzymatically via lysozyme. Additionally, enzymes like chitosanase and papain can degrade chitosan in vitro. The polymer is insoluble in organic solvents and in aqueous media at physiological pH. Chitosan solubilization can only be achieved under acidic media, wherein the protonation of the $-NH_2$ function on the C-2 position of the D-glucosamine repeat unit converts the polymer into a soluble polyelectrolyte form. The free hydroxyl and amino functionalities present in the chemical structure of chitosan make it amenable to chemical modification and crosslinking, which has been widely used to modulate the solubility, degradation behavior, and other physicochemical properties of the polymer. Furthermore, the positive charge generated due to the protonation of amino groups of chitosan polymeric chain, can result in significant charge interactions with negatively charged drugs or biomolecules as well as with negatively charged polymers for polyelectrolyte complexation. The hemostatic activity, mucoadhesion, cell permeation, and gene transfection ability of chitosan are directly related to the number of protonable amino groups in chitosan [150,151]. Mucoadhesion of chitosan occurs via the interaction of protonated amino groups with the negatively charged sialic acid residues in the mucin. Similarly, the negative charge on the red blood cell membranes is responsible for chitosan's hemostatic activity. Hence, increase in polymer molecular weight and degree of deacetylation, which ultimately increase the number of protonable amino groups, also lead to enhancement of the aforementioned properties. The same is true for the cell permeation effect and gene transfection capability of chitosan [152].

Chitosan has been fabricated in the form of porous sponges, foams, films, particulate scaffolds such as nanoparticles and microparticles; injectable hydrogels; nanofibers and composites, for drug delivery and as tissue engineering scaffolds for orthopedic applications [152–156]. A study investigated composite blend foams of chitosan and gelatin, with varying concentrations of bioactive glass, for bone regeneration [157]. The foams prepared by freeze-drying process were further crosslinked using genipin to improve the mechanical strength of the bioactive composites. The foams showed interconnected pores and improved bioactivity upon the addition of the bioactive glass. Additionally, the composites containing 70 wt% of glass showed an elastic modulus comparable to alveolar bone.

Our group and others have reported fabrication of injectable chitosan thermogels, via neutralization of chitosan chains with inorganic phosphate salts such as ammonium hydrogen phosphate (AHP) as well as polyol counterionic monohead salts such as β-glycerophosphate (β-GP) [158–162]. These pH and thermosensitive hydrogels have been investigated as delivery vehicles for cells, small molecules, bioactive lipids, and growth factors, alike. For instance, Chi-AHP hydrogels were shown to successfully deliver rhBMP-2 and BMSC combination in vivo and could result in significantly higher bone regeneration in a rat critical-sized, calvarial defect model with the combination group, when compared to BMSC alone. A composite matrix composed of Chi-AHP hydrogels and microspheres has been used for delivering sphingosine-1-phosphate analog (FTY720) to enhance the recruitment of endogenous progenitor cells for bone regeneration [163]. Furthermore, injectable thermosensitive composite hydrogels fabricated via sol–gel method by combining zinc-doped chitosan, *n*-HA, and β-GP (Zn-CS/*n*HA/β-GP) have also been investigated [155]. The sol–gel transition temperature of this system was 37°C and the hydrogel did not show any cytotoxicity toward mesenchymal stem cells. The presence of *n*-HA was found to enhance the swelling, protein adsorption, exogenous mineralization, in vitro osteoblast differentiation, as well as in vivo bone formation.

In addition to thermogelling hydrogels, we have also developed enzymatically crosslinkable hydrogel platform based on glycol chitosan. The injectable hydrogel, developed using 3-(4-hydroxyphenyl)propionic acid-modified glycol chitosan has been successfully utilized for the localized delivery of rhBMP-2 [154]. Gelation was initiated by the oxidative coupling of the substituted phenol groups within the polymer, in the presence of hydrogen peroxide and horse radish peroxidase. These porous hydrogels could maintain the viability of encapsulated 7F2 osteoblasts indicating the nontoxicity of the gelation process. The encapsulated BMP-2 could be localized

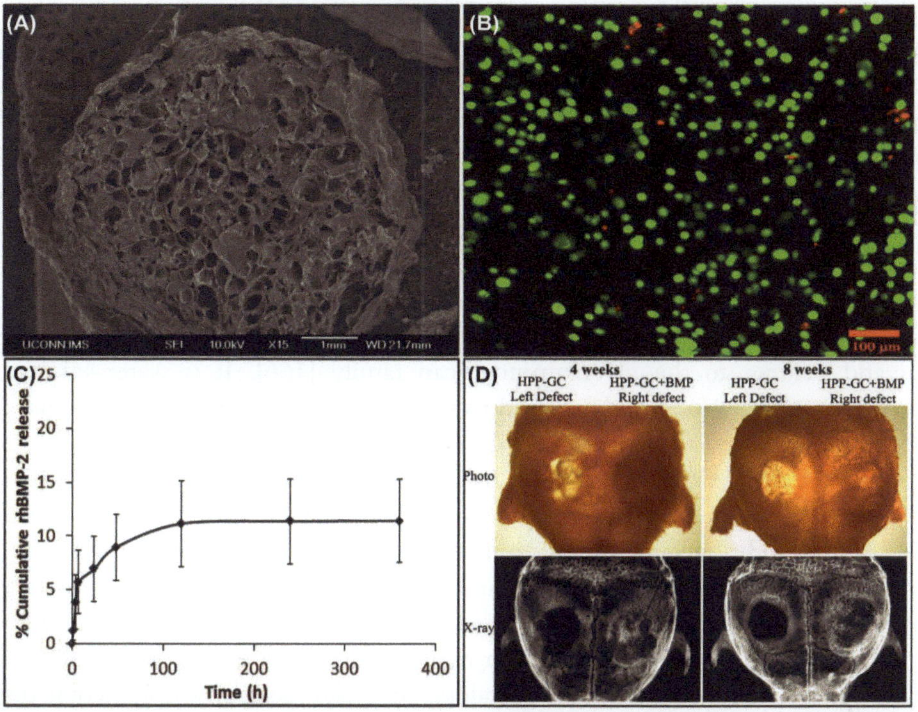

Figure 8.3 (A) SEM image showing morphology of HPP–GC hydrogels, (B) Z-stacked confocal image showing viability of 7F2 osteoblasts after 3 h of in situ gelation, (C) cumulative percent release of rhBMP-2 from HPP–GC hydrogel, (D) whole calvaria and X-ray images of calvaria implanted with HPP–GC hydrogels with and without rhBMP-2, at 4 and 8 weeks postimplantation.

within the hydrogel with only 11% release in 360 hours. Furthermore, the in vivo bioactivity of the encapsulated rhBMP-2 was maintained and the rhBMP-2 encapsulated hydrogels resulted in complete regeneration of critical-sized mouse calvarial defects at the tested time points of 4 and 8 weeks (Fig. 8.3).

A recent study showed the beneficial effect of chitosan nanofiber scaffolds on in vivo bone healing [153]. Here, metaphyseal bone defects were created in the femurs of C57BL/6 mice, implanted with either chitosan nanofiber scaffolds or left empty (controls) and analyzed by microCT and histomorphometry. The chitosan nanofiber scaffolds were found to increase new trabecular bone formation, and led to a significant increase in the trabecular bone thickness but a reduction in the trabecular parameter factor. The trabecular bone production observed upon implantation of these scaffolds was attributed to the upregulation of Runx2-mediated ALP and osteocalcin gene expressions. A biomimetic nanocomposite, nanofibrous scaffold prepared by in situ precipitation of HA on electrospun chitosan nanofibers has also been investigated for bone tissue engineering applications [164]. The study utilized a two-step approach and combined in situ coprecipitation synthesis route with electrospinning process. Ultrahigh-molecular-weight poly(ethylene oxide) was used as a fiber-forming additive to achieve composite nanofibers from an aqueous acetic acid-dominant solvent system, with uniform distribution of HA. The composite nanofibers showed excellent osteoconductivity and enhanced cell proliferation and mineral deposition of hFOB (osteoblast) cells in vitro. Other porous composite scaffold composed of chitosan–gelatin/HA and chitosan–*n*-HA, prepared by freeze-drying method, have also been reported [156,165].

Hyaluronic acid or hyaluronan is made up of repeating disaccharide units of D-glucuronic acid and *N*-acetyl glucosamine linked by β(1,4) and β(1,3) glucosidic bonds and belongs to the glycosaminoglycan family [166]. It is water-soluble, can form viscoelastic solutions, and is found in many body tissues including synovial fluid, vitreous humor, articular cartilage, and glycocalyx of endothelial cells. It is an essential component of extracellular matrix and has been shown to play a predominant role in various processes including tissue morphogenesis, cell migration, differentiation, and adhesion [167]. Hyaluronic acid is approved by the FDA for viscosupplementation treatment of osteoarthritic knee, as its injection in the arthritic joint is expected to facilitate movement and reduce pain. In addition, it is also used as a dermal filler and in various skin products to improve skin hydration. Baldini et al. [168] evaluated the potential of hyaluronic acid matrix (Hyaloss) to repair postextraction dental defects. Here, the Hyaloss matrix was mixed with autologous bone, implanted in postextractive sockets, and analyzed clinically and histologically after 4 months of grafting. Due to the gel-like consistency, Hyaloss was found to improve the injectability and placement of the composite in to the defect site. Bone deposition, angiogenesis, and remodeling were also found to be accelerated in the system. Another study showed accelerated new bone formation in the infrabone defects on using low-molecular-weight hyaluronic acid as a coadjuvant during grafting when employing autologous bone [169]. In one study, hyaluronan hydrogel was covalently crosslinked to bisphosphonate ligands (HA–BP) in an attempt to sequester BMP-2 in the hydrogel [170]. The HA–BP hydrogels released around 10% BMP-2 in 2 weeks, in contrast to 100% release with hyaluronan gel alone. The bioactivity of the sequestered BMP-2 could be maintained in the HA–BP hydrogel and the BMP-2 could be released by enzymatic degradation of the hydrogel. Another group investigated the potential of acrylated hyaluronic acid to serve as a carrier for BMP-2 and human mesenchymal stem cells and to regenerate calvarial bone defects in male Sprague–Dawley albino rats [171]. Briefly, the amine group was first introduced into the polymer chains by reacting with adipic acid dihydrazide, which was followed by acrylation by *N*-acryloxysuccinimide. Gelation was initiated by Michel-type addition using tetrathiolated poly(ethylene) glycol (PEG-SH) as a crosslinker. As expected, the hydrogels with BMP-2 and human mesenchymal stem cells showed the highest expression of osteocalcin and mature in vivo bone formation with vascular markers, after 4 weeks of implantation, indicating the potential of the system for combination delivery of cells and growth factor for bone regeneration. Methacrylated hyaluronic acid has also been used to fabricate bioactive hydrogels for localized drug delivery and bone repair [172]. Here, crosslinked hydrogels composed of methacrylated hyaluronic acid and poly(VPAc) were synthesized, which could act as a calcium-binding site during biomineralization via urea-mediation method. The hydrogels showed high water content ($>84\%$) which can be modulated by polymer composition, crosslinking density, biomineralization, and ionic strength of the medium.

Alginic acid is a nonbranched, binary, block copolymer of β-D-mannuronic acid and α-L-guluronic acid monomers linked via a 1−4-glycocidic bond. It is a biodegradable, nontoxic, and biocompatible material obtained mainly from brown algae such as *Laminaria hyperborea* and *Lessonia* and has been extensively used as a food additive and a thickener [173]. The presence of a large number of reactive carboxyl functionalities facilitates spontaneous and mild gelation of the polymer solution in the presence of divalent cations (e.g., calcium ions) and also makes the polymer amenable to chemical modifications. Due to the absence of enzyme alginate lyase, mammals cannot degrade alginates. The slow in vivo degradation of alginates can, however, be improved by irradiation with gamma rays which cleaves the mannuronic-guluronic glycoside bond or by oxidation with periodate which forms a hemiacetal ring changing the urinate residue to a hydrolytically labile open chain [174]. A study evaluated and compared alginate and high-molecular-weight hyaluronic acid hydrogels in terms of their biocompatibility and bioactivity [175]. Although both hydrogels showed good biocompatibility and supported the long-term viability of MC3T3-E1 cells, alginate hydrogels induced higher ALP levels and osteocalcin mRNA levels and also increased the intracellular calcium content in cells, suggesting that alginate could induce matrix mineralization directly proportional to the polymer concentration.

8.3.2.3 Natural polyesters (polyhydroxyalkanoates)

Polyesters of natural origin include those synthesized via bacterial bioprocess routes. The most common bacterial polyesters include poly(3-hydroxybutyrate) (PHB) and its copolymers with 3-hydroxyvalerate (PHBV). Various bacteria such as *Wautersia eutropha*, *Bacillus megaterium*, *Rhodospirillum rubrum*, *Alcaligenes eutrophus*, *Azotobacter chroococcum*, and bacteria from genus *Pseudomonas* have been used for synthesis of bacterial polyesters [176]. Random bulk hydrolysis of ester bonds in the polymer chain is responsible for the in vitro degradation of these polymers in aqueous media, as is the case with their synthetic counterparts. In addition, more than 300 microbial strains from soil, including denitrifying bacteria, are known to degrade polyhydroxyalkanoates [177]. Due to their biocompatibility and environment-friendly synthesis, over the past years, these natural polyesters have been used to develop devices including sutures, wound dressings, orthopedic pins, tendon and articular cartilage repair devices, drug delivery systems, and as scaffolds for tissue regeneration [178]. A study reported the feasibility of using macroporous PHBV foams for bone regeneration by testing the in vitro cell attachment, growth, and differentiation of rat marrow stromal osteoblasts [179]. Neat and RF oxygen plasma (100 W, 10 minutes)-modified matrices were tested. Both matrices were found to exhibit good cell attachment, growth, mineralization, ALP, and osteocalcin production in vitro, however, the plasma-treated matrix showed improvement over the nontreated matrices. A hybrid porous scaffold, prepared by embedding PHBV microspheres into PLGA matrix followed by salt leaching, was also investigated for its ability to repair bone defects. The addition of PHBV microspheres led to an enhancement of compressive strength of the scaffold (~1.48 MPa). The scaffolds also possessed good pore interconnectivity and allowed cell ingrowth within the macropores [180]. Larsson et al. developed PHB nanocomposites by incorporating nanogels of lithium-neutralized polyacrylic acid into the PHB polymer matrix [181]. The nanogels were prepared by microemulsion-templated polymerization and uniformly distributed in the matrix. The nanocomposite released around half the loaded lithium in around 3 hours and the remaining lithium was slowly released during the biodegradation. The observed controlled release and improved tolerance of the nanocomposites toward deformation implies their suitability for bone tissue engineering. A recent study utilized pearl powder to enhance the mineralization capacity of electrospun, PHBV nanofiber scaffolds [182]. The scaffolds were cytocompatible and the mineralization was found to be directly proportional to the pearl powder concentration, as it could act as a nucleation site for HA deposition. These studies indicate the potential of bacterial polyesters as biodegradable materials for some orthopedic applications.

8.4 MAJOR APPLICATIONS OF POLYMERS AND THEIR COMPOSITES FOR ORTHOPEDIC APPLICATIONS

As discussed earlier, both degradable and nondegradable materials, as well as their composites with other polymers, ceramics, and metals, have been investigated for orthopedic applications. Tables 8.2 and 8.3 present a compilation of some of the medical devices and products based on the polymer type and highlight the composition and key features. These products are being used for a variety of applications including, but not limited to, as cements, fillers, fixation devices, interspinous devices, intervertebral replacement devices, and as devices for bone repair, regeneration, or replacement (Fig. 8.4). The present section elaborates on the major applications of various polymers and their composites in the field of orthopedics, along with representative examples from each category.

Table 8.2 Nondegradable polymer-based products for orthopedic applications

Biomaterial	Product/ application	Remarks	Company, location
PMMA	Bone cement filler	Bone replacement for load-bearing sites, fixation of prostheses, vertebroplasty	Heraeus Medical, USA
PEAK	Joint arthoscopy	Strong mechanical properties generally used as parts in joint replacements, implants	Invibio Ltd., UK
	Wallis Posterior Dynamic Stabilization System	Low moisture absorption, good chemical resistance, radiation resistance	Zimmer, Netherlands
UHMWPE	Biomedical fibers	Articulating component for orthopedic prostheses, load-bearing sites, lubricating capacity	DSM Biomedical, USA
	GENESIS II Knee Replacement System	Knee replacement, load-bearing system, low elasticity, good tactile feedback	Smith and Nephew, New Zealand
	STAR Ankle Replacement	Ankle replacement, high-strength load-bearing system, facilitated articulation	Small Bone Innovations, USA
	ProDisc-L Total Disc Replacement	Replacement of lumbar intervertebral discs, minimizes the impact on surrounding tissue	DePuy Synthes, USA

(*Continued*)

Table 8.2 (Continued)

Biomaterial	Product/ application	Remarks	Company, location
Polypropylene	Rods for bone fixation	Ultrahigh-strength rods for bone fixation, high mechanical strength	Nationwide Plastics, USA
	MultiLoc Proximal Humeral Nails	Provide stability in treatment of humeral fractures	DePuy Synthes, USA
	DIAM Spinal Stabilization System	Excellent fatigue resistance, high melting temperature, low density	Medtronic, USA
Polysulfone	Silicone Implant Duplicator Kit	Stable, biocompatible, bone ingrowth mimics natural healing, bone fixation devices, total joint arthroplasties	Lang Dental, USA
Polydimethylsiloxane	Silicone molding material	Hand and food joints, bone implants, plastic surgery implants and orthopedics, characterized by flexibility, easy spread and flow, all temperature functionality	Albright Technologies, USA

8.4.1 Bone-related applications

8.4.1.1 Bone cements

Successful joint replacement depends on the sound fixation of the prosthesis to the bone. The bone cement serves as a space-filler to hold the implant against the bone and thereby acts as a "grout" [183]. PMMA, a nondegradable polymer, is commonly used as bone cement (see Section 8.2.1). PMMA-based bone cements are usually available as a two-component system consisting of a liquid MMA monomer and

Table 8.3 Degradable synthetic polymer-based products for orthopedic applications

Biomaterial	Products/applications	Remarks	Company, location
Synthetic polymers			
Poly(α-ester)	Resorbable biomaterial platform for regenerative medicine	Drug delivery, controllable degradation rates, high structural integrity	Secant Medical, USA
	Bioabsorbable scaffolds	pH-sensitive degradation, scaffolds for bone tissue engineering	ATEX Technologies Inc, USA
	chronOS Bone Graft Substitute	Radiopaque, resorbable, and osteoconductive, for posterolateral spinal fusion and as bone void filler	DePuy Synthes, USA
	BioScrew	PLLA-based bioabsorbable interference screws	ConMed, USA
	Cranios Reinforced Bone Cement	Reinforced by PLGA fibers, bone repair	DePuy Synthes, USA
Polyurethanes	Customized prosthetics	Scaffolds for tissue engineering, prostheses, grafts, permanent implants, drug delivery devices, good biocompatibility, excellent mechanical properties	Orthopaedic Motion, Inc., USA
Poly(anhydride-*co*-imide)	Biodegradable polymer for orthopedic applications	Drug delivery, hard and soft tissue repair, erosion degradation mechanism favorable to long-term stability of the implant	Sigma Aldrich Corporation, USA
Polyfumurates	Assorted injectable microspheres	Injectable polymeric biomaterial scaffolds, varying chemical compositions	Spherotech, USA
	OSSIF-i sem Mineralized Cancellous Bone Allograft (Patterson Dental)	Injectable polymeric biomaterial scaffolds, bone regeneration, superior biocompatibility	Patterson Dental, USA Surgical Esthetics, USA
Pseudo poly (amino acid)	General products	Drug delivery, tissue engineering, orthopaedic applications and grafts	–
Polyphosphazenes	Load-bearing hydrogel	Drug delivery, erosion degradation mechanism favorable to long-term stability of the implant, hydrogels and membranes for coating of bone implants, strong lubricating properties	Cambridge Polymer Group Inc., USA

(Continued)

Table 8.3 (Continued)

Biomaterial	Products/applications	Remarks	Company, location
Polydioxanone	TriStar Bone Graft Fixation System	Bioabsorbable fixation devices, bone regeneration, fracture fixation in nonload-bearing bones, sutures, wound clips	Impladent Ltd., USA
Polycarbonates	Makrolon Rx2530 Polycarbonate Bone Fixation Device	Bioabsorbable fixation devices and bone regeneration, drug delivery, strong mechanical properties, also used in scaffolds in orthopedic applications	Metric Medical Devices, Inc., USA
Natural polymers			
Collagen	Infuse Bone Graft	Hard and soft tissue repair, high compatibility, bioresorbable growth factor carrier, sinus augmentation and tibial shaft fracture repair, strength and flexibility	Medtronic, USA
	Integra Mozaik	Bioresorbable structure and compression resistance in lumbar fusions	Integra Life Sciences, USA
	NovaBone MacroFORM	Collagen and bioactive glass, is moldable and bioactive, can be mixed with bone marrow aspirate to enhance bone growth	NovaBone Products, LLC., USA
Albumin	BoneAlbumin, albumin-coated bone allograft serum	Joint and bone replacement (knee, shoulder, dental), highest tensile strength, resistance to fatigue, nonbone bonding, lubricating capacity	OrthoSera GmbH, Hungary
Fibrin	Macrofix, self-hardening bone void filler	Soft tissue healing, bone void fillers, strong sealing capacity, excellent biocompatibility	Citagenix Medical, Canada
	CERAMENT, bone void filler	Bioresorbable, used for bony defects, favor cell adhesion and proliferation	Bone Support AB, Sweden
Chitosan	Chi2Gel Hybrid Hydrogel	Hybrid gel of chitosan and hyaluronic acid for viscosupplementation, under preclinical testing	Chi2Gel Ltd., Israel
Hyaluronic acid	ORTHOVISC/MONOVISC	Injections for osteoarthritic knee pain treatment by viscosupplementation	Anika Therapeutics, DePuy Synthes, USA
	InQu bone substitute	Hyaluronic acid interwoven into a network of PLGA, various spinal and orthopedic procedures	Isto Technologies, USA

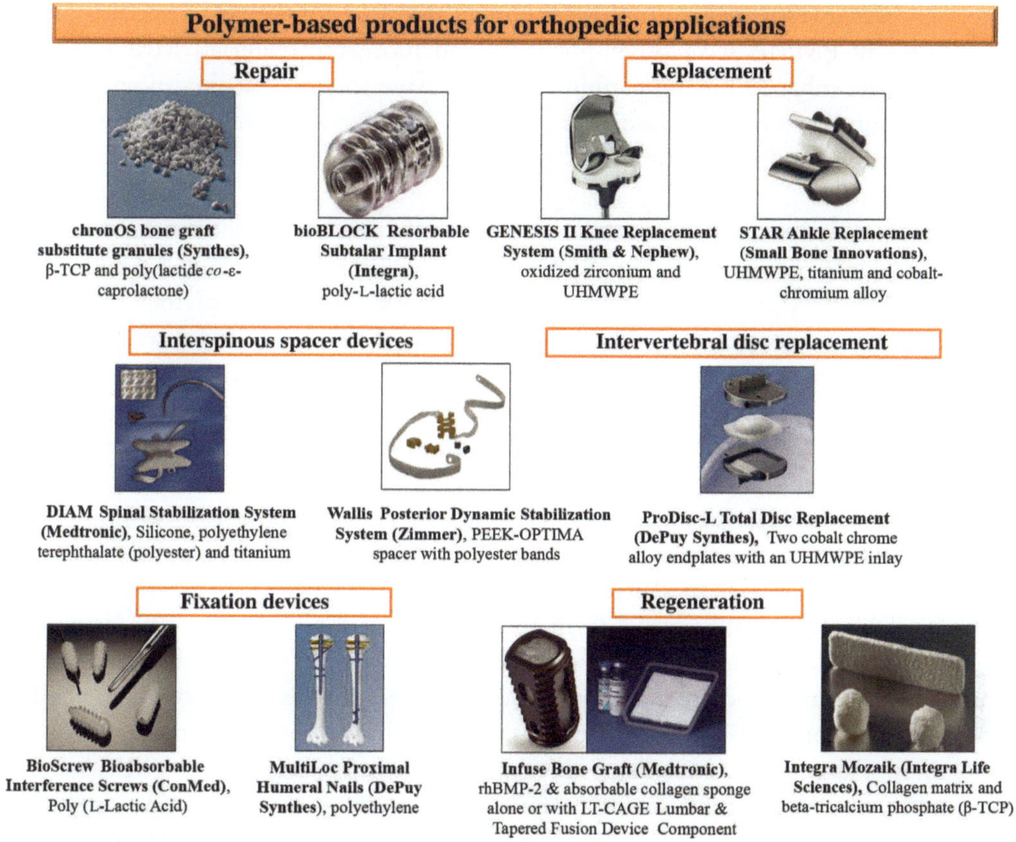

Figure 8.4 Schematic showing applications and representative examples of polymer-based products for orthopedic applications.

polymer beads consisting of MMA copolymers, BP (as an initiator), and possibly zirconium or barium to provide radio-opacity. When mixed together, the liquid monomer polymerizes around the polymer beads to form hardened PMMA cement [184]. Bone cements generally do not possess intrinsic adhesive properties and therefore mainly depend on mechanical interlock between the irregular bone surface and the prosthetic device [185].

In addition to the mechanical stability, the bioactivity and biocompatibility of the polymeric materials play a key role in determining its suitability for biomedical applications. For instance, elevated local temperature due to the exothermic polymerization reaction of PMMA has been shown to cause temperature changes leading to local bone necrosis [183,185]. The deterioration of the interfaces between the cement and the implant, or the cement and the bone, due to fatigue failure can lead to undesirable outcomes. The addition of stainless steel, Ti alloy wires, or UHMWPE nanofibers was investigated to improve the mechanical performance of cements [185]. Composites of PMMA with other polymers and inorganic materials have also been investigated to enhance biocompatibility. Studies have shown that incorporating bioactive substances in PMMA-based bone cements can increase bone-bonding strength, although high ceramic concentrations can diminish the mechanical properties of the cement [184].

A variety of bone cements and fillers are currently available in the market for clinical use. Exactech designed Cemex Bone Cement, composed of PMMA and liquid monomer MMA. Cemex employs a patented process, to create polymer spheres of consistent size and shape, which decreases the amount of liquid monomer needed to create the cement, thereby decreasing risks to patients and operating staff, as high levels of exposure to liquid monomer can be toxic. Another advantage of this system is the reduction in heat generated by the polymerization reaction, which can significantly reduce local tissue necrosis. Cemex Bone Cement has also been reported to show reduced shrinkage upon hardening, which in turn can reduce loosening of the prosthesis and therefore implant failure.

Cobalt Bone Cement, marketed by DJO Global, is PMMA-based cement, which is also available as an antibacterial form that incorporates gentamicin. The cement is reported to harden after 14 minutes of mixing and has a compressive strength of nearly 100 MPa and fracture toughness above 2 MPa. Cobalt MV bone cement has been designed for arthroplasty procedures, specifically of the hip, knee, and upper extremities. Palacos Bone Cement, developed by Zimmer, is also a PMMA-based cement enriched with gentamicin. It has shown to exhibit higher fatigue strength, and presents a viable option for drug delivery. The formulation is available in high and low viscosities and the high-viscosity formulation presents the additional advantage of ease of handling. Simplex P Bone Cement is another PMMA-based cement, originally designed in 1971 for total knee surgery but has expanded its applications to pathological fractures and prosthetic fixation over time. Tobramycin, an antibiotic, was added to the composition in 2003 and Stryker designed a faster-setting composition in 2006. Tobramycin was incorporated due to its ability to withstand the exothermic polymerization process. The medium viscosity of Simplex P Bone Cement formulation has shown the ability to support enhanced penetration into the pores of cancellous bone to provide better fixation.

8.4.1.2 Bone replacements

Bone replacements are typically needed in surgical procedures involving missing bone that has to be replaced. Bone graft materials are necessary for many orthopedic procedures, including but not limited to total joint replacement, trauma, nonunions, oral and craniofacial and other defect-filling purposes [49]. Structurally and mechanically, the ideal bone replacement is one that closely mimics the structure and mechanical properties of surrounding bone [184]. To this end, synthetic bone graft substitutes such as HA, calcium phosphate, and various polymers have been investigated [49]. Polymers provide orthopedic researchers the unique ability to proactively customize composition and therefore tailor properties based on their specific intended bone replacement application [184]. Based on its usage in hip and knee joint replacements, polyethylene is considered biocompatible; however, its stiffness and strength are significantly lower than that of native bone. In order to enhance load-bearing properties of polyethylene, HA particles have been added, which in turn has also been shown to increase its bioactivity [185]. Incorporation of other highly bioactive materials such as bioglass, have also been explored.

GENESIS II Knee replacement system by Smith and Nephew utilizes the company's VERILAST-Technology, which is a combination of oxidized zirconium alloy and a highly crosslinked polyethylene, or UHMWPE, materials chosen for their biocompatibility and mechanical properties. In this implant design, UHMWPE is used to reduce contact stress at the articular surface of the tibial baseplates.

STAR Ankle replacement system created by Small Bone Innovations is a three-piece mobile bearing nonconstrained, uncemented total ankle replacement approved by the FDA, for replacement of painful arthritic ankle joint due to osteoarthritis, post-traumatic arthritis, or rheumatoid arthritis. The three components of the system include a tibial plate, a talar component, and mobile bearing. The mobile bearing is made up of a UHMWPE sliding core, which articulates with the tibial component. The mobile bearing is sterilized using gamma sterilization, which creates crosslinks for enhanced wear performance. The talar component of the implant also features a polyethylene stabilizer fin which guides the motion of polyethylene without excessive friction. UHMWPE is also used for fabrication of sutures, for various biomedical applications, since it can provide uncompromising strength and minimize the impact on surrounding tissue.

Integra has created a resorbable arthroereisis device called bioBLOCK Resorbable Subtalar Implant, using PLLA, which can provide temporary support and also serve as an alternative to metal devices for patients with metal sensitivity. The application of this device is as internal support to surgical interventions in the treatment of flatfoot, and provides support for at least the first 3 months of healing. The device's size can range from 8 to 120 mm in 1-mm increments, which allows for a customized approach and minimally invasive surgical procedure.

8.4.1.3 Bone repair and regeneration

Due to the fact that bone is highly vascularized and dynamic, and that bone tissue constantly and naturally remodels, bone has a high natural regenerative ability. Large bone defects, however, often require surgical repair. Products that are created with the goal of regenerating bone are osteogenic, osteoconductive, and/or osteoinductive.

The combination of these properties has the potential to promote rapid bone healing. Both, natural and synthetic polymers have been investigated to support bone repair and regeneration. Inorganic–organic composites have raised significant interest in this respect due to their ability to mimic the composition as well as mechanical properties of bony tissue [49]. Furthermore, the addition of bioactive molecules, such as growth factors and use of stem cell technologies, has led to significant improvement in the bone repair and regeneration strategies. A few examples of commercially available products for these applications are discussed below.

A number of bone repair products utilize collagen to facilitate osteoconductivity. Mem-Lok by Biohorizons is a membrane barrier made up of highly purified Col-1 fibers for bone regeneration. The high density of collagen fibers allows for enhanced mechanical strength. The resorption period is between 26 and 38 weeks, and its macromolecular pore size ensures permeability to promote the exchange of nutrients during healing. The moldability of this product makes it easily adaptable to various bone defects. The recommended applications of Mem-Lok are ridge preservation, bone and sinus augmentation, and regeneration of bony defects. Novabone MacroFORM is another bioactive, moldable composite bone graft made up of collagen (10%) and highly purified bioactive glass granules (90%), with an open porous structure which encourages the absorption of bone marrow aspirate. The infusion of bone marrow into this device promotes bone growth, while collagen provides sites for cell and protein adhesion. The pore size of this product closely mimics the pore size of cancellous bone and the texture prevents implant displacement after implantation. INFUSE Bone Graft manufactured by Medtronic is one of the most widely used products for bone. It consists of the growth factor rhBMP-2 and an absorbable collagen sponge, which acts as a resorbable carrier. INFUSE has been approved by the FDA for use as an autograft alternative in the augmentation of the sinus and local alveolar ridge augmentation and for treatment of tibial shaft fractures. The usage of rhBMP-2 encourages natural bone growth through osteoinduction.

chronOS strip bone graft substitute, a product of synthes, is a synthetic bone void filler composed of β-TCP granules and PLCL, and is resorbable, osteoconductive, porous, and has a compressive strength of ~5 MPa, which is similar to that of human cancellous bone. chronOS bone graft substitute has been reported to be resorbed and replaced by bone in 6–18 months and has been used clinically in Europe for more than 20 years under the name CEROS 82. chronOS β-TCP has a total porosity of ~60% in its granule form and 70% in the preforms (strips and blocks), thus providing a good balance between promoting osteoconduction, without compromising the mechanical strength.

InQu bone substitute by Isto Technologies, Inc., has been designed to impart biocompatibility and osteoconductivity by incorporating hyaluronic acid into the structural network of PLGA, a resorbable polymer. This composite material has been shown to support new bone formation and achieve bony fusion faster than traditional ceramic bone grafts. The hydrophilic properties of InQu have been shown to facilitate absorption of blood and other bodily fluids during surgical procedures. The implant has been shown to be replaced with mature woven bone after 9 months, which is faster than the traditional ceramic products (more than 1 year). Moreover, it has been reported to possess good cohesiveness, handling, and molding properties, and is appropriate for a variety of spinal and orthopedic procedures.

Cranios Reinforced bone cement is a biocompatible, biodegradable, self-setting calcium phosphate bone cement, reinforced by randomly oriented and uniformly distributed PLGA polymer fibers, and is used for cranial applications. This material is highly conformable as the polymer reinforcement resists cracking during the setting process. During the healing process, Cranios is gradually absorbed and replaced by bone. This material sets in 3–6 minutes, and within 24 hours achieves a maximum compressive strength of approximately 25 MPa.

8.4.1.4 Plates, pins, nails, and screws

Nonresorbable composite plates consist of materials that are stable in the body and their strength and stiffness do not change in vivo. Such plates are typically made of thermoset or thermoplastic composite materials which are relatively stiff, fatigue-resistant, and biocompatible. PLA and related polymers undergo degradation in the body and thus loose mechanical integrity over time. Composites of fibers and resorbable materials, which provide reinforcement, typically make up fully resorbable bone plates. Partially resorbable plates can achieve improved mechanical properties through reinforcement by nonresorbable material such as carbon fibers [183]. The Rapisorb rapid resorbable fixation system by DePuy Synthes is fabricated using PLGA (LA:GA ratio 85:15) and consists of resorbable plates, meshes, screws, and tacks. It resorbs in 12 months and is used for craniofacial reconstruction.

Polymer-based screws are particularly advantageous as they can overcome the issue of corrosion, a major problem with their metallic counterparts. Researchers have developed carbon-fiber/carbon and carbon-fiber/PEEK composite screws for this purpose [185]. Similarly, intramedullary nails are used in the treatment of long bone fractures. Synthes MultiLoc Humeral Nails consist of a comprehensive system of both short and long nails with multiple screw options, for the treatment of humeral fractures. These titanium nails utilize a polyethylene inlay for secure fixation of proximal screws. BioScrews from ConMed are PLA-based interface screws for use in graft/knee fixation procedures, which are gradually absorbed in the body. The slow absorption of the screw helps in ensuring secure fixation of the graft throughout the healing process. Since composite materials are typically more biocompatible and show better mechanical properties in their interactions with bone, stainless steel, and GF/PEEK composite have also been commonly used to manufacture nails for orthopedic applications. Carbon fiber-reinforced crystalline polymers are also used as intramedullary nails as they can achieve an elastic modulus closer to that of the native bone [183].

8.4.2 Spinal applications

The main function of the spine is to protect the spinal cord and provide mobility and stability to the human body. The spine is made up of vertebra and intervertebral discs (IVDs), which provide cushion and flexibility to the spine [186]. When vertebrae or IVDs are damaged, spinal surgery is often necessary to repair or replace them, alleviating pain, discomfort, and immobility. One of the most encountered spinal disorders is degenerative disc disease. Either arthroplasty or spinal fusion could be used to tackle degenerative disc disease and other adverse spinal conditions. The complexity of the IVD, functionally and structurally, causes a complex challenge in developing artificial discs for replacement [187]. Bone grafting can further augment bone healing as it can provide enhanced stability following spinal surgery. Hence, bioabsorbable implants commonly used in sports medicine, are now expanding into spinal reconstructive surgery applications as well [188]. The spine-specific applications of polymeric materials can be classified as IVD replacement and regeneration systems or interspinous spacer devices.

8.4.2.1 Intervertebral disc replacement and regeneration

The IVD is a structure composed of an external collagenous band or annulus fibrous, which unites the articulating vertebral endplates. The center of the IVD is a core or nucleus pulposus composed of mucopolysaccharide gel and proteoglycans. The hydrophilic core generates tension on the annulus, which enhances resistance to external forces, increasing the capacity of the IVD to take on compressive force. Due to the structural and functional complexity of IVD and the presence of associated pathogenic factors, development of a reliable replacement or regeneration alternative can be quite challenging [187]. There are two main principles which inform the design of IVD replacement with consideration of the aforementioned constraints. One design goal is to achieve optimum mobility, usually carried out by metallic/polyethylene composite mechanical devices. Another design goal is to reproduce the viscoelastic properties, typically achieved by the implementation of silicones or polymers [187]. Some recent devices and technologies are now attempting to combine both these principles.

Many research groups are also investigating biological repair of the IVD through the application of tissue engineering principles and techniques. Cell delivery is expected to enhance the regeneration by repopulating disc tissue with cells, which will restore functional and structural characteristics of the tissue. Biomaterials applied for treatment of degenerated discs include, but are not limited to, hydrogels, electrospun fibers, and implantable scaffolds [186]. In particular, hydrogels present relevant properties for the replacement of the nucleus pulposus within the IVD. Hydrogels are hydrophilic, can potentially withstand cycles of loading and unloading, are injectable and have the capacity to be a vehicle for drug and cellular delivery [186]. Injection of cells in the absence of biomaterial often results in decreased cell survival and cellular organization. By specific selection of polymer composition and protein incorporation, parameters like viscosity, stiffness, gelation rate, degradation time, adhesivity, and other properties of the hydrogels can be easily controlled [186]. Hydrogels made up of natural polymers, including collagen, fibrin, and hyaluronic acid have been investigated for IVD regeneration due to their capability to mimic the native extracellular matrix. Biomechanical properties, however, are limited by crosslinking methods; therefore efforts are being made to increase the biomechanical capabilities of natural materials as implants. Synthetic materials can be used to combat the biomechanical limitations of natural materials. Synthetic materials present a host of advantages, including reproducibility, elimination of contamination risk, and availability. Many synthetic biomaterials are currently being investigated for the application of drug and cellular delivery, including PEG, PLGA, polyvinyl alcohol, and hydroxyethyl methacrylate. Despite efforts to develop methods for disc repair and regeneration and success in vitro and small animal models, many challenges inhibit scaling up to clinically viable solutions. Ideally, viable solutions would reduce pain, increase flexibility and tissue integrity, while maintaining motor functionality of the spine [186].

Infuse bone graft is also commonly used for anterior lumbar interbody fusion spine surgical procedures, in combination with Medtronic's LT-CAGE Lumbar Tapered Fusion Device, INTER FIX Threaded Fusion Device, or INTER FIX RP Threaded Fusion Device. The clinical indication includes treatment of skeletally mature patients with degenerative disc disease at a single level from L2–S1. The DIAM (device for intervertebral assisted motion) spinal stabilization system is a new device currently awaiting premarket approval and is indicated for lumbar surgery treatment of arthropatic facet syndrome, posterior prosthesis for discal assistance, transitional osteosynthesis, and foraminal stenosis. The materials used for fabricating the system include silicone, polyester (polyethylene terephthalate), and titanium, and the device is expected to provide flexible support of the lumbar spine while treating spinal degeneration. The Wallis posterior dynamic stabilization system from Zimmer is meant for treating lower back pains accompanied with degenerative disc disease and herniated discs. It is composed of a spacer made from PEEK-OPTIMA and polyester bands for distributing stress on bone after implantation. It serves as a reversible option for preserving mobility, anatomy, and stability of the spine, while keeping other therapeutic options open. Another product on the market for restoring the health of the spine is the Integra Mozaik Osteoconductive Scaffold, intended for use in posterolateral lumbar fusion. The Integra Mozaik is a formulation of 80% β-TCP and 20% crosslinked Col-1 that provides the material with structure and compression resistance. The matrix has an interconnected pore structure that can absorb bone marrow aspirate, in order to incorporate vital cells and proteins for bone formation. Integra Mozaik is offered in three configurations; strip, putty, and moldable morsels providing a customizable approach.

8.4.2.2 Spacer in intervertebral artificial disc replacement

A number of artificial IVD replacements have been developed, starting in the 1950s with Fernstrom's metal ball and Harmon's Vitalium spheres, with the goal of reproducing the "ball joint" function of the disc [187]. Later on, Fassio patented an elastic flying saucer shape implant, which, upon implantation, created intraspongious hernia and immobility [187]. More recently, engineers attempt to better control biocompatibility and mechanical properties by incorporating polymers into their designs [187].

Pro-Disc is an artificial disc replacement, which has a UHMWPE core and cobalt–chromium alloy cobalt chromium molybdenum endplates which are plasma-sprayed with titanium. A report shows that more than 80% of patients who participated in the Pro-Disc implantation clinical trial were "satisfied" or "completely satisfied" with the results. ACIS (Anterior Cervical Interbody Spacer) by DePuy Synthes is a comprehensive system of PEEK cervical interbody spacers. This product is indicated for use in skeletally mature patients with degenerative disc disease, and requires the incorporation of autogenous bone graft prior to implantation. The ACIS spacer has a large axial lumen to maximize fusion area as well as lateral windows to increase surface area for bone ingrowth. With various heights, DePuy Synthes provides surgeons with a number of options depending on the size and degree of damage. Octane Straight PEEK Interbody Spacer System made by Exactech Spine supports both biocompatibility and a minimally invasive approach. Octane Straight, similar to the ACIS design, features a large graft window, and also has an angular teeth design to prevent spacer migration.

8.5 CONCLUSIONS

Polymeric materials belonging to both degradable and nondegradable classes have positively impacted the progression of the field of orthopedics. Recent advances in the synthesis of novel tailor-made polymeric materials and the application of regenerative engineering principles for fabrication of scaffolds, as well as advanced delivery carriers, have provided a much-needed push to the advancement of healthcare related to musculoskeletal diseases. Furthermore, combination products utilizing stem cells and the use of composite materials have resulted in development of instructive environments suitable for achieving the desired levels of tissue replacement, repair, and regeneration. It is expected that the use and convergence of multidisciplinary approaches in the future would lead to the development of more successful and economical polymeric and composite orthopedic biomaterials.

REFERENCES

[1] Services USDoHaH. The surgeon general's report on bone health and osteoporosis: what it means to you. In: U.S. Department of Health and Human Services OotSG, editor. NIH Publication No 12−78272012.

[2] Global market study on orthopedic trauma devices: external fixator to witness highest growth by 2020. New York, NY: Persistence Market Research, 2014. p. 91.

[3] Persidis A. Tissue engineering. Nat Biotechnol 1999;17:508−10.

[4] Salgado AJ, Coutinho OP, Reis RL. Bone tissue engineering: state of the art and future trends. Macromol Biosci 2004;4:743−65.

[5] Brydone AS, Meek D, Maclaine S. Bone grafting, orthopaedic biomaterials, and the clinical need for bone engineering. Proc Inst Mech Eng H 2010;224:1329−43.

[6] Clinical Applications of Biomaterials. NIH Consens Statement. 1982 Nov 1−3 4:1−19.

[7] Nair LS, Laurencin CT. Biodegradable polymers as biomaterials. Prog Polym Sci 2007;32:762−98.

[8] Laurencin CT, Khan Y. Regenerative engineering. Sci Transl Med 2012;4:ed9.

[9] Yu X, Tang X, Gohil S, Laurencin C. Biomaterials for bone regenerative engineering. Adv Healthcare Mater 2015;4:1268−85.

[10] Laurencin C.T., Nair L.S. The quest towards limb regeneration: a regenerative engineering approach. Regen Biomater. 2016;3:123-5.

[11] Laurencin CT, Nair LS. Regenerative engineering: approaches to limb regeneration and other grand challenges. Reg Eng Trans Med 2015;1:1−3.

[12] Arora P, Jain R, Mathur K, Sharma A, Gupta A. Synthesis of polymethyl methacrylate PMMA by batch emulsion polymerization. Afr J Pure Appl Chem 2010;4:152−7.

[13] Gupta P, Elkins C, Long T, Wilkes G. Electrospinning of linear homopolymers of poly(methyl methacrylate): exploring relationships between fiber formation, viscosity, molecular weight and concentration in a good solvent. Polymer 2005;46:4799−810.

[14] Chen X-P, Qiu K-Y. Synthesis of well-defined poly(methyl methacrylate) by radical polymerization with a new initiation system TPED†/FeCl3/PPh3. Macromolecules 1999;32:8711−15.

[15] Wang G-A, Wang C-C, Chen C-Y. Preparation and characterization of layered double hydroxides—PMMA nanocomposites by solution polymerization. J Inorg Organomet Polym Mater 2005;15:239−51.

[16] Arora M, Chan EK, Gupta S, Diwan AD. Polymethylmethacrylate bone cements and additives: a review of the literature. World J Orthop 2013;4:67−74.

[17] Vaishya R, Chauhan M, Vaish A. Bone cement. J Clin Orthop Trauma 2013;4:157−63.

[18] Webb JCJ, Spencer RF. The role of polymethylmethacrylate bone cement in modern orthopaedic surgery. Bone Joint J 2007;89:851−7.

[19] Mendez JA, Aguilar MR, Abraham GA, Vazquez B, Dalby M, Di Silvio L, et al. New acrylic bone cements conjugated to vitamin E: curing parameters, properties, and biocompatibility. J Biomed Mater Res 2002;62:299−307.

[20] Nien Y-H, Chen J. Studies of the mechanical and thermal properties of cross-linked poly (methylmethacrylate-acrylic acid-allylmethacrylate)-modified bone cement. J Appl Polym Sci 2006;100:3727−32.

[21] Ormsby RW, Modreanu M, Mitchell CA, Dunne NJ. Carboxyl functionalised MWCNT/polymethyl methacrylate bone cement for orthopaedic applications. J Biomater Appl 2014;29:209−21.

[22] He Q, Chen H, Huang L, Dong J, Guo D, Mao M, et al. Porous surface modified bioactive bone cement for enhanced bone bonding. PLoS One 2012;7:e42525.

[23] Tan HL, Lin WT, Tang TT. The use of antimicrobial-impregnated PMMA to manage periprosthetic infections: controversial issues and the latest developments. Int J Artif Organs 2012;35:832−9.

[24] Tan H, Peng Z, Li Q, Xu X, Guo S, Tang T. The use of quaternised chitosan-loaded PMMA to inhibit biofilm formation and downregulate the virulence-associated gene expression of antibiotic-resistant *Staphylococcus*. Biomaterials 2012;33:365−77.

[25] Perni S, Thenault V, Abdo P, Margulis K, Magdassi S, Prokopovich P. Antimicrobial activity of bone cements embedded with organic nanoparticles. Int J Nanomed 2015;10:6317−29.

[26] Salamone JC. Concise polymeric materials encyclopedia. Boca Raton, FL: CRC Press; 1999.
[27] McKeen LW. High-temperature/high-performance polymers. The Effect of UV light and weather on plastics and elastomers. 3rd ed Amsterdam: Elsevier Inc; 2013. p. 271–98.
[28] Pritchard G. Anti-corrosion. In: Dolby R, editor. Polymers: PEEK, PEKK and other polyaryls. Rapra Review Reports; 1995.
[29] Meister JJ. Polymer modification: principles, techniques and applications. New York, NY: Marcel Dekker Inc.; 2000.
[30] Katti KS. Biomaterials in total joint replacement. Colloids Surf B Biointerfaces 2004;39:133–42.
[31] Kelly JM. Ultra-high molecular weight polyethylene. J Macromol Sci C Polym Rev 2002;3:355–71.
[32] Navarro M, Michiardi A, Castano O, Planell JA. Biomaterials in orthopaedics. J R Soc Interface 2008;5:1137–58.
[33] Ahmad M, Wahit M, Kadir M, Dahlan K, Jawaid M. Thermal and mechanical properties of ultra-high molecular weight polyethylene/high-density polyethylene/polyethylene glycol blends. J Polym Eng 2013;33:599–614.
[34] Kurtz SM. UHMWPE biomaterials handbook: ultra high molecular weight polyethylene in total joint replacement and medical devices. 2nd ed Burlington, MA: Academic Press; 2009.
[35] Bracco P, Oral E. Vitamin E-stabilized UHMWPE for total joint implants: a review. Clin Orthop Relat Res 2010;469:2286–93.
[36] Maier C, Calafut T. Polypropylene: the definitive user's guide and databook. New York, NY: William Andrew Publishing/Plastics Design Library; 1998.
[37] Akinci A. Mechanical and structural properties of polypropylene composites filled with graphite flakes. Arch Mater Sci Eng 2009;35:91–4.
[38] Shahriar A. Investigation of spatial configuration of polypropylene and the influence of molecular weight distribution, catalyst type and tacticity on mechanical, thermal and optical properties of polymers. IOSR J Polym Text Eng 2014;1:37–45.
[39] Degernes LA, Lind PJ, Redig PT. Raptor orthopedics using methyl methacrylate and polypropylene rods. In: Redig PT, Cooper JE, Remple D, Hunter DR, editors. Raptor biomedicine. Minneapolis, MN: University of Minnesota Press; 1993. p. 122–7.
[40] Liao C, Li K, Wong H, Tong W, Yeung K, Tjong C. Novel polypropylene biocomposites reinforced with carbon nanotubes and hydroxyapatite nanorods for bone replacements. Mater Sci Eng C 2013;33:1380–8.
[41] Chan K, Wong H, Yeung K, Tjong S. Polypropylene biocomposites with boron nitride and nanohydroxyapatite reinforcements. Materials 2015;8:992–1008.
[42] Dizman C, Tasdelen MA, Yagci Y. Recent advances in the preparation of functionalized polysulfones. Polym Int 2013;62:991–1007.
[43] Shabani I, Haddadi-Asl V, Soleimani M, Seyedjafari E, Hashemi SM. Ion-exchange polymer nanofibers for enhanced osteogenic differentiation of stem cells and ectopic bone formation. ACS Appl Mater Interfaces 2014;6:72–82.
[44] Wang M, Yue CY, Chua B. Production and evaluation of hydroxyapatite reinforced polysulfone for tissue replacement. J Mater Sci Mater Med 2001;12:821–6.
[45] Fearon FWG, Owen MJ. Silicon surface science opportunities. In: Prasad PN, Mark JE, Kandil SH, Kafafi ZH, editors. Science and technology of polymers and advanced materials: emerging technologies and business opportunities. New York, NY: Springer Science & Business Media; 2013. p. 873–8.
[46] Curtis J, Colas A. Medical applications of silicones. In: Ratner BD, Hoffman AS, Schoen FJ, Lemons JE, editors. *Biomaterials science: an introduction to materials in medicine*, 3rd ed. California, USA: Academic Press; 2013. p. 1–11.
[47] Thomas NP, Tran N, Tran PA, Walters JL, Jarrell JD, Hayda RA, et al. Characterization and bioactive properties of zirconia based polymeric hybrid for orthopedic applications. J Mater Sci Mater Med 2014;25:347–54.
[48] Lung CYK, Heinonen M, Kukk E, Matinlinna JP. Surface modification of titanium with thermally treated polydimethylsiloxane coating and the effect on resin to titanium adhesion. Surf Interface Anal 2014;47:105–12.

[49] Verma S, Garkhal K, Mittal A, Kumar N. Biodegradable polymers for emerging clinical use in tissue engineering. In: Domb AJ, Kumar N, Ezra A, editors. Biodegrdable polymers in clinical use and clinical development. Hoboken, NJ: John Wiley and Sons, Inc; 2011. p. 555–619.
[50] Ulery BD, Nair LS, Laurencin CT. Biomedical applications of biodegradable polymers. J Polym Sci B Polym Phys 2011;49:832–64.
[51] Tian H, Tang Z, Zhuang X, Chen X, Jing X. Biodegradable synthetic polymers: preparation, functionalization and biomedical application. Prog Polym Sci 2012;37:237–80.
[52] Rahman CV, Ben-David D, Dhillon A, Kuhn G, Gould TW, Müller R, et al. Controlled release of BMP-2 from a sintered polymer scaffold enhances bone repair in a mouse calvarial defect model. J Tissue Eng Regen Med 2014;8:59–66.
[53] Ko E, Yang K, Shin J, Cho SW. Polydopamine-assisted osteoinductive peptide immobilization of polymer scaffolds for enhanced bone regeneration by human adipose-derived stem cells. Biomacromolecules 2013;14:3202–13.
[54] Kim IG, Hwang MP, Du P, Ko J, Ha CW, Do SH, et al. Bioactive cell-derived matrices combined with polymer mesh scaffold for osteogenesis and bone healing. Biomaterials 2015;50:75–86.
[55] Yu NY, Gdalevitch M, Murphy CM, Mikulec K, Peacock L, Fitzpatrick J, et al. Spatial control of bone formation using a porous polymer scaffold co-delivering anabolic rhBMP-2 and anti-resorptive agents. Eur Cell Mater 2014;27:98–109.
[56] Tayton E, Fahmy S, Purcell M, Aarvold A, Smith JO, Kalra S, et al. An analysis of polymer type and chain length for use as a biological composite graft extender in impaction bone grafting: a mechanical and biocompatibility study. J Biomed Mater Res A 2012;100:3211–19.
[57] Zhang X, Chang W, Lee P, Wang Y, Yang M, Li J, et al. Polymer-ceramic spiral structured scaffolds for bone tissue engineering: effect of hydroxyapatite composition on human fetal osteoblasts. PLoS One 2014;9:e85871.
[58] Tayton E, Purcell M, Aarvold A, Smith JO, Briscoe A, Kanczler JM, et al. A comparison of polymer and polymer-hydroxyapatite composite tissue engineered scaffolds for use in bone regeneration. An in vitro and in vivo study. J Biomed Mater Res A 2014;102:2613–24.
[59] Minton J, Janney C, Akbarzadeh R, Focke C, Subramanian A, Smith T, et al. Solvent-free polymer/bioceramic scaffolds for bone tissue engineering: fabrication, analysis, and cell growth. J Biomater Sci Polym Ed 2014;25:1856–74.
[60] Baker KC, Maerz T, Saad H, Shaheen P, Kannan RM. In vivo bone formation by and inflammatory response to resorbable polymer-nanoclay constructs. Nanomedicine 2015;11:1871–81.
[61] Igwe JC, Mikael PE, Nukavarapu SP. Design, fabrication and in vitro evaluation of a novel polymer-hydrogel hybrid scaffold for bone tissue engineering. J Tissue Eng Regen Med 2014;8:131–42.
[62] Fujikura K, Lin S, Nakamura J, Obata A, Kasuga T. Preparation of electrospun fiber mats using siloxane-containing vaterite and biodegradable polymer hybrids for bone regeneration. J Biomed Mater Res B Appl Biomater 2013;101:1350–8.
[63] Kutikov AB, Song J. An amphiphilic degradable polymer/hydroxyapatite composite with enhanced handling characteristics promotes osteogenic gene expression in bone marrow stromal cells. Acta Biomater 2013;9:8354–64.
[64] Kutikov AB, Skelly JD, Ayers DC, Song J. Templated repair of long bone defects in rats with bioactive spiral-wrapped electrospun amphiphilic polymer/hydroxyapatite scaffolds. ACS Appl Mater Interfaces 2015;7:4890–901.
[65] Matsumoto T, Toyoda H, Dohzono S, Yasuda H, Wakitani S, Nakamura H, et al. Efficacy of interspinous process lumbar fusion with recombinant human bone morphogenetic protein-2 delivered with a synthetic polymer and β-tricalcium phosphate in a rabbit model. Eur Spine J 2012;21:1338–45.
[66] Tayton E, Purcell M, Smith JO, Lanham S, Howdle SM, Shakesheff KM, et al. The scale-up of a tissue engineered porous hydroxyapatite polymer composite scaffold for use in bone repair: an ovine femoral condyle defect study. J Biomed Mater Res A 2015;103:1346–56.
[67] Bagchi A, Meka SR, Rao BN, Chatterjee K. Perovskite ceramic nanoparticles in polymer composites for augmenting bone tissue regeneration. Nanotechnology 2014;25:485101.

[68] Lu W, Ji K, Kirkham J, Yan Y, Boccaccini AR, Kellett M, et al. Bone tissue engineering by using a combination of polymer/bioglass composites with human adipose-derived stem cells. Cell Tissue Res 2014;356:97–107.
[69] Nooeaid P, Li W, Roether JA, Mouriño V, Goudouri OM, Schubert DW, et al. Development of bioactive glass based scaffolds for controlled antibiotic release in bone tissue engineering via biodegradable polymer layered coating. Biointerphases 2014;9:041001.
[70] Brooks BD, Sinclair KD, Davidoff SN, Lawson S, Williams AG, Coats B, et al. Molded polymer-coated composite bone void filler improves tobramycin controlled release kinetics. J Biomed Mater Res B Appl Biomater 2014;102:1074–83.
[71] Brooks BD, Sinclair KD, Grainger DW, Brooks AE. A resorbable antibiotic-eluting polymer composite bone void filler for perioperative infection prevention in a rabbit radial defect model. PLoS One 2015;10:e0118696.
[72] Baker RM, Tseng LF, Iannolo MT, Oest ME, Henderson JH. Self-deploying shape memory polymer scaffolds for grafting and stabilizing complex bone defects: a mouse femoral segmental defect study. Biomaterials 2016;76:388–98.
[73] Xie M, Wang L, Ge J, Guo B, Ma PX. Strong electroactive biodegradable shape memory polymer networks based on star-shaped polylactide and aniline trimer for bone tissue engineering. ACS Appl Mater Interfaces 2015;7:6772–81.
[74] Zhang D, George OJ, Petersen KM, Jimenez-Vergara AC, Hahn MS, Grunlan MA. A bioactive "self-fitting" shape memory polymer scaffold with potential to treat cranio-maxillo facial bone defects. Acta Biomater 2014;10:4597–605.
[75] Bao M, Lou X, Zhou Q, Dong W, Yuan H, Zhang Y. Electrospun biomimetic fibrous scaffold from shape memory polymer of PDLLA-co-TMC for bone tissue engineering. ACS Appl Mater Interfaces 2014;6:2611–21.
[76] Ray JA, Doddi N, Regula D, Williams JA, Melveger A. Polydioxanone (PDS), a novel monofilament synthetic absorbable suture. Surg Gynecol Obstet 1981;153:497–507.
[77] Kricheldorf HR, Damrau D. Polylactones 42: Zn l-lactate-catalyzed polymerizations of 1,4-dioxan-2-one. Macromol Chem Phys 1998;199:1089–98.
[78] Tang H, Wu B, Qin X, Zhang L, Kretlow J, Xu Z. Tissue engineering rib with the incorporation of biodegradable polymer cage and BMSCs/decalcified bone: an experimental study in a canine model. J Cardiothorac Surg 2013;8:1–9.
[79] Xu J, Feng E, Song J. Renaissance of aliphatic polycarbonates: new techniques and biomedical applications. J Appl Polym Sci 2014;131:39822.
[80] Yu F, Zhuo R. Synthesis, characterization and degradation behaviors of end-group-functionalized poly(trimethylene carbonate)s. Polym J 2003;35:671–6.
[81] Le Hellaye M, Fortin N, Guilloteau J, Soum A, Lecommandoux S, Guillaume SM. Biodegradable polycarbonate-b-polypeptide and polyester-b-polypeptide block copolymers: synthesis and nanoparticle formation towards biomaterials. Biomacromolecules 2008;9:1924–33.
[82] van Leeuwen AC, Huddleston Slater JJR, Gielkens PFM, de Jong JR, Grijpma DW, Bos RRM. Guided bone regeneration in rat mandibular defects using resorbable poly(trimethylene carbonate) barrier membranes. Acta Biomater 2012;8:1422–9.
[83] van Leeuwen AC, van Kooten TG, Grijpma DW, Bos RR. In vivo behaviour of a biodegradable poly(trimethylene carbonate) barrier membrane: a histological study in rats. J Mater Sci Mater Med 2012;23:1951–9.
[84] Shuo T, Jingjing Z, Shuyun X, Jingfeng L, Yu T, Daping Q, et al. Bone induction through controlled release of novel BMP-2-related peptide from PTMC 11-F127-PTMC 11 hydrogels. Biomed Mater 2012;7:015008.
[85] Neut D, Kluin OS, Crielaard BJ, van der Mei HC, Busscher HJ, Grijpma DW. A biodegradable antibiotic delivery system based on poly-(trimethylene carbonate) for the treatment of osteomyelitis. Acta Orthopaed 2009;80:514–19.
[86] Wang X, Yang Y, Jia H, Jia W, Miller S, Bowman B, et al. Peptide decoration of nanovehicles to achieve active targeting and pathology-responsive cellular uptake for bone metastasis chemotherapy. Biomater Sci 2014;2:961–71.

[87] Lewandrowski KU, Bondre SP, Wise DL, Trantolo DJ. Enhanced bioactivity of a poly(propylene fumarate) bone graft substitute by augmentation with nano-hydroxyapatite. Biomed Mater Eng 2003;13:115–24.

[88] Mistry AS, Cheng SH, Yeh T, Christenson E, Jansen JA, Mikos AG. Fabrication and in vitro degradation of porous fumarate-based polymer/alumoxane nanocomposite scaffolds for bone tissue engineering. J Biomed Mater Res A 2009;89:68–79.

[89] Mistry AS, Pham QP, Schouten C, Yeh T, Christenson EM, Mikos AG, et al. In vivo bone biocompatibility and degradation of porous fumarate-based polymer/alumoxane nanocomposites for bone tissue engineering. J Biomed Mater Res A 2010;92:451–62.

[90] Hile DD, Kowaleski MP, Doherty SA, Lewandrowski KU, Trantolo DJ. An injectable porous poly (propylene glycol-*co*-fumaric acid) bone repair material as an adjunct for intramedullary fixation. Biomed Mater Eng 2005;15:219–27.

[91] Henslee AM, Gwak DH, Mikos AG, Kasper FK. Development of a biodegradable bone cement for craniofacial applications. J Biomed Mater Res A 2012;100:2252–9.

[92] de Girolamo L, Niada S, Arrigoni E, Di Giancamillo A, Domeneghini C, Dadsetan M, et al. Repair of osteochondral defects in the minipig model by OPF hydrogel loaded with adipose-derived mesenchymal stem cells. Regen Med 2015;10:135–51.

[93] Lim CT, Ren X, Afizah MH, Tarigan-Panjaitan S, Yang Z, Wu Y, et al. Repair of osteochondral defects with rehydrated freeze-dried oligo[poly(ethylene glycol) fumarate] hydrogels seeded with bone marrow mesenchymal stem cells in a porcine model. Tissue Eng Part A 2013;19:1852–61.

[94] Kim J, Sharma A, Runge B, Waters H, Doll B, McBride S, et al. Osteoblast growth and bone-healing response to three-dimensional poly(epsilon-caprolactone fumarate) scaffolds. J Tissue Eng Regen Med 2012;6:404–13.

[95] Fernandez JM, Molinuevo MS, Cortizo AM, McCarthy AD, Cortizo MS. Characterization of poly(epsilon-caprolactone)/polyfumarate blends as scaffolds for bone tissue engineering. J Biomater Sci Polym Ed 2010;21:1297–312.

[96] Bodakhe S, Verma S, Garkhal K, Samal SK, Sharma SS, Kumar N. Injectable photocrosslinkable nanocomposite based on poly(glycerol sebacate) fumarate and hydroxyapatite: development, biocompatibility and bone regeneration in a rat calvarial bone defect model. Nanomedicine 2013;8:1777–95.

[97] Giannitelli SM, Basoli F, Mozetic P, Piva P, Bartuli FN, Luciani F, et al. Graded porous polyurethane foam: a potential scaffold for oro-maxillary bone regeneration. Mater Sci Eng C Mater Biol Appl 2015;51:329–35.

[98] Li L, Zuo Y, Zou Q, Yang B, Lin L, Li J, et al. Hierarchical structure and mechanical improvement of an n-HA/GCO-PU composite scaffold for bone regeneration. ACS Appl Mater Interfaces 2015;7:22618–29.

[99] Dumas JE, Prieto EM, Zienkiewicz KJ, Guda T, Wenke JC, Bible J, et al. Balancing the rates of new bone formation and polymer degradation enhances healing of weight-bearing allograft/polyurethane composites in rabbit femoral defects. Tissue Eng Part A 2014;20:115–29.

[100] Prieto EM, Talley AD, Gould NR, Zienkiewicz KJ, Drapeau SJ, Kalpakci KN, et al. Effects of particle size and porosity on in vivo remodeling of settable allograft bone/polymer composites. J Biomed Mater Res B Appl Biomater 2015;103:1641–51.

[101] Mi HY, Palumbo S, Jing X, Turng LS, Li WJ, Peng XF. Thermoplastic polyurethane/hydroxyapatite electrospun scaffolds for bone tissue engineering: effects of polymer properties and particle size. J Biomed Mater Res B Appl Biomater 2014;102:1434–44.

[102] Beauty D, Pronobesh C, Somnath M, Aadesh U, Manashi Das P, Charu lata M, et al. Bio-functionalized MWCNT/hyperbranched polyurethane bionanocomposite for bone regeneration. Biomed Mater 2015;10:025011.

[103] Yoshii T, Hafeman AE, Nyman JS, Esparza JM, Shinomiya K, Spengler DM, et al. A sustained release of lovastatin from biodegradable, elastomeric polyurethane scaffolds for enhanced bone regeneration. Tissue Eng Part A 2010;16:2369–79.

[104] Liu H, Zhang L, Shi P, Zou Q, Zuo Y, Li Y. Hydroxyapatite/polyurethane scaffold incorporated with drug-loadedethyl cellulose microspheres for bone regeneration. J Biomed Mater Res B Appl Biomater 2010;95B:36–46.
[105] Gogolewski S, Gorna K, Turner AS. Regeneration of bicortical defects in the iliac crest of estrogen-deficient sheep, using new biodegradable polyurethane bone graft substitutes. J Biomed Mater Res A 2006;77:802–10.
[106] Kumar N, Langer RS, Domb AJ. Polyanhydrides: an overview. Adv Drug Deliv Rev 2002;54:889–910.
[107] Katti DS, Lakshmi S, Langer R, Laurencin CT. Toxicity, biodegradation and elimination of polyanhydrides. Adv Drug Delivery Rev 2002;54:933–61.
[108] Lucas PA, Laurencin C, Syftestad GT, Domb A, Goldberg VM, Caplan AI, et al. Ectopic induction of cartilage and bone by water-soluble proteins from bovine bone using a polyanhydride delivery vehicle. J Biomed Mater Res 1990;24:901–11.
[109] Wada K, Yu W, Elazizi M, Barakat S, Ouimet MA, Rosario-Melendez R, et al. Locally delivered salicylic acid from a poly(anhydride-ester): impact on diabetic bone regeneration. J Controll Release 2013;171:33–7.
[110] Li H-Y, Chen Y-F, Xie Y-S. Nanocomposites of cross-linking polyanhydrides and hydroxyapatite needles: mechanical and degradable properties. Mater Lett 2004;58:2819–23.
[111] Lai P-L, Hong D-W, Chu I-M, Chen W-J, Chen L-H, Niu C-C, et al. Polyanhydride copolymer and bioceramic composites as bone substitutes. Formosan J Musculoskel Disord 2013;4:6–10.
[112] Lee HS, Kwon SY, Seo EM, Kim Y-H, Kim SS. Preparation and characterization of alpha-tricalcium phosphate cements incorporated with polyamino acids. Macromol Res 2011;19:90–6.
[113] Li H, Tao S, Yan Y, Lv G, Gu Y, Luo X, et al. Degradability and cytocompatibility of tricalcium phosphate/poly(amino acid) composite as bone tissue implants in orthopaedic surgery. J Biomater Sci Polym Ed 2014;25:1194–210.
[114] Wang J., Li H., Fan X., Li T., Lv G., Yan Y. Bone substitute of poly(amino acid)/β-Ca2SiO4 biocomposite: degradability and bioactivity. Polym Compos. 2014;37:1335–1341.
[115] Yang X, Li Y, Huang Q, Yang J, Shen B, Pei F. Evaluation of a biodegradable graft substitute in rabbit bone defect model. Indian J Orthop 2012;46:266–73.
[116] Yan L, Jiang DM. Study of bone-like hydroxyapatite/polyamino acid composite materials for their biological properties and effects on the reconstruction of long bone defects. Drug Des Devel Ther 2015;9:6497–508.
[117] Dai Z, Li Y, Lu W, Jiang D, Li H, Yan Y, et al. In vivo biocompatibility of new nano-calcium-deficient hydroxyapatite/poly-amino acid complex biomaterials. Int J Nanomed 2015;10:6303–16.
[118] Lee HJ, Koo AN, Lee SW, Lee MH, Lee SC. Catechol-functionalized adhesive polymer nanoparticles for controlled local release of bone morphogenetic protein-2 from titanium surface. J Control Release 2013;170:198–208.
[119] Teasdale I, Bruggemann O. Polyphosphazenes: multifunctional, biodegradable vehicles for drug and gene delivery. Polymers (Basel) 2013;5:161–87.
[120] Lakshmi SN, Katti DS, Laurencin TC. Biodegradable polyphosphazenes for drug delivery applications. Adv Drug Deliv Rev 2003;55:467–82.
[121] Ibim SE, El-Amin SF, Goad MEP, Ambrosio AMA, Allcock HR, Laurencin CT. In vitro release of colchicine using poly(phosphazenes): the development of delivery systems for musculoskeletal use. Pharm Dev Technol 1998;3:55–62.
[122] Krogman NR, Steely L, Hindenlang MD, Nair LS, Laurencin CT, Allcock HR. Synthesis and characterization of polyphosphazene-block-polyester and polyphosphazene-block-polycarbonate macromolecules. Macromolecules 2008;41:1126–30.
[123] Deng M, Nair LS, Nukavarapu SP, Jiang T, Kanner WA, Li X, et al. Dipeptide-based polyphosphazene and polyester blends for bone tissue engineering. Biomaterials 2010;31:4898–908.
[124] Deng M, Kumbar SG, Nair LS, Weikel AL, Allcock HR, Laurencin CT. Biomimetic structures: biological implications of dipeptide-substituted polyphosphazene–polyester blend nanofiber matrices for load-bearing bone regeneration. Adv Funct Mater 2011;21:2641–51.

[125] Laurencin CT, El-Amin SF, Ibim SE, Willoughby DA, Attawia M, Allcock HR, et al. A highly porous 3-dimensional polyphosphazene polymer matrix for skeletal tissue regeneration. J Biomed Mater Res 1996;30:133–8.
[126] Nukavarapu SP, Kumbar SG, Brown JL, Krogman NR, Weikel AL, Hindenlang MD, et al. Polyphosphazene/nano-hydroxyapatite composite microsphere scaffolds for bone tissue engineering. Biomacromolecules 2008;9:1818–25.
[127] Cunniffe GM, O'Brien FJ. Collagen scaffolds for orthopedic regenerative medicine. JOM 2011;63:66–73.
[128] Ramshaw JA, Shah NK, Brodsky B. Gly-X-Y tripeptide frequencies in collagen: a context for host-guest triple-helical peptides. J Struct Biol 1998;122:86–91.
[129] Shoulders MD, Raines RT. Collagen structure and stability. Ann Rev Biochem 2009;78:929–58.
[130] Chen S, Osaka A, Ikoma T, Morita H, Li J, Takeguchi M, et al. Fabrication, microstructure, and BMP-2 delivery of novel biodegradable and biocompatible silicate–collagen hybrid fibril sheets. J Mater Chem 2011;21:10942–8.
[131] Lee SS, Huang BJ, Kaltz SR, Sur S, Newcomb CJ, Stock SR, et al. Bone regeneration with low dose BMP-2 amplified by biomimetic supramolecular nanofibers within collagen scaffolds. Biomaterials 2013;34:452–9.
[132] Moreau JL, Weir MD, Xu HHK. Self-setting collagen-calcium phosphate bone cement: mechanical and cellular properties. J Biomed Mater Res A 2009;91:605–13.
[133] Socrates R, Sakthivel N, Rajaram A, Ramamoorthy U, Kalkura SN. Novel fibrillar collagen–hydroxyapatite matrices loaded with silver nanoparticles for orthopedic application. Mater Lett 2015;161:759–62.
[134] Kawamura M, Urist MR. Human fibrin is a physiologic delivery system for bone morphogenetic protein. Clin Orthop Relat Res 1988;302–10.
[135] Martino MM, Briquez PS, Ranga A, Lutolf MP, Hubbell JA. Heparin-binding domain of fibrin (ogen) binds growth factors and promotes tissue repair when incorporated within a synthetic matrix. Proc Natl Acad Sci U S A 2013;110:4563–8.
[136] Martino MM, Tortelli F, Mochizuki M, Traub S, Ben-David D, Kuhn GA, et al. Engineering the growth factor microenvironment with fibronectin domains to promote wound and bone tissue healing. Sci Transl Med 2011;3:100ra89.
[137] Yang HS, La WG, Bhang SH, Jeon JY, Lee JH, Kim BS. Heparin-conjugated fibrin as an injectable system for sustained delivery of bone morphogenetic protein-2. Tissue Eng Part A 2010;16:1225–33.
[138] Yang HS, La W-G, Cho Y-M, Shin W, Yeo G-D, Kim B-S. Comparison between heparin-conjugated fibrin and collagen sponge as bone morphogenetic protein-2 carriers for bone regeneration. Exp Mol Med 2012;44:350–5.
[139] Schutzenberger S, Schultz A, Hausner T, Hopf R, Zanoni G, Morton T, et al. The optimal carrier for BMP-2: a comparison of collagen versus fibrin matrix. Arch Orthop Trauma Surg 2012;132:1363–70.
[140] Park K-H, Kim H, Moon S, Na K. Bone morphogenic protein-2 (BMP-2) loaded nanoparticles mixed with human mesenchymal stem cell in fibrin hydrogel for bone tissue engineering. J Biosci Bioeng 2009;108:530–7.
[141] van der Stok J, Koolen MK, de Maat MP, Yavari SA, Alblas J, Patka P, et al. Full regeneration of segmental bone defects using porous titanium implants loaded with BMP-2 containing fibrin gels. Eur Cell Mater 2015;29:141–53. discussion 53-4.
[142] Yamaguchi M, Igarashi A, Misawa H, Tsurusaki Y. Enhancement of albumin expression in bone tissues with healing rat fractures. J Cell Biochem 2003;89:356–63.
[143] Horvathy DB, Vacz G, Szabo T, Szigyarto IC, o IT, Vamos B, et al. Serum albumin coating of demineralized bone matrix results in stronger new bone formation. J Biomed Mater Res Part B Appl Biomater 2016;104B:126–32.
[144] Skaliczki G, Schandl K, Weszl M, Major T, Kovács M, Skaliczki J, et al. Serum albumin enhances bone healing in a nonunion femoral defect model in rats: a computer tomography micromorphometry study. Int Orthop 2013;37:741–5.

[145] Gallego L, Junquera L, Garcia E, Garcia V, Alvarez-Viejo M, Costilla S, et al. Repair of rat mandibular bone defects by alveolar osteoblasts in a novel plasma-derived albumin scaffold. Tissue Eng Part A 2010;16:1179–87.
[146] Li P-S, Liang Lee I, Yu W-L, Sun J-S, Jane W-N, Shen H-H. A novel albumin-based tissue scaffold for autogenic tissue engineering applications. Sci Rep 2014;4:5600.
[147] Zhang S, Wang G, Lin X, Chatzinikolaidou M, Jennissen HP, Laub M, et al. Polyethylenimine-coated albumin nanoparticles for BMP-2 delivery. Biotechnol Prog 2008;24:945–56.
[148] Cui Z, Nair LS. Chitosan: a versatile biomedical polymer. Recent Pat Biomed Eng 2010;3:129–37.
[149] Dutta PK, Dutta J, Tripathi VS. Chitin and chitosan: chemistry, properties and applications. J Sci Ind Res 2004;36:20–31.
[150] Dash M, Chiellini F, Ottenbrite RM, Chiellini E. Chitosan—a versatile semi-synthetic polymer in biomedical applications. Prog Polym Sci 2011;36:981–1014.
[151] Croisier F, Jérôme C. Chitosan-based biomaterials for tissue engineering. Eur Polym J 2013;49:780–92.
[152] Bernkop-Schnürch A, Dünnhaupt S. Chitosan-based drug delivery systems. Eur J Pharm Biopharm 2012;81:463–9.
[153] Ho M-H, Yao C-J, Liao M-H, Lin P-I, Liu S-H, Chen R-M. Chitosan nanofiber scaffold improves bone healing via stimulating trabecular bone production due to upregulation of the Runx2/osteocalcin/alkaline phosphatase signaling pathway. Int J Nanomed 2015;10:5941–54.
[154] Gohil SV, Brittain SB, Kan H-M, Drissi H, Rowe DW, Nair LS. Evaluation of enzymatically crosslinked injectable glycol chitosan hydrogel. J Mater Chem B 2015;3:5511–22.
[155] Dhivya S, Saravanan S, Sastry TP, Selvamurugan N. Nanohydroxyapatite-reinforced chitosan composite hydrogel for bone tissue repair in vitro and in vivo. J Nanobiotechnol 2015;13:40.
[156] Wattanutchariya W, Changkowchai W. Characterization of porous scaffold from chitosan-gelatin/hydroxyapatite for bone grafting. Proceedings of the International MultiConference of Engineers and Computer Scientists, Vol. II, March 12–14, IMECS, Hong Kong; 2014.
[157] Gentile P, Mattioli-Belmonte M, Chiono V, Ferretti C, Baino F, Tonda-Turo C, et al. Bioactive glass/polymer composite scaffolds mimicking bone tissue. J Biomed Mater Res A 2012;100:2654–67.
[158] Gohil SV, Kuo C-L, Adams DJ, Maye P, Rowe DW, Nair LS. Evaluation of the donor cell contribution in rhBMP-2 mediated bone formation with chitosan thermogels using fluorescent protein reporter mice. J Biomed Mater Res A 2016;104:928–41.
[159] McLaughlin SW, Cui Z, Starnes T, Laurencin CT, Kan H-M, Wu Q, et al. Injectable thermogelling chitosan for the local delivery of bone morphogenetic protein. J Mater Sci Mater Med 2012;23:2141–9.
[160] Stephan SJ, Tholpady SS, Gross B, Petrie-Aronin CE, Botchway EA, Nair LS, et al. Injectable tissue-engineered bone repair of a rat calvarial defect. Laryngoscope 2010;120:895–901.
[161] Nair LS, Starnes T, Ko J-W, Laurencin CT. Development of injectable thermogelling chitosan–inorganic phosphate solutions for biomedical applications. Biomacromolecules 2007;8:3779–85.
[162] Wang L, Stegemann JP. Thermogelling chitosan and collagen composite hydrogels initiated with beta-glycerophosphate for bone tissue engineering. Biomaterials 2010;31:3976–85.
[163] Das A, Barker DA, Wang T, Lau CM, Lin Y, Botchwey EA. Delivery of bioactive lipids from composite microgel-microsphere injectable scaffolds enhances stem cell recruitment and skeletal repair. PLoS One 2014;9:e101276.
[164] Zhang Y, Venugopal JR, El-Turki A, Ramakrishna S, Su B, Lim CT. Electrospun biomimetic nanocomposite nanofibers of hydroxyapatite/chitosan for bone tissue engineering. Biomaterials 2008;29:4314–22.
[165] Thein-Han WW, Misra RDK. Biomimetic chitosan–nanohydroxyapatite composite scaffolds for bone tissue engineering. Acta Biomater 2009;5:1182–97.
[166] Schanté CE, Zuber G, Herlin C, Vandamme TF. Chemical modifications of hyaluronic acid for the synthesis of derivatives for a broad range of biomedical applications. Carbohydr Polym 2011;85:469–89.

[167] Collins MN, Birkinshaw C. Hyaluronic acid based scaffolds for tissue engineering—a review. Carbohydr Polym 2013;92:1262–79.
[168] Baldini A, Zaffe D, Nicolini G. Bone-defects healing by high-molecular hyaluronic acid: preliminary results. Ann Stomatol (Roma) 2010;1:2–7.
[169] Ballini A, Cantore S, Capodiferro S, Grassi FR. Esterified hyaluronic acid and autologous bone in the surgical correction of the infra-bone defects. Int J Med Sci 2009;6:65–71.
[170] Hulsart-Billstrom G, Yuen PK, Marsell R, Hilborn J, Larsson S, Ossipov D. Bisphosphonate-linked hyaluronic acid hydrogel sequesters and enzymatically releases active bone morphogenetic protein-2 for induction of osteogenic differentiation. Biomacromolecules 2013;14:3055–63.
[171] Kim J, Kim IS, Cho TH, Lee KB, Hwang SJ, Tae G, et al. Bone regeneration using hyaluronic acid-based hydrogel with bone morphogenic protein-2 and human mesenchymal stem cells. Biomaterials 2007;28:1830–7.
[172] Kim SY, Park J-S. Biomineralized hyaluronic acid/poly(vinylphosphonic acid) hydrogel for bone tissue regeneration. J Appl Polym Sci 2014;131:41194.
[173] Augst AD, Kong HJ, Mooney DJ. Alginate hydrogels as biomaterials. Macromol Biosci 2006;6:623–33.
[174] Boontheekul T, Kong H-J, Mooney DJ. Controlling alginate gel degradation utilizing partial oxidation and bimodal molecular weight distribution. Biomaterials 2005;26:2455–65.
[175] Rubert M, Alonso-Sande M, Monjo M, Ramis JM. Evaluation of alginate and hyaluronic acid for their use in bone tissue engineering. Biointerphases 2012;7:1–11.
[176] Lenz RW, Marchessault RH. Bacterial polyesters: biosynthesis, biodegradable plastics and biotechnology. Biomacromolecules 2005;6:1–8.
[177] Bonartsev AP, Myshkina VL, Nikolaeva DA, Furina EK, Makhina TA, Livshits VA, et al. In: Mendez-Vilas V, editor. Biosynthesis, biodegradation, and application of poly(3-hydroxybutyrate) and its copolymers—natural polyesters produced by diazotrophic bacteria. Communicating current research and educational topics and trends in applied microbiology: ©FORMATEX; 2007. p. 295–307.
[178] Chen G-Q, Wu Q. The application of polyhydroxyalkanoates as tissue engineering materials. Biomaterials 2005;26:6565–78.
[179] Köse GT, Korkusuz F, Korkusuz P, Purali N, Özkul A, Hasırcı V. Bone generation on PHBV matrices: an in vitro study. Biomaterials 2003;24:4999–5007.
[180] Huang W, Shi X, Ren L, Du C, Wang Y. PHBV microspheres—PLGA matrix composite scaffold for bone tissue engineering. Biomaterials 2010;31:4278–85.
[181] Larsson M, Bergstrand A, Mesiah L, Van Vooren C, Larsson A. Nanocomposites of polyacrylic acid nanogels and biodegradable polyhydroxybutyrate for bone regeneration and drug delivery. J Nanomater 2014;2014:9.
[182] Bai J, Dai J, Li G. Electrospun composites of PHBV/pearl powder for bone repairing. Prog Nat Sci Mater Int 2015;25:327–33.
[183] Praveen Kumar A, Jackson Irudhayam S, Naviin D. A review on importance and recent applications of polymer composites in orthopaedics. Int J Eng Res Dev 2012;5:40–3.
[184] Puska M, Aho AJ, Vallittu P. Polymer composites for bone reconstruction. In: Těšinova P, editor. *Advances in composite materials——analysis of natural and man-made materials*. In Tech; 2011. p. 55–72.
[185] Ramakrishna S, Mayer J, Wintermantel E, Leong K. Biomedical applications of polymer-composite materials: a review. Compos Sci Technol 2001;61:1189–224.
[186] O'Connell GD, Leach JK, Klineberg EO. Tissue engineering a biological repair strategy for lumbar disc herniation. Biores Open Access 2015;4:431–45.
[187] Szpalski M, Gunzburg R, Mayer M. Spine arthroplasty: a historical review. Eur Spine J 2002;11: S65–84.
[188] Vaccaro AR, Chiba K, Heller JG, Patel T, Thalgott JS, Truumees E, et al. Bone grafting alternatives in spinal surgery. Spine J 2002;2:206–15.

CHAPTER 9

Surface Modifications and Surface Characterization of Biomaterials Used in Bone Healing

V.G. Varanasi[1], M.F. Velten[2], T. Odatsu[3], A. Ilyas[1], S.M. Iqbal[2] and P.B. Aswath[1]
[1]Texas A&M University, Dallas, TX, United States
[2]University of Texas at Arlington, Arlington, TX, United States
[3]Nagasaki University, Nagasaki, Japan

Contents

9.1 INTRODUCTION

Biocompatibility has been broadly defined by the IUPAC as the ability of a material to perform with an appropriate host response in a specific application [1]. In practice, the application of this concept requires knowledge of the host tissue, particularly in the case of diseased or disordered tissues, and the biomaterial in order to develop biocompatibility in a given host tissue. Biomaterials are generally classified into one of four categories: toxic, inert, resorbable, and bioactive [2].

In the context of bone as the host tissue system, the biocompatibility of a biomaterial is defined by the type of bond bone forms with the biomaterial surface. Inert biomaterials do not form a bond with host bone tissue and tend instead to form a fibrous encapsulation in vivo. Resorbable biomaterials degrade in vivo into nontoxic products and are replaced over time by host bone tissue. Though the process seems ideal in theory, in the sense that it appears to mimic the natural bone remodeling process, in practice it is difficult to control the rate of dissolution of the biomaterial to match the rate of replacement of the host bone tissue. These types of biomaterials are therefore rarely used in load-bearing tissue applications. Bioactive biomaterials form a strong chemical bond with local bone host tissue through a series of chemical reactions at the bioceramic—bone interface that results in the formation of a carbonated apatite layer at the interface surface [2]. This strong interface makes them ideal for use in load-bearing bone implant applications, such as hip stems and dental screws; however, most bioactive biomaterials used in bone tissue applications do not have the necessary mechanical strength required to replace load-bearing bone.

The current state-of-the-art materials used in dental, craniofacial, and orthopedic bone healing are metals such as titanium (commercially pure Ti or Ti6Al4V alloy). These bioinert metals are used in load-bearing bone implant applications, but they do not bond to local bone tissue and have a finite fatigue life in vivo. Previous attempts to improve the biocompatibility of titanium implants have included the use of calcium phosphate-based coatings. These coatings have been shown to slightly improve the healing rate of bone, however, at the cost of compromising the coating—Ti interface. The resultant implant system endures resorption of the ceramic coating and separation of the bone from the implant. These limitations are due to (1) the use of high-temperature processes that can compromise bioactivity of the coating, (2) poor interfacial adhesion due to thermal expansion mismatch that manifest interfacial stresses upon cooling after coating fabrication, and (3) inhomogeneity of the coating chemical, physical, and mechanical properties in support of bone healing. Therefore, there is a need to explore the possibility of creating a new type of bioactive coating that is capable of forming a strong bond to both host bone tissue and a titanium implant.

9.1.1 Objective of this chapter

The objective of this chapter is to illustrate the use of novel bioactive materials for applications in healing healthy or disordered bone. We will focus discussion on improving the biomaterial—bone interface by using concepts in material science and engineering combined with molecular and cellular biology. The chapter will incorporate principles of evidence-based medicine and dentistry with an "eye-to-the-future" presentation of new fabrication and testing methods to tailor biomedical devices to meet patient needs. We present current load-bearing and nonload-bearing applications that manifest as a result of disorder or disease and the use of current biomaterials including synthetic and autologous materials. We will then discuss the use of surface modification and surface characterization to improve these materials for bone attachment. Then, we will describe future applications in which new surface modification modalities can be used for the detection or diagnosis of disease by measuring biomaterial surface—cellular interactions.

9.2 CURRENT BIOMATERIALS FOR BONE HEALING

9.2.1 Load-bearing

A biomaterial is any material designed to elicit (or prevent) a specific host tissue response for the repair or replacement of the host tissue [3]. As noted previously, biomaterials are generally classified by host tissue response into one of four categories: toxic, inert, resorbable, and bioactive [2,3]. Toxic biomaterials elicit unfavorable tissue responses and damage or kill surrounding tissue. Inert biomaterials tend to form a fibrous encapsulation in vivo but otherwise interact with surrounding tissue only in a limited sense. Most metals, polymers, ceramics, and composites used in biomedical applications fall into this category. Resorbable materials dissolve or break down in vivo into nontoxic products and are eventually replaced by the host tissue. Some specifically designed polymers and a few specific ceramics fall into this category.

Bioactive materials react with the host tissue and form a strong interfacial bond with the surrounding host tissue. A few types of ceramics including some silicate glasses and some calcium phosphates fall into this category. Inert, resorbable, and bioactive materials are all used in bone biomaterial applications [3].

For load-bearing bone applications, neither polymers nor porous ceramics have the necessary compressive strength to replace cortical bone tissue. A few dense (>99.8%) hydroxyapatite and beta-tricalcium phosphate ceramic materials have been observed to meet or exceed the compressive strength of bone [4,5]; however, these materials lack the necessary fracture toughness for therapeutic use in human load-bearing bone tissues [4]. Fig. 9.1 compares the elastic modulus and compressive strength of biopolymer and bioceramics materials with the material properties of trabecular and cortical bone.

Currently, metals are used to achieve the necessary material compressive strength and fracture toughness for the replacement of cortical bone. Some metals commonly used for load-bearing bone applications include 316L stainless steel, cobalt—chromium alloys, titanium, and titanium alloys (particularly Ti-6A1-4V). These materials are generally considered bioinert due to the spontaneous formation of a passivating oxide layer after exposure to the bone tissue environment. The application of these bioinert metals in vivo, however, is not without some complications at the bone—metal interface.

Yet, the elastic moduli of bioinert metals are higher than those of cortical bone. Differences in the stiffness of the bone and the metal implant can result in an effect

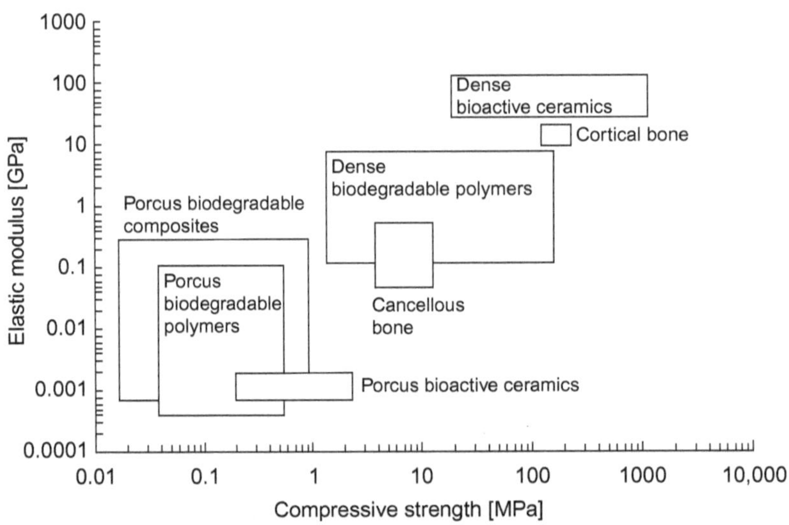

Figure 9.1 Mechanical properties of biomaterials for bone tissue applications compared with cortical and trabecular bone properties [6].

known as stress shielding, where the stiffer implant material reduces the load on surrounding bone [7]. This transfer of load from the bone to the implant interferes with the bone remodeling process, which is triggered by loading via a mechanism that is still not well understood [8]. Metals with relatively low stiffness—on the order of bone—are therefore more attractive in load-bearing osseoapplications. Titanium and titanium alloys have some of the lowest elastic moduli of all bioinert metals and have consequently found widespread use in load-bearing osseoimplant applications such as dental screws and hip stems (Table 9.1).

Since bioinert titanium implants do not bond to the bone tissue directly, but are instead mechanically fixed in place; Ti implants are susceptible to micromotion due to the fibrous lining that coats foreign materials as a part of the long-term immune response [11]. This small-scale motion simultaneously promotes the acute immune response to wear-debris created by fretting of the passivating surface and corrosion of the underlying base metal in a scheme shown in Fig. 9.5. Briefly, micromotion at the bone–implant surface (due to cyclic loading from physiological movement such as walking or chewing) results in damage to both the passivating oxide layer on the Ti metal implant surface and to the underlying metal. Metallic ions and wear-debris are released from the implant surface, which incites an acute immune response. The acute immune response results in the clearing of fretting debris and the formation or thickening of a fibrous encapsulation network around the implant surface as the passivating oxide layer reforms. The fibrous encapsulation and change in implant surface topography compromise the mechanical fixation of the implant, which can ultimately lead to implant loosening [11].

9.2.2 Metal implants

Long-term clinical success of titanium dental implants is largely a factor of initial bone host tissue response. Recent studies have focused on adapting the surface chemistry, roughness, and topography of titanium [12–14] to enhance the formation of bone around the implant, generally either through the creation of a calcium phosphate-based coating [15] or incorporation of relevant ions like Ca^{2+} and Mg^{2+} [16] directly into titanium dioxide. Of particular interest is investigation into early-stage (from 0 to

Table 9.1 Comparison of elastic moduli of some common bioinert metals with cortical bone

Material	Elastic modulus (GPa)	References
Cortical bone	12–20	[9]
316L stainless steel	190	[9,10]
Vitallium (Co-Cr-Mo-W alloy)	248	[10]
Ti-6Al-4V	106	[10]
Titanium	110	[9,10]

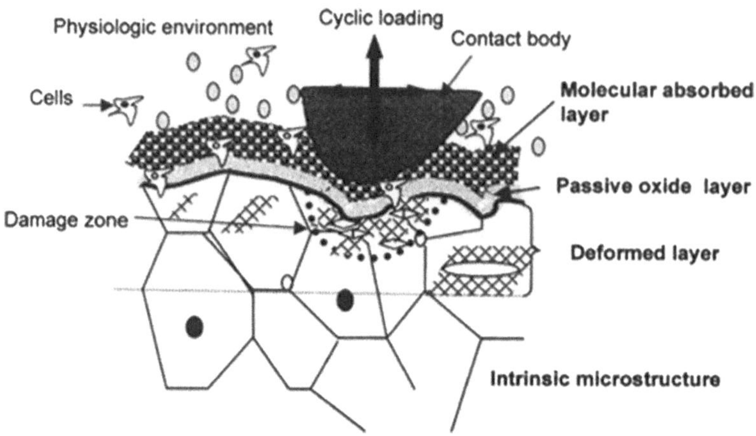

Figure 9.2 Fretting mechanism observed in load-bearing bone metallic implants [11].

3 days) osseointegration. Despite these bare metal implants exhibiting the strength needed to stabilize the fracture site, they have long healing times, do not resorb, and have not shown any antioxidant effect [17] and thus are considered inadequate for rapid healing of the fracture. Therefore, alternative materials and surface modifications have been explored to hasten the healing response (Fig. 9.2).

9.2.3 Bioactive ceramics

To prevent loosening of Ti implants, various Ti surface modifications and coating strategies have been employed. The use of bioactive ceramic coatings is a particularly promising solution to the fixation problem of Ti implants, since bioactive ceramics can be used not only to chemically bond to local bone tissue and improve the mechanical strength of the bone–implant interface, they can also be used to deliver therapeutic ionic products to the surrounding bone tissue. To better understand the ability of bioceramics to bond to local tissue and deliver therapeutic agents to local tissues, a deeper understanding of bioceramic chemistry and dynamic response in vivo is instructive.

Bioceramics, like the broader category of biomaterials, are classified according to the type of host tissue response. These responses are separated into four types. Type 1, or nearly inert bioceramics, do not form a bond with host bone tissue and tend instead to form a fibrous encapsulation in vivo. An example of this type of bioceramic would be alumina or zirconia. Type 2, or porous inert bioceramics, do not form a chemical bond with local bone, both allow for bony in-growth for a better mechanical fixation of the surface in vivo. An example of this type of bioceramic would be a porous membrane or structure coated with a relatively unreactive

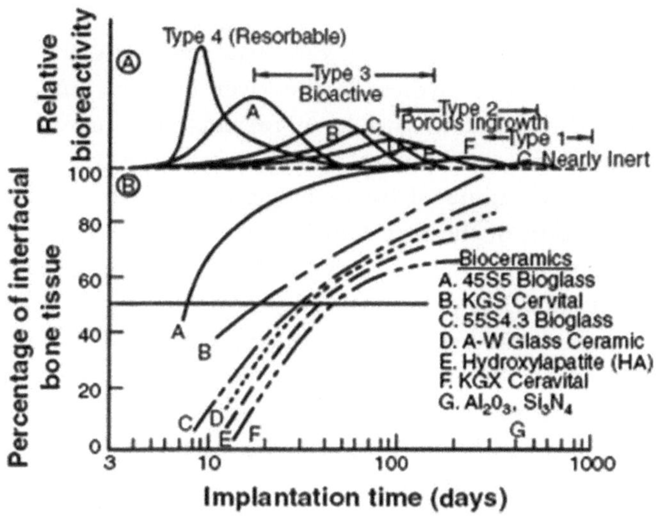

Figure 9.3 The four types of bioceramics and the timescale over which each forms a bond with surrounding host bone tissue [18].

calcium phosphate ceramic like stoichiometric hydroxyapatite. Type 4, or resorbable bioceramics, degrade over time in vivo into nontoxic products and are replaced over time by host bone tissue. Though this process seems ideal in theory in the sense that it appears to mimic the natural bone remodeling process, in practice it is difficult to control the rate of dissolution of the bioceramic material to match the rate of replacement of the host bone tissue. These types of bioceramics are therefore rarely used in load-bearing tissue applications. An example of this type of bioceramic would be certain dissolvable silica-based bioglasses or amorphous calcium phosphate, which dissolves readily in physiological conditions. Type 3, or bioactive ceramics, form a strong chemical bond with local bone host tissue through a series of chemical reactions at the bioceramic—bone interface that results in the formation of a carbonated apatite layer at the interface surface. An example of this type of bioceramic would be 45S5 Bioglass or beta-tricalcium phosphate, which has a dissolution rate in vivo intermediate to pure hydroxyapatite and amorphous calcium phosphate (Fig. 9.3) [2,3].

9.2.4 Bioactive glasses

Bioactive glasses, a class of type 3 bioceramics, are amorphous silicate-based biomaterials that react with bone tissue to form a strong chemical bond through the formation of a carbonated hydroxyapatite layer at the bone—bioglass interface. This carbonated hydroxyapatite layer is almost chemically identical to the mineral phase of bone, and the carbonate content observed in this structure has been seen to vary anywhere from 4% to 12% of phosphate replacement by carbonate. With its chemical similarity to bone mineral, this carbonated hydroxyapatite layer develops an adherent interface with the host bone tissue that is capable of resisting the micromechanical motion effects that are generally observed in implant–bone interface systems. This interface is so strong that mechanical failure of bone–bioglass interfaces is virtually unheard of [2]. The glass composition of the first commercially available bioactive glass, Bioglass 45S5, was developed back in 1969 by Larry Hench and is composed of 45 wt% SiO_2, 6 wt% P_2O_5, 24.5 wt% CaO, and 24.5 wt% Na_2O [19].

After Hench's initial discovery, interest in bioactive glasses has grown tremendously, and there are now over 20 different bioglass formulations in clinical use. In addition to SiO_2, P_2O_5, CaO, and Na_2O, some newer bioactive glass compositions also contain small (>5 wt%) amounts of MgO, K_2O, Al_2O_3, TiO_2, and Ta_2O_5 [20]. Extensive research has been done on the SiO_2-P_2O_5-CaO-Na_2O bioactive glass system to determine the effect of each component on bioactivity as well as the range of chemical compositions that are bone-bonding and nonbonding. Fig. 9.4 summarizes this research and shows a compositional diagram of a ternary SiO_2-CaO-Na_2O system with 6% P_2O_5.

Bone-bonding bioglass formulations (region A) are comprised of approximately 40–60 wt% of SiO_2. At concentrations above 60%, the material is no longer bioactive, and instead acts as inert bioceramic and forms a fibrous encapsulation in vivo (region B). Glasses in region C act like type 3 resorbable ceramics, and completely dissolve without forming a bond at the glass–bone interface. Region D consists of

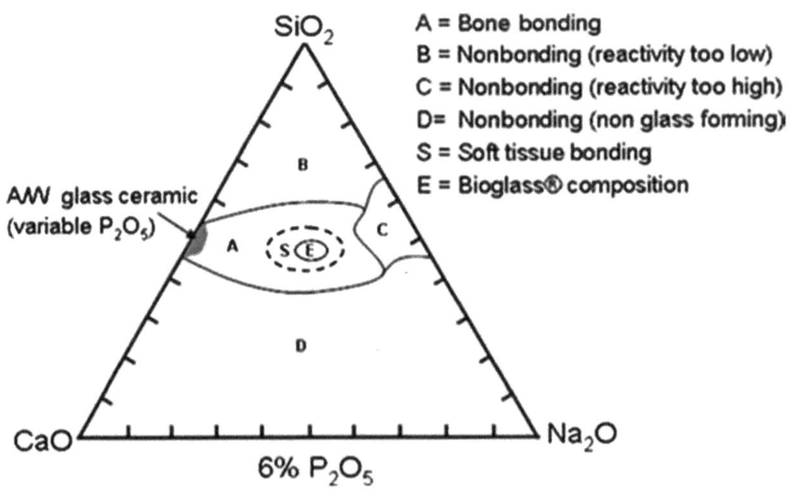

Figure 9.4 Composition diagram of bioactive glasses [21].

Table 9.2 Concentration of inorganic salt species found in blood plasma

Ion	Plasma (mM)
Na^+	142
K^+	5.0
Mg^{2+}	1.5
Ca^{2+}	2.5
Cl^-	103.0
HCO_3^-	27.0
HPO_4^{2-}	1.0
SO_4^{2-}	0.5

compositions that are nonglass-forming and therefore have not been studied. Region S glass formulations, which include 45S5 Bioglass, are a subset of region A, where the bioglass forms a strong bond to both the mineral and organic soft tissue phases of bone. The initial sequence of events that result in a strong bioglass–bone bond occurs due to the reaction of the bioglass with ionic salts in physiological solution (blood plasma) rather than with the host bone tissue itself. Table 9.2 lists the concentration of inorganic salt species found in physiological solution.

The fact that bone-bonding bioglass reacts with these inorganic salt species to form a carbonated apatite layer independent of any host tissue response has one interesting implication for the study of bioactive glasses, namely, that the initial response in vivo can be well-modeled by an in vitro study with a soaking solution that contains inorganic salt concentrations similar to those of blood plasma. The initial stages of the interaction of bioglass and a simulated body fluid (SBF) similar to human blood plasma have been well documented and confirmed in vivo. Fig. 9.5 summarizes the initial set of reactions that occur at the bioactive glass–bone (or more precisely physiological solution) interface. The process involves five basic steps. (1) There is a rapid exchange of cations (Na^+ or Ca^{2+}) with H^+ from the physiological environment which results in the formation of silanol bonds (Si–OH) on the glass surface. The local pH of the dissolving environment increases and a silica-rich layer forms near the exposed glass surface. Phosphate ions (PO_4^{3-}) are also lost from the surface region during this step. (2) The high pH leads to the breakdown of the silica network via Si–O–Si bond attack by hydroxide ions (OH^-). The soluble silicon (Si^{4+}) is lost in the form of $Si(OH)_4$ which again results in Si–OH bonds at the glass surface. (3) These silanol groups condense to form a silica-rich layer at the glass surface. (4) Calcium Ca^{2+} and phosphate ions (PO_4^{3-}) start to migrate through this surface layer to form an amorphous film of calcium oxide (CaO) and phosphate on the silica-rich layer. (5) Hydroxyl (OH^-) ions and carbonate ions (CO_3^{2-}) from the environment begin to incorporate within the Ca-P layer to form a carbonated apatite.

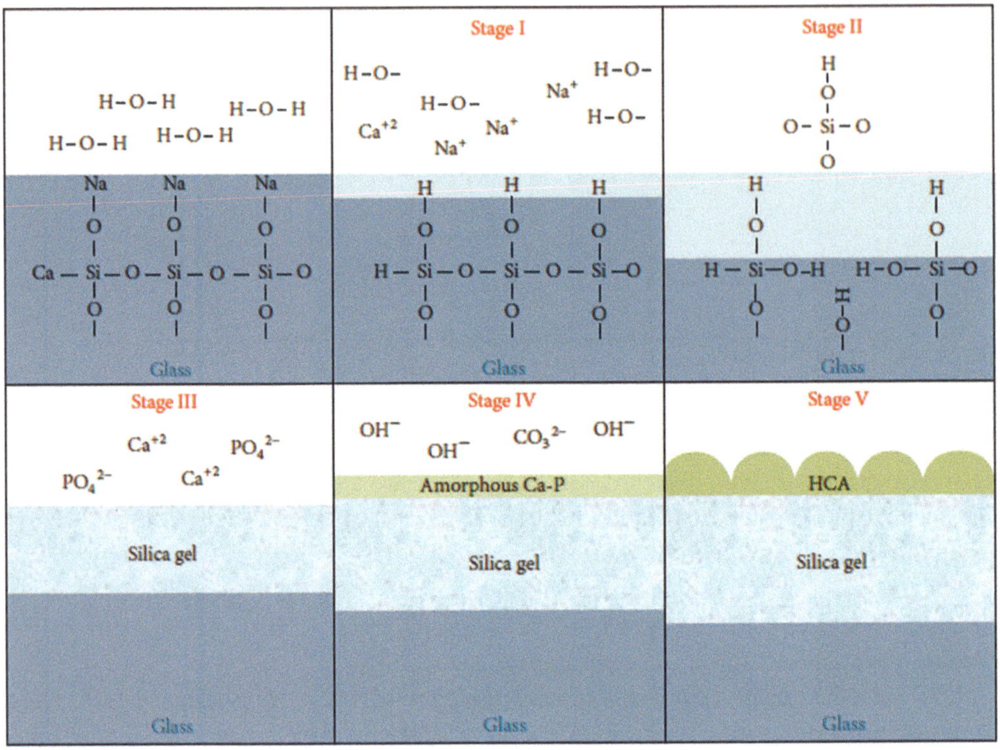

Figure 9.5 Mechanism of bioglass dissolution and carbonated hydroxyapatite formation in physiological solution [22].

9.2.5 Bone substitute used in oral and maxillofacial bone disorders

In the case of alveolar bone loss, which can result from trauma, tumor, infection, or periodontal disease, an autogenic bone graft is used for "bone reconstruction." It is difficult for these bone substitutes to regenerate the bone and maintain the form at the site of massive severe bone loss (Fig. 9.6). Autogenic bone grafting remains the "gold standard" due to its osteoinductive, osteoconductive, and osteogenic properties. However, it has significant limitations, including donor site morbidity, and limited quantities, inappropriate forms for the graft site.

For bone "augmentation," bone substitute materials have been used in order to compensate for the drawbacks caused by autogenic bone grafting, especially in the dental implant field. Bone substitute materials are divided into three main classes according to their source: "allograft," "xenograft," or "alloplast" (Fig. 9.7).

Allografts are harvested from cadaver donors and chemically processed, such as freeze-dried (freeze-dried bone allograft: FDBA) or demineralized (demineralized freeze-dried bone allograft: DFDBA). Although both FDBA and DFDBA are

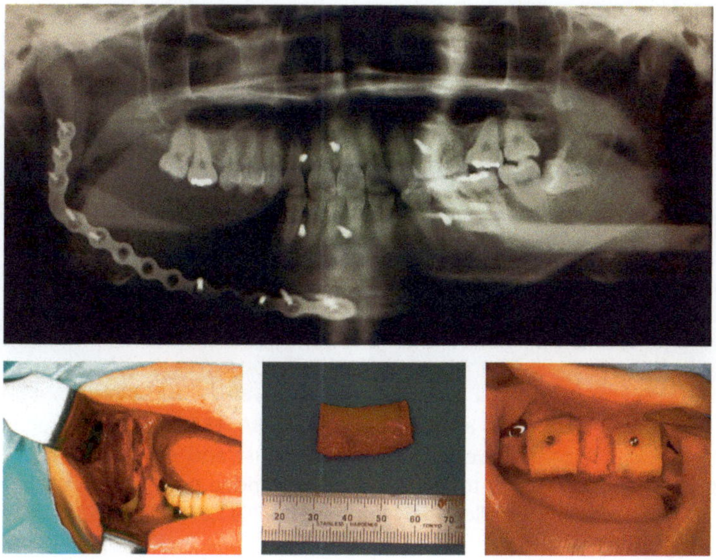

Figure 9.6 Reconstruction harvested from iliac bone after segmentectomy (top). Bone grafting from mandibular ramus for dental implants (bottom).

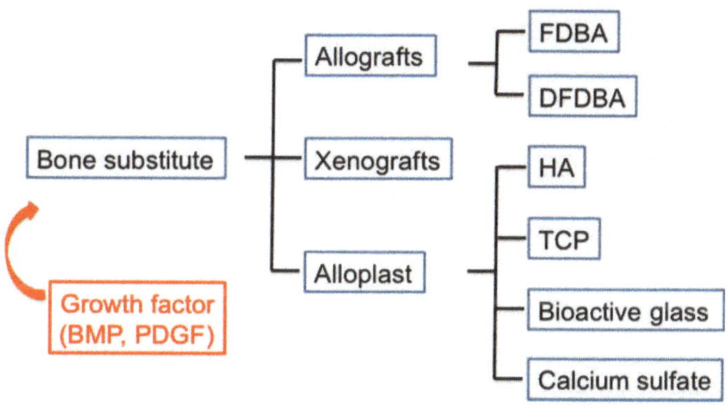

Figure 9.7 Types of bone substitute materials.

osteoconductive, only DFDBA has shown osteoinductivity, due to the release of bone morphogenetic proteins (BMPs) [23]. Although FDBA has the same BMP content in its organic matrix, it does not have the same osteoinductive property. BMPs in the FDBA are mineral-bounded, thus demineralization by osteoclasts is necessary to release BMP from its matrix [24]. Both FDBA and DFDBA have similar bioabsorption and new bone formation (Fig. 9.8A, B). Although either FDBA or DFDBA have been reported as bioabsorbable materials, Kolerman et al. reported that 20% of residual was indicated in the biopsy 9 months after implantation [24]. Their limitation is the

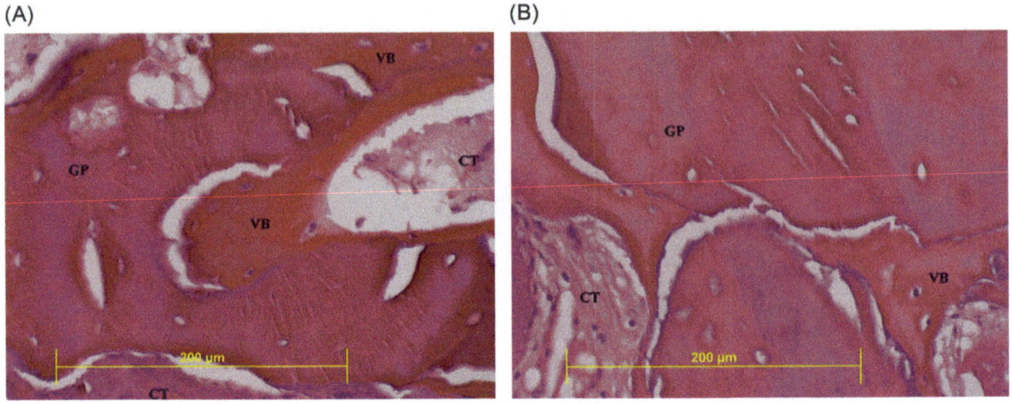

Figure 9.8 (A) DFDBA 18–20 weeks after grafted. (B) FDBA 18–20 weeks after grafted. *VB*, vital bone; *GP*, graft particle; *CT*, connective tissue with fibroblast and collagen. Wood, RA, Mealey BL. Histologic comparison of healing after tooth extraction with ridge preservation using mineralized versus demineralized freeze-dried bone allograft. J Periodontol 2012;83(3):329–336 [25].

potential risk of crossinfection or immunologic reaction due to their residual donor protein (although no cases have yet been reported by using FDBA and DFDBA [26]).

Xenografts are the graft materials from nonhuman donors, such as bovine, equine, and coral. Above all, deproteinized bovine bone (DPBB, Bio-Oss, Geistlich Pharmaceutical, Wolhusen, Switzerland) has been mainly used in oral and maxillofacial sites and has shown good biocompatibility and osteoconductivity. Bovine bone is deproteinized for the organic components to prevent the possibility of immunologic reaction while maintaining the original porous trabecular structure and inorganic bone mineral compositions. However, reports on bioabsorption of DPBB indicate a lack of consistency [27–30]. Furthermore, there have been reports of the presence of osteoclast around DPBBs [28,31]. Others have reported the lack of osteoclasts around DPBBs [32]. Sartori et al. reported the amount of DPBB ossification by comparing histomorphometric data 8 months, 2 and 10 years after surgery [33]. Unchanged DPBBs were identified surrounded by newly formed lamellar bone (Fig. 9.9). Mordenfeld et al. also reported the presence of DPBBs, showing no significant changes in particle size after 11 years surgery [34].

Alloplasts are the synthetic bone substitutes made from hydroxyapatite (HA) [35], tricalcium phosphate (TCP) [36], bioactive glass [37], or biopolymers. The Ca/P ratio of HA is 1.67, which is equal to the inorganic phase of crystallographic structure of bone. On the other hand, the Ca/P ratio of TCP is 1.5 and occurs in two phases (α and β), which is closer to the composition of the amorphous biological precursor to bone [36]. Physical properties and degradation rates of HA and TCP depend on their processing and sintering condition (porosity, sintering time, temperature, etc.).

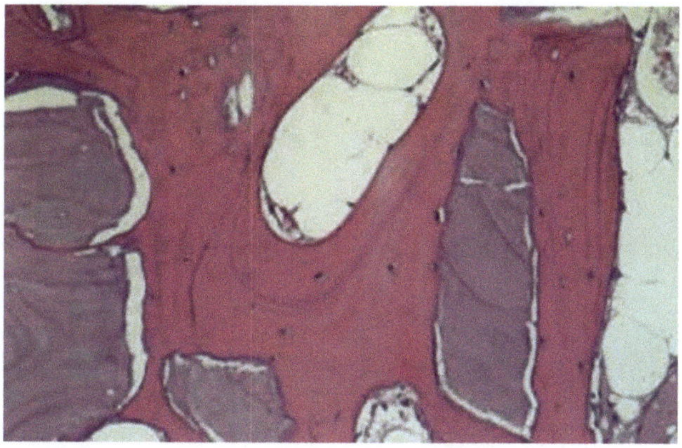

Figure 9.9 Section from 10 years biopsy revealing DPBBs surrounded by lamellar bone.

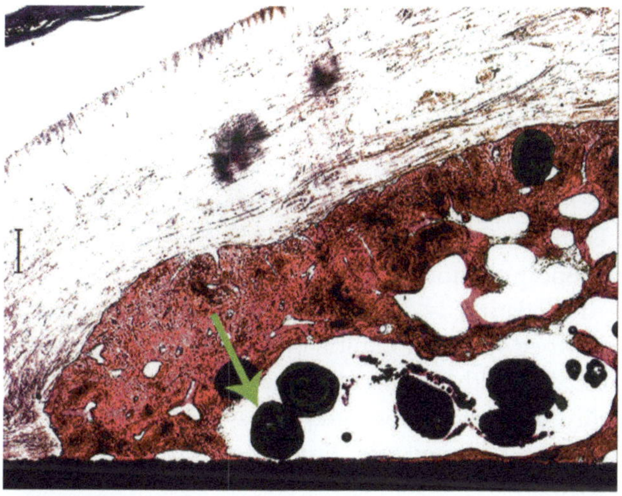

Figure 9.10 HA granules remained minimally degraded after 10 years. Bone tissue is present around the granules (*arrow*).

In general, HA is considered to resorb slowly, and hence would limit new bone formation and remodeling. Beekmans et al. reported that HA granules grafted with autologous bone in sinus had only minimally degraded after 10 years (Fig. 9.10) [38].

Conventional bioactive glass is made from SiO_2, Na_2O, CaO, and P_2O_5. Bioactive glass is considered to have an osteoinductivity due to its ability to form the biological-like hydroxycarbonate apatite layer on to the material surface. This mechanism starts with a rapid ion exchange between the alkali ions from the glass surface and the hydrogen ions from the solution, followed by the formation of silanols, which then develop a silica gel layer and nucleation of amorphous calcium phosphate occurs,

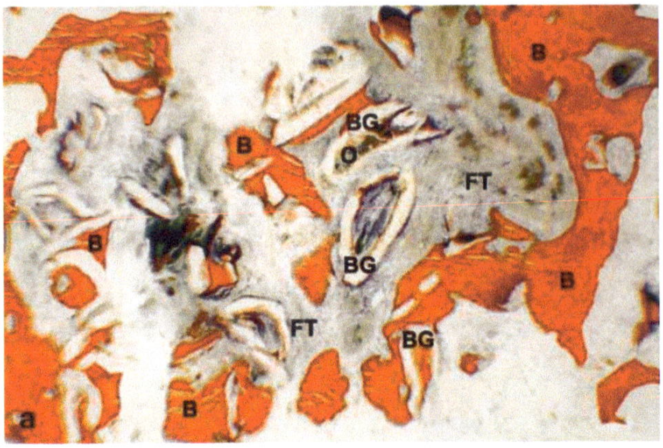

Figure 9.11 The granules of bioactive glass are surrounded by fibrous tissue (*FT*, fibrous tissue; *B*, bone; *O*, osteoid)

resulting in hydroxycarbonate apatite layer on crystallization. Furthermore, dissolved ions from bioactive glass play an active role in osteoblast behavior, alter the expression of osteoblast differentiation markers associated with bone matrix formation. Although, Cordioli et al. reported that residual bioglass particles grafted into the sinus appeared to be surrounded by fibrous tissue [39]. Kobayashi et al. also reported issues related to bioactive glass microencapsulation (Fig. 9.11) [40].

The period of degradation is different for each bone substitute, some show slow absorption or unabsorbed. From a clinical point of view, this delay has some advantages, especially to maintain the space for bone regeneration. On the other hand, this might be a possibility that bone substitutes act as a source of infection, even if once allowed and organized by recipient site. From the above, the ideal bone substitute has the following properties:

1. Maintain the space during bone formation and completely replace bone;
2. Osteoinductivity should be an advantage for rapid bone formation;
3. No risk of crossinfection or immunologic reaction.

Alloplasts have been studied for modifying their crystalline, micro- to nanostructure and surface topography, in order to improve the absorbing ratio, cell attachment. Biopolymers, such as poly-L-lactic acid (PLLA), poly-ε-caprolactone (PCL), [41] and chitosan, have been studied for their bioactivity [42]. Furthermore, growth factors (BMP, fibroblast growth factor, platelet-derived growth factor) [43,44] and some metallic ions (Zn, Sr, Si, Mg) have been studied for the combination use of bone substitutes in order to enhance and/or invest osteoinductivity [45–47]. Such aspects of surface modifications of some of these alloplasts will be discussed in the following sections.

9.3 USE OF PRECISION MANUFACTURING TO IMPROVE BIOMATERIALS FABRICATION AND BIOLOGICAL RESPONSE

Despite the progress that was just described, the lack of nanoscale precision and atomic-scale understanding of the bone–biomaterial interface is still a limitation to realizing the potential of healing bone using biomaterials. From this point forward, we will delve into the use of new methods of precision manufacturing that can potentially improve the robustness of host responses to hasten bone healing. We consider two approaches for precision manufacturing methods to modify surfaces of biomaterials used for bone healing. One approach involves the use of nano-phase material for use in coating applications for fixative devices for load-bearing bone fracture healing. In the following sections, we outline these methods for fabrication, characterization, and their current uses in research and clinical translation. We will focus our attention to biosilica-based biomaterials since these materials have shown an innate ability to rapidly promote the bone-healing response. We focus on materials used for applications in both load-bearing and nonload-bearing. These materials also lend themselves to be used in precision manufacturing processes as we describe below.

9.3.1 Nano-phase methods of biomaterials fabrication

In this section, we describe various methods of surface modification used for biomaterials. This section describes the methodology and gives examples of tools used for fabrication. Before delving into various surface modification methods, it is worth noting the biological process and cell-surface markers that can respond to surface modifications.

9.3.2 Surface adhesion molecules on cell membranes

Cells attach to a surface via proteins, which are also called cell adhesion molecules, and cell-response to a surface is controlled via an integrin pathway. Integrin receptors interact with the extracellular environment and direct signaling molecules to the cell's cytoskeleton at adhesion sites, which are also referred to as focal adhesions. The cytoskeleton, which is comprised primarily of actin fibers, tubulin microtubules, and vimentin, desmin or keratin microfilaments, then interacts with the surface via the focal adhesion [48]. A recent study conducted a time-lapse observation of cell migration on a "nanograting" surface (Fig. 9.12) [49]. Findings suggest the ability of this type of surface to direct cell migration depends on the focal adhesion of a cell's actin filaments. Actin filaments parallel to the grating have the opportunity to form a continuous focal adhesion while filaments perpendicular to the grating form discontinuous connections with the surface that result in their eventual retraction. Although cell protrusions are generally formed isotropically, protrusions that form perpendicular

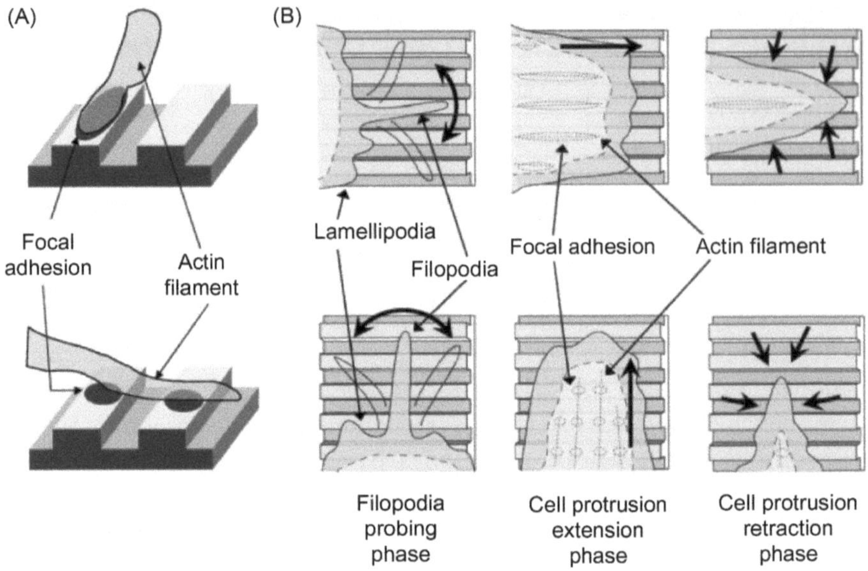

Figure 9.12 Ability of a nanograting surface to direct cell migration depends on the topographical effect on (A) focal adhesion points, while remaining relatively independent of (B) filipodia probing [49].

to the grating tend to retract more readily than those that form protrusions isotropically, suggesting that the effect on the local focal adhesion is responsible for the cell-directing capability of the surface [50].

9.3.3 Examples of surface modification

As described in the above illustration of cellular–material interactions, there are various structural and signaling mechanisms that regulate these interactions. Thus, surface modifications can be rather complex to handle the nanoscale and microscale hierarchy of such cell–material interactions. In general, surface modifications involve a single or multistep process. Broadly speaking, a biomedical device material, such as metals, ceramics, polymers, glasses, or their composites, can be surface-modified to improve bone attachment or even biosensing. For example, metal (e.g., Ti) or ceramic (e.g., silicon wafer) can be patterned via a photolithography process and dry or wet etching. These surfaces can also be coated with bioactive chemistries to induce altered cellular activity. In some applications, the surface can be "pitted" with nanoscale or microscale pores that do not alter greatly the overall biomedical device mechanical or structural properties, but greatly enhance the device's biosensing or surface functionalization properties. An example of a multistep process in which a biomedical device surface is patterned, etched, and coated can be seen in Fig. 9.13.

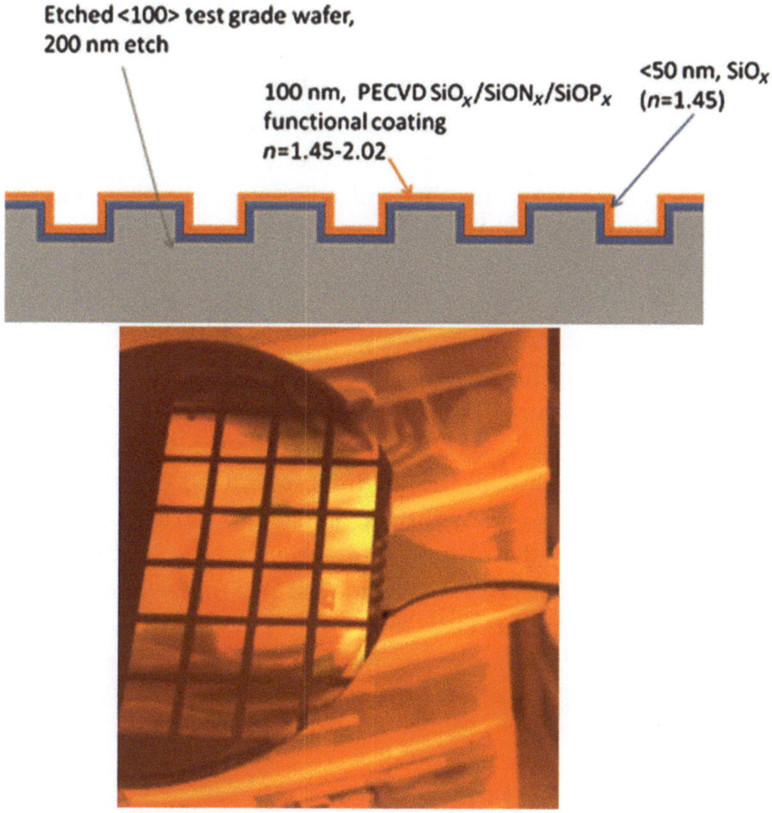

Figure 9.13 Material surface 12 × 12 mm sample cross section and wafer patter.

This micro/nano-"grating" pattern was selected to aid in cell attachment, and for its ability to direct cell migration, which may help to form a more consistent bond between the proposed bioactive surface and native bone tissue.

9.3.4 Photolithography processing

Photolithography is a staple of the microfabrication industry, and, as a relatively mature technology, it is well understood and allows for precise control of process variables and process design to achieve the desired micro- and nanoarchitecture. After the constraints of the material surface selection and mask design, the photolithography process can be premeditated. Parameters of the final surface features can be designed, such as dimension, depth, shape, and overall pattern.

For example, an etch depth that was originally designed to be 2 μm with the smallest feature size on a metal surface to aid in cell attachment have been updated with subsequent designs that employed a shallower etch that still allowed for cell attachment

[51]. To then create such a design, a proper resist must be selected that can help controllably create such a feature or pattern under the highly reactive wet, plasma, or ion etching process. This also plays a role in the mask that will be used to transpose the etch features or pattern onto the material surface. The pattern in turn plays a role in the developer solution used to develop the pattern and the material surface to be etched plays a role in the resist processing and subsequent cleaning. Therefore, careful planning must go into the photolithography process prior to creating surface nanofeatures and/or patterns.

Typically, one follows an example from a publication or manufacturer's recommendation on standard material surfaces (e.g., Ti or Si). However, issues with resultant feature resolution can hinder effective feature fabrication. To increase the resolution of the mask features, several process adjustments can be considered. A primer can be coated on the material surface prior to spin-coating the resist. This primer can be used to increase photoresist adhesion and aid in prewetting of the surface for a more uniform coating. As for the actual exposure process, a vacuum can be applied to the backside of the material to improve surface placement for the contact printing method selected. Finally, the smallest 365-nm I-line wavelength of the Hg-Xe source can be used to expose the resist. These processes are typical steps used in the photolithography process where high-resolution features can be fabricated.

9.3.5 Deep reactive ion etching

Once the pattern has been transferred to the resist, the resist and material can then be etched to form the pattern or feature on the material surface. This can involve a method of dry etching in which an ionized gas at various temperatures is used to control the etching depth into the resist and underlying material. Ideally, the etch rate of the resist and underlying material should be identical for reliable etching. This is termed "selectivity". This requires proper selection of the primer and resist for the underlying material to be etched. If the material is completely exposed to an unpatterned, and uncoated surface with no resist, then the etching process would simply remove layers of material conformally over the surface cross section and not form any features (except for the etchant profile). The selection of the etchant depends on the material. For standard metals, a boron trichloride or chloride ion plasma is used. For silicon wafers, sulfur hexafluoride or argon plasma is typically used. The selection of the etchant also plays a role in the ability to form anisotropic or isotropic etched patterns. Anisotropic etches result in etched features that form nearly 90 degrees side-wall trenches. Therefore, one must be careful in planning the etch process for formation of the nanofeatures. We provide an example of anisotropic etching by deep reactive ion etching below.

Deep reactive ion etching allows for the combination of two distinct etching regimes which results in a higher-quality anisotropic etch ideal for cell attachment concerns. The original etch design was a >1-μm anisotropic etch. Though both a wet-etch bench and dry plasma etching instruments were available, a dry etch process was selected over a wet etch process for better anisotropy. An anisotropically etched "nanograting" has been demonstrated to aid not only in cell attachment, but also in cell migration, which may ultimately prove useful in predict the characteristics of a bone–implant interface [52,53]. Such anisotropy—particularly in the context of small feature size—can be better achieved through a dry etching process. There are two types of dry etching processes. One is based on ion bombardment of the surface, which physically removes material. This process is often referred to as ion etching. The second type of dry etch process relies on a chemical process to etch the surface. This process, that is often referred to as plasma etching, relies on the generation of an etchant species from the reaction of a so-called etchant gas and energetic electrons found in the plasma. DRIE is a mixture of the two dry etching processes and allows for relatively high etch rate, anisotropic etch while minimizing the risk of damage to the wafer or material surface that might result from a purely physical dry etch.

The selection of a cryogenic plasma gas is critical to control the etch rate and profile (anisotropic vs isotropic). For example, tetrafluoromethane (CF_4) can be selected for its ability to anisotropically etch the base silicon substrate via the formation of fluorine radicals (F) which then react with silicon to form silicon tetrafluoride (SiF_4) [54]. Silicon tetrafluoride is a volatile gas and results in the removal of silicon from the substrate as shown in the mechanism below:

$$CF_4 + e^- \rightarrow CF_3^+ + F + 2e^-$$
$$CF_4 + e^- \rightarrow CF_3 + F + e^-$$
$$Si + 4F \rightarrow SiF_4(gas)$$

Argon and helium can also be used during the etch process. Argon gas is introduced into the chamber during the etch process to form a plasma to simultaneously physically etch the surface. This physical etching process can cause damage to the substrate, which results in a rough surface that may not be ideal for later deposition processing of the material surface. Therefore the pressure in the chamber is kept sufficiently low to ensure the mean free path of the argon plasma allowed for an orthogonal angle of incidence with the substrate. Helium can be used as a carrier gas to transport heat from the photoresist surface to adjust the selectivity of the exposed silicon surface of the wafer to the resist close to parity.

9.3.6 Surface modification by overlays or coatings

9.3.6.1 *Plasma-enhanced chemical vapor deposition coating*

Plasma-enhanced chemical vapor deposition (PECVD) is a thin-film deposition technique that allows for tunable control over the chemical composition of a thin film. Generally speaking, the energetic conditions in a PECVD reactor allow for the creation of high-energy, relatively unstable bonding states as compared to more traditional thin-film techniques [55]. While such chemical instability is often seen as detrimental in the microelectronics industry, for eventual application in physiological conditions, it could be considered beneficial in terms of enabling ionic release of components from the film. As an example, we will discuss the use of PECVD to fabricate coatings of amorphous silica-based bioactive coatings below.

PECVD-generated silicon dioxide, silicon nitride, and silicon oxynitride films designed for use in the microelectronics industry have been well studied [55–61]. Considering that silicon dioxide is one of the primary components of commercial bioglass, as well as the understanding that ionic silicon release from bioactive glasses is believed to enhance osteogenesis, such films may also show promise for osseoapplications.

In light of the currently available body of research of $SiON_x$ films for microelectronics, it is important to note the difference in several key design criteria between a $SiON_x$ film for use as a waveguide or a thin-film transistor and a $SiON_x$ coating for the proposed use in an osseointegration application. One major difference is the desirability of hydrogen incorporation into the film. In general, N-H and Si-H are undesirable in optical waveguides; for osseointegration, they provide likely sites for hydrolysis attack of the coating [62]. Another main distinct difference is the need for uniformity. While a preliminary understanding of coating chemistry and process validation is more easily achieved in a uniform system, this is by no means a stringent requirement for eventual in vivo application. Use of energetic plasma to "damage" the substrate surface could result in an appreciable surface roughness that aids in cell attachment—a one-step processing method for achieving desirable surface roughness and chemistry.

In the generation of thin silicon oxynitride and phosphorous-containing silicon oxynitrides, silane (SiH_4), nitrous oxide (N_2O), ammonia (NH_4), and nitrogen (N_2) can be used as reactant gases. Argon (Ar) can also be used as a carrier gas and a dilutant gas to prevent undesirable gas-phase reactions. For the majority of samples, the N_2O gas flow rate can be varied to adjust the proportion of N:O in the final film composition while all other gas flow rates can be kept constant. In the chamber, the pressure, temperature, radio frequency power, and plasma power for generating the initial ionized carrier gas can be adjusted to ensure proper reaction efficiency. PECVD process provides uniform and conformal layer that adheres well with the underlying metal surface [63,64].

9.3.7 Surface modification of solid-state micropores for selective cell surface binding

Micropores on solid-state devices can be used for selective cell binding. It is a method to present a surface with features that are attractive to one cell type over another. These pores can be left on their own or can be combined with a biomolecule motif that can further enhance cell selectivity.

The micropore fabrication process starts with thermal oxidation of a double-sided polished silicon wafer or other selected biomaterial. The material can be placed in an oxidation furnace to grow an oxide layer (~200 nm) on both sides of the material, as explained in Fig. 9.14. After piranha cleaning, a positive photoresist is spin-coated on one side of the material and conventional g-line photolithography can be used to open windows of desired shape (square in the case of Fig. 9.14). The photoresist layer can be manually applied to the other side (bottom) of the material to protect the oxide layer against buffered hydrofluoric (BHF) acid. The window pattern is transferred to the underside oxide layer using BHF etching followed by removing all the

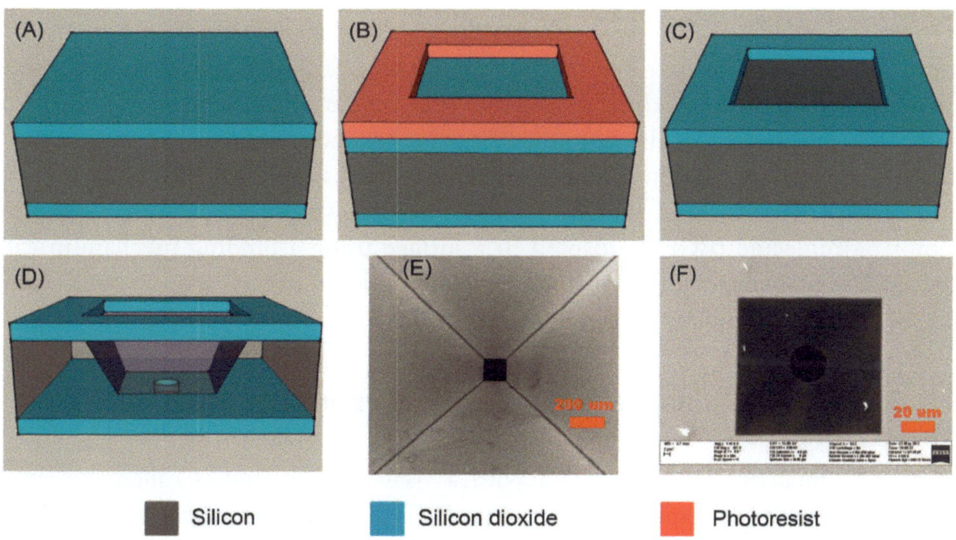

Figure 9.14 Process flow for solid-state micropores fabrication: (A) 200-nm-thick oxide layer grown on both sides of double-sided polished silicon wafer. (B) Photolithography to open square windows in the spin-casted photoresist layer. (C) Transfer of square window pattern to the underlying oxide layer by using BHF etching. (D) Anisotropic etching of Si using TMAH which performs V-groove etching to get oxide membrane on the other side of the wafer (bottom side). FIB is used to drill micropore in the membrane diaphragm. (E) SEM micrograph shows slanted sidewalls of Si ending at oxide membrane resulted from TMAH etching. (F) SEM micrograph of a thermally annealed micropore drilled in the oxide membrane.

remaining photoresist in acetone. Anisotropic etching can be performed using diluted (~25%) tetramethylammonium hydroxide (TMAH) at 90°C during the etching process. The material substrate can be etched through its thickness until it reaches the other oxide layer side. This yields free-standing SiO_2 membranes as shown in Fig. 9.14E. A focused ion beam (FIB) is then deployed to mill 20-μm-sized micropores in each of the membranes. The diameter of the milled micropore can be controlled by the FIB dose (milling current, drilling time). Membrane material and the thickness of the membrane also affect the diameter of the micropore [65,66]. A higher dose can yield a larger pore for oxide membranes of similar thickness. The scanning electron microscope (SEM) analysis can be used to image the surface and inner periphery to determine whether the micropore is not smooth, which could potentially rupture cell membranes while translocating through the micropore. Secondly, observation of crimped topography of the membrane can confirm residual stress in the oxide membrane. Therefore, the SiO_2 membranes can be annealed at 1050°C for 5 minutes to smoothen the inner pore walls and reduce residual stress in the membrane. Fig. 9.14F shows an SEM micrograph of a micropore after thermal treatment.

9.3.8 Surface biomolecular functionalization

Surface functionalization is a helpful tool in also selecting certain cell types for adhesions. Other applications could use such surfaces in drug delivery. This usually involves the preparation of the biomolecule prior to device or material surface preparation. A primer layer is administered and the desired biomolecule is passivated over the material surface to bind the biomolecule. Below, we use an example of a cancer receptor biomolecule (EGFR) adapted to a surface using a binding mechanism called an anti-EGFR aptamer to give more detailed understanding on how such surface functionalization is implemented.

9.3.9 Surface functionalization example: preparation of anti-EGFR aptamers

Anti-EGFR aptamers are synthesized with a well-known process called "systematic evolution of ligands by exponential enrichment" (SELEX) as reported earlier [67,68]. An iterative selection of binding species against purified human EGFR is used to isolate anti-EGFR RNA aptamers [3,4]. The high-affinity (K_d = 2.4 nM) anti-EGFR RNA aptamer and a nonfunctional mutated aptamer can be extended with a capture sequence. The extended anti-EGFR aptamer (5′-GGC GCU CCG ACC UUA GUC UCU GUG CCG CUA UAA UGC ACG GAU UUA AUC GCC GUA GAA AAG CAU GUC AAA GCC GGA ACC GUG UAG CAC AGC AGA **GAA UUA AAU GCC CGC CAU GAC CAG**-3′); extended mutant aptamer (5′-GGC GCU CCG ACC UUA GUC UCU GUU CCC ACA UCA UGC ACA AGG ACA AUU CUG

UGC AUC CAA GGA GGA GUU CUC GGA ACC GUG UAG CAC AGC AGA **GAA UUA AAU GCC CGC CAU GAC CAG**-3′) and amino-modified substrate-anchored probe oligonucleotide (5′-amine-CTG GTC ATG GCG GGC ATT TAA TTC-3′) can be used. The capture sequence is used to modify anti-EGFR aptamer and the mutant aptamer by extending the DNA template at its 3′ end with a 24-nucleotide sequence. The extended capture sequence does not disrupt the aptamer structure and immobilizes aptamers on the surface through duplex-formation with the surface-bound single-stranded DNA (ssDNA) probe molecules.

9.3.10 Immobilization of aptamers on SiO_2 substrate

A thermally oxidized silicon wafer is initially cleaned in oxygen plasma (15 minutes, Ar + O_2, 200 W) to create a hydrophilic SiO_2 surface. The substrates are immediately immersed in a solution of 2% APTES in ethanol for 1 hour at room temperature to silanize the surface. The surface is sequentially rinsed with 2-propanol and deionized (DI) water and then dried under nitrogen gas, followed by curing at 115°C for 30 minutes to ensure absence of contaminants. The surface is submerged in a solution of 1 mM phenyldiisothiocyanate (PDITC) in dimethyl sulfoxide containing 10% pyridine for 5–7 hours at 45°C in order to get PDITC cross-linker molecules attached onto the silanized surface. Subsequent washing sequentially with ethanol and DI water and drying in nitrogen flow for further surface preparation. After that, the substrate is incubated in a humidity chamber with a small volume of amine-modified ssDNA solution (5 μM concentration of DNA in DI water with 50% DMSO, 1% pyridine) overnight at 45°C to attach amino-modified DNA to PDITC cross-linker molecules. After ssDNA attachment, surfaces are rinsed sequentially with ethanol and DEPC-treated DI water and dried with nitrogen. The functionalized surface is then deactivated by capping unbound reactive groups of PDITC and submerging the surface in a blocking buffer solution that contained 50 mM 6-amino-1-hexanol with 150 mM DIPEA in DMF for 1 hour. The surface was then rinsed with DMF, ethanol, DEPC-treated DI water and dried under nitrogen stream. After that, anti-EGFR RNA aptamer hybridization is carried out by incubating the surface in a buffer solution (100 nM concentration of anti-EGFR aptamer with 5:1 DI water and hybridization buffer solution) at 42°C for 1 hour. The surface is washed thoroughly with DEPC-treated DI water and dried with nitrogen gas. The anti-EGFR RNA aptamer can also have an extension that can be hybridized with the surface-bound complementary ssDNA. As controls, the mutant aptamer is hybridized to surface-bound ssDNA on separate surfaces using identical protocol. The presence of ssDNA and RNA aptamers immobilized on the SiO_2 surface is determined by fluorescence measurements of acridine orange stain at an excitation wavelength of 460 nm and the emission wavelength of 650 nm using a confocal microscope.

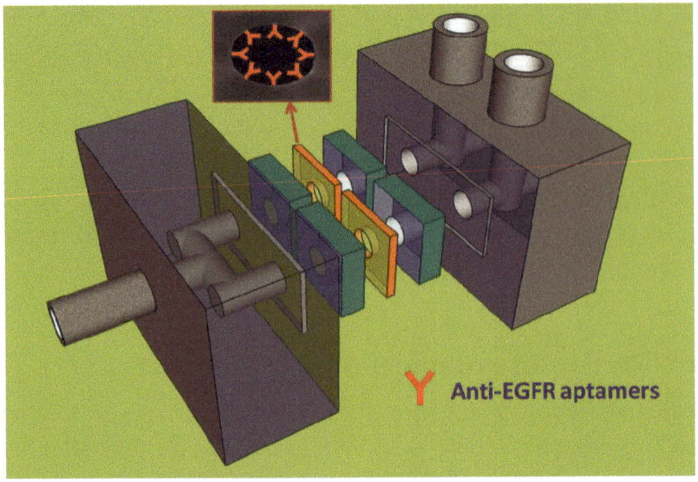

Figure 9.15 Schematic representation for system modification where the micropore is chemically activated with anti-EGFR aptamers for enhanced discrimination of cancer cells.

9.3.11 Protein binding and electrical detection

Surfaces with the attached RNA aptamer are then incubated in 50 ng/μL of EGFR protein prepared in phosphate-buffered saline (PBS) with 5 mM Mg^{2+} solution at 37°C for 45 minutes. The surface is washed thoroughly with PBS and DEPC-treated DI water and dried under nitrogen flow. The surface is analyzed for the captured EGFR protein by optical detection of fluorescent SYPRO ruby protein blot stain at 488 nm wavelength. The fluorescence intensity analysis is conducted using ImageJ software for bound ssDNA to immobilize an anti-EGFR aptamer and subsequently the aptamer is used to capture the EGFR protein. A sample device with solid-state micropores and anti-EGFR aptamers attached on the micropore surfaces is shown in Fig. 9.15.

9.4 SURFACE CHARACTERIZATION OF BIOMINERAL AND BIOMATERIAL SURFACES

The characterization of mineral on bone and biomaterial surfaces can be carried out through the use of traditional biological methods—μCT scanning and histology—as well as techniques that are more commonly associated with materials research—Raman and XANES spectroscopy, along with SEM and nanoindentation measurements. The combination of techniques is designed to focus exclusively on the hard tissue of the bone, and, in particular, on both the atomic and ultrastructural levels of the bone hierarchy since the bone morphology at this scale could help predict the formation of chemical bonding structures in a bone–implant interface.

9.4.1 Microcomputed tomography measurements

X-ray scanning has been used in the diagnosis of bone pathologies almost since the discovery of the X-ray itself. It was only 3 months between Röntgen's initial discovery and the first publication of a bone X-ray in 1896 [69]. Computed tomography (CT) scanning, or the use of multiple X-ray scans to build a 3D X-ray image has become a widespread clinical technique; academically, however, a standard method of collecting and reporting microcomputed tomography results for rodent specimens has only been published recently [70]. Standardized methods for image acquisition and image processing have been used to determine cortical thickness (decreased cortical thickness can be used to help identify disorder phenotypes), cortical bone porosity and apparent/mineral density (as evidence of potential differences in bone chemistry), and moment of inertia (a measure of bone strength).

9.4.2 Raman spectroscopy analysis

Raman spectroscopy offers the ability to study bonding information, and, unlike the more common FTIR spectroscopy technique, it can be used to study materials where water is present, since water is Raman-inactive. Several Raman measures of bone quality have been developed. Most bands observed in a Raman spectrum of bone can be assigned to mineral-phase carbonate and phosphate or matrix collagen, and these bands can be used to assess relative measures of bone mineral quality. Three of the most common measures of bone quality that can be determined from a Raman spectrum include carbonate-to-phosphate ratio, mineral-to-matrix ratio, and mineral crystallinity. To determine carbon-to-phosphate ratio, the area of the 1070 cm^{-1} carbonate band is compared to the primary phosphate band at 959 cm^{-1} [71]. Likewise, the mineral-to-matrix ratio is generally determined by comparing the area of the amide I band near 1700 cm^{-1} to the 959 cm^{-1} phosphate band [72], though depending on embedding conditions and orientational sensitivity of the collagen, other matrix bands may be used for this comparison, such as the 921 and 855 cm^{-1} proline or 876 cm^{-1} hydroxyproline bands [73]. Determining a FWHM from a Gaussian fit to the primary 959 cm^{-1} phosphate peak can also provide a measure of mineral crystallinity. Though, in general, absolute measurements of bone mineral properties are difficult to obtain with Raman spectra [71], calibration with carbonated apatitic standards can be used to determine the carbonate content of bone via comparison of carbonate-to-phosphate ratio to wt% carbonate [74]. An example Raman bone spectrum with relevant peaks can be seen in Fig. 9.16.

9.4.3 Electron microscopy

SEM allows for creating high-resolution images with a relatively large depth of focus, and, by combining different detection methods (secondary electrons, backscattered

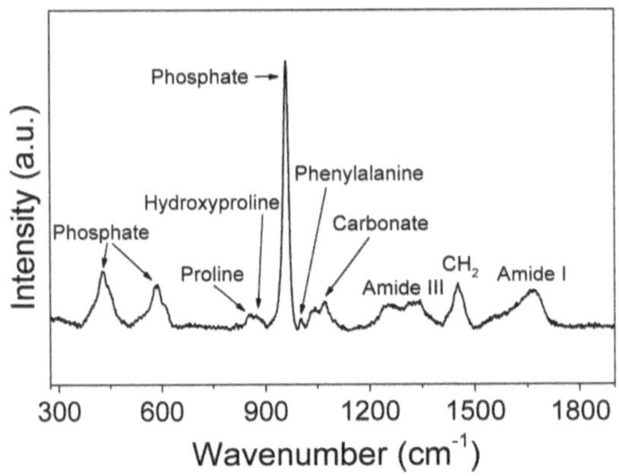

Figure 9.16 Typical Raman spectrum of a bone with major peaks identified.

electrons, and X-rays), can provide surface topography as well as compositional information about a sample. For bone in particular, bone mineral density distribution (BMDD), measured via SEM quantitative backscattered electron imaging (qBSEI), is thought to give a measure of bone health by providing an indirect method of measuring the local (on the order of 10 nm) calcium-to-phosphorous ratios in bone mineral [75]. Bone qBSE images can be processed, compared to standards with known Ca:P ratios, and evaluated by grayscale leveling software such as ImageJ, the NIH's publicly available image software. The Ca:P determination is possible due to the fact that elements with higher atomic number, *Z*, produce proportionately greater numbers of backscattered electrons. In bone, the primary constituent elements of the collagen matrix (H, C, N, O, P, S) and mineral phase (Ca, P, O, H, C, Mg) are, with the exception of Ca, found in the first three periods of the periodic table (i.e., they have small atomic numbers). Ca, found in relatively high concentrations, has an atomic number of $Z = 20$, and areas of high Ca concentration can be readily visualized by brighter sections on BSE images. Coupled with a material of known Ca:P ratio—a hydroxyapatite standard powder—as well as materials with average *Z* numbers both above and below that of the sample (pure aluminum, $Z = 13$, and carbon in the form of graphite, $Z = 6$, respectively) gray levels of qBSE images of cortical bone sections can be imaged.

9.4.4 X-ray diffraction

X-ray diffraction builds on the method for electron dispersive spectroscopy in which chemical characterization can be determined. However, in XRD, the crystal planes that make up the material surface are examined. The distance between interatomic planes is determined using Bragg's law. The distance between planes has three dimensions such that $d = (h^2 + k^2 + l^2)^{1/2}$, where *h*, *k*, and *l* are the Cartesian coordinates represented by Miller indices that are characteristic for a material with crystals that grow in characteristic directions. The specific X-ray method (Bragg–Brentano method) can be used to allow for the comparison of the relative intensities of the various hkl plane reflections. This comparison is very useful when qualitatively (or semi-quantitatively) determining the preferred orientation of a particular crystal plane or lattice, crystallite size, and mole fraction of a two-phase material (if applicable). In this method, the incident and diffracted beam angles, θ, were the same and the angle, 2θ, between the diffracted and transmitted beam was analyzed. Typical spectra are very similar in profile to most X-ray spectra generated from EDS analysis. However, the peaks in XRD represent the hkl plane reflections that are present in a material and these peaks can broaden depending on the number of crystallographic grains.

When analyzing a sample diffraction pattern, using the full-width at half maximum (*FWHM*) is advantageous in characterizing any peak broadening associated with the sample. The peak broadening in a sample pattern is comprised of the full-width instrumental broadening ($FW(U)$) and the full-width sample broadening ($FW(S)$). Thus,

$$FWHM = FW(I) + FW(S). \tag{9.1}$$

The instrumental broadening was obtained by using the NIST 340A LaB_6 powder standard for powder X-ray diffraction. From the sample pattern obtained, a resultant *FWHM* is observed; however, this broadening is typically miniscule. The sample broadening in this LaB_6 powder is usually simply owed to the instrumental broadening, thus the resulting *FWHM* becomes $FW(I)$. This sample is then profile fitted with a known LaB_6 PDF card to obtain the FWHM curve. This FWHM curve is used as a basis to subtract the instrumental broadening from future sample patterns. Thus, $FW(I)$ is defined as,

$$FW(I) = FWHM_{LaB_6} = A + B\cdot(2\theta) + C\cdot(2\theta)^2. \tag{9.2}$$

In Eq. (9.2), A, B, and C are least squares regression coefficients and 2θ is the diffraction angle for the Bragg–Brentano diffractometer. The sample broadening is defined by the Debye–Scherrer relation,

$$FW(S) = \frac{1}{\cos(\theta)}\left(\frac{K\lambda}{d} + 4\tau\sin(\theta)\right), \tag{9.3}$$

where K is the shape factor for the average crystallite, λ is the wavelength for the $CuK_{\alpha1}$ X-ray in nm, d is the average crystallite size in nm, and τ is the microstrain. The Debye–Scherrer equation is solved for the family of X-ray lines for a sample.

In general, the sample broadening is determined using the following relation,

$$FW(S)^D = FWHM^D - FW(I)^D, \tag{9.4}$$

where D is a deconvolution factor (set to 0 to 2.0). If small crystallites are assumed to be present, then the strain is neglected ($K\lambda/d >> 4\tau \sin(\theta)$). This means that Eq. (9.3) is simplified to the Scherrer relation and the average crystallite size is estimated by

$$d = \frac{K\lambda}{FW(S)\cos(\theta)}. \tag{9.5}$$

Once a sample pattern is profile fitted, it is analyzed for the relative abundance of a two-phase material (if necessary). This calculation was performed using the relative intensity ratio method. For a two-phase mixture that is profile fitted with known PDF cards (and hence, has a known reference intensity ratio, $RIR_{\alpha,standard}$, the weight fraction of phase αx_α is given by

$$x_\alpha = \frac{I_{i,\alpha} \cdot I^{rel}_{k,standard} \cdot x_{standard}}{I_{k,standard} \cdot I^{rel}_{i,\alpha} \cdot RIR_{\alpha,standard}}. \tag{9.6}$$

Since the sum of all the weight fractions must equal unity, then finding the weight fractions of each phase is relatively simple. For a polycrystalline phase with multiple resolvable and nonoverlapping peaks, an optimized weighted average is used for each phase to give more precision for this calculation. Note that the estimated values for the crystallite size, microstrain, and phase weight fraction are considered semiquantitative at best, since the values given from the PDF cards are not considered very accurate. If performed consistently, however, these calculations provided a wealth of information with regard to how various CVD process conditions influenced the coating crystallinity.

9.4.5 Surface compositional analysis

Electron probe microanalysis (EPMA), sometimes known as wavelength dispersive spectroscopy (WDS), was used in measuring the elemental composition in CVD coatings (>3 μm thick). EPMA uses an incident electron beam to excite a sample and produce X-rays of characteristic energy and wavelength. The EPMA spectrometer analyzes specimens at a range of incident angles such that Bragg's law is satisfied,

$$n\lambda = 2d\sin(\theta) \tag{9.7}$$

Although electron-dispersive spectroscopy is an easier tool to employ and is available with the SEM in situ, there are several advantages offered by EPMA. First, the EPMA has a resolution of approximately 10 eV as opposed to the EDS resolution of 150 eV. The EPMA resolution makes it easier to resolve elements with families of close X-ray lines since these lines can differ by as much as 80–120 eV. This means that the resolution of the EDS can be considered insufficient for resolving some elements' characteristic X-ray lines. In addition, the peak-to-background ratio for the EPMA detector is about 10 times greater than the EDS detector, making it easier to discern characteristic peaks from the continuum background.

Due to the large amount of X-ray lines that can be analyzed from a specimen, corrections are usually made to account for the interelement (matrix) effects. These matrix effects originate from the phenomenological effects of elastic and inelastic scattering and the propagation of X-rays through the sample to the detector. These matrix effects are classified into effects owed to atomic number (Z), absorption (A), and fluorescence (F). The product of these correction factors is known as the ZAF correction. The ZAF correction is the most accurate method to account for these matrix effects. The ZAF correction is performed sequentially for the family of X-ray lines generated from each element, i, in a specimen. This correction is used to adjust the weight fraction determination of each element, i, in the specimen by the following relation,

$$\frac{C_i}{C_{(i)}} = [ZAF]_i \cdot \frac{I_i}{I_{(i)}}, \tag{9.8}$$

where C_i is the weight fraction of element i in the specimen, $C_{(i)}$ is the weight fraction of element i in the standard, $[ZAF]_i$ is the correction factor for element, i, I_i is the X-ray intensity of element i in the specimen, and $I_{(i)}$ is the X-ray intensity of element i in the standard. The discussion with regard to the ZAF is truncated here as most software packages employ correction factors that are each unique.

9.4.6 Optical property characterization

Nano- and microfabrication methods allow for superior process control and reliability; this is particularly important given the variability of biological systems and the repeatability of biological experiments. Most microfabrication methods—and particularly the metrological measurements available in a microfabrication clean room—are designed to evaluate components based on electronic and optical properties. Process repeatability and reliability can be measured using the optical properties of the coatings in measures well accepted in the semiconductor industry. For a potential biomaterial, measures of film chemistry and microstructure can give insight into their potential performance in physiological environments. Thus, optical property measurements can help connect biomaterial physiological performance to the underlying chemical and ultrastructural composition.

Optical metrology tools are commonly found in clean-room environments and provide a method to evaluate thin films. They allow rapid evaluation of wafer processing methods, particularly with respect to within wafer uniformity and wafer-to-wafer uniformity. Optical investigation of the surfaces (i.e., process reliability and repeatability measurements) are performed by a thin-film reflectometer (250–850 nm, single-point reflection stage) and an ellipsometer (632.8 nm He-Ne source). Ellipsometry is performed to estimate the refractive index and thickness uniformity of the samples. Refractive indices determined via ellipsometry can then be used to verify thickness measurements using a nine-point testing matrix for each surface with the reflectometer.

9.4.7 Fourier transform infrared (FTIR) spectroscopy analysis

While Raman spectroscopy is a particularly useful technique for the study of bone and bone quality, as previously mentioned, compositional information about any surface or diffused hydrogen bonding in various chemical systems can be obtained through the use of Fourier transform infrared (FTIR) spectroscopy. The reliability of this method for surface characterization has been exemplified for silica-based materials. For example, the use of this technique for silicon oxynitride and phosphorous-doped silicon dioxide systems has been well established, and the primary peaks of interest have been identified [76–79]. Table 9.3 gives a summary of the relevant peak positions. Note that the exact peak position can be affected by film stress so a range of wavenumbers is given for each vibrational mode.

In addition to providing a qualitative analysis of sample chemistry, a method for the quantitative calculation of N–H bond concentration has been proposed by Lanford and Rand [79] and is given by the expression

$$[N-H] = \frac{1}{2.303 \times \sigma_{N-H}} \times \int \alpha(\omega) d\omega \tag{9.9}$$

where σ_{N-H} is the absorption cross section for the N–H bonds, the integral is the normalized area of the absorption band, and α is related to the absorption coefficient A and film thickness t by the expression $\alpha = 2.303\ A/t$. This expression can also be used to quantify other bond concentrations, if the absorption cross section for the bond is known. Table 9.4 gives values and references of absorption cross sections of some of the bond pairs considered.

Table 9.3 Vibration modes active in FTIR for Si-O-N-P systems with hydrogen

Vibrational mode	Peak position (cm^{-1})	References
Si–O bending	800–850	[40,42]
Si–O stretching	1000–1100	[40,41]
P=O stretching	1300–1350	[42,43]
Si–H stretching	2150–2300	[40,41]
N–H stretching	3300–3400	[40,41]

Table 9.4 Values for absorption cross sections in Si-O-N-P-H systems

Bond	Absorption cross section (cm^2)	References
σ_{N-H}	5.3×10^{-18}	[46]
σ_{Si-H}	7.4×10^{-18}	[47]
σ_{Si-N}	2.1×10^{-18}	[48]

9.4.7.1 Biological surface characterization

9.4.7.1.1 In vitro bioactivity testing of $SiON_x$ and $SiONP_x$ coatings

For any surface, in vitro testing can be further studied to evaluate its potential for bioactivity. While the term "bioactivity" can be applied quite broadly, in the context of biomineralization, it is taken to mean the formation of a carbonate-substituted hydroxyapatite layer on the material which is known to allow for cell adhesion and collagen formation on the surface—which results in the formation of a strong bond between the native bone tissue and the implant surface [2]. Such carbonated apatite formation is known to occur in both bioactive calcium phosphate ceramic systems as well as bioactive glass systems [80,81]. In order to evaluate biomaterial surface potential for osseointegration, some preliminary evaluation of coating response to the physiological environment must be performed. The formation of the aforementioned carbonated hydroxyapatite layer is one such metric that can be used to investigate bioactivity, but the dissolution rate and surface energy are also important in determining suitability in the biological environment [82].

After preliminary studies of the chemical reactions and dissolution kinetics involved, in vitro studies of the surface with a model cell line can be considered. The selection of a cell line for study often represents a series of trade-offs: primary cells from a human patient are often favored in terms of establishing clinical relevance, while commercially available animal cell lines such as the MC3T3-E1subclone 4 line allow for increased repeatability of an experimental setup. With the wealth of research available for the commercial cell lines, there is also the potential for increased understanding of the cellular response to a given material and a more direct comparison between different material systems such as bioactive calcium phosphates and more traditional bioactive glasses. Many gene expression studies, in particular, have been performed with these cell line/material systems combinations [83–86].

9.4.8 SBF dissolution test

In most systems, a strong bond at the interface between a bioactive material and native bone tissue is achieved via the formation of a calcium phosphate layer [87]. Some studies have suggested that this layer can be described as an amorphous calcium phosphate layer, but most agree that this calcium phosphate layer that helps cement a bioactive material in place is a carbonated hydroxyapatite layer [87]. Therefore, in any new candidate bioactive material, evidence of the formation of a calcium phosphate layer is an essential component in the consideration of a new candidate bioactive material. In vivo conditions that allow for the formation of this calcium phosphate layer can be modeled through the use of a salt solution that closely mimics the pH and salt concentrations of blood plasma, which is often referred to as an SBF [88]. Cell culture media are another option for modeling the behavior of a bioactive surface exposed to plasma, however, with the added benefit of the ability to more directly relate material behavior in the acellular environment to the material behavior in cell culture.

Cell culture media can be prepared through the combination of a commercially available minimum essential media (MEM), a blood serum, and an antibiotic/antimycotic. The MEM provides the necessary inorganic salts, amino acids, vitamins, and sugars for cell viability. It also generally contains a buffer to maintain pH and an indicator, such as phenol red, to aid in the monitoring of pH. Several types of MEM are commercially available, including Eagle's MEM, Dulbecco's modified Eagle's Medium (DMEM), and alpha-modified minimum essential media (αMEM). Each was developed with a particular cell line in mind, however, αMEM, which contains no phosphorus-containing nucleotides and can be well adapted for the culture of MC3T3-E1 cells, could be considered ideal for this study [89]. The serum supplies proteins, vitamins, hormones, trace elements, and growth/adhesion factors to aid in cell viability and proliferation. The antibiotic/antimycotic inhibits bacterial growth in the culture media. Gentamicin, amphotericin B, penicillin, and streptomycin are commonly used for this purpose. In fact, a mixture of penicillin and streptomycin is commercially available and is often referred to as pen-strep. A typical culture media would be 90% αMEM, 10% FBS, and 1% pen-strep (by volume). Of these components, αMEM is the most important source of passive ion exchange with the bioactive material surface [90]. Therefore a first approximation of biomaterial response to both the blood plasma and cell culture media environment can be achieved via a study based on biomaterial response to αMEM. Table 9.5 lists the inorganic components of αMEM and their relative concentrations, while Table 9.6 compares the concentrations of inorganic salts found in human blood plasma and αMEM.

9.4.9 Inductively coupled plasma-optical emission spectra (ICP-OES) analyses

ICP-OES analysis is capable of detecting concentrations and changes in the concentrations of analyte elements on the order of parts per billion and is well known for its ability to quantify individual analyte elements in complex matrices with minimal interferences. Thus, it is a technique useful for both rapid dissolution and longer dissolution kinetic studies in a relatively complex environment meant to simulate a biological system of even greater complexity.

Table 9.5 Components of α-modified minimum essential media

Components	Molecular formula	Molecular weight	Concentration (mg/L)	mM
Inorganic salts				
Calcium chloride (anhyd)	$CaCl_2$	111	200	1.8
Magnesium sulfate (anhyd)	$MgSO_4$	120	97.67	0.814
Potassium chloride	KCl	75	400	5.33
Sodium bicarbonate	$NaHCO_3$	84	2200	26.19
Sodium chloride	NaCl	58	6800	117.25
Sodium phosphate monobasic	NaH_2PO_4	138	140	1.01
Other components				
D-glucose (dextrose)	$C_6H_{12}IO_6$	180	1000	5.56
Lipoic acid	$CgH_{14}O_2S_2$	206	0.2	0.001
Phenol red	$C_{19}H_{14}O_5S$	376.4	10	0.0266
Sodium pyruvate	$C_3H_3NaO_3$	110	110	1.00

Table 9.6 Comparison of the concentration of inorganic salt species in human blood plasma and α-modified minimum essential media [91]

Ion	Plasma (mM)	αMEM (mM)
Na^+	142	144
K^+	5.0	5.3
Mg^{2+}	1.5	0.8
Ca^{2+}	2.5	1.8
Cl^-	103.0	122.5
HCO_3^-	27.0	26.2
HPO_4^{2-}	1.0	1.0
SO_4^{2-}	0.5	0.8

9.4.10 Thermodynamics of surfaces: surface energy and surface tension

9.4.10.1 Goniometric analysis

Hydrophilicity, or wettability, of a biomaterial surface is known to have a strong effect on cell response and biocompatibility [92]. In bone/implant systems, increased hydrophilicity has been shown to increase both the rate and the extent of new bone formation around the implant, which is thought to be due to faster cell adhesion and spreading through the adsorbed protein layer [93]. The relative hydrophilicity of a biomaterial surface can be investigated via a sessile drop technique with a goniometer. This technique involves the use of apolar and dispersive solvent used to measure the relative change in the surface contact angle.

Distilled water (polar solvent) is dropped onto the surface and an image taken of the surface/droplet system after a 24-second delay. The images are then processed using image processing (e.g., ImageJ program) to measure the contact angle. The surface energy of the surface can be investigated using distilled, DI water and diiodomethane (dispersive solvent).

To analyze three-phase equilibrium and surface energy, the interfacial tensions of the solid—vapor, liquid—vapor, and solid—liquid interface, and the contact angle can be related through Young's equation (Eq. 9.10). Measurement of the two solid interfacial terms is difficult in practice and further treatment of the surface tension is considered in Good's equation which breaks the surface energy down into a dispersive and a polar component (Eq. 9.11).

$$\gamma_{LV} \cos\theta = \gamma_{SV} - \gamma_{SL} \tag{9.10}$$

$$\gamma = \gamma^d + \gamma^p \tag{9.11}$$

For relatively low energy surfaces, the Owens—Wendt—Kaeble equation, which treats the total surface energy as the geometric mean of the dispersive and polar terms (Eq. 9.12), is considered to be a relevant treatment of the system [91], and can be combined with Young's equation to determine the polar and dispersive components of a solid's surface energy, as long as the dispersive and polar components of the surface tension of at least two probing liquids are known (Eq. 9.13).

$$\gamma_{SL} = \gamma_S - \gamma_L - 2(\gamma_L^d \gamma_S^d)^{1/2} - 2(\gamma_L^p \gamma_S^p)^{1/2} \tag{9.12}$$

$$\gamma_{LV}(1 + \cos\theta) = 2(\gamma_L^d \gamma_S^d)^{1/2} + 2(\gamma_L^p \gamma_S^p)^{1/2} \tag{9.13}$$

9.4.11 Cell proliferation analysis

Outside of a substrate's or scaffold's ability to form a carbonated apatite layer, the cellular response to the surface must also be considered. Culture of the MC3T3-E1 subclone 4 osteoblast precursor cell line offers the ability to study cellular response to the surface. While the use of the MC3T3-E1 line has been well established, primary cells from a human source such as human periosteum cells offer the chance to better establish a path to clinical relevance [84,85].

As such, cellular response to surface properties can be investigated via the culture of both MC3T3-E1 and human periosteum cells. These cells are cultured in 150 cm^2 flasks with α-MEM (Life Technologies Corp.) containing 10% fetal bovine serum (VWR) and an antibiotic/antimyotic (1% streptomycin/penicillin) in a humidified atmosphere of 95% air and 5% CO_2 at 37°C. After they reached confluence, 50,000—100,000 cm^{-2} cells are seeded on the surface. Control surfaces must control for each property being investigated and they must be conducted in replicate number with replicate independent experiments for the most statistically powered results. Twenty-four hours after seeding, cells are serum starved (1% FBS) to allow them to synchronize. Ascorbic acid-2-phosphate (50 ppm) is then added to induce differentiation. For proliferation, cells can be cultured for up to 5−7 days; however, early, mid, and later timepoints must be used such that sufficient early time points give results significantly above background and to overcome limitations in the assay reagent effectiveness.

9.4.12 Cell differentiation analysis

Osteoblastic precursors can be forced into an osteogenic pathway through the use of a differentiation media which generally contains a phosphorus-containing material such as ascorbic acid-2-phosphate or beta-glycerophosphate [94]. Ideally, however, such forced differentiation should be unnecessary for a candidate osteoinductive and ultimately osteogenic material. To study cell differentiation, protein expression of MC3T3 cells can be assayed after 7, 14, 21, and 28 days of culture. Medium can be collected and assayed for extracellular osteocalcin enzyme activity.

Osteogenic markers can also be determined at the gene level to determine a surface's osteogenic potential. For gene expression assays, cells are lysed, their mRNA is collected, and reverse transcription polymerase chain reaction (RT-PCR) is used to evaluate the expression of osteogenic marker genes as compared to an internal reference housekeeping gene at each of the time points. The gene expression of glyseraldehyde-3-phosphate dehydrogenase (GAPDH), superoxide dismutase (SOD1), osteocalcin (OCN), core-bending factor (Cbfa1/Runx2), Osterix (Sp7), and collagen type 1 (Col(I)-α1) are detected by a real-time PCR machine. Typical RT-PCR amplification conditions are as follows: one cycle of 10 minutes at 95°C for activation of the polymerase, 50 cycles of 15 seconds at 95°C, and 1 minute at 60°C for amplification. The amount for each gene is calculated using a delta-delta C_T method and target gene expression is normalized relative to the expression of the GAPDH reference gene.

9.4.13 X-ray absorption near-edge structure analyses

X-ray absorption near-edge structure (XANES) spectroscopy is a powerful, relatively nondestructive technique that enables the study of the nature of the chemical bonding in a material as well as an element-by-element analysis of the local atomic environment (i.e., valence, coordination, and distortions in geometry due to nearest-neighbor atoms). This highly selective technique is possible through the use of synchrotron radiation as a beam source. A synchrotron facility generates an intense electromagnetic beam by accelerating charged particles at speeds close to that of light through magnetic fields in an electron or positron storage ring. There are several key advantages to generating a source beam in this manner. First, the beam collimation inherent in this set up allows for high resolution in the X-ray region. Secondly, the high resolution in conjunction with the high intensity of the beam enables the investigation of trace materials in the bulk. Finally, unlike X-ray diffraction, XANES can be used to probe amorphous materials.

A typical XANES spectra consists of three primary zones: a preedge, an absorption edge, and a postedge. The "edge" refers to the fact that each spectrum is taken around an element-specific core-electron excitation energy. Features in a XANES spectrum relate to the excitation of a core shell electron (K-edge or $L_{2,3}$-edge) from its bound state into the conduction band of the material. The preedge can be used to investigate the local geometry around an absorbing atom and can be shifted due to oxidation state or bonding characteristics. The main edge position is mainly used in the determination of oxidation state and can be shifted up to as much as 5 eV per one unit change. The postedge part of the spectrum gives information about interatomic distances and bond angles, though interpretation of this region remains difficult due to multiple scattering domains [95]. Fig. 9.17 shows features typical in a XANES spectra.

In the example spectra, the absorption is measured via the current or total electron yield (TEY). There are other types of detection methods, most of which rely on the fluorescence signal (FLY) of the material during absorption. These detectors are beamline-dependent. A beamline can be thought of as an endstation equipped to detect certain energy ranges of signals.

For amorphous silica-based materials, the edges of interest are the Si-K, Si-L, O-K, N-K, P-K, and P-L edges. For in vitro studies, the Ca-L edge may also be of interest. Though it is possible to collect the spectra for all these edges at one synchrotron facility, multiple beamlines must be used due to the large difference in energy

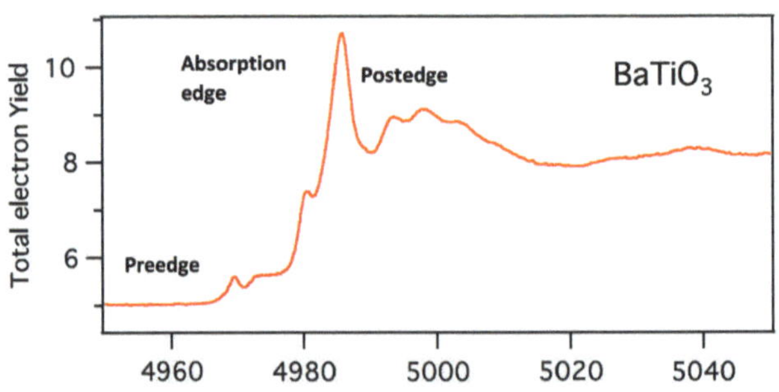

Figure 9.17 Typical XANES absorption spectra showing preedge, edge, and postedge features.

Table 9.7 Canadian light source beamline parameters

Beamline	SXRMB	SGM	VLS PGM
Energy range	1700–10,000 eV	250–2000 eV	5.5–250 eV
Edge(s)	P-K	N-K, O-K, Si-K, Ca-L	P-L, Si-L
Spot size	300 × 300 μm	1000 × 100 μm	500 × 500 μm
Source	Bending magnet	45-mm planar undulator	185-mm planar undulator
Resolution	0.5 eV	0.2 eV	0.1 eV

between the edges. All edges can be collected using synchrotron X-ray radiation at facilities such as the Canadian light source synchrotron using various beamlines: such as the soft X-ray microcharacterization beamline (SXRMB, 06B1-1), the high-resolution spherical grating monochromator (SGM, 11ID-1), and the variable line spacing plane grating monochromator (VLS PGM, 11ID-2). Table 9.7 summarizes relevant beamline parameters including available detectors, energy range, edge that can be collected, resolution, and beam spot size.

9.4.14 Histological staining for collagen elongation

Collagen visualization can be accomplished using polarized light microscopy and staining methods. First, the sample (must be optically transparent) can be extracted from culture or prepared as a slide section from tissue and prepared for fixation. The fixation process involves removal of excess proteinaceous species using saline washing and then fixation using low percentage ($<5\%$) of formaldehyde or glutaraldehyde for 1 hour. Once fixed, a secondary fixative that can be used to bind the stain for collagen can be used, such as Bouin's fixative solution. This fixation procedure is undertaken for an additional hour. After fixation, a background stain can be used to contrast the foreground collagen stain to improve contrast and white balancing during imaging. This can be a stain such as Fast Green at low concentration ($<1\%$) for a short time such that the stain permeates the ECM without overstaining. Removal of excess stain can be accomplished via DI water flushing. This can then be followed for the collagen-specific Picrosirius stain with acetic acid to remove excess red stain color. Once staining for 30 minutes is complete, the sample can be sequentially alcohol-dehydrated and imaged using a light microscope with 10 or 20 × objectives and two polarizers. The polarizers improve imaging of collagen by having the light path out of phase with the incident light into the microscope. This takes advantage of the collagen fiber's birefringent nature. The image can then be processes using ImageJ or another type of imaging software as observed in Fig. 9.18.

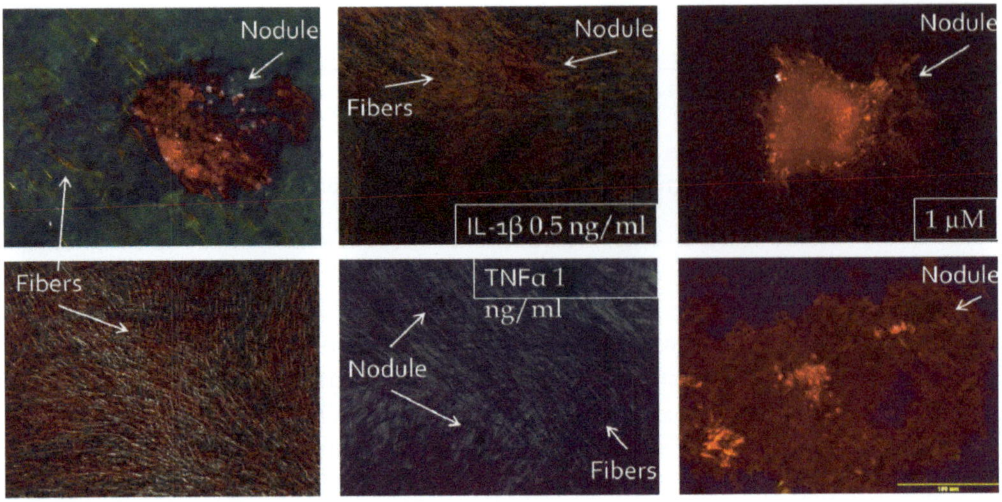

Figure 9.18 Picrosirius imaging of collagen in ECM synthesized by dental pulp stem cells. Collagen stained red in the foreground while ECM is unstained in the background. Background stain with Fast Green turns the ECM analine blue or hunder green-blue [96].

9.5 CURRENT CHALLENGES AND FUTURE TRENDS

The bone diseases described above and in other chapters remain silent at their earlier stages and are usually diagnosed at advanced stages where treatment strategies are difficult to implement. Early detection of diseases like cancer and bone disorders has an immediate and far-reaching impact on better prognosis of patients. Diseases are initially expressed at molecular and cellular levels and identification of these diseases at such small scales would be a great step toward early detection. The study of biological molecules and diseased cells requires efficient fabrication techniques to develop sensing devices with molecular size entrapment. Bionanotechnology and bioMEMs promise to fabricate devices not only down to the cellular scale but also down to the size of the biological molecules, such as proteins, bacteria, and viruses. The overall goal of this research is to develop robust and highly sensitive electronic biosensors for identification of bone diseases and disorders at the molecular and cellular levels. In this section, we describe two types of biosensors, break-junction biochemical biosensors and transduction biomechanical biosensors, that could potentially improve future development of diagnostics for potential bone disease detection and diagnosis.

9.5.1 Nanogap break junctions for molecular detection of cancer

Break junctions have emerged as an important tool to investigate electrical transport properties of molecules. Selective probe molecules are immobilized between the contact structures with nanometer-sized separation. Different process flows are employed for break-junction manufacturing. All approaches either suffer from time-consuming e-beam writing of the whole device or low yield that results from stochastic nature of electromigration process. We have deployed a new class of break-junction fabrication using FIB scratch followed by electromigration. The approach results in elegant, rapid, and controlled high-yield nanomanufacturing of break-junctions at exact locations with very narrow distribution of the gaps (between electrodes).

A variety of metal—molecule—metal structures have been developed for measuring electrical conductivity through molecules [97]. Metal—molecule—metal structures can be broadly classified as vertical device structures (VDSs) and lateral device structures (LDSs). VDSs utilize a self-assembled monolayer of molecules grown on a metal surface and second contact is made through conductive probe atomic force microscopy [98], crosswire [99], or scanning tunneling microscopy [100]. Whereas LDSs involve a pair of metal contacts with nanometer-sized separation and the probes selective to protein molecules are immobilized between the contact structures. Such devices that contain a thin metal strip, in which a gap is created by some technique, are known as break-junctions. This gap can be formed through e-beam lithography [101], mechanically controlled break-junctions [102], electrodeposition [103], and electromigration-induced break-junctions [104,105]. Most of these techniques are either slow and costly, mainly because of e-beam writing, or face lower yield of functional devices. Herein, we present a detection model for cancer biomarkers (EGFR molecules) by making use of a new class of break-junctions where a FIB is used to scratch a thin metal strip, followed by conventional microscale probing and electromigration in order to produce break-junctions with high throughput, greater yield, low cost, and at an exact spot, as reported earlier [106].

The break junctions are then employed as biological transducers to detect an important disease biomarker (as illustrated in Fig. 9.19). Biomarkers can include cell-surface biomarkers such as integrins that regulate collagen formation or phosphatases that regulate enzymatic production of alkaline phosphatase that are involved in bone matrix turnover. The silicon dioxide (SiO_2) surface between the nanoelectrodes can be functionalized with RNA aptamers that can selectively bind to cell-surface protein biomarkers. The selectivity was demonstrated by the mutated nonselective aptamers. The gold electrodes with nanometer-sized separation give a two orders of magnitude increase in current when selective capture of cell surface proteins occurs [107]. The surface chemistry for immobilization of RNA aptamers is verified by optical detection.

Recently researchers have shown significant effort toward introducing aptamers against several vital biomarkers [108,109]. Aptamers are reported to be as selective and sensitive as antibodies and are exceedingly stable over changing temperature, humidity, and ionic concentration [110]. Antibodies were previously used to functionalize nano-devices that were used for biomarker detection. These antibody-based devices are not

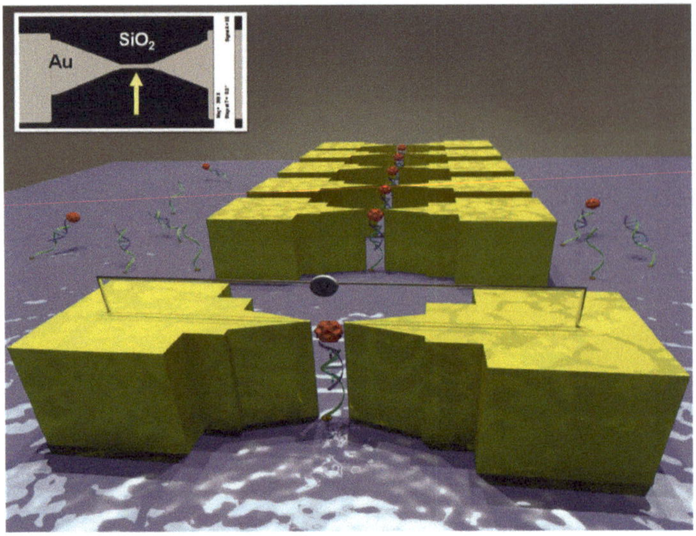

Figure 9.19 Schematic of the device that demonstrates the mechanism of the electronic detection (not to scale). Inset shows an SEM micrograph of the thin Au line on SiO_2 chip where an arrow points out the prospective location for nanogap to be induced [107].

capable of performing well for field-deployable or point-of-care modalities because antibodies require specific temperature, humidity, and low ionic strength of the buffer solution in order to retain their function [111]. Low ionic strength is necessitated to prevail over surface Debye screening but it causes poor interactions between target and surface probes [111].

9.5.2 Biomechanical discrimination of cancer cells using solid-state micropores

Osteosarcoma is a secondary cancer that is an indication of primary cancer metastasis from other organs such as the breast or prostate. This occurs as a result of cancer cells entering the bloodstream and arriving in the bone marrow. Cancer cells as compared to normal-functioning cells have different properties that can be detected in the bloodstream. Biomechanical properties (size, shape, stiffness, viscosity, deformability) of cells change significantly in unhealthy cells and can be used to indicate the physiological state of the cells. Cancer cells differ from normal cells in various aspects including size, shape, cellular functions and their biophysical properties. Although biopsy samples are the most valuable sources for cancer diagnosis, the analysis schemes are limited. High turnaround time, need for stains, lack of quantitative metrics, and failure to recognize diseased cells when these are very few in number are the major challenges in contemporary clinical pathology. We have developed a solid-state micropore sensor to discriminate cancer cells based on their biomechanical properties [112,113].

The detection scheme utilized a single solid-state micropore as the biological transducer which translated the cell's viscoelastic behavior into electrical signals. As a model, bladder cancer cells and normal urothelial cells were investigated. The approach did not require any staining, functionalization, or availability of any biomarkers, but merely relied on cellular mechanical properties. Temporal measurements of the ionic current were recorded across the micropore. Cancer cells gave distinctive pulse signals while passing through the micropore and showed one order of magnitude faster translocation time as compared to normal cells due to their softer nature [112]. The statistical analysis of each single cell present in the probed sample demonstrated its capability to identify cancerous cells when they were very few in number.

So far, only a few experimental systems have been deployed to study cellular mechanical properties. Micropipette aspiration is one of the prevailing techniques which applies negative pressure to the cell and records the aspiration distance as a function of time [114]. Optical deformability, scanning force microscopy, optical tweezers, microplate manipulation, and acoustic microscopy have also been reported for determining the cell rigidity [115–119]. All of these approaches revealed cancerous cells to be softer and less resistant to flow under applied forces. Oncogenically transformed fibroblast cells are known to have significantly different elasticity when compared to their complementary normal cells [114]. Human breast cancerous cell lines (MCF-7) also exhibit enhanced elasticity compared with their counterpart normal cell lines (MCF-10) due to the dissimilar viscoelastic nature of cells [115]. Metastatic cancer cells display even higher elasticity, which stems from their need to squeeze through the surrounding tissue matrix to make their way into the circulatory systems [114,120]. The micropore-based scheme can efficiently discriminate between metastatic and nonmetastatic cancer cells [121]. These discoveries advocate the use of cellular elasticity as a robust cell marker to diagnose the underlying disease. But all of the current techniques are limited by poor statistical differentiation, low throughput, high cost, special preparation, and nonphysiological handling or cell adhesion due to mechanical contact of the probe. Herein, we present a novel scheme of using a single solid-state micropore as a biological transducer that translates the cell mechanics to electrical signals (as illustrated in Fig. 9.20). A single micropore on a membrane sandwiched by a dual-compartment setup is used to record the electrical signature of the single cell translocated through the micropore. The specific pulse characteristics distinguish the cancerous cells from healthy cells and provide a statistical differentiation of each translocated cell in a cost-effective, high-throughput, and very reliable fashion.

Solid-state micropores have been used in a variety of sensor applications. These have been deployed for electroporation, patch clamp measurements, stability of lipid bilayers, monitoring bacterial activities, investigating cell deformability, size-based discrimination, cell counting, and measuring the electric properties of a single cell [122–127]. Chemical and thermal stability, mechanical strength, and capability to be

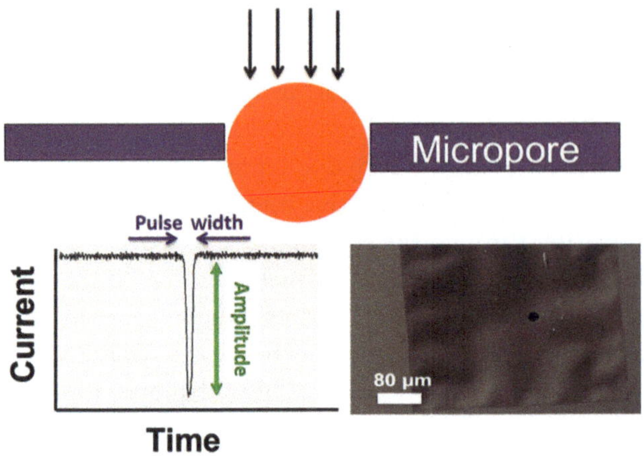

Figure 9.20 Schematic of the detection mechanism using solid-state micopore (shown in the SEM micrograph here) as a transducer component that translates a cell's biomechanical properties into an electrical profile using a resistive pulse signal [121].

integrated in a lab-on-a-chip locale enable micropores to be used for such diverse studies. Though micropores have been reported for investigating cell deformability or detecting large-size circulating tumor cells (CTCs) present in blood, these have never been deployed for diagnosing cancerous cells based merely on cell mechanics discrimination between similar-sized cells. Future research applications using such nanoporous devices with solid-state nanotechnology fabrication techniques will allow for rapid screening of various biomechanical sensors to help discern tumorigenic and normal cell types.

9.6 SUMMARY

Nanotechnology has rapidly emerged among other fields of science and engineering. The evolution and development of this field over the last few years has convinced researchers and scientists that it can sustainably overturn the existing technical models. Miniaturization of the probes, ultrasensitive interfaces, characterization, and prediction of the pathologic tendency of diseased cells are the essential enabling aspects of nanotechnology. Recent advancements in fabricating nanoscale devices and nanoobject-mediated modalities allowed nanoscale probing where detection and characterization of biological entities, their development and interactions, are carried out at the molecular level. The state of the art in microfabrication and nanotechnology has facilitated us with instruments, techniques, and skills to examine the presence or absence of a particular disease biomarker at the molecular and cellular level. Bionanotechnology broadly encircles cross-cutting research in engineering and biology. Much of current research focuses on the integration of biomedical engineering, nanoscience, and nanotechnology, with a particular focus toward their application in diverse areas such as nanomanufacturing of implant surfaces, characterization, molecular diagnostics, chip-based recognition of diseased cells, and site-specific controlled drug delivery systems. As we develop future advances in nanotechnology, some new avenues in their application in bone research could be implemented to diagnose disorders or diseases.

REFERENCES

[1] Doi Y, Vert M, Hellwich K-H, Hess M, Hodge P, Kubisa P, et al. Terminology for biorelated polymers and applications (IUPAC recommendations 2012). Pure Appl Chem 2012;84:377. Available: http://www.degruyter.com/view/j/pac.2012.84.issue-2/pac-rec-10-12-04/pac-rec-10-12-04.xml. http://dx.doi.org/10.1351/PAC-REC-10-12-04.

[2] Hench LL, Wilson J, editors. An introduction to bioceramics, Vol. 1. World Scientific; 1993.

[3] A. S. H. [35] B. D. Ratner, F. J. Schoen and J. E. Lemons. Biomaterials Science: an Introduction to Materials in Medicine 2004Available: http://books.google.com/books?id=9PMU1iYGe34C.

[4] Schaeverbeke T, Le Huec JC, Clement D, Faber J, Le Rebeller A. Influence of porosity on the mechanical resistance of hydroxyapatite ceramics under compressive stress. Biomaterials 1995;16 (2):113–18.

[5] Akao M, Aoki H, Kato K, Sato A. Dense polycrystalline β-tricalcium phosphate for prosthetic applications. J Mater Sci 1982;17(2):343–6.

[6] Ratner BD, Hoffman AS, Schoen FJ, Lemons JE. Biomaterials science: an introduction to materials in medicine. Amsterdam: Academic Press; 2004.

[7] Takeda J, Niinomi M, Akahori T. Effect of microstructure on fretting fatigue and sliding wear of highly workable titanium alloy, Ti–4.5 Al–3V–2Mo–2Fe. International journal of fatigue 2004;26(9):1003–15.

[8] Raggatt LJ, Partridge NC. Cellular and molecular mechanisms of bone remodeling. J Biol Chem 2010;285(33).

[9] Bureau MN, Legoux J-G, Denault J. Implantable biomimetic prosthetic bone. In Google Patents, editor; 2006.

[10] Cardarelli F. Composite metallic materials, uses thereof and process for making same. Google Patents, editor; 2007.

[11] Teoh SH. Fatigue of biomaterials: a review. Int J Fatigue 2000;22:825–37.

[12] Kim KH, Ramaswamy N. Electrochemical surface modification of titanium in dentistry. Dent Mater J 2009;28(1).

[13] Nasatzky E, Gultchin J, Schwartz Z. The role of surface roughness in promoting osteointegration. Refu'at ha-peh veha-shinayim (1993) 2003;20(3):8–19.

[14] Sul YT, Kang BS, Johansson C, Um HS, Park CJ, Albrektsson T. The roles of surface chemistry and topography in the strength and rate of osseointegration of titanium implants in bone. J Biomed Mater Res A 2009;89A(4):942–50. Available from: http://dx.doi.org/10.1002/jbm.a.32041.

[15] Alghamdi HS, van Oirschot BA, Bosco R, van den Beucken JJ, Aldosari AA, Anil S, et al. Biological response to titanium implants coated with nanocrystals calcium phosphate or type 1 collagen in a dog model. Clin Oral Implants Res 2013;24(5):475–83. Available from: http://dx.doi.org/10.1111/j.1600-0501.2011.02409.x.

[16] Kang BS, Sul YT, Johansson CB, Oh SJ, Lee HJ, Albrektsson T. The effect of calcium ion concentration on the bone response to oxidized titanium implants. Clin Oral Implants Res 2012;23 (6):690–7. Available from: http://dx.doi.org/10.1111/j.1600-0501.2011.02177.x.

[17] Iwai-Yoshida M, Shibata Y, Wurihan, Suzuki D, Fujisawa N, Tanimoto Y, et al. Antioxidant and osteogenic properties of anodically oxidized titanium. J Mech Behav Biomed Mater 2012;13:230–6.

[18] Hench LL, Wilson J. An introduction to bioceramics. Singapore: World Scientific; 1993. p. 223–38.

[19] Hench LL. Bioactive glasses and glass-ceramics. Materials Science Forum, Vol. 293. Trans Tech Publications; 1999.
[20] Bronzino JD. Biomedical Engineering Handbook, Vol. 2. CRC Press; 1999.
[21] Hench LL. The story of Bioglass®. J Mater Sci Mater Med 2006;17:967−78.
[22] Renno ACM, Bossini PS, Crovace MC, Rodrigues ACM, Zanotto ED, Parizotto NA. Characterization and in vivo biological performance of biosilicate. BioMed Res Int 2013;2013:141427.
[23] Shigeyama Y, D'Errico JA, Stone R, Somerman MJ. Commercially-prepared allograft material has biological activity in vitro. J Periodontol 1995;66:478−87.
[24] Kolerman R, Tal H, Moses O. Histomorphometric analysis of newly formed bone after maxillary sinus floor augmentation using ground cortical bone allograft and internal collagen membrane. J Periodontol 2008;79:2104−11.
[25] Wood RA, Mealey BL. Histologic comparison of healing after tooth extraction with ridge preservation using mineralized versus demineralized freeze-dried bone allograft. J Periodontol 2012;83 (3):329−36.
[26] Yukna RA. Synthetic bone grafts in periodontics. Periodontology 2000 1993;1:92−9.
[27] Berglundh T, Lindhe J. Healing around implants placed in bone defects treated with Bio-Oss. An experimental study in the dog. Clin Oral Implants Res 1997;8:117−24.
[28] Hurzeler MB, Quinones CR, Kirsch A, Gloker C, Schupbach P, Strub JR, et al. Maxillary sinus augmentation using different grafting materials and dental implants in monkeys. Part I. Evaluation of anorganic bovine-derived bone matrix. Clin Oral Implants Res 1997;8:476−86.
[29] Hallman M, Sennerby L, Lundgren S. A clinical and histologic evaluation of implant integration in the posterior maxilla after sinus floor augmentation with autogenous bone, bovine hydroxyapatite, or a 20:80 mixture. Int J Oral Maxillofac Implants 2002;17:635−43.
[30] Schlegel KA, Fichtner G, Schultze-Mosgau S, Wiltfang J. Histologic findings in sinus augmentation with autogenous bone chips versus a bovine bone substitute. Int J Oral Maxillofac Implants 2003;18:53−8.
[31] Karabuda C, Ozdemir O, Tosun T, Anil A, Olgac V. Histological and clinical evaluation of 3 different grafting materials for sinus lifting procedure based on 8 cases. J Periodontol 2001;72:1436−42.
[32] Artzi Z, Tal H, Dayan D. Porous bovine bone mineral in healing of human extraction sockets: 2. Histochemical observations at 9 months. J Periodontol 2001;72:152−9.
[33] Sartori S, Silvestri M, Forni F, Icaro Cornaglia A, Tesei P, Cattaneo V. Ten-year follow-up in a maxillary sinus augmentation using anorganic bovine bone (Bio-Oss). A case report with histomorphometric evaluation. Clin Oral Implants Res 2003;14:369−72.
[34] Mordenfeld A, Hallman M, Johansson CB, Albrektsson T. Histological and histomorphometrical analyses of biopsies harvested 11 years after maxillary sinus floor augmentation with deproteinized bovine and autogenous bone. Clin Oral Implants Res 2010;21:961−70.
[35] Bohner M. Calcium orthophosphates in medicine: from ceramics to calcium phosphate cements. Injury 2000;31(Suppl. 4):37−47.
[36] Midura RJ, Vasanji A, Su X, Wang A, Midura SB, Gorski JP. Calcospherulites isolated from the mineralization front of bone induce the mineralization of type I collagen. Bone 2007;41:1005−16.
[37] Kokubo T, Kim HM, Kawashita M. Novel bioactive materials with different mechanical properties. Biomaterials 2003;24:2161−75.
[38] Beekmans HC, Meijer GJ, Barkhuysen R, Blijdorp PA, Merkx MA, Jansen J. The hydroxylapatite-bone interface: 10 years after implant installation. Int J Oral Maxillofac Surg 2008;37:768−72.
[39] Cordioli G, Mazzocco C, Schepers E, Brugnolo E, Majzoub Z. Maxillary sinus floor augmentation using bioactive glass granules and autogenous bone with simultaneous implant placement. Clinical and histological findings. Clin Oral Implants Res 2001;12:270−8.
[40] Kobayashi H, Turner AS, Seim III HB, Kawamoto T, Bauer TW. Evaluation of a silica-containing bone graft substitute in a vertebral defect model. J Biomed Mater Res A 2010;92:596−603.
[41] Guarino V, Causa F, Taddei P, di Foggia M, Ciapetti G, Martini D, et al. Polylactic acid fibre-reinforced polycaprolactone scaffolds for bone tissue engineering. Biomaterials 2008;29:3662−70.
[42] Jiao Y, Liu Z, Zhou C. Fabrication and characterization of PLLA-chitosan hybrid scaffolds with improved cell compatibility. J Biomed Mater Res A 2007;80:820−5.

[43] Alam S, Ueki K, Marukawa K, Ohara T, Hase T, Takazakura D, et al. Expression of bone morphogenetic protein 2 and fibroblast growth factor 2 during bone regeneration using different implant materials as an onlay bone graft in rabbit mandibles. Oral Surg Oral Med Oral Pathol Oral Radiol Endod 2007;103:16−26.
[44] Santana RB, Santana CM. A clinical comparison of guided bone regeneration with platelet-derived growth factor-enhanced bone ceramic versus autogenous bone block grafting. Int J Oral Maxillofac Implants 2015;30:700−6.
[45] Beattie JH, Avenell A. Trace element nutrition and bone metabolism. Nutr Res Rev 1992;5:167−88.
[46] Gentleman E, Fredholm YC, Jell G, Lotfibakhshaiesh N, O'Donnell MD, Hill RG, et al. The effects of strontium-substituted bioactive glasses on osteoblasts and osteoclasts in vitro. Biomaterials 2010;31:3949−56.
[47] Varmette EA, Nowalk JR, Flick LM, Hall MM. Abrogation of the inflammatory response in LPS-stimulated RAW 264.7 murine macrophages by Zn- and Cu-doped bioactive sol-gel glasses. J Biomed Mater Res A 2009;90:317−25.
[48] Anselme K, Ponche A, Bigerelle M. Relative influence of surface topography and surface chemistry on cell response to bone implant materials. Part 2: biological aspects. Proceedings of the Institution of Mechanical Engineers, Part H. J Eng Med 2010;224(12):1487−507.
[49] Fujita S, Ohshima M, Iwata H. Time-lapse observation of cell alignment on nanogrooved patterns. J Royal Soc Interf 2009;S269−77.
[50] Gaind AK, Hearn EW. Physicochemical Properties of Chemical Vapor-Deposited Silicon Oxynitride from a SiH4-CO 2-NH 3-H 2 System. J Electrochem Soc 1978;125(1):139−45.
[51] Murphy CJ, Flemming RG, Abrams GA, Goodman SL, Nealey PF. Effects of synthetic micro- and nano-structured surfaces on cell behavior. Biomaterials 1999;20(6):573−88 doi:S0142-9612(98)00209-9 [pii].
[52] Bettinger CJ, Langer R, Borenstein JT. Engineering substrate topography at the micro-and nano-scale to control cell function. Angew. Chem. Int. Ed Engl 2009;48(30):5406−15.
[53] Clark P, Connolly P, Curtis AS, Dow JA, Wilkinson CD. Topographical control of cell behaviour: II. multiple grooved substrata. Development 1990;108(4):635−44.
[54] Hartney M, Hess D, Soane D. Oxygen plasma etching for resist stripping and multilayer lithography. J Vacuum Sci Technol B 1989;7(1):1−13.
[55] Sivaram S. Chemical vapor deposition: thermal and plasma deposition of electronic materials. Springer Science & Business Media; 2013.
[56] Kwok RWM, Gritsenko VA, Wong H, Xu JB. Short-range order in non-stoichiometric amorphous silicon oxynitride and silicon-rich nitride. J Non Cryst Solids 2002;297(1):96−101. Available from: <http://dx.doi.org/10.1016/S0022-3093(01)00910-3>.
[57] Liu Y, Jehanathan N, Walmsley B, Dell J, Saunders M. Effect of oxidation on the chemical bonding structure of PECVD SiNx thin films. J Appl Phys 2006;100(12). Available from: http://dx.doi.org/10.1063/1.2402581.
[58] Campmany J, et al. Optical, vibrational and compositional study of amorphous silicon oxynitride thin films grown by an RF plasma using N2O + SiH4 gas mixtures. Applied surface science 1993;70:695−700.
[59] Kok CW, Poon MC, Wong H, Chan PJ. Bonding structures of silicon oxynitride prepared by oxidation of si-rich silicon nitride. Thin Solid Films 2004;462−463(0):42−5. Available from: http://dx.doi.org/10.1016/j.tsf.2004.05.043.
[60] Wong H, Chan J, Poon MC, Kok CW. Oxynitride gate dielectric prepared by thermal oxidation of low-pressure chemical vapor deposition silicon-rich silicon nitride. Microelectr Reliabil 2003;43(4):611−16. Available from: http://dx.doi.org/10.1016/S0026-2714(03)00031-3.
[61] Klinkenberg E-D, Behrens K-M, Finster J, Meiwes-Broer K-H. Geometric structure of thin SiOxNy films on si(100). Surf Sci 1998;402−404:729−33. Available from: http://dx.doi.org/10.1016/S0039-6028(97)00998-9.
[62] Ay F, Aydinli A. Comparative investigation of hydrogen bonding in silicon based PECVD grown dielectrics for optical waveguides. Opt Mater 2004;26(1):33−46.

[63] Ilyas A, Lavrik NV, Kim HKW, Aswath PB, Varanasi VG. Enhanced Interfacial Adhesion and Osteogenesis for Rapid "Bone-like" Biomineralization by PECVD-Based Silicon Oxynitride Overlays. ACS Appl Mater Interf 2015;7(28):15368–79.
[64] Ilyas A, Odatsu T, Shah A, Monte F, Kim HKW, Kramer P, et al. Amorphous Silica, a New Antioxidant Role for Rapid Critical-Sized Bone Defect Healing. Advanced Healthcare Materials 2016;5(17):2199–213.
[65] Doulaverakis M, Tartaix PH, George A, Fisher LW, Butler WT, Qin C, et al. In vitro effects of dentin matrix protein-1 on hydroxyapatite formation provide insights into in vivo functions. J Biol Chem 2004;279(18):18115–20. Available from: http://dx.doi.org/10.1074/jbc.M314114200.
[66] Huang H, Feng JQ, Lu Y, Ye L, Xie Y, Tsutsui TW, et al. The dentin matrix protein 1 (Dmp1) is specifically expressed in mineralized, but not soft, tissues during development. J Dent Res 2003;82 (10):776–80.
[67] Mishina Y, Ye L, Chen D, Huang H, Dallas SL, Dallas MR, et al. Dmp1-deficient mice display severe defects in cartilage formation responsible for a chondrodysplasia-like phenotype. J Biol Chem 2005;280(7):6197–203. Available from: http://dx.doi.org/10.1074/jbc.M412911200.
[68] Rios HF, Ling Y, Myers ER, Lu Y, Feng JQ, Boskey AL. DMP1 depletion decreases bone mineralization in vivo: an FTIR imaging analysis. J Bone Miner Res 2005;20(12):2169–77. Available from: http://dx.doi.org/10.1359/JBMR.050815.
[69] Spiegel PK. The first clinical X-ray made in America—100 years. AJR Am J Roentgenol 1995;164 (1):241–3.
[70] Boyd SK, Bouxsein ML, Christiansen BA, Guldberg RE, Jepsen KJ, Muller R. Guidelines for assessment of bone microstructure in rodents using micro-computed tomography. J Bone Miner Res 2010;25(7):1468–86. Available from: http://dx.doi.org/10.1002/jbmr.141.
[71] Kent A, Wopenka B, Pasteris JD, Yoon Y, Thomopoulos S. The tendon-to-bone transition of the rotator cuff: a preliminary raman spectroscopic study documenting the gradual mineralization across the insertion in rat tissue samples. Appl Spectrosc 2008;62(12):1285–94. Available: http://www.ingentaconnect.com/content/sas/sas/2008/00000062/00000012/art00007. http://dx.doi.org/10.1366/000370208786822179>.
[72] Seeley DG, Stone KL, Lui LY, Cauley JA, Ensrud K, Browner WS, et al. BMD at multiple sites and risk of fracture of multiple types: long-term results from the study of osteoporotic fractures. J Bone Miner Res 2003;18(11):1947–54. Available from: http://dx.doi.org/10.1359/jbmr.2003.18.11.1947.
[73] Sahar ND, Kohn DH, Wallace JM, Golcuk K, Morris MD. Exercise alters mineral and matrix composition in the absence of adding new bone. Cells Tissues Organs 2009;189(1–4):33–7. Available: http://www.karger.com http://dx.doi.org/10.1159/000151452>.
[74] Awonusi A, Morris MD, Tecklenburg MMJ. Carbonate assignment and calibration in the Raman spectrum of apatite. Calcified Tissue Intern 2007;81:46–52.
[75] Fratzl P, Roschger P, Eschberger J, Klaushofer K. Validation of quantitative backscattered electron imaging for the measurement of mineral density distribution in human bone biopsies. Bone 1998;23(4):319–26.
[76] Bona G-L, Germann R, Offrein BJ. SiON high-refractive-index waveguide and planar lightwave circuits. IBM Journal of Research and Development 2003;47:239–49.
[77] Hussein MG, et al. Characterization of thermally treated PECVD SiON layers (2001).
[78] Thorsness AG, Muscat AJ. Moisture absorption and reaction in BPSG thin films. J Electrochem Soc 2003;150(12):F219–28.
[79] Lanford W, Rand M. The hydrogen content of plasma-deposited silicon nitride. J Appl Phys 1978;49(4).
[80] Cao W, Hench LL. Bioactive materials. Ceram Int 1996;22(6):493–507.
[81] Román J, Padilla S, Sánchez-Salcedo S, Vallet-Regi M. Hydroxyapatite/SiO < sub > 2–CaO–P < sub > 2 O < sub > 5 glass materials: in vitro bioactivity and biocompatibility. Acta Biomater 2006;2(3):331–42.
[82] Himeno T, Kim HM, Kokubo T, Nakamura T. Process and kinetics of bonelike apatite formation on sintered hydroxyapatite in a simulated body fluid. Biomaterials 2005;26(21):4366–73. Available from: http://dx.doi.org/10.1016/j.biomaterials.2004.11.022.

[83] Farina M, dos Santos EA, Soares GA, Anselme K. Chemical and topographical influence of hydroxyapatite and β-tricalcium phosphate surfaces on human osteoblastic cell behavior. J Biomed Mater Res A 2009;89(2):510–20.
[84] Edgar AJ, Xynos ID, Buttery LD, Hench LL, Polak JM. Gene-expression profiling of human osteoblasts following treatment with the ionic products of bioglass® 45S5 dissolution. J Biomed Mater Res 2001;55(2):151–7.
[85] Sfeir C, Kumta PN, Lee DH, Olton D, Choi D. Nanostructured calcium phosphates for biomedical applications: novel synthesis and characterization. Acta Biomater 2005;1(1):65–83.
[86] Ning CQ, Mehta J, El-Ghannam A. Effects of silica on the bioactivity of calcium phosphate composites in vitro. Journal of Materials Science: Materials in Medicine 2005;16:355–60.
[87] Splinter RJ, Hench LL, Allen WC, Greenlee TK. Bonding mechanisms at the interface of ceramic prosthetic materials. J Biomed Mater Res 1971;5(6):117–41.
[88] Kushitani H, Kokubo T, Sakka S, Kitsugi T, Yamamuro T. Solutions able to reproduce in vivo surface-structure changes in bioactive glass-ceramic A-W3. J Biomed Mater Res 1990;24 (6):721–34.
[89] Song J, Lee YK, Lee SB, Kim KM, Choi SH, Kim CK, et al. Proliferation, differentiation, and calcification of preosteoblast-like MC3T3-E1 cells cultured onto noncrystalline calcium phosphate glass. J Biomed Mater Res A 2004;69(1):188–95. Available from: http://dx.doi.org/10.1002/jbm.a.20137.
[90] Kokubo T, Takadama H. How useful is SBF in predicting in vivo bone bioactivity? Biomaterials 2006;27(15):2907–15.
[91] Chen JY, Feng B, Qi SK, He L, Zhao JZ, Zhang XD. Characterization of surface oxide films on titanium and bioactivity. J Mater Sci Mater Med 2002;13(5):457–64. Available from: http://dx.doi.org/10.1023/A%3A1014737831371. doi:10.1023/A:1014737831371.
[92] Razzouk S, Redey SA, Rey C, Bernache-Assollant D, Leroy G, Nardin M, et al. Osteoclast adhesion and activity on synthetic hydroxyapatite, carbonated hydroxyapatite, and natural calcium carbonate: relationship to surface energies. J Biomed Mater Res 1999;45(2):140–7. Available from: http://dx.doi.org/10.1002/(SICI)1097-4636(199905)45:2<140::AID-JBM9>3.0.CO;2-I.
[93] Murray DW, Rae T, Rushton N. The influence of the surface energy and roughness of implants on bone resorption. Bone & Joint. Journal 1989;71:632–7.
[94] Haynesworth SE, Jaiswal N, Caplan AI, Bruder SP. Osteogenic differentiation of purified, culture-expanded human mesenchymal stem cells in vitro. J Cell Biochem 1997;64(2):295–312. Available from: http://dx.doi.org/10.1002/(SICI)1097-4644(199702)64:2 < 295::AID-JCB12 > 3.0.CO;2-I [pii].
[95] Bare SR. XANES measurements and interpretation. University of Chicago; 2005.
[96] Foppiano S, Marshall SJ, Marshall GW, Saiz E, Tomsia AP. The influence of novel bioactive glasses on in vitro osteoblast behavior. J Biomed Mater Res A 2004;71A:242–9.
[97] Reed MA, Zhou C, Muller CJ, Burgin TP, Tour JM. Conductance of a molecular junction. Science 1997;278:252–4.
[98] Wold DJ, Frisbie CD. Fabrication and characterization of metal- molecule- metal junctions by conducting probe atomic force microscopy. J Am Chem Soc 2001;123:5549–56.
[99] Kushmerick JG, Holt DB, Yang JC, Naciri J, Moore MH, Shashidhar R. Metal-molecule contacts and charge transport across monomolecular layers: measurement and theory. Phys Rev Lett 2002;89:86802.
[100] Datta S, Tian W, Hong S, Reifenberger R, Henderson JI, Kubiak CP. Current-voltage characteristics of self-assembled monolayers by scanning tunneling microscopy. Phys Rev Lett 1997; 79:2530–3.
[101] Liu K, Avouris P, Bucchignano J, Martel R, Sun S, Michl J. Simple fabrication scheme for sub-10 nm electrode gaps using electron-beam lithography. Appl Phys Lett 2002;80:865.
[102] Zhou C, Muller CJ, Deshpande MR, Sleight JW, Reed MA. Microfabrication of a mechanically controllable break junction in silicon. Appl Phys Lett 1995;67:1160.
[103] Li CZ, He HX, Tao NJ. Quantized tunneling current in the metallic nanogaps formed by electrodeposition and etching. Appl Phys Lett 2000;77:3995.

[104] Park H, Lim AKL, Alivisatos AP, Park J, McEuen PL. Fabrication of metallic electrodes with nanometer separation by electromigration. Appl Phys Lett 1999;75:301.

[105] Strachan DR, Smith DE, Johnston DE, Park TH, Therien MJ, Bonnell DA, et al. Controlled fabrication of nanogaps in ambient environment for molecular electronics. Appl Phys Lett 2005;86:043109.

[106] Asghar W, Ramachandran PP, Adewumi A, Noor MR, Iqbal SM. Rapid nanomanufacturing of metallic break junctions using focused ion beam scratching and electromigration. J Manufact Sci Eng 2010;132:030911.

[107] Ilyas A, Asghar W, Allen PB, Duhon H, Ellington AD, Iqbal SM. Electrical detection of cancer biomarker using aptamers with nanogap break-junctions. Nanotechnology 2012;23:275502.

[108] Song S, Wang L, Li J, Fan C, Zhao J. Aptamer-based biosensors. TrAC Trends Analyt Chem 2008;27:108–17.

[109] Zhang H, Wang Z, Li XF, Le XC. Ultrasensitive detection of proteins by amplification of affinity aptamers. Angew Chemie 2006;118:1606–10.

[110] Bunka DHJ, Stockley PG. Aptamers come of age—at last. Nat Rev Microbiol 2006;4:588–96.

[111] Ramachandran, Priyanka P., Shawn M. Christensen, and Samir M. Iqbal. Electronic detection of selective proteins using non antibody-based CMOS chip. Life Science Systems and Applications Workshop, 2009. LiSSA 2009. IEEE/NIH. Ieee, 2009.

[112] Ilyas A, Asghar W, Ahmed S, Lotan Y, Hsieh J-T, Kim Y-t, et al. Electrophysiological analysis of biopsy samples using elasticity as an inherent cell marker for cancer detection. Analyt Methods 2014;6:7166–74.

[113] Ilyas A, Asghar W, Kim Y-t, Iqbal SM. Parallel recognition of cancer cells using an addressable array of solid-state micropores. Biosen Bioelectr 2014;62:343–9.

[114] Ward KA, Li WI, Zimmer S, Davis T. Viscoelastic properties of transformed cells: role in tumor cell progression and metastasis formation. Biorheology 1991;28:301.

[115] Guck J, Schinkinger S, Lincoln B, Wottawah F, Ebert S, Romeyke M, et al. Optical deformability as an inherent cell marker for testing malignant transformation and metastatic competence. Biophys J 2005;88:3689–98.

[116] Radmacher M. Measuring the elastic properties of living cells by the atomic force microscope. Methods Cell Biol 2002;68:67–90.

[117] Sleep J, Wilson D, Simmons R, Gratzer W. Elasticity of the red cell membrane and its relation to hemolytic disorders: an optical tweezers study. Biophys J 1999;77:3085–95.

[118] Thoumine O, Ott A. Comparison of the mechanical properties of normal and transformed fibroblasts. Biorheology 1997;34:309–26.

[119] Kundu T, Bereiter-Hahn J, Karl I. Cell property determination from the acoustic microscope generated voltage versus frequency curves. Biophys J 2000;78:2270–9.

[120] Wyckoff JB, Jones JG, Condeelis JS, Segall JE. A critical step in metastasis: in vivo analysis of intravasation at the primary tumor. Cancer Res 2000;60:2504–11.

[121] Ali W, Ilyas A, Bui L, Sayles B, Hur Y, Kim Y-T, et al. Differentiating metastatic and non-metastatic tumor cells from their translocation profile through solid-state micropores. Langmuir 2016;32:4924–34.

[122] Ul Haque A, Zuberi M, Diaz-Rivera RE, Marshall Porterfield D. Electrical characterization of a single cell electroporation biochip with the 2-D scanning vibrating electrode technology. Biomed Microdevices 2009;11:1239–50.

[123] Matthews B, Judy JW. Design and fabrication of a micromachined planar patch-clamp substrate with integrated microfluidics for single-cell measurements. J Microelectromechan Sys 2006;15:214–22.

[124] Kitta M, Tanaka H, Kawai T. Rapid fabrication of Teflon micropores for artificial lipid bilayer formation. Biosen Bioelectr 2009;25:931–4.

[125] Niu X, Yan Z. The expression of red blood cell deformability in micropore filtration tests. J Biomed Eng 2001;18:615.

[126] Chang H, Ikram A, Kosari F, Vasmatzis G, Bhunia A, Bashir R. Electrical characterization of micro-organisms using microfabricated devices. J Vacuum Sci Technol B 2002;20:2058–64.

[127] Asghar W, Wan Y, Ilyas A, Bachoo R, Kim Y, Iqbal SM. Electrical fingerprinting, 3D profiling and detection of tumor cells with solid-state micropores. Lab Chip 2012;12:2345–52.

CHAPTER 10

Predictive Methodologies for Design of Bone Tissue Engineering Scaffolds

D.R. Katti, A. Sharma and K.S. Katti
North Dakota State University, Fargo, ND, United States

Contents

10.1 INTRODUCTION

Tissue engineering combines the fields of life sciences and engineering with a purpose of developing biological substitutes that can repair/replace damaged tissues and organs of the human body. Over the years, significant progress has been made in designing implants/scaffolds for bone tissue regenerations. In general, tissue-engineered scaffolds should have: (1) suitable porosity for cell migration, nutrient delivery, and removal of biodegraded materials; (2) adequate mechanical properties that can support and stimulate tissue formation; and (3) controllable biodegradation rate. However, designing a hierarchical tissue-engineered polymer scaffold is a complex process and requires consideration of factors such as biomaterial selection and design, structural integrity, and mechanical properties evolution during degradation and tissue regeneration. These parameters, if not properly optimized in the synthesis process, may result in a final product with the mismatched mechanical properties which eventually lead to severe wear and even in damage to implants inside the body. Therefore, it is important to investigate the role of these parameters in the successful design of a polymer scaffold for bone tissue regeneration.

Many of the scaffold designs for bone tissue engineering applications in literature are investigated in vitro. These models are often studied for specific scale and process and, thus, fail to capture complex multiscale processes involved in the bone tissue formation. Also, these models are inadequate to predict the scaffold behavior in in vivo conditions. Likewise, in vivo models are tested with animal models and, therefore, lack translatability to human. In this context, an in silico modeling technique has emerged as a powerful tool for simulations and prediction of highly complex multiscale processes of scaffold design. An "in silico" approach implies any biological experiment performed on the computer or via computer simulations. This approach is based on linking modeling with experiments in a multiscale regime. This technique can bridge the gap between in vitro and in vivo modeling by simulating the model using in vitro parameters in in vivo conditions.

In silico approaches are limited and few in literature. The deformation, perfusion, and revascularization of human mesenchymal cells seeded porous β-tricalcium phosphate (TCP) scaffold was investigated using the in silico approach. The deformation and perfusion processes were combined into the computational model, and mechanical forces that acted on the cells due to scaffold–cell interactions, nutrient supply, and cellular glucose consumption were modeled. Additionally, the model was preloaded with proangiogenic factors such as vascular endothelial growth factor (VEGF) to induce angiogenesis. The computational model integrated mechanical, fluid, nutrient, glucose consumption, and vascular growth situations in the bone tissue regeneration [1]. A numerical micro–macro model was proposed that predicted the effect of bone regeneration on the evolution of mechanical properties and scaffold microstructure [2]. Similar, multiscale computational techniques were applied to design a nonlinear elastic model for soft tissue [3], bone microstructure for scaffold design [4], and scaffold microstructure for tissue engineering [5]. A new atomic-scale finite element method (AFEM) was proposed that combines molecular dynamics (MD) and finite element techniques. In this method, the interatomic potential energy functions in MD were represented by the FEs and computational demands were significantly reduced compared to the MD method [6]. In a separate study, they used AFEM to calculate the effect of polymer chain scission on the Young's modulus of the amorphous poly(lactide) structure at the atomic level [7]. The computational models provide a framework for an in-depth understanding of the underlying mechanism during complex scaffold design.

The overall objective of this chapter is to provide sufficient background about the methodologies used in multiscale modeling techniques applied to tissue engineered biomaterial systems. The first section provides a background about the common materials and methods used in the fabricating the scaffolds. The complexity of the material systems and nanocomposites requires advanced modeling techniques for modeling the molecular behavior of these nanocomposites. Section 10.2 discusses modeling methods used to understand the in vitro mechanical properties of scaffolds. Section 10.3 reviews the use of molecular modeling in understanding the role of molecular interactions on the mechanical properties of clay-based polymer nanocomposite. Section 10.4 provides a review of the use of FE methods for predicting scaffold properties. Section 10.5 reviews the degradation of scaffolds in cell culture media and mathematical modeling of mechanical properties evolution in polymer scaffold during degradation and tissue formation. Section 10.6 reviews the state of the art in multiscale modeling strategies for scaffold mechanics. Finally, Section 10.7 provides some perspectives on in silico approaches used in scaffold design.

10.1.1 Bio and synthetic polymers and nanoscale additives

Materials selection is the initial and most important step in the fabrication of a bone tissue-engineered scaffold. Hydroxyapatite (HAP) is the main mineral phase in the human bone and thus is widely used for fabrication of tissue-engineered scaffolds. HAP is known for its good osteoconductivity, biocompatibility, and high biological affinity to proteins [8—10]. HAP has been used to control the pH in the vicinity of biodegrading polylactic acid (PLA)—polyglycolic acid (PGA) implants [11]. Nano-HAP is also used due its improve cell-adhesive properties [12]. The mechanical strength, stoichiometry, and size of HAP can be controlled by changing the synthesis methods of HAP [13—16]. Due to all these properties, HAP is also used as a nanofiller to enhance the properties of nanocomposites [17,18]. In an earlier study, we have used in situ biomineralized HAP using amino acid-modified nanoclays to enhance the mechanical properties and bone regeneration [19].

Montmorillonite (MMT) is the most commonly used clay mineral, and it demonstrates good biocompatibility and biodegradability in combination with good mechanical properties. Sodium montmorillonite (Na-MMT) clay unit cells consist of two silica tetrahedral layers with a sandwiched alumina octahedral layer. The negative charge is created in the clay sheets due to the isomorphous substitution of Al^{3+} by Mg^{2+} or Fe^{2+} in the octahedral layer. The negatively charged clay sheets are stacked in the crystalline phase by the positive counter cations such as Na^{+} placed between the clay sheets. The MMTclay sheets are up to 1 μm in lateral dimension and 1 nm in thickness. Nano-size MMTclay has been widely used to improve the mechanical properties of polymer nanocomposites. The mechanical strength of Gel/MMT-CS nanocomposite scaffold increased with the increase of MMT% in nanocomposite from 0% to near 11%. Also, nanocomposite showed a highly porous surface within this range [20]. It has been reported that the small amount of MMTclay enhanced the nanomechanical properties of polymer nanocomposites [21]. MMTclay-based nanocomposite system was first introduced by the Katti et al. for bone tissue engineering applications [22]. Further studies have demonstrated the use of nanoclay as a good viable system for bone tissue engineering [23].

Carbon nanotubes showed a wide range of practical applications due to their good mechanical, sensor, and medical properties [24]. Biocompatibility studies have enhanced their potential use in biomaterials application [25]. Although lacking superior mechanical properties of synthetic polymers, natural polymers are used in tissue engineering due to their improved biological properties. Collagen is widely used as a natural polymer in the fabrication of tissue engineering scaffold because it is a component of extracellular matrices. It shows good biocompatibility. Results of in vitro studies as well as in vivo studies showed that addition of collagen in scaffolds supports the regeneration of the articular cartilage tissues [24], cardiovascular tissues [26], as well as other tissues [27]. Naturally derived polymers like collagen are also added to synthetic biodegradable polymers like PLGA, PGA for fabricating 3D scaffolds with high mechanical strength, high porosity, and improved biocompatibility. Such hybrid scaffolds also provide suitable surface properties for cell growth, cell proliferation, and cell distribution. A common biopolymer investigated is chitosan. Chitosan (Chi) and polygalactouronic acid (Pga) were used in a polyelectrolyte formulation to produce ChiPga scaffold polyelectrolyte complex formed due to strong electrostatic interactions between chitosan and PGA. The effects of initial concentration of ChiPga on freeze-dried tissue engineer scaffolds were studied. Negative-charge ChiPga does not support osteoblast adhesion. Similar results were also shown in our previous work [28]. Some other natural polymers used in the fabrication of tissue engineering scaffold are gelatin, silk fibroin, and starch.

Synthetic polymers such as PLA, polycaprolactone (PCL), poly(glycolic acid), and poly(lactic-co-glycolic acid) (PLGA) belong to the class of aliphatic polyesters. Due to the good biodegradability and high molecular weight, these polymers are extensively investigated for bone tissue engineering applications. PLA exists in two optical isomers; D-lactide, also referred as Poly(L-lactic acid) (PLLA), is a semicrystalline polymer and L-lactide, as PLDA, is an amorphous polymer [29]. Among these two, PLLA is a transparent polymer and has high modulus. On the other hand, PLA has poor thermal stability and is brittle. The PLLA is often used in biodegradation due to its hydrolysis degradation product, which is also found in the human body [30,31]. The addition of MMT nanosized platelets in PLLA polymer exhibited an improvement in mechanical strength and structural integrity of nanocomposite scaffold during biodegradation compared to pristine polymer scaffold [32]. Modified PLLA surface by incorporating HAP particles has been used for tissue engineering applications [33]. PGA is a highly crystalline polymer and has good mechanical properties but exhibits poor solubility in organic solvents due to high crystallinity. Although PGA has an improved hydrolysis-based degradation rate compared to PLA, the degradation product of PGA is acidic and, therefore, its use in scaffold fabrication is limited [29,31]. Nanoparticulate HAP/PLGA composite material has also been designed to enhance the natural bone regeneration and sustained drug release [34]. Highly porous and interconnected PGA/β-TCP composite 3D scaffolds were fabricated that improved osteogenesis, mineralization, and biodegradation during the bone replacement process [35]. PCL is the most extensively used and studied biopolymer in tissue engineering applications. It has a low melting point, good solubility, blending, viscoelastic properties, rheological properties, and lower degradation rate compared to PLA and PGA [36,37]. These numerous advantages over other biopolymers make PCL a suitable candidate for bone tissue engineering applications [36,38–40]. Various techniques to improve the hydrophilicity and biological properties of PCL nanofibrous scaffolds have been applied. An alkaline hydrolysis method has been used to investigate in vitro cell adhesion and proliferation study on nerve precursor cells [41].

10.1.2 Polymer scaffold manufacturing methods in laboratory and manufacturing technologies

10.1.2.1 Particulate leaching

The particulate leaching method was introduced for the fabrication of highly porous scaffolds for tissue engineering applications [42]. Using this technique the amount of pores can be controlled, and highly porous membrane scaffolds can be achieved [43]. Some of the major disadvantages of this method are the use of toxic solvents, poor pore interconnectivity, and long processing time (evaporation can take a longer time). Over the years, many similar shaping methods which involve compression molding were tested [44–46]. This technique provides highly porous scaffolds and higher productivity, but the thermal properties of scaffolds degrade due to a high processing temperature. A novel room-temperature injection molding (RTIM/PL) was developed to fabricate three-dimensional PLGA and PCL-based tissue engineered composite scaffolds with high porosity and interconnectivity [47].

10.1.2.2 Freeze-drying

The freeze-drying method is widely used to fabricate polymer scaffolds with high porosity and pore interconnectivity. This method is very inexpensive and only requires basic laboratory equipment. Here, a solution of desired concentration of polymer and solvent (usually organic) is prepared. After that, the solvent is removed by freezing the solution at very low temperature leaving a highly porous scaffold. The pore size of the polymer scaffold can be controlled by adjusting the freezing rate and pH. The freeze-drying method also depends on freezing temperature, time period, and initial solution concentration [48]. In other studies, very high porosity nanoclay-based composite scaffolds with different polymers were fabricated via the freeze-drying technique [23,28].

10.1.2.3 Electrospinning

The electrospinning technique is used for fabricating high nanofibrous scaffolds [49,50]. Some of the advantages of electrospinning are the achievement of high mechanical properties, high surface area to mass ratio, and a reduction in the use of toxic components in the process. Many studies in the literature have reported improvement in cell adhesion and cell growth due to the large surface area in electrospun nanofiber scaffolds [51–54]. However, due to the size of fibers, it is difficult to achieve large pore sizes in the scaffold. Also, the use of polar solvents with high dielectric constant may limit their use as a biological material. A novel hybrid electrospinning process to fabricate 3D scaffolds with millimeter-scale thickness has been developed. These nano-/microfibrous scaffolds exhibited very high cell adhesion and cell growth compared to microfibrous scaffolds without nanofibers [55].

10.1.2.4 Textiles techniques

Textile technologies have great potential to be used in highly porous fabrics. Fibers have a naturally large surface area to volume ratio which enhances the properties of scaffold materials. Nonwoven textiles composed of polymer fibers lack structural stability that is important to withstand the biomechanical loading. Even though biomechanical loading is a problem with textile-based techniques, some of the major techniques used in tissue engineering in bone, cartilage, heart valves, bladder, and liver have used nonwoven composed textiles. These techniques include but are not limited to PGA, PGA/PDLA, and PGA/PLLA. Since biomechanical loading proves to be quite a bit of a challenge, some techniques have been developed to overcome this issue. Fiber bonding techniques were developed to prepare interconnecting fiber networks with different shapes [56]. Alternative methods involve coating a nonbonded mesh of PGA fiber with solutions of PLLA or PLGA [57].

10.1.2.5 Solid free-form (SFF) fabrication

In recent times, there have been a lot of advances in manufacturing technologies. Advanced manufacturing technologies also known as rapid prototyping (RP) or solid free-form (SFF) fabrication technologies are now being explored [58,59]. With rapid prototyping, one can create a 3D object through repeatedly depositing and processing the material layer by layer. This technology has wide use in research where we quickly need to see the actual prototype from a computer-aided design. This technique has gained importance in the medical domain where patient data from MRI and CT scans are often converted to 3D models and then prototyped. There are several RP methods available, such as selective laser sintering, laminated object manufacturing, etc. [60–63]. RP finds extensive use in early verification of product design. Tissue engineering applications require greater control over pore interconnections, microstructure, and reproducible morphology, which is the subject of current studies using rapid prototyping techniques.

10.1.2.6 Three-dimensional printing

Three-dimensional (3D) printing technology involves making free-form solids by using ink-jet printing as a binder into sequential powder layers [64]. The technique involves first obtaining a thin layer of powder on the surface. A computer algorithm then computes the slicing information for the model. A binder is then ejected using ink-jet technology on to the powder where the object is to be formed. This step is repeated until the entire product is fabricated. The packing density of the powder particles plays a very crucial role in the entire process. The aggregation of binder and powder is governed by the mechanical properties of the powder, which in turn is affected by the packing density of the powder. These agglomerates of powder and binder can spread to multiple layers, and if such an effect is undesirable, the product quality will be reduced. Several studies have been done on the mechanical properties of biomaterial components made using 3D printing. For example, in one study, mechanical properties of PLLA made using 3D printing are reported [65]. The tensile strength for the low-molecular weight PLLA (53000) was reported as 17.40 ± 0.71 MPa and for a molecular weight PLLA (312000) as 15.94 ± 0.71 MPa. Various methods, such as cold isostatic printing, variations in binder strength, etc., were used to increase the overall mechanical properties of the product. An indirect three-dimensional printing method is also investigated in which molds were printed with 3D printing and then this mold was use for casting the final desired product [66]. PLGA solution was cast into a mold to fabricate tissue engineered scaffolds with uniform and highly interconnected pores [67].

10.1.2.7 Fused deposition modeling

Fused deposition modeling (FDM) is another of the latest advances in manufacturing technology [68,69]. Similar to 3D printing, this technology also involves a layer-by-layer concept of manufacturing. The process takes in data from a CAD model and virtually draws layer-by-layer. The source of the CAD data could be a geometric conceptual model that may be derived from MRI/CT data [70]. The FDM extrusion head moves in X and Y axes, while the platform is lowered in the Z direction. The FDM extrusion head feeds on the thermoplastic polymer filaments which are fed in a temperature-controlled fashion. The layer deposition is done ultrathin and the direction of the heat is very critical for placing the material directly into place. After a layer is completed, the platform is lowered, and another layer is constructed. In this manner, layer-by-layer, the entire 3D model is generated. The materials used for FDM have increased in number over the last few years. Biocompatible products with good mechanical properties and interconnectivity of pores with high porosity can be achieved.

10.2 IN VITRO MECHANICAL PROPERTIES: METHODS AND CHALLENGES

10.2.1 Ab initio

Ab initio calculations, also known as the first principles method, are used to solve the Schrödinger equation. This method allows to investigate the structure and material properties of different materials at the atomistic level [71–73]. Hartree–Fock (HF) and density functional theory (DFT) methods are often used for ab initio calculations to obtain the energy levels. With an appropriate wavefunction, ab initio calculations can be used to investigate various polymers, large macromolecules, and minerals including HAP structure. HAP is a main mineral phase of the bone and critical for the mechanical strength of bone. Thus, it is important to calculate the electronic structure and lattice parameters of HAP. Also, MD methods that are used for solving complex biological phenomena such as apatite growth on surfaces, interactions between proteins and HAP, surface ion exchange in simulated body fluids, and nucleation of HAP, strongly depend on reliable interatomic potential. In an earlier study, ab initio calculations to derive partial charges, lattice constants, interatomic distances, vibrational spectra, and bond parameters of different surfaces of HAP structure have been reported [74]. Similarly, the interatomic potential of the hexagonal structure of HAP was also reported where the geometric parameters, such as unit cell size, bond lengths, lattice dynamics, and internal coordinates were derived with excellent agreement with the experimental results [75]. Depending on the nature of interacting atoms/molecules, many different force fields have been developed over the years. The derived HAP structures enable further studies of complex biological phenomena in the design of polymer scaffolds for tissue engineering applications.

Similar studies have also been done on natural bone. Human bone is a composite of water, an organic/protein phase and a mineral phase. Ab initio methods have been applied to study the interactions between these phases of the bone. DFT calculations of adsorption of monosaccharides onto HAP showed that the adsorption process depends on crystallographic faces of HAP [76]. Conversely, binding of peptides to HAP was also affected by the orientations of the HAP surfaces [77]. In both studies, organic phases preferred (0110) compared to (0001) for the adsorption process, indicating the role of the HAP surface in the bone formation. Ab initio modeling of surface interactions between HAP and protein has revealed that the polar proteins (basic and/or acidic side chains) strongly adsorb to the HAP surfaces and the adsorption

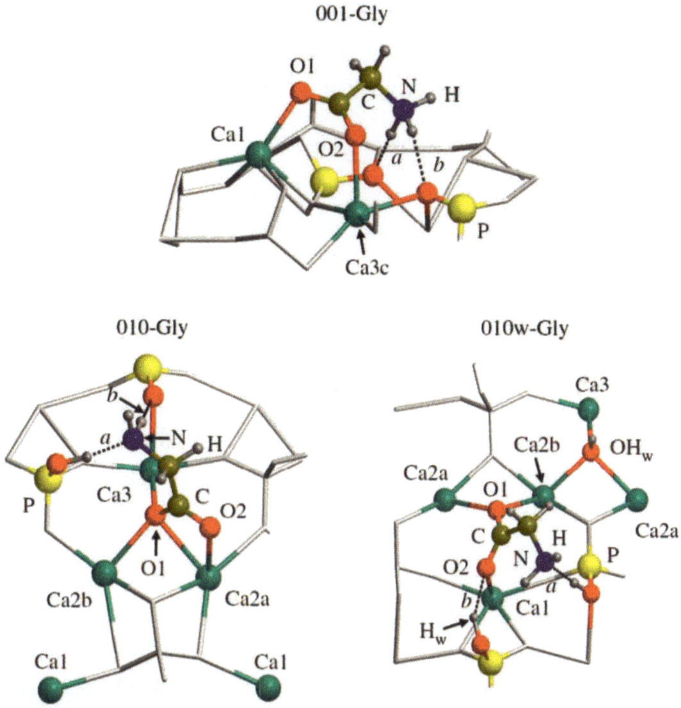

Figure 10.1 B3LYP-optimized geometries of Gly with the considered HAP surfaces. *Reproduced with permission from [78].*

strength is affected by the type of side chains and the crystal face of HAP surface. The calculations showed hydrogen bonding between surface oxygen atoms of HAP and strong electrostatic interactions between NH_3^+ protons and strong electrostatic interactions between calcium ions of HAP and COO^- (Fig. 10.1) [78–80].

10.2.2 Molecular modeling

MD simulation is a useful methodology to determine the molecular structure, dynamics, and thermodynamic properties of the system. It allows evaluation of the interactions/relationship between molecular structure and biological function at nanoscale length and time. In this method, classical mechanics is used to predict the trajectory of atoms in terms of positions and velocities over time. The MD technique is a step-by-step, numerical solution of the Newton's second law of motion for a set of "N" number of atoms. The Newton's equation of motion for the system of N atoms can be written as:

$$F_i = m_i a_i = m_i \frac{d^2x}{dt^2} \tag{10.1}$$

where m_i is mass, a_i is the acceleration, x_i is a position, and F_i is a force exerted on an atom i in the direction of x_i. The force, F_i acting on an atom is obtained from the potential energy function of the system, $E(x)$ as follows:

$$F_i = \frac{dE}{dx_i} \tag{10.2}$$

Therefore, from Eqs. (10.1) and (10.2), we obtain:

$$\frac{dE}{dx} = m_i \frac{d^2x}{dt^2} \tag{10.3}$$

Furthermore, the potential energy function of the system can be represented in the form of a "force field." The force field is a set of parameters needed to define the behavior of the atoms and bonds. These parameters are divided into two energy sets (Eq. 10.1): (1) bonded energy: comprised of the bond, angle, dihedral, and torsional energy and (2) nonbonded energy, including electrostatic and van der Waals energy.

$$E = E_{Bond} + E_{Angle} + E_{Dihedral} + E_{Torsional} + E_{Electrostatic} + E_{vanderWaals} \tag{10.4}$$

Depending on the nature of interacting atoms/molecules, many different force fields have been developed over the years. One of the widely used force fields for protein, large macromolecules, and organic molecules is CHARMm (Chemistry at Harvard Macromolecular Mechanics) [81]. The potential equation of the CHARMm force field is as follows:

$$\begin{aligned} E = & \sum_{bond} K_b(b-b_0)^2 + \sum_{angle} K_a(\theta-\theta_0)^2 + \sum_{dihedral} K_\Phi[1+\cos(n\Phi+\delta)] \\ & + \sum_{electrostatic} \sum_{i \neq j} \frac{q_i q_j}{r_{ij}} + \sum_{vanderWaals} \sum_{i \neq j} 4\varepsilon_{ij}\left[\left(\frac{\sigma_{ij}}{r_{ij}}\right)^{12} - \left(\frac{\sigma_{ij}}{r_{ij}}\right)^{6}\right] \end{aligned} \tag{10.5}$$

where K_b is the force constant of bonds, K_a is the force constant of angles, and K_Φ is the force constant of dihedrals, and b_0 and θ_0 are the equilibrium bond length and bond angle, respectively. The terms n, Φ, and δ are the dihedral angles, a multiplicity of dihedral angle, and phase angle of the dihedral cosine function. The Lenard–Jones potential parameters are represented as σ_{ij} and ε_{ij}. The distance between atoms is represented by r_{ij} and the partial charges of atoms are denoted as q_i and q_j.

The steered molecular dynamics (SMD) simulation approach is used to determine the binding/unbinding mechanisms of biomaterials and mechanical properties of different molecules [82]. There are two types of SMD techniques: (1) the constant force method, where a constant force of the order of picoNewtons (pN) is applied to selected atoms in a given direction and (2) the constant velocity method, in which one end or center of mass of a virtual spring is attached to the molecule, and the other end of the spring is pulled with a constant velocity. The force exerted on the pulling atoms can be calculated from the constant velocity:

$$F = K(x_0 + vt - x) \tag{10.6}$$

where K is force constant, v is pulling velocity, x_0 is the initial position, and x is the position at time t of the end attached to pulled atom.

MD and SMD simulations have been widely used for investigating molecular-level mechanics in bone. The role of hierarchy [83], mineralization [84], crosslink densities [85], mineral proximity [86], water [87], and direction of mineral–collagen interactions [88] in the nanomechanics of collagen fibrils were evaluated using SMD simulations. Recently, an MD model of a full-length (~300 nm) collagen molecule was built and revealed that the mechanics of collagen is controlled by the three-level helical hierarchy of collagen [89]. In another MD modeling approach, for biomaterials applications, the interactions between the HAP surface and biopolymers such as polyacrylic acid, collagen, and PCL in the nanocomposite biomaterials were investigated in detail by Katti's research group [74,86,90–93]. The modeling results showed the biomineralization process through the unidentate calcium bridge between calcium atoms at the bulk HAP surface and carbonyl atoms of the polymer. Furthermore, the effect of HAP mineral–polymer molecular interactions on the mechanical properties of the nanocomposite was analyzed using SMD simulations. The load-deformation behavior of polymer indicated high stiffness in the close proximity of the mineral compared to in the absence of mineral due to the high molecular interactions between the polymer and mineral surface.

MD simulations were also used in evaluating the mechanical properties during the degradation process of the polymers. It was shown that a change in Young's modulus of semicrystalline biopolymer (similar to PGA and polyethylene) was caused by polymer chain scission using MD [94]. The modeling results indicated two different mechanisms of Young's modulus degradation during the polymer scissions. Below the glass transition temperature, the Young's modulus of the polymer was reduced simultaneously with chain scissions and controlled by the van der Waals interactions between polymer chains. On the other hand, above the glass transition temperature, there was a significant lag between chain scissions and a decrease in Young's modulus. This delay was attributed to the insufficient scissions of polymer chains and, consequently, insignificant entropy change during the deformation of the polymer [95].

10.2.3 FE methods

The FE method is a numerical technique that can be used for finding solutions for complex engineering problems such as structural mechanics, fluid mechanics, electromagnetics, and thermal analysis. The complex engineering problem is considered as a continuum mathematical model which consists of differential equations. The differential equations have an infinite number of degrees of freedom, and thus, the analytical solution of the model may not be available. The concept of discretization is employed to limit the number of degrees of freedom and solve the field variables such as pressure, velocity, temperature, and displacement. In the FE method, a model is represented as a collection of a smaller finite number of elements also knows as "FEs." These elements are interconnected with each other at specified finite number of points called "nodes" or "nodal points." Since the variation of field variable within the FE is unknown, an interpolation or shape function is defined in terms of the value of the field variables at the nodes to approximate the variation over the continuum model. The shape function is described as follows:

$$u_i(x) = N_i(x)\widetilde{u_i} \tag{10.7}$$

where $u_i(x)$ and $\tilde{u}_i$ are values of field variable at x and nodes, respectively, and $N_i(x)$ is a shape function. For the FE models with general continuum and structural elements such as truss, plane stress, axisymmetric elements, and hexahedral element, the procedure for FE method is as follows.

Step 1: The first step involves dividing the structure or body into the FE with the suitable type, size, and number of elements. The selection of these parameters for FE analysis primarily depends on the engineering/analyst judgment and how closely the FE model can describe the actual physical behavior of the structure.

Step 2: The next step is to define displacement function within the element in terms of nodal values of the FE. Then, the displacement function within an element is described as nodal unknowns. This function should satisfy certain requirements so that the obtained numerical solution can converge to correct results. For deformation problems, the function is strain and expressed as:

$$\{\varepsilon(x) = [B]\{q\}\} \tag{10.8}$$

where $[B]$ is a strain-displacement transformation matrix, ε and $\{q\}$ are nodal displacement vector and strain vector, respectively. After that, the constitutive relations of a material and geometrical properties are used to relate the stress and strain within the element,

$$\{\sigma(x)\} = [C]\{\varepsilon(x)\} \tag{10.9}$$

where $[C]$ is the material and geometric properties (elastic) matrix and $\{\sigma(x)\}$ is the stress vector.

Step 3: For an element, the displacements of the nodal points are linked to the applied nodal forces and stiffness matrix of element using force equilibrium conditions and are given by:

$$\{f\} = [k]\{q\} \tag{10.10}$$

where $\{f\}$ is a nodal load (force) vector, $[k]$ is an element property (stiffness) matrix, and $\{q\}$ is a nodal displacement vector. The element stiffness matrix can be calculated as:

$$[k] = \int_{v} [B]^{T}[\mathrm{C}][\mathrm{B}]d\mathrm{V} \tag{10.11}$$

Then, the nodal equilibrium equation of complete structure is calculated by assembling the element nodal equilibrium equations of each element. The global nodal equilibrium equation can be written as:

$$\{F\} = [K]\{q\} \tag{10.10}$$

where $\{F\}$ is the global nodal force matrix, $[K]$ is the global stiffness matrix of the complete structure, and $\{q\}$ is the generalized global nodal displacement matrix.

Step 4: Finally, the boundary conditions are imposed to global equilibrium equations and then are solved for any unknown using numerical methods.

FE modeling is by far the most widely used technique to study the mechanical behavior of all structures and is also used for biomaterial scaffolds. Several FE models have been developed to understand and predict the degradation mechanism in polymer scaffolds under different conditions. An in vitro degradation kinetics model of poly(DL-lactide-*co*-glycolide) scaffolds has been reported [96]. The effect of scaffold porosity under static and fluid flow conditions on degradation rate were predicted from the model and successfully validated by using experimental results. Others have used an FE modeling approach to study the hydrolytic degradation and time-dependent behavior of biodegradable polymers [97–99]. The hyperelastic constitutive models as a function of time were proposed, and mechanical properties evolution during the in vitro degradation of biodegradable polymers were described. In another study, the time-dependent mechanical behavior of PLA-PCL fiber was simulated by adapting the Bergstrom–Boyce viscoplastic model [99]. The success of a scaffold is significantly dependent on the compatibility of mechanical properties of the scaffold with its surrounding tissues inside the body. A mismatch between the load-bearing strength of replaced scaffold/implant and surrounding tissues during the degradation and tissue formation process will lead to implant failure. Therefore, it is critical to capture the evolution of the biomechanical properties of bone tissue around the replaced scaffold. The Young's modulus and crystallinity of PCL/HAP scaffolds were predicted over time during the degradation process using a representative volumes FE modeling approach. The FEM-predicted results showed reasonably good agreement with experimental results [100].

10.2.4 Degradation of polymers and nanocomposites

Synthetic linear polyesters, such as PGA, PCL, PLA, and their copolymers, have been commonly used in tissue engineering applications due to their wide range of mechanical properties and biodegradation rates. Their degradation in aqueous and accelerated conditions involves cleavage of chain bonds of polymers and results in degradation products that are present in metabolic pathways of the body. Degradation studies of polymer and nanocomposite biomaterials are usually performed in in vitro or in vivo conditions [39]. The in vitro experiments are generally carried out under aqueous, accelerated (basic medium), different physiological conditions or with different kinds of cell lines. In the case of PCL, it degrades in two phases; initially, the ester groups in the PCL chains undergo hydrolytic cleavage for a long time, followed by loss of polymer due to its low molecular weight and high crystallinity, thus, loss of molecular weight and mechanical strength of the polymers [101].

Furthermore, modified MMTclay nanoparticles with quaternary ammonium salts and nanoparticles of fumed silica enhance the degradation rate via aminolysis and hydrolysis of the polymer. On the other hand, unmodified MMTclay nanoparticles and carbon nanotubes reduce the thermal degradation of polymers due to shielding effect [102]. The rate of hydrolytic degradation in polymer composite scaffolds can be accelerated by using alkaline conditions during degradation studies. In a recent hydrolytic degradation study of PCL/in situ HAPclay composite scaffolds under alkaline conditions (0.1 M NaOH), a significant increase in weight loss from 7 (<2%) to 18 (>12%) days of degradation was observed. However, the overall structure of composite scaffolds remained intact during the degradation period, indicating the surface degradation pathway in the scaffolds [23]. The degradation of porous PLGA-based scaffold in distilled water (dH_2O), phosphate-buffered saline (PBS) solution, and human promyelocytic leukemia cells (HL-60) was investigated [103]. In this study, under the wet condition, the porosity and pore size of the scaffolds decreased in all degradation media. However, the mechanical properties of scaffolds were affected differently with different degradation media. It was observed that the Young's modulus of scaffold increased in HL-60 cells and decreased in dH_2O and PBS medium. Other studies have compared the in vitro degradation of PCL-based scaffolds under alkaline accelerated and simulated physiological conditions [104]. The results revealed that under accelerated conditions scaffolds degrade via a surface degradation pathway and bulk degradation pathway under long-term physiological conditions.

Thus, although the in vitro degradation studies of polymers are performed to mimic the clinical situation of the body;, it is however observed that the in vivo degradation exhibits a faster degradation process compared to in vitro conditions. This may be owing to the complex dynamic processes such as enzymatic degradation, the autocatalytic effect due to the accumulation of acidic products near implants, phagocytosis, and reactive species generated by inflammatory cells during in vivo degradation compared to in vitro degradation. Collectively, the in vitro and in vivo degradation studies of polymer-based composite scaffolds demonstrate that the degradation mechanisms depend significantly on the degradation medium and, thus, the medium selection is critical while replicating the actual environment that would be experienced by scaffolds.

10.3 MOLECULAR MODELING FOR DESIGN OF SCAFFOLDS

10.3.1 Successful material design in polymer clay nanocomposite

Polymer clay nanocomposite (PCN) is synthesized by adding/dispersing nanoclay particles in polymers. The Toyota research group in the 1990s for the first time used MMTclay with nylone-6 to synthesize nylone-6-clay nanocomposite [105]. Since then, PCN has been widely studied to significantly increase the properties of polymers. It has been observed that the addition of a small amount of modified clay nanoparticles in polymer matrix improves the thermal, mechanical, liquid/gas barrier properties, biodegradability, and biocompatibility of PCN [22,106–110]. These modified clay nanoparticles act as reinforcement and polymer as a matrix in the PCN. Based on the type of polymers, modifiers, and clay minerals; the PCNs are basically of two types (Fig. 10.2): (1) exfoliated PCN in which clay structure is delaminated in the polymer matrix due to individual dispersion of clay layers and (2) intercalated PCN in which clay interlayer spacing maintains its periodicity and structure of clay expand due to the insertion of polymer into the clay interlayer. Computational methodologies, such as molecular modeling, have been used to investigate the structure, dynamics, and interactions of PCN. This technique allows evaluation of the role of clay, organic modifier, and polymer in the enhancement of physical properties of PCN at the molecular level. Tanaka et al. predicted the binding energies for the PCN comprising nylon6,6 resin (polymer) and exfoliated clay layers treated with 12 different ammonium salts (organic modifiers) using MD simulations [112].

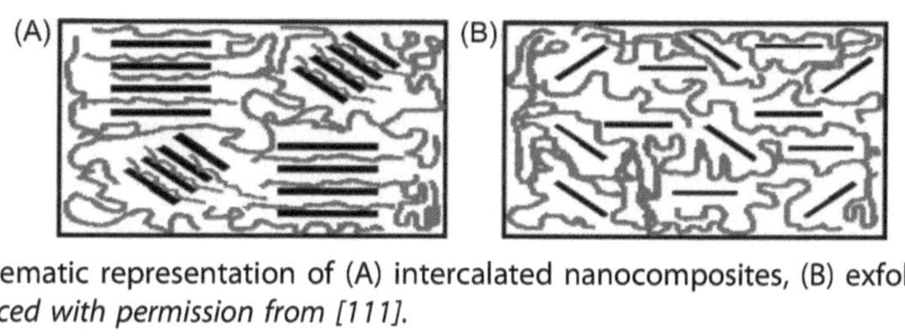

Figure 10.2 Schematic representation of (A) intercalated nanocomposites, (B) exfoliated nanocomposites. *Reproduced with permission from [111].*

The MD results revealed a significant role of the organic modifier volume on the binding energies of the PCN. The binding energy between clay and polymer linearly decreases with increasing volume of the organic modifiers. On the other hand, binding energy between organic modifier and clay, and organic modifier and polymer increases with increasing volume. In separate studies, a similar effect on the binding energies between polymer, clay, and organic modifier due to increasing concentration of organic modifier in PCN [113,114] was also observed. MD simulations were used to calculate the modulus of PCN, indicating good agreement between experimental and predicted results [115]. MD was also used for the ε-caprolactone-based PCN to understand the intercalation process of caprolactone into Na-MMT clay [116]. The MD simulations of nylon-6-based PCN showed that the length of the polymer chains has no significant effect on the bulk modulus, density, and basal spacing of PCN [117]. Using MD simulations, realistic models of organically modified MMT (OMMT) and PCN containing MMTclay, polyamide-6 polymer, and organic modifiers was developed [111,118,119]. The constructed models were then successfully validated by using minimum energy conformation of the models, X-ray diffraction (XRD), and Fourier transform infrared spectroscopy (FTIR) results of OMMT and PCN. The nonbonded interactions between different constituents of PCN were quantitatively calculated in terms of electrostatic and van der Waals energies, and consequently, the intercalation mechanism, nature, and contribution of specific molecular interaction in the molecular system were investigated. The simulations revealed significant attractive nonbonded interactions among clay, polymer, and organic modifiers in PCN. It was observed that the final orientation of organic modifiers does not depend on their initial orientation and is flat and parallel with respect to the interlayer clay surface.

The effect of organic modifiers on the crystallinity and nanomechanical properties of PCN was studied by evaluating molecular nonbonded interactions between different constituents. The molecular interaction energies map was drawn to understand the interaction mechanisms in detail (Fig. 10.3). It was found that the backbone and functional groups of the polymer and organic modifiers interact differently in the PCN system, and these molecular interactions control the mechanical properties of PCN. The molecular interactions between functional groups of modifiers and polymer were attractive in nature. On the other hand, interactions between modifiers and polymer backbone were repulsive. These strong attractive and repulsive interactions resulted in the disruption of polymer conformation in the clay gallery of PCN and appeared to create a "ripple action" in the polymer. The higher the level of "ripple action," the higher the disruption of crystallinity of the polymer. This leads to lower crystallinity and, consequently, the higher elastic modulus in PCNs. Furthermore, MD simulations of PCNs indicated that the molecular interactions between intercalated nanoclay and polymer create a localized zone of influence surrounding the clay gallery, and the crystallinity of the polymer is significantly altered inside the zone of influence compared to outside. The AFM phase imaging showed that this influence

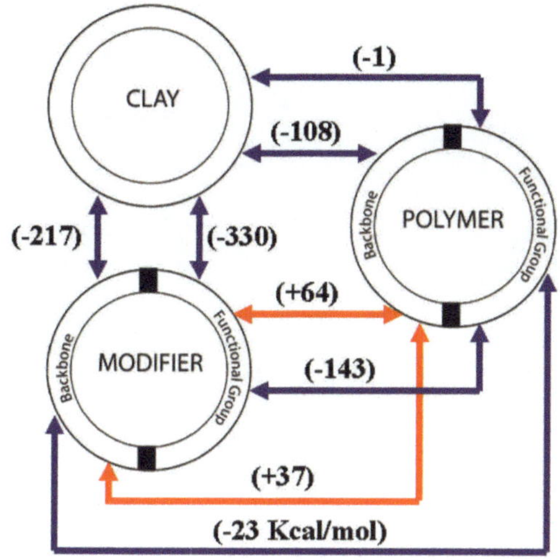

Figure 10.3 Schematic representation of nonbonded interactions in PCN. *Reproduced with permission from [120].*

zone in the PCN exists up to 200–300 Å from the clay surface. Based on these results, the concept of "altered phase theory" in the PCN system was developed. Furthermore, nanoindentation tests and SMD simulation results revealed that the elastic modulus of the polymer in "altered phase" is significantly higher than the bulk unaltered polymer (Fig. 10.4). Furthermore, the molecular structure and interactions between different constituents can be controlled or tailored for the different applications of PCN by using this new molecular modeling approach.

10.3.2 MD for tissue engineering scaffolds

Recently a novel MD-based in silico approach for the design of biomaterial nanocomposite systems was proposed [121]. The nanocomposite system involved MMT nanoclay (MMTclay), aminovaleric acid, HAP, and PCL polymer. MMTclay was modified using protonated aminovaleric acid (OMMT) to mineralize HAP. Furthermore, PCL/in situ HAPclay nanocomposite scaffold system was synthesized by adding 10% mineralized HAP into PCL (OMMT-HAP-PCL). Representative molecular models of OMMT, OMMT with HAP (OMMT-HAP), and OMMT-HAP-PCL were systematically developed to investigate the underlying interaction mechanism of the nanocomposite system. First, the OMMT model was constructed by replacing Na^+ ions of MMTclay with protonated aminovaleric acid molecules (modifier). The final OMMT representative model was selected on the basis of XRD results (d-spacing), balanced charge system, and minimum energy conformation in the system (Fig. 10.5). The MD simulations revealed that the molecular interactions between modifier and MMTclay are attractive in nature.

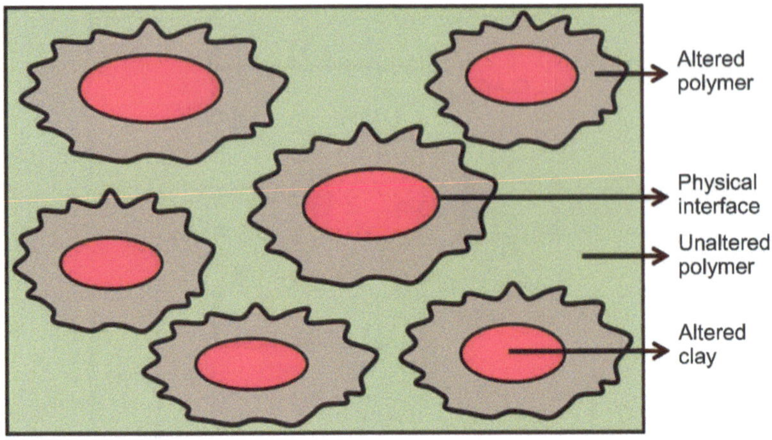

Figure 10.4 Schematic representation showing the influence zone of nanoclay blocks in PCNs. *Reproduced with permission from [122].*

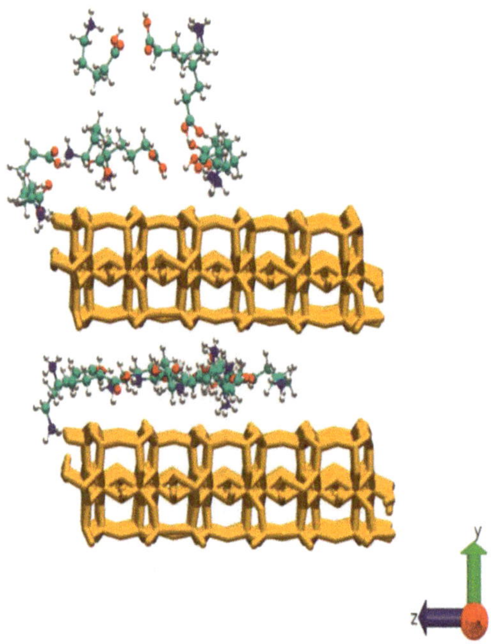

Figure 10.5 Structure of final representative model of organically. *Modified MMTclay at a temperature of 300 K and 1 atm pressure (d-spacing = 14.08 Å) [121].*

The van der Waals energy, which depends only on the distance between the two atoms was found to be similar between MMTclay and modifier backbone $(CH_2)_5$ and MMTclay and functional groups (COOH and NH_3^+) of modifier. This results in parallel and flat orientation of modifiers to the MMTclay surface in OMMT. After that, two representative OMMT-HAP models were constructed by placing an OMMT model in perpendicular and parallel orientation to the HAP (001) surface. The two OMMT-HAP models were based on the TEM analysis that observed that the MMTclay sheets were perpendicular and parallel to the mineralized HAP surfaces. Both OMMT-HAP models were validated using the XRD results, chelate formation between calcium ions of HAP and carbonyl oxygen atoms of modifiers and minimum energy conformation of the models. The molecular interaction energy calculations between modifiers, HAP, and MMTclay, showed strong attractive interactions with each other and were found to be largely electrostatic in nature. It was observed that some modifiers of OMMT have moved out from MMTclay interlayer toward the HAP surface in the OMMT-HAP models, indicating that the HAP surface interacts with MMTclay mainly via modifiers (Fig. 10.6). To further understand the molecular interactions mechanism in OMMT-HAP models, interaction energies between different constituents of MMTclay, modifiers (backbone, COOH, and NH_3^+), and HAP (Ca, PO_4, and OH) were evaluated (Fig. 10.7). It was found that change in backbone conformation of modifiers in OMMT-HAP compared to OMMT was due to the new interactions between HAP and backbone. The strong attractive and repulsive interactions between PO_4 and Ca groups with different constituents of modifiers and MMTclay in OMMT-HAP and change in the high attractive interaction between functional H atoms of modifiers and MMTclay surface oxygen atoms in OMMT-HAP compared to OMMT indicated the influence of HAP in the OMMT-HAP system. Furthermore, the molecular interaction results of OMMT-HAP models were

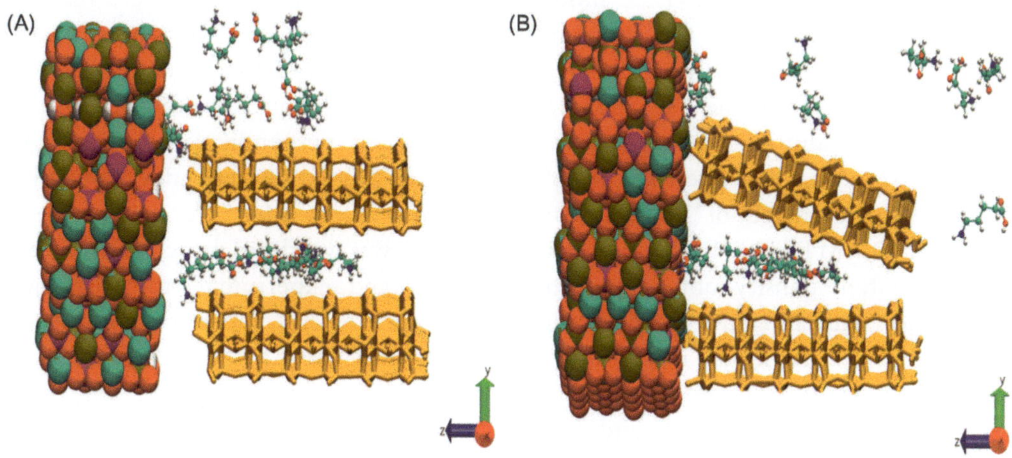

Figure 10.6 (A) Structure of OMMT-HAP perpendicular before minimization (initial d-spacing = 14.08 Å). (B) Structure of OMMT-HAP perpendicular at 300 K and 1 atm (final d-spacing = 13.92 Å). HAP represented as ball model, aminovaleric molecules as ball and stick model, and MMTclay as a stick model [121].

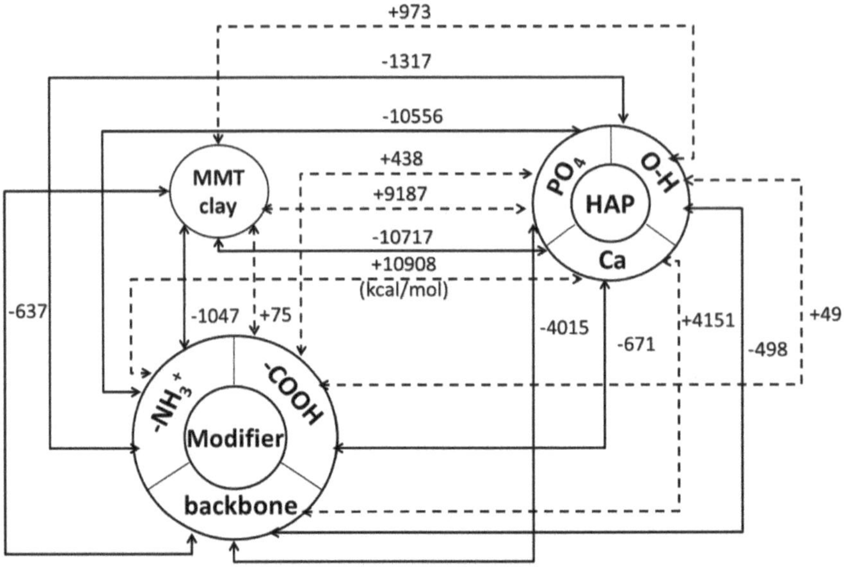

Figure 10.7 Map of total nonbonded interactions between different constituents of HAP, aminovaleric acid, and MMTclay in OMMT-HAP perpendicular. Negative values indicate attractive interactions and positive values indicate repulsive interactions [121].

compared to the FTIR results of experimentally mineralized in situ HAPclay. The comparison study showed good synergy between experiments and modeling results, validating that these models are the representative models of OMMT-HAP.

Next, the OMMT-HAP-PCL model was developed to investigate the molecular interaction mechanism in the PCL/in situ HAPclay nanocomposite system [123]. The XRD and TEM analysis of the nanocomposite showed that MMTclay sheets were well dispersed in the PCL polymer. Therefore, to design an exfoliated system, nine modifiers and one MMTclay sheet were placed perpendicular to the HAP surface (001). After that, the total of 261 PCL chains (90 wt.%) were added following the weight percentage of PCL polymer used in PCL/in situ HAPclay synthesis. The final OMMT-HAP-PCL representative model was validated by comparing the material system density obtained from simulation and experiment, the formation of chelation indicating the mineralization of in situ HAPclay and minimum energy conformation of the model (Fig. 10.8). Similar to OMMT-HAP models, modifiers in the OMMT-HAP-PCL model were also shifted toward the surface calcium atoms at the HAP surface. The nonbonded interactions energy calculations showed strong interactions between MMTclay, modifiers, HAP, and PCL. The modifier was further divided into COOH, NH_3^+ and backbone, HAP into Ca, OH, and PO_4 and PCL into the functional group, and backbone to understand the molecular interactions mechanism of the OMMT-HAP-PCL system (Fig 10.9).

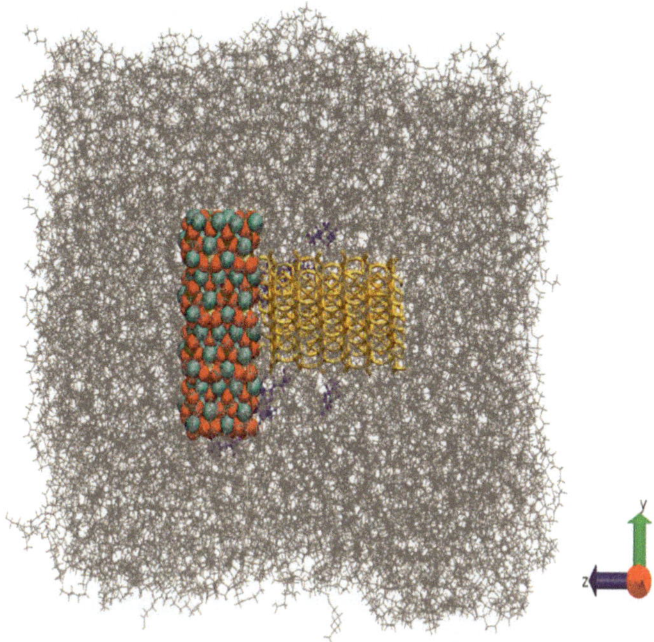

Figure 10.8 Structure of final representative model of OMMT-HAP-PCL at a temperature of 300 K and 1 atm pressure after 50 ns. HAP represented as a ball model, aminovaleric molecules as a ball and stick model, and MMTclay as a stick model [123].

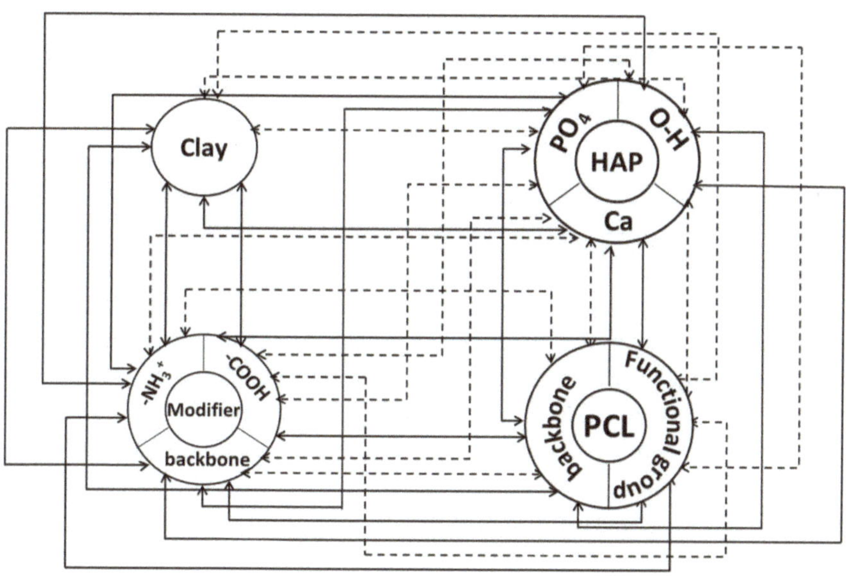

Figure 10.9 Map of total nonbonded interactions between different constituents of MMTclay, aminovaleric acid modifier, HAP, and PCL in OMMT-HAP-PCL. Solid lines indicate attractive interactions and dotted lines indicate repulsive interactions [123].

The detailed analysis of a complex molecular interaction energies map showed that the high interactions between MMTclay and different constituents of modifiers and HAP were mainly electrostatic in nature. These interactions resulted in the shift of the MMTclay sheet toward the HAP surface. On the other hand, the interaction energy calculations between MMTclay and PCL chains revealed the significant contribution of the van der Waals interactions. The high partial atomic charges of Ca and PO_4 constituents significantly contributed to the large repulsive and attractive molecular interactions between the constituents of HAP and PCL chains. Similarly, attractive interactions between Ca and COOH, PO_4, and modifier backbone and PO_4 and NH_3^+ were due to the electrostatic energy. The high repulsive interactions between modifier backbone and PCL backbone as well as NH_3^+ and PCL backbone resulted in the total repulsive interactions between PCL and modifiers in the OMMT-HAP-PCL system. The overall strong molecular interactions of PCL chains with HAP, modifiers, and MMTclay indicated the significant role of PCL polymer in the PCL/in situ HAPclay nanocomposite system.

10.4 USE OF FE METHODS FOR PREDICTIVE CAPABILITIES OF SCAFFOLD PROPERTIES

One of the major challenges in the optimized design of scaffold is to maintain a strength–porosity relationship comparable to the damaged tissue/organ. The high porosity facilitates the cell migration and increases the permeability, however, this also leads to a decrease in the mechanical strength of scaffolds. Similarly, an increase in mechanical strength at the expense of porosity might inhibit the tissue growth and biological performance of the scaffolds. Therefore, it is important to optimize these material parameters in scaffolds for successful tissue engineering applications.

The concept of combined use of microcomputed tomography (μCT) and FE modeling, also known as μCT-FE modeling, has emerged as a powerful tool for design optimization and mechanical behavior prediction of scaffolds [124]. This technique has been used to optimize the design of porous scaffolds for tissue engineering applications [125]. It was concluded that the nonregular porosity distribution within the scaffolds significantly affects the mechanical stimuli experienced by seeded cells. The μCT-FE modeling technique was applied by Lacroix et al. to study the relationship between mechanical properties and porosity of highly porous scaffolds of calcium phosphate (CaP)-based bone cement and glass ceramic materials. The FE simulations predict a linear relationship between effective Young's modulus and scaffold porosity. The strain distributions in scaffolds showed tension in many parts of struts linking pores during the FE compressive loading of scaffolds. The areas of stress concentrations were observed owing to the nonuniformity of the scaffold architecture [125]. In another study, the μCT-FE modeling approach was used to predict the mechanical stimuli behavior in the CaP-based scaffolds [126]. The 3D mesh models were developed for fluid flow distribution analysis within the pores of the scaffolds. The FE simulation results showed that a wide range of pore sizes have influenced the fluid pressure, fluid shear stress, and fluid velocity in the scaffolds. The mechanical stimuli caused by interstitial fluid flow within the internal walls of scaffolds were sensed by the cells during the migration process and thus affected the cell attachment, cell differentiation, and subsequently, bone formation in the scaffolds [126]. Similarly, μCT images were employed to create 3D high-resolution FE models of implanted interconnected porous hydroxyapatite (IPHA) and time-dependent changes of mechanical properties of IPHA were estimated. The FE analysis revealed that the in vivo biomechanical changes in IPHA are strongly influenced by bone ingrowth. The increase in predicted elastic modulus with bone mineral density and evolution of strain energy density distribution over the period of time provided an insight into the mechanobiological mechanisms of porous ceramic scaffolds [127].

Computer-aided fabrication methods such as SFF techniques allow detailed control over the microstructure, porosity, pore interconnectivity, and pore size in the design of tissue engineering scaffolds [58,59,128]. The high degree of control and layer-by-layer additive process in the SFF technique also enables the design of anisotropic and heterogeneous scaffolds that can match the mechanical properties of bone defects. These factors significantly influence the internal and external architectures of scaffolds and, subsequently, the cell proliferation, flow of nutrients, tissue growth, and mechanical properties of scaffolds. Therefore, it is critical to understand and predict the mechanical behavior in designing a complex multilayer structure and highly porous scaffold for tissue engineering applications. In recent years, FE methods have been employed to investigate and predict the mechanical behavior and optimization of scaffolds. The FE method was used to predict the fracture modes of robocast HAP and β- TCP 3D scaffolds [129]. The prototype structures of the 3D tetragonal lattice of interpenetrating rods of HAP or β-TCP were subjected to different loading conditions for compression, tension, and shear testing. The fracture strength of scaffolds was evaluated and successfully validated with experimental compression tests. The predicted FE modeling results showed the critical locations of stresses acting on the scaffolds and thereby further optimization of design and mechanical performance of scaffolds [129]. The potential use of FE methods to analyze the mechanical performance of SLS-fabricated PA and PCL scaffolds was also shown [130]. The FE predicted, and experimental results showed, that the microdefects such as micropores and surface roughness present within the scaffold struts can have a significant effect on the mechanical properties of scaffolds. Thus, these features should be taken into account to design scaffolds with suitable and desirable pore size and strut thickness [130]. Recently, geometrical parameters of an open-porous titanium scaffold were systematically optimized using FE modeling to match the mechanical properties of cortical bone [131]. In another FE analysis study, the micromechanical model was developed to predict the reinforcement effect of HAP loading on the mechanical properties of PCL-HAP composite scaffolds. The FE predicted, and experimental compressive tests results showed, good agreement [132].

10.5 DEGRADATION OF SCAFFOLDS IN CELL CULTURE MEDIA AND MODELING DEGRADATION

Generally, the mechanical properties of degraded scaffolds are measured in the dry state and room temperature, however, such conditions are different to the actual body conditions where scaffolds are to be implanted. Hence, it is important to understand the degradation mechanical properties under "wet-state" (tissue fluid and 37°C). The compressive modulus and compressive strength at 10% strain decrease by 10–35% and 10–25%, respectively, under the simulated "wet" physiological environment as compared with the usual "dry/25°C" condition [133]. In addition to material degradation, one must also consider the effect of cell culture media and cell viability on the in vitro biodegradability of scaffolds. Scaffold materials, such as calcium alginate hydrogel, have shown different degradation behavior in the cell culture media as compared to water. This is attributed to the exposure of phosphate ions and monovalent cations (present in cell culture media) dissipating the cross-linked calcium ions in alginate hydrogels. Hunt at al. investigated the effect of cell encapsulation on alginate hydrogel degradation (28 days). The mechanical properties of degraded encapsulating hydrogels significantly decreased in the first 7 days due to the high release of calcium ions in the early stages of culture. The rate of degradation of alginate slowed down after 7 days, and this was attributed to the proliferation of cells and secretion of extracellular matrix (ECM) due to the release of encapsulated cells with the alginate degradation [134]. In another study, cell-seeded PCL-based scaffolds showed lower degradation and, thus, no significant change in mechanical properties compared to scaffolds without cells. This may be due to the deposition of cell-secreted ECM molecules in the cell-seeded scaffolds, which was not present in the acellular scaffolds. The new tissue regeneration initiated by seeded cells may have compensated the reduction in mechanical properties owing to the degradation [135]. Similar improvement in mechanical properties of cell-seeded polymer scaffolds due to the deposition of new ECM molecules was reported recently [136]. The Human Osteoblast (hOB) cells are known to play an important role in the initiation of mineralization and ECM synthesis. The ECM in turn aided bone nodule formation. A 28-day study of hOB cell viability on the PCL/in situ HAPclay scaffolds in culture media showed significant growth in cell proliferation. The characteristic stress–strain curves for PCL/in situ HAPclay scaffolds seeded with hOB in culture media is presented in Fig. 10.10B. The increase in mechanical properties of seeded scaffolds over

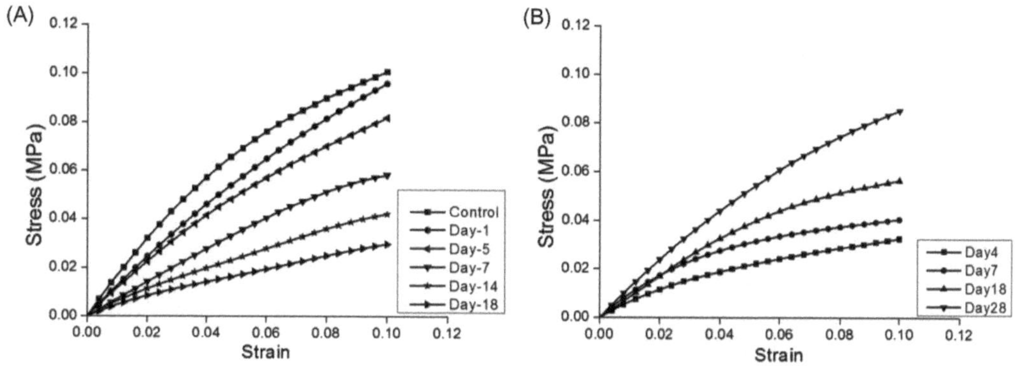

Figure 10.10 (A) Compressive mechanical properties of undegraded (control) and degraded (Days 1, 5, 7, 14, and 18) PCL/in situ HAPclay scaffolds in alkaline condition (0.1 M NaOH). The compressive mechanical properties of PCL/in situ HAPclay scaffold decreases with degradation time. (B) Compressive mechanical properties of PCL/in situ HAPclay scaffolds seeded with hOB cells (Days 4, 7, 18, and 28). The compressive mechanical properties of PCL/in situ HAPclay scaffold increase with cell culture time.

cell culture time is found to be similar to the increase in cell proliferation. This indicated the possible contribution of the hOB cell growth in the mechanical properties of hOB-seeded PCL/in situ HAPclay scaffolds.

Considerable efforts have been made in recent years to use computational modeling techniques to predict the mechanical behavior of polymer composite scaffolds during degradation over a period of time. The hydrolysis process is the most common degradation mechanism in polymer biomaterials [137]. During the degradation of the polymer via the hydrolysis process, long chains in the bulk of polymer react with water molecules and subsequently break into shorter chains (oligomers). The cleaving of chains into smaller chains decreases the molecular weight of a polymer and successively its mechanical properties. Several mathematical models of scissions of polymer chains due to a hydrolysis reaction have been reported to predict the evolution in molecular weight and mechanical properties of biodegradable polymers. Comprehensive coverage on degradation modeling of biodegradable polymers and composites is presented in a recent new book [138]. The authors summarized mathematical degradation models incorporating the rate of chain scission in the amorphous and semicrystalline phase of the polymer. The numerical equations were further extended by considering crystallinity and diffusion of short chains during the degradation process. Molecular scale models of bioresorbable polymer were simulated to understand the changes in mechanical properties during degradation due to polymer chain scission. In another study, the FE method was used to demonstrate the use of mathematical equations for polymer chain scission during hydrolysis degradation of the amorphous polymer. The results revealed the effect of pore size and porosity of scaffolds on the degradation rate [139].

In a very recent work, the disturbed state concept (DSC) was used to predict the mechanical behavior of polymer scaffolds during in vitro degradation and tissue formation [136]. The DSC was first proposed by Desai and coworkers to provide a hierarchical and simplified framework for characterization of the behavior of material from its undisturbed/undeformed (intact) to disturbed/deformed state [140]. Due to its simple parameter determination, validation, and implementation approach, DSC is used in a wide range of material systems [141–143]. A new scaffold degradation modeling technique was proposed [136] that effectively captures the mechanical properties evolution during tissue formation and degradation of the polymer scaffolds. The degradation modeling is described for a specific material system but can be easily expanded for degradable metals (such as magnesium) or degradable ceramics (such as TCP). The degradation experiments will guide the choice of the degradation function. The formulation of degradation theories would be similar to as presented here. The degradation is calculated with the following equation:

$$D = 1 - (S_t/S_0) \tag{10.11}$$

where D is the polymer scaffold sample degradation; S_0 is the strain energy of the undegraded (intact) sample; S_t is the strain energy of degraded sample at time t.

The mathematical form of predictive degradation of polymer scaffold with time derived [136] is based on the idea of damage mechanics by Katti et al. [141].

$$D = D_u(1-\exp(-\mathrm{A}t^Z)) \tag{10.12}$$

where D is the predictive mechanical degradation function, t is the time of degradation, A and Z are the critical parameters obtained from experimental mechanical tests on polymer scaffolds, and D_u is the residual degradation value if degradation does not lead to a complete loss of mechanical properties. For this work, the value of D_u is 1. The fluid flow rate and pressure influence the critical parameters. However, the mechanical tests performed for this work are at no flow condition and atmospheric pressure. Therefore, Eq. (10.12) can be expressed as

$$D = (1-\exp(-At^Z)) \tag{10.13}$$

Furthermore, take natural log on the right- and left-hand side of Eq. (10.3),

$$\ln[-\ln(1-D)] = \ln(A) + z\ln(t) \tag{10.14}$$

Critical parameters A and z can be obtained by substituting degradation values at a different time in Eq. (10.4) using the least-square method. Here, Z is the slope, and $\ln(A)$ is the intercept of the $\ln[-\ln(1 - D)]$ vs $\ln(t)$ line. Finally, predictive mechanical degradation function, D, can be calculated by substituting the value of A and Z in Eq. (10.3).

Fig. 10.10A shows the stress–strain response from the compressive test experiments of the PCL/in situ HAPclay scaffolds that were degraded in a 0.1 M NaOH solution at 37°C for 0, 1, 5, 7, 14, and 18 days. Fig. 10.10A indicates a decrease in mechanical properties of the PCL/in situ HAPclay scaffolds with the degradation time. The degradation values for days 1, 5, 7, and 18 were calculated using the stress–strain response of the PCL/in situ HAPclay scaffolds and Eq. (10.1). The calculated degradation data were then substituted in Eq. (10.4) to obtain the values of A and Z. Subsequently, predictive mechanical degradation function, D, was obtained for degraded PCL/in situ HAPclay scaffolds in 0.1 M NaOH solution and can be expressed as:

$$D = 1 - \exp(-0.1205t^{0.8253}) \tag{10.15}$$

Finally, the predictive mechanical degradation function, D, proposed in Eq. (10.3) was validated by back predicting the stress–strain response and strain energy values that were not used in critical parameters calculations (Day 14). The predicted stress values for 14 days degraded PCL/in situ HAPclay scaffold can be calculated by substituting predictive degradation function, D from Eq. (10.14) into the following equation:

$$\sigma = (1 - D)\sigma_0 \tag{10.16}$$

where σ_0 is the stress of the undegraded scaffold, σ is the stress of degraded scaffold at the same strain, and D is the degradation function value at day t.

The comparison of the stress–strain response of the degraded PCL/in situ HAPclay scaffold (14 days) obtained from the predicted model and experimental compression tests showed a good agreement with each other (Fig. 10.11A). The strain energy values of the degraded PCL/in situ HAPclay scaffold (14 days) at 5% and 10% strains were also

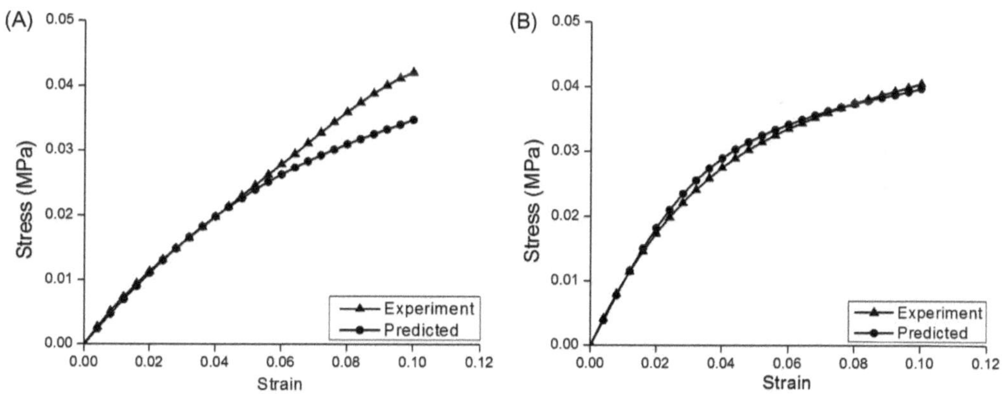

Figure 10.11 Model verification. (A) Experimental compressive stress–strain curve of PCL/in situ HAPclay scaffolds degraded in alkaline conditions (0.1 M NaOH) at 14 days and compared to the model predicted compressive stress–strain curve. (B) Experimental compressive stress–strain curve of PCL/in situ HAPclay scaffolds seeded with hOB cells at 7 days and compared to the model predicted compressive stress–strain curve.

calculated from the predicted model and compared with the compression test results. The comparison of the strain energy values showed satisfactory agreement.

A similar predictive mechanical degradation function, D was proposed for the PCL/in situ HAPclay scaffolds seeded with hOB cells for 4, 7, 18, and 28 days. In this case, the degradation values were calculated for 4, 18, and 28 days using the stress–strain response of the PCL/in situ HAPclay scaffolds seeded with hOB cells and found to be decreasing with time (due to improving mechanical properties). The predictive mechanical degradation function, D, for the PCL/in situ HAPclay scaffolds seeded with hOB cells can be expressed as:

$$D = 1 - \exp(-1.9644t^{-0.4786}) \tag{10.17}$$

Here also, the comparison of the stress–strain response and strain energy values of the PCL/in situ HAPclay scaffolds seeded with hOB cells (7 days) obtained from the predicted model and experimental compression tests showed good agreement with each other (Fig. 10.11B).

10.6 DEVELOPMENT OF MULTISCALE MODELING STRATEGIES FOR SCAFFOLD MECHANICS

Human bone is a hierarchical composite that consists of mineral and organic phases linked to each other at different lengths of the scale. The structural hierarchy promotes and controls biological functions and biomechanical properties of bone at each scale. The hierarchical design allows the bone to sustain different mechanical loads by distributing stresses to different levels of bone structure. However, designing a hierarchical tissue-engineered polymer scaffold with desirable mechanical properties is a complex process. In this context, multiscale modeling strategies are used to understand and predict the scaffold mechanics at the different levels of hierarchy. Significant improvement in computational resources and modeling software in the last two decades has allowed simulation of complex and large scaffold structures for bone tissue engineering applications. Several different multiscale techniques were studied.

Most of the multiscale mechanics models use specific mechanical properties, such as Young's modulus, to capture mechanical behavior evolution of biological materials and biomaterials. However, these models often failed to simulate the hierarchically organized and highly complex structure of these materials system and, therefore, need the entire stress–strain material response [144]. In this work, a truly multiscale biomechanics methodology is presented to predict the evolution of mechanical properties of biomaterials. The mechanical properties at the molecular scale are used as material parameters for multiscale modeling of polymer scaffolds. Here, a multiscale model of PCL/in situ HAPclay scaffold is developed for bone tissue engineering and summarized in Fig. 10.12.

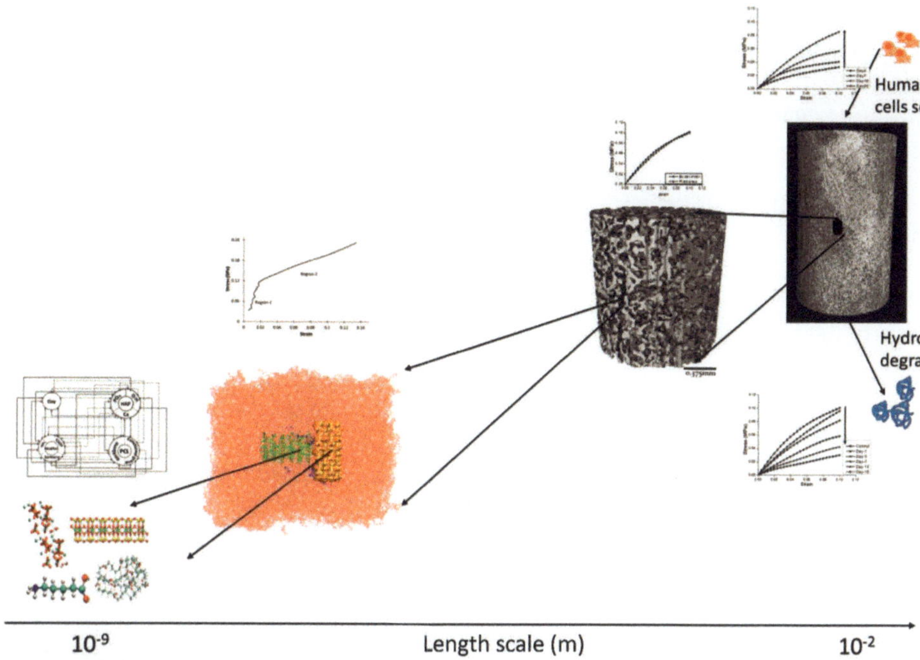

Figure 10.12 Multiscale and multiprocess schematic of PCL/in situ HAPclay scaffold.

At the molecular scale, a representative model of PCL/in situ HAPclay nanocomposite scaffold was constructed using an MD technique and mechanical properties of the model were calculated using constant-force steered molecular dynamics (F-SMD) simulations [123]. For F-SMD simulations, the OMMT-HAP-PCL model was used. The PCL chain atoms were identified from the upper and bottom surface (z direction) of the model. The atoms of the bottom surface were fixed in all directions, and different magnitudes of compressive point load were applied on each upper surface atom. The deformation in the model corresponding to every compressive point load was determined. Finally, stress–strain values were calculated for the OMMT-HAP-PCL model (Fig. 10.13). The mechanical response of the molecular model showed two distinct regions in the stress–strain plot, high modulus (6.03 GPa) at lower strain (<1.8%) and a significantly low modulus (0.98 GPa) at higher strain (>1.8%). This two-phase nanomechanical behavior of the nanocomposite scaffold was incorporated in the multiscale modeling of polymer scaffold (Fig. 10.13).

At the macroscale, the high porosity, irregular pore size, and connectivity, varying material properties and fabrication techniques cause highly irregular and complex

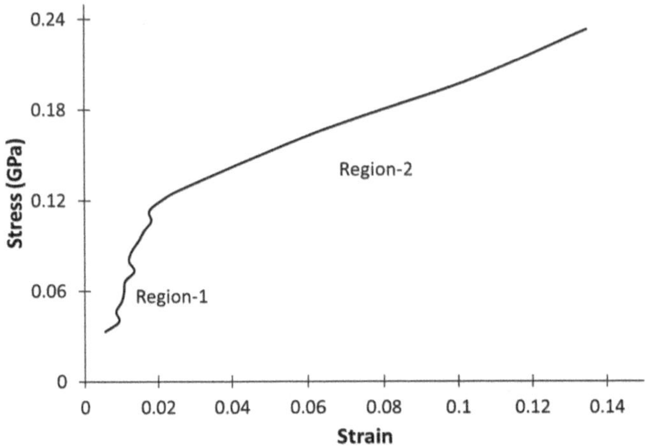

Figure 10.13 Stress–strain characteristics in the OMMT-HAP-PCL obtained from steered MD [123].

geometry of the polymer scaffolds. The μCT imaging technique allows the nondestructive characterization of complex microstructure of the scaffolds. In μCT-FE modeling method, a 3D representative model of the scaffold is reconstructed from high-resolution images of μCT data. After that, a 3D volume mesh of representative model is generated for the FE modeling. This volume-meshed model then can be used to predict the mechanical properties of the scaffold in different conditions. Following this method, a multiscale model of PCL/in situ HAPclay scaffold was developed [136]. The μCT images were acquired for the real 3D reconstruction of the highly porous polymer scaffold geometry. The acquired images were reconstructed into a 3D volume of the scaffold using image analysis software MIMICS (Materialise). After that, representative cylindrical shape (1.5 mm diameter and 1.5 mm height) models were extracted from the complete scaffold and subsequently, meshed into a 3D tetrahedral mesh using 3-Matic software (Materialise). Furthermore, these meshed models were imported into Mentat (MSC software) to simulate the mechanical behavior of the scaffold under unconfined compression loading conditions. The stress–strain response of the nanocomposite scaffold obtained from the aforementioned F-SMD simulations was used as the material parameters in the multiscale modeling simulations. The 3D volume reconstructed from the acquired μCT images contains pore interconnectivity, macrosize pores (100–300 μm), and high porosity of the PCL/in situ HAPclay scaffold. However, due to the limitation of the μCT resolution, the micron-size pores (10–30 μm or less) in the scaffold walls could not be acquired in the μCT imaging and, thus, the 3D reconstructed volume and tetrahedral mesh obtained from the μCT images have lower porosity.

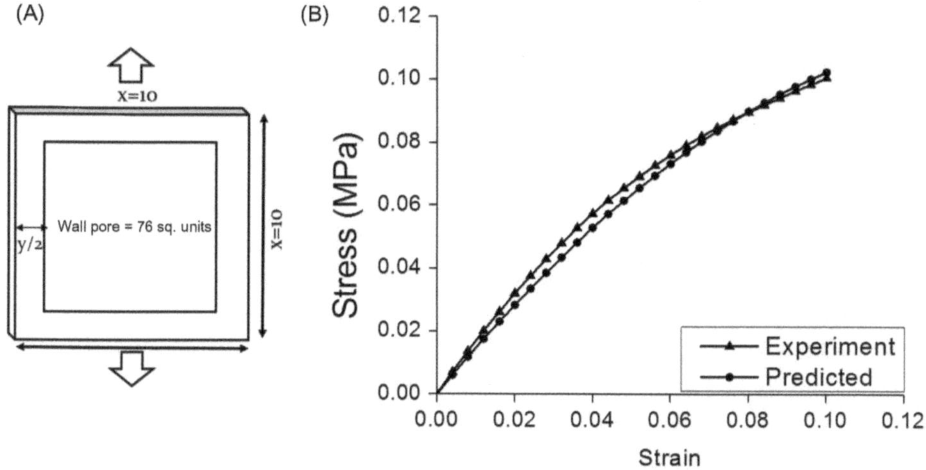

Figure 10.14 (A) Wall porosity correction (reduction factor) applied to FE analysis stress due to wall porosity = K = total wall length/material length = x/y = 8, and (B) comparison of mechanical behavior obtained from experiments and FE analysis.

As a result, the absence of the scaffold wall porosity in the models leads to higher stress predicted from the multiscale modeling analysis compared to stress calculated from the compression test experiments. Therefore, a new reduction factor, K, was introduced to include the wall porosity effect on the mechanical behavior prediction of the scaffold. The reduction factor is defined as:

$$K = \frac{x}{y} \tag{10.17}$$

where x is the total wall length and y is the material length in the scaffold. The values of x and y can be obtained by calculating wall porosity from the SEM imaging of the scaffold walls. The wall porosity in the PCL/in situ HAPclay scaffolds walls was 76%, and consequently, K was 8 (Fig. 10.14A). Finally, the predicted stress values obtained from the multiscale modeling simulations were multiplied by the reduction factor to incorporate the effect of wall porosity. The stress–strain behavior obtained from the multiscale simulations (after wall porosity correction) and compression test experiments were compared to validate the representative multiscale model of the PCL/in situ HAPclay scaffold (Fig. 10.14B). The experimentally calculated and simulation-predicted results showed good agreement with each other. Overall, the proposed multiscale model integrates and quantitatively predicts the molecular interactions, mechanical properties at the molecular and structural level, and mechanical behavior evolution in the polymer scaffold.

10.7 SUMMARY

The highly complex process of bone tissue regenerations involves the interactions and regulations of different biochemical, biophysical, and mechanical factors at multiple lengths and time scales. Several computational and experimental methodologies have been developed to design the scaffolds, which attempt to mimic the material and mechanical behavior of bone at the multiscale level. The in vitro experimental models have shown great control over the design of scaffolds. However, they lack the complexities present inside the human body during the different biological processes. On the other hand, in vivo studies are often carried out on animal models and, therefore, their results for the human body are not completely reliable. In this context, computational modeling or in silico modeling can be used as a potential tool in designing scaffolds for bone tissue engineering. The computational in silico methodologies not only improve the understanding of mechanisms involved in the complex multiscale biological system but also help in predicting the various properties of the system under different environmental conditions. The predictive in silico models can be used in developing in vitro scaffolds that can also withstand the in vivo conditions.

This chapter covered the various methodologies used in multiscale modeling techniques applied to tissue engineering scaffolds. The complexity of material systems necessitates the use of advanced modeling techniques to accurately predict the scaffold and regenerated tissue behavior in vivo. A review of various modeling techniques from ab initio methods to FE modeling is presented as also is the use of hierarchical multiscale modeling approach for scaffold–tissue mechanical behavior prediction. Degradation experiments are presented for a specific material system and incorporated into general-purpose degradation modeling theories using damage mechanics. Essentially, this procedure may be easily implemented for other biomaterial systems including degradable metals and ceramics.

10.8 PERSPECTIVES AND FUTURE DIRECTIONS ON THE IN SILICO APPROACH TO SCAFFOLD DESIGN

Several attempts have been made to use in silico methods for designing scaffolds and predicting the biomechanical and biochemical properties for bone tissue engineering applications. Recently a multiscale in silico perfusion bioreactor to investigate the influence of stresses and flow properties in the pores of the porous polymer scaffold has been developed. The proposed model incorporated the dynamics of the different species involved during the growth of bone tissues in the scaffold [145]. An integrative model approach was developed to investigate the biological processes of in vivo bone formation in the CaP scaffolds. The multiscale modeling results were further used to design the optimal cell-customized CaP scaffold for enhancing the bone tissue regeneration [146]. Recently, an integrative in silico approach to predict the mechanical properties evolution in PCL/in situ HAPclay scaffold during degradation and tissue regeneration for critical-size bone defects was also developed. The developed multiscale mechanics model captured the microstructure and time-dependent mechanical behavior of scaffold at multiscale level [136].

In silico modeling techniques combine mathematics with biology and offer potential solutions for designing scaffolds with desirable properties for bone tissue engineering applications. However, the complexity of the processes and limitations of computational resources only allow addressing the problems in separation (length−time scale, biological-mechanical-physical-chemical process) and not fully coupled as true biological processes are. This makes it extremely challenging to model the tissue formation and its impact on the design of scaffolds in its entirety. Therefore, there is a tremendous opportunity for designing biomaterials using efficient and reliable multiscale methodologies, which can provide reliable predictions and an in-depth understanding of the materials structure/property relationship in scaffolds for bone tissue engineering applications. There is also interest and need to develop multiscale physics of the biological processes. Synergy between the physical and biological sciences with advanced engineering and computational technologies could overcome the current limitations in modeling coupled biological phenomena. Another goal of in silico modeling is to provide solutions for patient-specific problems in tissue engineering. In the future, this technique has tremendous potential to replace in vitro techniques by reducing the laboratory testing cost and time, reducing animal testing, and enabling further improvement of biological substitutes for regenerative medicine. The availability of massively parallel computing capabilities makes the multiscale in silico approach a real possibility for advancing biomaterials design in tissue engineering for various regenerative medicine applications.

REFERENCES

[1] Kalig A, Hansmann J, Groeber F. In silico approaches for the identification of optimal culture condition for tissue engineered bone substitutes. Curr Anal Chem 2013;9:16−28.
[2] Sanz-Herrera JA, García-Aznar JM, Doblaré M. Micro−macro numerical modelling of bone regeneration in tissue engineering. Computer Methods in Applied Mechanics and Engineering 2008;197:3092−107.
[3] Hollister SJ, Jeong CG, Schwiedrzik JJ, Mitsak AG, Kang H, Migneco F. Nonlinear elastic scaffold design, modeling and fabrication for soft tissue engineering. Advances on Modeling in Tissue Engineering. Springer; 2011. p. 35−53.
[4] Holdstein Y, Podshivalov L, Fischer A. Geometric modeling and analysis of bone micro−structures as a base for scaffold design. Advances on modeling in tissue engineering. Springer. 2011. p. 91−109.
[5] Rodrigues HC, Coelho PG, Fernandes PR. Multiscale Modelling of Bone Tissue−Remodelling and Application to Scaffold Design. Advances on modeling in tissue engineering. Springer. 2011. p. 15−33.

[6] Gleadall A, Pan J, Ding L, Kruft M-A, Curcó D. An atomic finite element model for biodegradable polymers. Part 1. Formulation of the finite elements. Journal of the Mechanical Behavior of Biomedical Materials 2015;51:409–20.
[7] Gleadall A, Pan J, Kruft M-A. An atomic finite element model for biodegradable polymers. Part 2. A model for change in Young's modulus due to polymer chain scission. Journal of the Mechanical Behavior of Biomedical Materials 2015;51:237–47.
[8] Wang H, Li Y, Zuo Y, Li J, Ma S, Cheng L. Biocompatibility and osteogenesis of biomimetic nano-hydroxyapatite/polyamide composite scaffolds for bone tissue engineering. Biomaterials 2007;28:3338–48.
[9] Li X, Wang L, Fan Y, Feng Q, Cui FZ, Watari F. Nanostructured scaffolds for bone tissue engineering. Journal of Biomedical Materials Research Part A 2013;101:2424–35.
[10] Ong J, Appleford M, Oh S, Yang Y, Chen W-H, Bumgardner J, et al. The characterization and development of bioactive hydroxyapatite coatings. Jom 2006;58:67–9.
[11] Agrawal CM, Athanasiou KA. Technique to control pH in vicinity of biodegrading PLA-PGA implants. Journal of Biomedical Materials Research 1997;38:105–14.
[12] Lee HJ, Kim SE, Choi HW, Kim CW, Kim KJ, Lee SC. The effect of surface-modified nano-hydroxyapatite on biocompatibility of poly (ε-caprolactone)/hydroxyapatite nanocomposites. European Polymer Journal 2007;43:1602–8.
[13] Liu D-M. Influence of porosity and pore size on the compressive strength of porous hydroxyapatite ceramic. Ceramics International 1997;23:135–9.
[14] Pramanik S, Agarwal AK, Rai K, Garg A. Development of high strength hydroxyapatite by solid-state-sintering process. Ceramics International 2007;33:419–26.
[15] Charriere E, Lemaitre J, Zysset P. Hydroxyapatite cement scaffolds with controlled macroporosity: fabrication protocol and mechanical properties. Biomaterials 2003;24:809–17.
[16] Daniels Y, Alexandratos SD. Design and synthesis of hydroxyapatite with organic modifiers for application to environmental remediation. Waste and Biomass Valorization 2010;1:157–62.
[17] Lyons FG, Gleeson JP, Partap S, Coghlan K, O'Brien FJ. Novel microhydroxyapatite particles in a collagen scaffold: a bioactive bone void filler? Clinical Orthopaedics and Related Research® 2014;472:1318–28.
[18] Khanna R, Katti KS, Katti DR. Nanomechanics of surface modified nanohydroxyapatite particulates used in biomaterials. Journal of Engineering Mechanics 2009;135:468–78.
[19] Ambre A, Katti KS, Katti DR. In situ mineralized hydroxyapatite on amino acid modified nanoclays as novel bone biomaterials. Materials Science and Engineering: C 2011;31:1017–29.
[20] Zheng JP, Wang CZ, Wang XX, Wang HY, Zhuang H, Yao KD. Preparation of biomimetic three-dimensional gelatin/montmorillonite-chitosan scaffold for tissue engineering. Reactive and Functional Polymers 2007;67:780–8.
[21] Sikdar D, Katti D, Katti K, Mohanty B. Effect of organic modifiers on dynamic and static nanomechanical properties and crystallinity of intercalated clay–polycaprolactam nanocomposites. Journal of Applied Polymer Science 2007;105:790–802.
[22] Katti KS, Katti DR, Dash R. Synthesis and characterization of a novel chitosan/montmorillonite/hydroxyapatite nanocomposite for bone tissue engineering. Biomedical Materials 2008;3:034122.
[23] Ambre AH, Katti DR, Katti KS. Biomineralized hydroxyapatite nanoclay composite scaffolds with polycaprolactone for stem cell-based bone tissue engineering. Journal of Biomedical Materials Research Part A 2015;103:2077–101.
[24] Balaji S, Kumar R, Sripriya R, Rao U, Mandal A, Kakkar P, et al. Characterization of keratin–collagen 3D scaffold for biomedical applications. Polymers for Advanced Technologies 2012; 23:500–7.
[25] Smart SK, Cassady AI, Lu GQ, Martin DJ. The biocompatibility of carbon nanotubes. Carbon 2006;44(6):1034–47.
[26] Shi C, Li Q, Zhao Y, Chen W, Chen B, Xiao Z, et al. Stem-cell-capturing collagen scaffold promotes cardiac tissue regeneration. Biomaterials 2011;32:2508–15.
[27] Dai W, Kawazoe N, Lin X, Dong J, Chen G. The influence of structural design of PLGA/collagen hybrid scaffolds in cartilage tissue engineering. Biomaterials 2010;31:2141–52.

[28] Ambre AH, Katti KS, Katti DR. Nanoclay based composite scaffolds for bone tissue engineering applications. Journal of Nanotechnology in Engineering and Medicine 2010;1:031013.
[29] Vroman I, Tighzert L. Biodegradable polymers. Materials 2009;2:307–44.
[30] Agrawal C, Ray RB. Biodegradable polymeric scaffolds for musculoskeletal tissue engineering. Journal of Biomedical Materials Research 2001;55:141–50.
[31] Ulery BD, Nair LS, Laurencin CT. Biomedical applications of biodegradable polymers. Journal of Polymer Science Part B: Polymer Physics 2011;49:832–64.
[32] Lee YH, Lee JH, An I-G, Kim C, Lee DS, Lee YK, et al. Electrospun dual-porosity structure and biodegradation morphology of Montmorillonite reinforced PLLA nanocomposite scaffolds. Biomaterials 2005;26:3165–72.
[33] Luong ND, Moon I-S, Lee DS, Lee Y-K, Nam J-D. Surface modification of poly(l-lactide) electrospun fibers with nanocrystal hydroxyapatite for engineered scaffold applications. Materials Science and Engineering: C 2008;28:1242–9.
[34] Ignjatović N, Uskoković V, Ajduković Z, Uskoković D. Multifunctional hydroxyapatite and poly (d,l-lactide-co-glycolide) nanoparticles for the local delivery of cholecalciferol. Materials Science and Engineering: C 2013;33:943–50.
[35] Cao H, Kuboyama N. A biodegradable porous composite scaffold of PGA/β-TCP for bone tissue engineering. Bone 2010;46:386–95.
[36] Dash TK, Konkimalla VB. Poly-є-caprolactone based formulations for drug delivery and tissue engineering: A review. Journal of Controlled Release 2012;158:15–33.
[37] Woodruff MA, Hutmacher DW. The return of a forgotten polymer—polycaprolactone in the 21st century. Progress in Polymer Science 2010;35:1217–56.
[38] Nitya G, Nair GT, Mony U, Chennazhi KP, Nair SV. *In vitro* evaluation of electrospun PCL/nanoclay composite scaffold for bone tissue engineering. Journal of Materials Science: Materials in Medicine 2012;23:1749–61.
[39] Yeo A, Rai B, Sju E, Cheong J, Teoh S. The degradation profile of novel, bioresorbable PCL–TCP scaffolds: an in vitro and *in vivo* study. Journal of Biomedical Materials Research Part A 2008;84:208–18.
[40] Yahiaoui F, Benhacine F, Ferfera-Harrar H, Habi A, Hadj-Hamou A, Grohens Y. Development of antimicrobial PCL/nanoclay nanocomposite films with enhanced mechanical and water vapor barrier properties for packaging applications. Polymer Bulletin 2014;1–20.
[41] Ghasemi-Mobarakeh L, Prabhakaran MP, Morshed M, Nasr-Esfahani MH, Ramakrishna S. Bio-functionalized PCL nanofibrous scaffolds for nerve tissue engineering. Materials Science and Engineering: C 2010;30:1129–36.
[42] Mikos AG, Thorsen AJ, Czerwonka LA, Bao Y, Langer R, Winslow DN, et al. Preparation and characterization of poly (L-lactic acid) foams. Polymer 1994;35:1068–77.
[43] Engelberg I, Kohn J. Physico-mechanical properties of degradable polymers used in medical applications: a comparative study. Biomaterials 1991;12:292–304.
[44] Thomson RC, Yaszemski MJ, Powers JM, Mikos AG. Fabrication of biodegradable polymer scaffolds to engineer trabecular bone. Journal of Biomaterials Science, Polymer Edition 1996;7: 23–38.
[45] Thomson RC, Yaszemski MJ, Powers JM, Mikos AG. Hydroxyapatite fiber reinforced poly (α-hydroxy ester) foams for bone regeneration. Biomaterials 1998;19:1935–43.
[46] Wu L, Zhang H, Zhang J, Ding J. Fabrication of three-dimensional porous scaffolds of complicated shape for tissue engineering. I. Compression molding based on flexible-rigid combined mold. Tissue Engineering 2005;11:1105–14.
[47] Wu L, Jing D, Ding J. A "room-temperature" injection molding/particulate leaching approach for fabrication of biodegradable three-dimensional porous scaffolds. Biomaterials 2006;27:185–91.
[48] Verma D, Katti KS, Katti DR. Polyelectrolyte-complex nanostructured fibrous scaffolds for tissue engineering. Materials Science and Engineering: C 2009;29:2079–84.
[49] Ngiam M, Liao S, Patil AJ, Cheng Z, Chan CK, Ramakrishna S. The fabrication of nano-hydroxyapatite on PLGA and PLGA/collagen nanofibrous composite scaffolds and their effects in osteoblastic behavior for bone tissue engineering. Bone 2009;45:4–16.

[50] Venugopal J, Ramakrishna S. Applications of polymer nanofibers in biomedicine and biotechnology. Applied Biochemistry and Biotechnology 2005;125:147–57.

[51] Zhou Z, Wu X-F, Fong H. Electrospun carbon nanofibers surface-grafted with vapor-grown carbon nanotubes as hierarchical electrodes for supercapacitors. Applied Physics Letters 2012;100: 023115.

[52] Gaharwar AK, Mukundan S, Karaca E, Dolatshahi-Pirouz A, Patel A, Rangarajan K, et al. Nanoclay-enriched poly (ε-caprolactone) electrospun scaffolds for osteogenic differentiation of human mesenchymal stem cells. Tissue Engineering Part A 2014;20:2088–101.

[53] Li WJ, Laurencin CT, Caterson EJ, Tuan RS, Ko FK. Electrospun nanofibrous structure: a novel scaffold for tissue engineering. Journal of Biomedical Materials Research 2002;60:613–21.

[54] Sill TJ, von Recum HA. Electrospinning: applications in drug delivery and tissue engineering. Biomaterials 2008;29:1989–2006.

[55] Kim SJ, Jang DH, Park WH, Min B-M. Fabrication and characterization of 3-dimensional PLGA nanofiber/microfiber composite scaffolds. Polymer 2010;51:1320–7.

[56] Mikos AG, Sarakinos G, Leite SM, Vacant JP, Langer R. Laminated three-dimensional biodegradable foams for use in tissue engineering. Biomaterials 1993;14:323–30.

[57] Mooney DJ, Baldwin DF, Suh NP, Vacanti JP, Langer R. Novel approach to fabricate porous sponges of poly (D, L-lactic-co-glycolic acid) without the use of organic solvents. Biomaterials 1996;17:1417–22.

[58] Leong K, Cheah C, Chua C. Solid freeform fabrication of three-dimensional scaffolds for engineering replacement tissues and organs. Biomaterials 2003;24:2363–78.

[59] Sachlos E, Czernuszka J. Making tissue engineering scaffolds work. Review: the application of solid freeform fabrication technology to the production of tissue engineering scaffolds. Eur Cell Mater 2003;5:39–40.

[60] Lohfeld S, Cahill S, Doyle H, McHugh P. Improving the finite element model accuracy of tissue engineering scaffolds produced by selective laser sintering. Journal of Materials Science: Materials in Medicine 2015;26:1–12.

[61] Williams JM, Adewunmi A, Schek RM, Flanagan CL, Krebsbach PH, Feinberg SE, et al. Bone tissue engineering using polycaprolactone scaffolds fabricated via selective laser sintering. Biomaterials 2005;26:4817–27.

[62] L.G. Cima, M.J. Cima. Computer aided design; stereolithography, selective laser sintering, three-dimensional printing. Google Patents, 1996.

[63] Tan K, Chua C, Leong K, Cheah C, Cheang P, Bakar MA, et al. Scaffold development using selective laser sintering of polyetheretherketone–hydroxyapatite biocomposite blends. Biomaterials 2003;24:3115–23.

[64] Wu BM, Borland SW, Giordano RA, Cima LG, Sachs EM, Cima MJ. Solid free-form fabrication of drug delivery devices. Journal of Controlled Release 1996;40:77–87.

[65] Giordano RA, Wu BM, Borland SW, Cima LG, Sachs EM, Cima MJ. Mechanical properties of dense polylactic acid structures fabricated by three dimensional printing. Journal of Biomaterials Science, Polymer Edition 1997;8:63–75.

[66] Lee M, Dunn JC, Wu BM. Scaffold fabrication by indirect three-dimensional printing. Biomaterials 2005;26:4281–9.

[67] Kim SS, Utsunomiya H, Koski JA, Wu BM, Cima MJ, Sohn J, et al. Survival and function of hepatocytes on a novel three-dimensional synthetic biodegradable polymer scaffold with an intrinsic network of channels. Annals of surgery 1998;228:8.

[68] Zein I, Hutmacher DW, Tan KC, Teoh SH. Fused deposition modeling of novel scaffold architectures for tissue engineering applications. Biomaterials 2002;23:1169–85.

[69] Hutmacher DW, Schantz T, Zein I, Ng KW, Teoh SH, Tan KC. Mechanical properties and cell cultural response of polycaprolactone scaffolds designed and fabricated via fused deposition modeling. Journal of Biomedical Materials Research 2001;55:203–16.

[70] Tellis B, Szivek J, Bliss C, Margolis D, Vaidyanathan R, Calvert P. Trabecular scaffolds created using micro CT guided fused deposition modeling. Materials Science and Engineering: C 2008;28: 171–8.

[71] Christie JK, Ainsworth RI, de Leeuw NH. Ab initio molecular dynamics simulations of structural changes associated with the incorporation of fluorine in bioactive phosphate glasses. Biomaterials 2014;35:6164–71.
[72] Dubey DK, Tomar V. Ab Initio Investigation of Strain Dependent Atomistic Interactions at Two Tropocollagen-Hydroxyapatite Interfaces. Journal of Engineering Materials and Technology 2013; 135:021015.
[73] Ren F, Leng Y, Xin R, Ge X. Synthesis, characterization and ab initio simulation of magnesium-substituted hydroxyapatite. Acta Biomaterialia 2010;6:2787–96.
[74] Bhowmik R, Katti KS, Katti D. Molecular dynamics simulation of hydroxyapatite–polyacrylic acid interfaces. Polymer 2007;48:664–74.
[75] Pedone A, Corno M, Civalleri B, Malavasi G, Menziani MC, Segre U, et al. An ab initio parameterized interatomic force field for hydroxyapatite. Journal of Materials Chemistry 2007;17: 2061–8.
[76] Streeter I, de Leeuw NH. Binding of glycosaminoglycan saccharides to hydroxyapatite surfaces: a density functional theory study. In: Proceedings of the royal society of London A: mathematical, physical and engineering sciences. The Royal Society (London, UK); 2011. p. rspa20100559.
[77] Almora-Barrios N, de Leeuw NH. A density functional theory study of the interaction of collagen peptides with hydroxyapatite surfaces. Langmuir 2010;26:14535–42.
[78] Rimola A, Corno M, Garza J, Ugliengo P. Ab initio modelling of protein–biomaterial interactions: influence of amino acid polar side chains on adsorption at hydroxyapatite surfaces. Phil. Trans. R. Soc. A 2012;370:1478–98.
[79] Rimola A, Corno M, Zicovich-Wilson CM, Ugliengo P. Ab initio modeling of protein/biomaterial interactions: glycine adsorption at hydroxyapatite surfaces. Journal of the American Chemical Society 2008;130:16181–3.
[80] Rimola A, Corno M, Zicovich-Wilson CM, Ugliengo P. Ab initio modeling of protein/biomaterial interactions: competitive adsorption between glycine and water onto hydroxyapatite surfaces. Physical Chemistry Chemical Physics 2009;11:9005–7.
[81] Brooks BR, Bruccoleri RE, Olafson BD, States DJ, Swaminathan S, Karplus M. CHARMM: A program for macromolecular energy, minimization, and dynamics calculations. Journal of Computational Chemistry 1983;4:187–217.
[82] Isralewitz B, Gao M, Schulten K. Steered molecular dynamics and mechanical functions of proteins. Current opinion in structural biology 2001;11:224–30.
[83] Gautieri A, Vesentini S, Redaelli A, Buehler MJ. Hierarchical structure and nanomechanics of collagen microfibrils from the atomistic scale up. Nano letters 2011;11:757–66.
[84] Buehler MJ. Molecular nanomechanics of nascent bone: fibrillar toughening by mineralization. Nanotechnology 2007;18:295102.
[85] Buehler MJ. Nanomechanics of collagen fibrils under varying cross-link densities: atomistic and continuum studies. Journal of The Mechanical Behavior of Biomedical Materials 2008;1: 59–67.
[86] Bhowmik R, Katti KS, Katti DR. Mechanisms of load-deformation behavior of molecular collagen in hydroxyapatite-tropocollagen molecular system: steered molecular dynamics study. Journal of Engineering Mechanics 2009;135:413–21.
[87] Bhowmik R, Katti KS, Katti DR. Mechanics of molecular collagen is influenced by hydroxyapatite in natural bone. Journal of Materials Science 2007;42:8795–803.
[88] Katti DR, Pradhan SM, Katti KS. Directional dependence of hydroxyapatite-collagen interactions on mechanics of collagen. Journal of Biomechanics 2010;43:1723–30.
[89] Pradhan SM, Katti KS, Katti DR. Structural hierarchy controls deformation behavior of collagen. Biomacromolecules 2012;13:2562–9.
[90] Ghosh P, Katti DR, Katti KS. Mineral proximity influences mechanical response of proteins in biological mineral-protein hybrid systems. Biomacromolecules 2007;8:851–6.
[91] Bhowmik R, Katti KS, Verma D, Katti DR. Probing molecular interactions in bone biomaterials: Through molecular dynamics and Fourier transform infrared spectroscopy. Materials Science and Engineering: C 2007;27:352–71.

[92] Bhowmik R, Katti KS, Katti DR. Molecular interactions of degradable and non-degradable polymers with hydroxyapatite influence mechanics of polymer-hydroxyapatite nanocomposite biomaterials. International Journal of Nanotechnology 2009;6:511−29.
[93] Ghosh P, Katti DR, Katti KS. Mineral and protein-bound water and latching action control mechanical behavior at protein-mineral interfaces in biological nanocomposites. Journal of Nanomaterials 2008;2008.
[94] Ding L, Davidchack RL, Pan J. A molecular dynamics study of Young's modulus change of semi-crystalline polymers during degradation by chain scissions. Journal of the Mechanical Behavior of Biomedical Materials 2012;5:224−30.
[95] Wang Y, Han X, Pan J, Sinka C. An entropy spring model for the Young's modulus change of biodegradable polymers during biodegradation. Journal of the Mechanical Behavior of Biomedical Materials 2010;3:14−21.
[96] Heljak MK, Swieszkowski W, Kurzydlowski KJ. Modeling of the degradation kinetics of biodegradable scaffolds: the effects of the environmental conditions. Journal of Applied Polymer Science 2014;131.
[97] Vieira AC, Vieira JC, Ferra JM, Magalhães FD, Guedes RM, Marques AT. Mechanical study of PLA−PCL fibers during in vitro degradation. Journal of the Mechanical Behavior of Biomedical Materials 2011;4:451−60.
[98] Vieira A, Marques A, Guedes R, Tita V. Material model proposal for biodegradable materials. Procedia Engineering 2011;10:1597−602.
[99] Vieira AC, Guedes RM, Tita V. Constitutive modeling of biodegradable polymers: hydrolytic degradation and time-dependent behavior. International Journal of Solids and Structures 2014;51: 1164−74.
[100] Bawolin N, Li M, Chen X, Zhang W. Modeling material-degradation-induced elastic property of tissue engineering scaffolds. Journal of Biomechanical Engineering 2010;132:111001.
[101] Woodward SC, Brewer P, Moatamed F, Schindler A, Pitt C. The intracellular degradation of poly (ε-caprolactone). Journal of Biomedical Materials Research 1985;19:437−44.
[102] Chrissafis K, Antoniadis G, Paraskevopoulos K, Vassiliou A, Bikiaris D. Comparative study of the effect of different nanoparticles on the mechanical properties and thermal degradation mechanism of in situ prepared poly (ε-caprolactone) nanocomposites. Composites Science and Technology 2007;67:2165−74.
[103] Perron JK, Naguib HE, Daka J, Chawla A, Wilkins R. A study on the effect of degradation media on the physical and mechanical properties of porous PLGA 85/15 scaffolds. Journal of Biomedical Materials Research Part B: Applied Biomaterials 2009;91B:876−86.
[104] Lam CX, Savalani MM, Teoh S-H, Hutmacher DW. Dynamics of in vitro polymer degradation of polycaprolactone-based scaffolds: accelerated versus simulated physiological conditions. Biomedical Materials 2008;3:034108.
[105] Okada A, Kawasumi M, Usuki A, Kojima Y, Kurauchi T, Kamigaito O, et al. Polymer based molecular composites. MRS symposium proceedings, 171. Pittsburgh, Pennsylvania, USA: Materials Research Society; 1990. p. 45.
[106] Gupta N, Lin TC, Shapiro M. Clay-epoxy nanocomposites: processing and properties. JOM 2007;59:61−5.
[107] Picard E, Vermogen A, Gérard JF, Espuche E. Barrier properties of nylon 6-montmorillonite nanocomposite membranes prepared by melt blending: Influence of the clay content and dispersion state: consequences on modelling. Journal of Membrane Science 2007;292:133−44.
[108] Mieszawska AJ, Llamas JG, Vaiana CA, Kadakia MP, Naik RR, Kaplan DL. Clay enriched silk biomaterials for bone formation. Acta Biomaterialia 2011;7:3036−41.
[109] Maiti P, Batt CA, Giannelis EP. New biodegradable polyhydroxybutyrate/layered silicate nanocomposites. Biomacromolecules 2007;8:3393−400.
[110] Yano K, Usuki A, Okada A, Kurauchi T, Kamigaito O. Journal of Polymer Science Part A: Polymer Chemistry 1993;31:2493−8.
[111] Sikdar D, Katti DR, Katti KS, Bhowmik R. Insight into molecular interactions between constituents in polymer clay nanocomposites. Polymer 2006;47:5196−205.

[112] Tanaka G, Goettler LA. Predicting the binding energy for nylon 6,6/clay nanocomposites by molecular modeling. Polymer 2002;43:541–53.
[113] Fermeglia M, Ferrone M, Pricl S. Computer simulation of nylon-6/organoclay nanocomposites: prediction of the binding energy. Fluid Phase Equilibria 2003;212:315–29.
[114] Fermeglia M, Ferrone M, Pricl S. Estimation of the binding energy in random poly (butylene terephtalate-co-thiodiethylene terephtalate) copolyesters/clay nanocomposites via molecular simulation. Molecular Simulation 2004;30:289–300.
[115] Luo J-J, Daniel IM. Characterization and modeling of mechanical behavior of polymer/clay nanocomposites. Composites Science and Technology 2003;63:1607–16.
[116] Gaudel-Siri A, Brocorens P, Siri D, Gardebien F, Brédas J-L, Lazzaroni R. Molecular dynamics study of ε-caprolactone intercalated in wyoming sodium montmorillonite. Langmuir 2003;19: 8287–91.
[117] Anoukou K, Zaoui A, Zaïri F, Naït-Abdelaziz M, Gloaguen JM. Molecular dynamics study of the polymer clay nanocomposites (PCNs): elastic constants and basal spacing predictions. Computational Materials Science 2013;77:417–23.
[118] Katti KS, Sikdar D, Katti DR, Ghosh P, Verma D. Molecular interactions in intercalated organically modified clay and clay–polycaprolactam nanocomposites: experiments and modeling. Polymer 2006;47:403–14.
[119] Sikdar D, Katti DR, Katti KS. A molecular model for ε-caprolactam-based intercalated polymer clay nanocomposite: integrating modeling and experiments. Langmuir 2006;22:7738–47.
[120] Sikdar D, Katti DR, Katti KS. The role of interfacial interactions on the crystallinity and nanomechanical properties of clay–polymer nanocomposites: a molecular dynamics study. Journal of applied polymer science 2008;107:3137–48.
[121] Katti DR, Sharma A, Ambre AH, Katti KS. Molecular interactions in biomineralized hydroxyapatite amino acid modified nanoclay: In silico design of bone biomaterials. Materials Science and Engineering: C 2015;46:207–17.
[122] Sikdar D, Pradhan SM, Katti DR, Katti KS, Mohanty B. Altered phase model for polymer clay nanocomposites. Langmuir 2008;24:5599–607.
[123] Sharma A, Payne S, Katti KS, Katti DR. Evaluating molecular interactions in polycaprolactone-biomineralized hydroxyapatite nanocomposites using steered molecular dynamics. JOM 2015;67: 733–43.
[124] Jaecques SVN, Van Oosterwyck H, Muraru L, Van Cleynenbreugel T, De Smet E, Wevers M, et al. Individualised, micro CT-based finite element modelling as a tool for biomechanical analysis related to tissue engineering of bone. Biomaterials 2004;25:1683–96.
[125] Lacroix D, Chateau A, Ginebra M-P, Planell JA. Micro-finite element models of bone tissue-engineering scaffolds. Biomaterials 2006;27:5326–34.
[126] Sandino C, Planell J, Lacroix D. A finite element study of mechanical stimuli in scaffolds for bone tissue engineering. Journal of Biomechanics 2008;41:1005–14.
[127] Ren L-M, Arahira T, Todo M, Yoshikawa H, Myoui A. Biomechanical evaluation of porous bioactive ceramics after implantation: micro CT-based three-dimensional finite element analysis. Journal of Materials Science: Materials in Medicine 2012;23:463–72.
[128] Danforth C, Agarwala M, Bandyopadhyay A, Langrana N, Jamalabad VR, Safari A, Van Weeren R. Solid freeform fabrication methods. Google Patents, US Patent #5,738,817S, 1998.
[129] Miranda P, Pajares A, Guiberteau F. Finite element modeling as a tool for predicting the fracture behavior of robocast scaffolds. Acta biomaterialia 2008;4:1715–24.
[130] Cahill S, Lohfeld S, McHugh P. Finite element predictions compared to experimental results for the effective modulus of bone tissue engineering scaffolds fabricated by selective laser sintering. Journal of Materials Science: Materials in Medicine 2009;20:1255–62.
[131] Wieding J, Wolf A, Bader R. Numerical optimization of open-porous bone scaffold structures to match the elastic properties of human cortical bone. Journal of the Mechanical Behavior of Biomedical Materials 2014;37:56–68.

[132] Eshraghi S, Das S. Micromechanical finite-element modeling and experimental characterization of the compressive mechanical properties of polycaprolactone–hydroxyapatite composite scaffolds prepared by selective laser sintering for bone tissue engineering. Acta Biomaterialia 2012;8: 3138–43.
[133] Wu L, Zhang J, Jing D, Ding J. "Wet-state" mechanical properties of three-dimensional polyester porous scaffolds. Journal of Biomedical Materials Research Part A 2006;76:264–71.
[134] Hunt NC, Smith AM, Gbureck U, Shelton RM, Grover LM. Encapsulation of fibroblasts causes accelerated alginate hydrogel degradation. Acta Biomaterialia 2010;6:3649–56.
[135] Sant S, Iyer D, Gaharwar AK, Patel A, Khademhosseini A. Effect of biodegradation and de novo matrix synthesis on the mechanical properties of valvular interstitial cell-seeded polyglycerol sebacate–polycaprolactone scaffolds. Acta Biomaterialia 2013;9:5963–73.
[136] Sharma A, Molla MDS, Katti KS, Katti DR, Multiscale model of degradation and healing of bone tissue engineering nanocomposite scaffolds. Under review
[137] Göpferich A. Mechanisms of polymer degradation and erosion. Biomaterials 1996;17:103–14.
[138] Pan J. Modelling Degradation of Bioresorbable Polymeric Medical Devices. Sawston, Cambridge, UK: Elsevier; 2014.
[139] Han X, Pan J. Finite element analysis of degradation of biodegradable medical devices, OA. Biotechnology 2013;2:10.
[140] Desai C. A consistent finite element technique for work-softening behavior. Proc., Int. Conf. on Computational Methods in Nonlinear Mechanics: University of Texas, Austin, 1974.
[141] Katti DR, Desai CS. Modeling and testing of cohesive soil using disturbed-state concept. Journal of Engineering Mechanics 1995;121:648–58.
[142] Kwak C, Park I, Park J. Evaluation of disturbance function for geosynthetic–soil interface considering chemical reactions based on cyclic direct shear tests. Soils and Foundations 2013;53:720–34.
[143] Kwak C, Park I, Park J. Chemical and cyclic degradation of geosynthetic-soil interface. Asian Journal of Chemistry 2014;26.
[144] Hellmich C, Katti D. Multiscale mechanics of biological, bioinspired, and biomedical materials. MRS Bulletin 2015;40:309–13.
[145] Spencer T, Hidalgo-Bastida L, Cartmell S, Halliday I, Care C. In silico multi-scale model of transport and dynamic seeding in a bone tissue engineering perfusion bioreactor. Biotechnology and Bioengineering 2013;110:1221–30.
[146] Carlier A, Chai YC, Moesen M, Theys T, Schrooten J, Van Oosterwyck H, et al. Designing optimal calcium phosphate scaffold–cell combinations using an integrative model-based approach. Acta Biomaterialia 2011;7:3573–85.

CHAPTER 11

Ethical Issues in Biomaterials Research

A. Kashi[1,2] and S. Saha[3]
[1]Private Practice, Rochester, NY, United States
[2]Biomedical Research and Services, Brooklyn, NY, United States
[3]SUNY Downstate Medical Center, Brooklyn, NY, United States

Contents

11.1 INTRODUCTION

Biomedical engineering is currently the fastest growing and the most rapidly evolving field among all engineering disciplines. It is an applied science that utilizes the principles of engineering to solve medical problems and improve the quality of life of our patients. Due to its interdisciplinary nature, biomedical engineering presents unique ethical challenges. Presently, the results from only a very small percentage of in vitro research can be directly applied to in vivo human performance. For instance, there are significant differences between the in vitro and in vivo performance of many new biomaterials and implant devices. One of the main goals of biomedical engineering research is aimed toward providing solutions to improve currently available clinical treatments by designing new devices and utilizing new biomaterials to solve clinical problems [1]. Clinicians have recognized the need for collaborative efforts to solve biomedical problems faced by humanity, and this has not only fueled the growth of biomedical engineering research but their resultant ethical challenges as well [2–4]. Some of these ethical concerns include questions related to emerging technologies (e.g., nanobiotechnology, stem cell research, tissue engineering, and telemedicine), animal research, and clinical trials [5,6]. Many materials and techniques that were once strictly reserved or rather utilized for traditional engineering applications are being increasingly adopted for biomedical uses (e.g., industrial ceramics modified to be used as bioceramics for medical uses in orthopedics and dentistry). These previously mentioned examples can raise ethical questions in terms of their safety, efficacy, and long-term survival when used in humans. Furthermore, issues related to conflict of interest issues, authorship, intellectual property, disease burden, and cost versus benefit analysis are going to become increasingly important topics of discussion in the future (Fig. 11.1) [7–9].

11.2 ETHICAL ISSUES WITH EMERGING TECHNOLOGIES

Some of the most promising areas of emerging technologies include application of nanotechnology in medicine, tissue engineering, stem cell research, and new imaging techniques for better diagnosis [10]. Although many theoretical scientific ideas were proposed in the past, they were not proven in laboratory experiments due to the

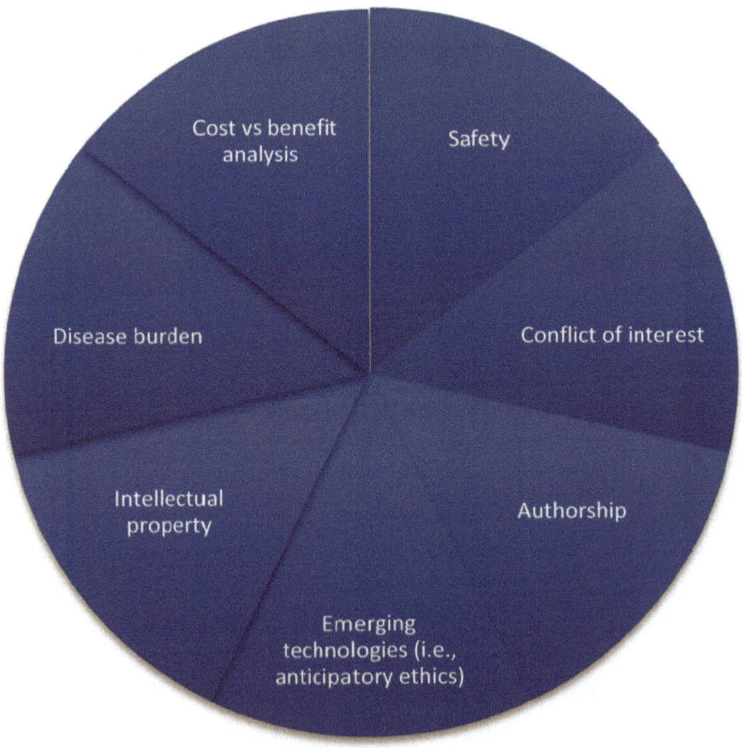

Figure 11.1 Ethical challenges related to biomaterials research.

absence of advanced manufacturing, characterization, and/or imaging techniques, until recently. Moreover, globalization has brought to the forefront some ethical issues that are due to differences in the cultural and social norms among nations. Due to the globalization of our economy, taking into account the moral beliefs and theories of other cultures and nations into decision-making when conducting research is ever more important in current scientific research when compared to earlier times. An emerging area of discussion related to ethics in biomaterials research includes anticipatory ethics where researchers are encouraged to be in a position to anticipate ethical challenges and solutions to problems with emerging technologies. Although this might not always be possible and can be challenging at times, the idea that one can be encouraged to anticipate challenges from newer technologies will be paramount to understanding how to tackle them from a societal and scientific perspective.

11.2.1 Nanobiotechnology and ethics

Researchers have only recently been able to visualize, characterize, and even fabricate materials at the nanoscale level [11]. One might envision a future where nanorobots may be injected into our bloodstream to remove plaques from blood vessels and repair other defects. The science of nanotechnology holds promise in providing solutions to many biomedical problems. A few examples include the development of nanoparticles that are capable of delivering drugs to target tissues, fabrication of biomaterials at the nanoscale for the manufacture of devices to enhance their mechanical properties, improve survival times in vivo, and modify biological substances to lead to enhanced efficacy when utilized in vivo. Many ideas that were theoretical or hypothetical in the past have recently materialized into actual devices in the field of nanotechnology. This can be attributed to advances in materials processing, fabrication, and improved imaging technologies.

Nanotechnology research has raised the issue of safety, specifically related to nanomaterials when used for human applications, although it is fair to assume that the science is progressing at a faster pace when compared to its related ethical guidelines [12–14]. There is very little information available to show the short- or long-term effects of many nanoparticles when applied in human tissues or organs for treating illnesses. For instance, if nanoparticles are used to clear circulatory obstructions and infections when administered in humans, the possibility that they might lead to clots in the microvasculature and other unforeseen consequences is yet to be thoroughly investigated. The environmental effects of nanoparticles (i.e., the failure of existing filters to remove the nanoparticles) have not been examined fully. Many of these aforementioned concerns stress the need for discussing emerging technologies in an ethical framework, for it is not only the responsibility of the scientific community to be answerable to their employers and colleagues, but to the general public as well as they might be prone to the effects of nanotechnology unknowingly or unwillingly. Some of the other issues that need further discussion include equity and privacy with respect to nanodevices research.

Whether emerging technologies and inventions such as nanotechnology will be available for only a select group of people to use or if they will be distributed across nations to be used widely needs to be debated. Budinger and Budinger mention that restrictions related to the use of pharmaceutical drugs (e.g., for the treatment of AIDS) that are developed and patented in Western nations but are not transferred to be used in other populations in developing countries where certain diseases are prevalent is a matter of ethical concern [15]. These are but a few of the ethical concerns that need to be addressed. A lack of specialists to address ethical issues related to nanotechnology needs to be taken into consideration by academic institutions, government and international agencies, and industry alike. This will insure that as the field progresses, their related ethical issues will also be adequately addressed. It should also be the responsibility of journalists to report correctly the safety and benefits of nanotechnology along with their dangers in the 21st century. This will constitute ethical journalism and a need for conveying the impact of these emerging technologies such that they can be evaluated and appropriately received by the public. A revision of definitions pertaining to intellectual property and the possibility of whether nanotechnology can be distributed to other nations in a more widespread manner compared to current practices need to be considered in the future.

11.2.2 Stem cell research and ethics

Stem cell research is another promising area of science and biomedical engineering that proposes to offer solutions to many medical problems. The main ethical considerations associated with stem cell research include the source of the cells (i.e., whether they are embryonic stem cells from 5- to 7-day-old embryos, adult stem cells from adult tissues, or stem cells derived from aborted fetuses), the safety and viability of the cells when used for human applications. It is a highly interdisciplinary field of science that is bound to face numerous ethical challenges in the future [16–20]. Successful growth of this scientific discipline will be possible due to the collaboration between professionals including molecular and cellular biologists, physicians, and biomedical engineers. Such collaborative efforts are needed to advance the science of stem cell research and produce biologically viable products. As a consequence of these unique collaborations, it will become essential that scientists with different backgrounds be in a position to address ethical issues that may arise from their combined research efforts. As an example, if stem cell therapies are going to be devised by cell biologists in collaboration with bioengineering/biomaterials scientists, the expertise of cell biologists might be significantly different, including their ethical norms when compared to bioengineering scientists [9]. The cell biologists may have expertise to choose the appropriate stem cell(s) and to provide appropriate cues so that they can grow in certain fashion and biomedical engineering scientists typically may have expertise in designing nanomaterial scaffolds to seed cells onto the scaffolds so that they may be grown optimally. Both these disciplines have to be in a position to be able to address ethical concerns related to their colleagues' scientific work, i.e., the source of the cells (e.g., animal, human, embryonic, adult) and biomaterials concerns (e.g., safety and long-term survival from a mechanical perspective) [21]. In the United States, there has also been significant political and religious debate related to stem cell research from the scientific and nonscientific communities. Most of these debates have focused on one or more of the previously mentioned ethical dilemmas. Although there are strong opinions, there has never been any unanimous guideline(s) that is acceptable to all, thus warranting further debate in this emerging area of science [16].

11.2.3 Tissue engineering

Tissue engineering aims to replace lost or diseased tissue(s) with laboratory-engineered tissue constructs. Although there might be different clinical indications for tissue engineered materials, their end result is aimed toward the replacement of lost tissue with satisfactory outcomes. Similar to stem cell research, tissue engineering is also a highly interdisciplinary field of study and one that needs to take into account emerging ethical challenges. Some of these include the safety and long-term effects, the source of the cells used for the fabrication of the tissue constructs, the costs, and intellectual property issues. Inadequate avenues for discussing and/or resolving one or more of these previously mentioned factors can potentially slow the advances in tissue engineering research. The use of cells from animal sources for tissue engineered constructs poses safety concerns including their viability in the long term when used in humans. If tissue engineered structures will utilize cells from animal sources that are seeded onto artificially constructed constructs, whether it will be ethical to obtain intellectual property protection on such constructs needs further discussion. Addressing whether the cells themselves can be patented or if the combination of cells and artificial materials used to create tissue engineered constructs can be patented is yet to be resolved. However, many issues might be complex and may be solved only when crisis situations arise. Cost versus benefit analysis to determine if the tissue engineered constructs are feasible from an economic standpoint is going to become important given the increasing costs of health care. The expertise of biomedical engineers might be needed in the future to determine if the tissue engineered constructs are adequate in their physical properties (e.g., strength) if they are going to be used for load-bearing applications in vivo. Creating a structure that might be biologically viable but not necessarily suitable for long-term patient use in terms of adequate strength and fatigue properties will create an inferior and/or unacceptable end product. When these materials need to be used for longer durations in vivo, it will be essential that they are capable of surviving within the biological milieu as well as sustaining the biomechanical stresses of the human physiological system. Failure to do so might prompt some individuals to question its use from an ethical standpoint. Further research needs to be carried out to refine many processes so that tissue engineering can produce solutions to replace lost tissues. There might be promising solutions to many clinical problems, but they might not reach fruition unless adequate attention is paid to these previously mentioned factors. Some patients may also refuse cells or tissue products from animal sources due to religious reasons.

11.3 COST VERSUS BENEFIT ANALYSIS

When conducting biomedical engineering research, scientists must consider that their products are suitable from a cost–benefit perspective similar to any other research. Specifically, this means that the research will lead to solutions that are not only scientifically valid but are also cost-effective. For instance, the introduction of electronic medical records for healthcare data management of patients by individual clinicians will take a longer time when compared to the larger institutions that might be able to afford them from a cost-effectiveness perspective. Another example that can be discussed in this context can be related to the research and development of many biomedical implants (e.g., stents, hip and knee replacements, and dental implants). These previously mentioned implants need to be tested in laboratory experiments for their endurance and long-term survival in terms of their fatigue strength prior to their testing in animal models. These experiments may require significant financial resources to be carried out in sufficient numbers so that statistically significant results can be obtained. Besides, federal laws mandate that new biomedical devices, if significantly different from other equivalent devices, be tested by such experiments to prove their effectiveness. In the long term, it may be realized that a new design for a hip implant might last twice as long in duration when compared to an existing design, thus leading to better outcomes in patients. Since the United States and most other countries in the world have an aging population, it is likely that there will be a greater need for such devices in the future. From a cost–benefit analysis, it may be seen that prostheses that last longer will reduce long-term healthcare costs and improve the quality of life for patients, while also making them more productive and independent. This will lead to a positive cost–benefit situation. On the other hand, if the newer design of a medical device lasts similar to or even less in duration compared to an existing device, this would lead to a negative cost–benefit ratio and would thus not be a motivating factor to further carry on research. Although some ethicists, scientists, and clinicians believe that equating health and health care in terms of costs and benefits seems unacceptable, the reality of current health care is that it is measured in such terms by governments and large institutions (e.g., insurance companies). The experimental results, long-term survival, and the cost—benefit data are further utilized by insurance companies to provide or deny medical devices and coverage for certain illnesses in specific populations. When conducting biomedical engineering research, scientists need to take into consideration and strive to make sure that the product(s) or solution(s) that are being developed to improve the quality of life of mankind will be done in a cost-effective manner.

11.4 RESOURCE ALLOCATION FOR BIOMEDICAL RESEARCH

Biomedical engineering research aims to apply the principles of engineering to solve medical problems, thus benefiting mankind. The progress of a nation should be judged not only by its economic growth but also by the health of its population. Thus, it only makes sense that biomedical engineering research be encouraged to reach this objective. In other developing countries (e.g., India, China, Brazil), the uplifting of societies from poverty and disease will be possible when cost-effective healthcare solutions are developed and implemented. Governments and nations must realize that allocating resources toward research that produces such results will benefit everyone in the long term. There are several real-world examples to support the fact that a healthy nation is a more productive nation. In the United States, federal funding for biomedical research has remained stagnant or only slightly increased in recent years, although the population and the number of senior citizens has been increasing significantly [22]. Furthermore, senior citizens will soon comprise, if they are not already, the fastest-growing segment of the population in the United States. Thus, in order to sustain an aging population in the United States, biomedical research needs to be supported. The judicious allocation of resources for healthcare research is paramount to insure that meaningful studies are carried out in the future. Research projects that improve the understanding of the disease processes and/or create new knowledge for medical treatments need to be encouraged. This will help future scientists to achieve breakthroughs in biomedical engineering research and thus improve the health of our nation.

11.5 ETHICAL ISSUES WITH AUTHORSHIP

Since biomedical engineering research is increasingly interdisciplinary in nature, several ethical issues that cross the disciplines of medicine and engineering can arise as a consequence [23]. Some of these include concerns related to authorship of publications and conflicts of interests when conducting research. In the case of authorship, one needs to consider several factors including the intellectual contributions from specific individuals when publishing. This topic has been debated among many important research groups worldwide. Failure to address these issues can have trickle-down effects in terms of withholding research data due to an inability to publish them soon, thus hindering the progress of science. Currently, many peer-reviewed journals require that authors specify in detail about the exact nature of work or contribution to the specific research experiments or studies. It is only after fulfilling these criteria that journals accept a manuscript for publication. Some of the other concerns include the order of the authors' names listed on a manuscript. In many instances, one or more authors involved in a research project might have contributed a great deal to the actual experiments, while other authors might have formulated and conceptualized the idea for the research. In such scenarios, the order in which authors need to be listed on a manuscript can be controversial.

Conflicts of interest issues include another very important aspect of research and may introduce bias in reporting the results [23]. Many times, this can include the source of the funding (e.g., industry) and the eventual ownership of the research results. For example, if company "X" funds a study in an animal model to evaluate a new device such as a dental implant, the scientist(s) involved in the study need to disclose specifically while publishing their results that they have a conflict of interest (i.e., receiving funding from the company "X") in this particular situation. This will allow readers of the research results to make their own decisions about the influence that funding might have produced on the study. It was often thought that, in many instances, having a conflict of interest in a research study was enough to have deemed the results as biased. However, on the other hand, if a company funds a study and the results of the research reveal that their product(s) are indeed better than their competitors', it would be absolutely justified in publishing and defending these results. The onus would then lie on the readers and other researchers to disprove the results or to agree with the existing results. Some of the other conflicts of interests include financial conflicts, nonfinancial conflict of interest (e.g., publishing data too early to advance one's career), and institutional conflict of interest (e.g., universities having conflicts with a faculty's activities). To avoid such biases, double-blind studies should be the standard for clinical trials.

11.6 DISCUSSION

The concerns regarding the ownership of experimental results and intellectual property rights, although ubiquitous in almost all research might however, present new challenges in a highly interdisciplinary field of science such as nanotechnology, stem cell research, and tissue engineering. The current accepted standard in medicine that most clinicians follow is the results from double-blind randomized controlled trials. Further evidence-based data have become universal in their acceptance by clinicians worldwide to implement therapies and treatments for the benefit of their patients [24]. As a caveat it will be interesting to note that although evidence-based data are acceptable on many levels at the same time it must be understood that the limitations of evidence-based techniques need further discussion. There could be outliers in populations in whom evidence-based results may not apply. For example, it is rarely seen when 100% of treatment outcomes can be attributed to evidence-based results and a segment of the population might not fall into the studied treatments. This has to be considered when evaluating evidence-based criteria and adopting them.

11.7 CURRENT CHALLENGES AND FUTURE DIRECTIONS

Biomedical engineering and biomaterials research has been built on the foundation of employing or utilizing engineering principles to solve medical problems. Since biomedical engineering is a relatively new field compared to other traditional engineering disciplines and due to its highly interdisciplinary nature, an emphasis on introducing the concept of ethics in every aspect of research in this field should be encouraged. Although there may be many unforeseen ethical concerns that will arise as the field progresses, a constant readiness to face and address these issues needs to be in place. Several solutions including the formulation of a code of ethics pertaining to biomedical engineering research that can be likened to an ethical code taken by medical professionals might be worthwhile considering as proposed by some authors [25]. There have been some promising starts toward this direction including the formulation of a Code of Ethics by the Biomedical Engineering Society in 2004 [25]. However, there still needs to be a consensus among other major societies and organizations toward formulating a universal code of ethics for biomedical and biological engineering. Introduction of this code of ethics during graduate study or once an individual graduates from a biomedical engineering program might be considered. This will help future research to progress on par with the ethical challenges that might be expected. In addition, a moral basis for conducting research in this new and exciting discipline will be emphasized earlier in the evolution of this field and help young scientists face ethical challenges readily. This will also ensure that the public confidence in biomedical engineering research will be maintained.

11.8 GUIDELINES FOR ETHICAL PRACTICE IN BIOMATERIALS RESEARCH

Researchers working in the field of biomaterials research and practice, that includes manufacturing and evaluation of new materials, should follow the best ethical practices as mentioned in this chapter and references. They need to follow the directives included in the code of ethics of many engineering societies (i.e., IEEE, ASME, and BMES) as well as in the Declaration of Helsinki: Recommendations for Conduct of Clinical Research and other similar documents. Such research engineers and scientists should be aware of all ethical, legal, and regulatory requirements on animals and humans. The research protocols must be approved by the appropriate IACUC (for animal study) and IRB (for human study) before starting the experiments.

The bioengineers and scientists should work with physicians and other appropriate healthcare professionals who have adequate backgrounds in the treatment of patients for the use of investigative devices and implants. Such research should only be conducted after careful assessment of the risks and benefits to the patient and others. The populations selected for the clinical trial should benefit from the results of the research. The subjects must be volunteers and they should only be enrolled after obtaining informed consent. If the research subject is a minor or mentally or physically incapable of giving an informed consent, the consent must be obtained from an authorized legal representative. If a biological tissue is obtained from the patient or the healthy volunteer, then the future use of the tissue material should also be described in the informed consent.

The participants in clinical trials should be informed about the goals and methods of the study. Any possible harms and benefits to the subjects should be discussed. The sources of funding and any possible conflicts of interest should also be disclosed. In publications from the research study such conflicts of interest as well as the approval of the IACUC and IRB committees should be mentioned.

REFERENCES

[1] Bhatia SK. Biomaterials for Clinical Applications. New York: Springer; 2010.
[2] Musib M, Saha S. Ethical considerations in biomaterials research and development. In: Hench LL, Jones JR, Fenn MB, editors. New Materials and Technologies for Healthcare. London: Imperial College Press; 2012. p. 483–92 [chapter 33].
[3] Saha S, Saha P. Biomedical ethics and the biomedical engineer: a review. Critical Reviews in Biomed. Eng. 1997;Vol. 25(No. 2):163–201.
[4] Saha S, Saha P. Ethical issues in the development of new biomaterials. In: Ratner BD, et al., editors. Biomaterials Science. 2nd Ed. Academic Press; 2004. p. 793–7.
[5] Saha P, Saha S. Ethical issues on the use of animals in the testing of medical implants. J. Long-Term Effects of Med. Imp 1991;Vol. 1(No. 2):127–34.
[6] Saha S, Saha P. Ethical issues of animal and human experimentation in the development of medical devices. In: Bronzino J, editor. Biomedical Engineering Handbook. 2nd ed. Boca Raton: CRC; 2000. p. 191.1–191.8.
[7] Bertolami CN. Why does our ethics curricula don't work. Journal of Dental Education 2004;68:414–25.
[8] Cuomo AV, Lieberman JR. Ch. 29 Musculoskeletal Tissue Regeneration. Pietrzak WS. Totowa, NJ: Humana Press; 2008.
[9] Yeszemski MJ, Trantolo DJ, Lewandrowski KU, Hasirci V, Altobelli DE, Wise DL. Biomaterials in Orthopaedics. New York: Marcel Dekker, Inc; 2004.
[10] Malsch I, Emond C. Nanotechnology and Human Health. Boca Raton, FL: CRC Press; 2013.
[11] Lee S, Henthorn D. Materials in Biology and Medicine. Boca Raton, FL: CRC Press; 2012.
[12] Florczyk SJ, Saha S. Ethical issues in nanotechnology. J. Long-Term Effects of Med. Imp 2007; Vol. 17(No. 3):107–13.

[13] Kashi A, Saha S. Ethics in biomaterials research. Journal of Long-Term Effects of Medical Implants 2009;19:19–30.
[14] Mnyusiwalla A, Daar AS, Singer PA. "Mind the gap": science and ethics in nanotechnology. Nanotechnology 2003;14:R9–13.
[15] Budinger TF, Budinger MD. Ethics of emerging technologies. In: Budinger TF, Budinger MD, editors. Ethics of Emerging Technologies. Hoboken: John Wiley & Sons, Inc; 2006.
[16] Bhatia SK. Engineering Biomaterials for Regenerative Medicine. New York: Springer; 2012.
[17] Kashi A, Saha S. Ethical and legal aspects of tissue engineered products. In: Vishwakarma A, Sharpe P, Shi S, Wang X-P, Ramalingam M, editors. Stem Cell Biology and Tissue Engineering in Dental Sciences. Elsevier; 2015. p. 865–70. Chapter 64.
[18] Nestor MW, Artimovich E, Wilson RL. The ethics of gene editing technologies in human stem cells. Ethics in Biology, Engineering and Medicine 2014;5(4):323–38.
[19] Ramalingam M, Ramakrishna S, Best S. Biomaterials and Stem Cells in Regenerative Medicine. Boca Raton, FL: CRC Press; 2012.
[20] Stephens N. Ethics and emerging laws in stem cell science Ch. 63 In: Vishwakarma A, Sharpe P, Shi S, Ramalingam M, editors. Stem Cell Biology and Tissue Engineering in Dental Research. London: Academic Press; 2015. p. 855–63
[21] Saha S, Saha P. Bioethics and applied biomaterials. J. Biomed. Mat. Res.: Applied Biomat 1987;Vol. 21(No. A2):181–90.
[22] United Nations, Department of Economic and Social Affairs, World Population Prospects: 2012 Revision, June 2013. available from <http://esa.un.org/unpd/wpp/index.htm>.
[23] Gordon SL, Gordon LE. Ethical dilemmas in medicine in the 21st century. Ethics in Biology, Engineering and Medicine: An International Journal 2010;1:101–6.
[24] Kashi A, Saha S. Evidence based techniques to assess the performance of dental implants. J. Oral Implantology 2013;39(6):655–61.
[25] Voigt HF. Editorial: a need for a universal code of ethics for medical and biological engineers. Ethics in Biology, Engineering and Medicine: An International Journal 2010;1:79–81.

CHAPTER 12

Research on Bone Disorders—From Ideas to Clinical Use Product—The Path to Commercialization*

M. Kumar
Zimmer Biomet, Warsaw, IN, United States

Contents

12.1 INTRODUCTION

The author has over 17 years of experience in the orthopedic device industry—first as an applied researcher at the orthopedic device manufacturer (ODM) facility and later managing research and development activities at the ODM. The author has been instrumental in taking various products to market and has evaluated multiple technologies as potential acquisition targets. Consequently, the examples in this chapter are mostly pertinent to the field of orthopedics but the concepts could be applied to almost any field. The author has been a reviewer in a few National Science Foundation (NSF) grant review sessions as well. The addressing of issues raised in this chapter may help the reader in obtaining research support as well. The chapter is not about what research helps with cutting-edge publications but more about how to determine research topics that get the

* The views expressed in this chapter are solely of the author and not of his current employer.

attention of ODMs and what additional information may give the potential investor at the ODM comfort in embracing the technology.

Just to put things in perspective, the orthopedic device industry is fairly mature with an exemplary product success rate. It is commonly understood that 95% of implants will functional well in vivo for over 10 years—such is the track record for many kinds of orthopedic devices. For this kind of success to be common place, a lot of research and product development efforts must have happened already. Therefore, any research team must consider two fundamental questions: will the learning from their current research (and or development effort) solve a clinical issue and move the financial needle for the ODM? Another reason to answer these questions is to identify which ODMs may be a potential client of your research. The orthopedic industry is fairly mature—and quite profitable. As the industry is mature, larger and well-established ODMs have a reasonably strong product portfolio, with product offerings that span the gamut of devices used in orthopedic surgery today. To illustrate the point, most of these larger companies have products that address the surgeon's needs in say primary implant setting (i.e., where the recipient patient is getting an implant at that affected diseased site for the first time) and in the revision setting (where an implant is extracted and a new implant is used to replace it). However, as the orthopedic device industry is still quite profitable and the nature of the regulations that govern these products are well understood, there are a growing number of smaller companies who are entering the market place. As these smaller and newer companies may not have a vast product portfolio, there is a possibility that such companies may show interest on research that may be of little interest to the larger well-established ODMs. As an example, the orthopedic device industry has many calcium phosphate-based cements (or grout material) that are used to fill bony defects. Most ODMs may not have any more appetite to bring another one of these to the market. However, a smaller or newer company could show interest in this research as they may not have such biomaterials in their product portfolio. The understanding of where a potential product fits in the product portfolio of a device manufacturer may have researchers target their ideas to appropriate companies and thus better their chances to commercialization.

12.2 WHAT IS THE PATH TO COMMERCIALIZATION?

An understanding of this will help researchers understand what companies look at when evaluating new technologies. And perhaps answering these may help researchers address some of the questions that would be asked at ODMs during internal review when evaluating this technology. If some of these are already addressed or at least considered, the evaluators at the ODM naturally would have a sense that they are not just buying an idea but are buying an idea that is well baked and well researched. The question to answer is—if a company were to show interest buying your research, what would they get in addition to the Big Idea? So a few questions to consider when working on the Big Idea are:

1. The Big Idea—what is it? Does it solve a clinical problem? Is this a big enough clinical problem that ODMs would spends millions in bringing this technology to the market?
2. Does this idea/product differentiate ODM from competition or can fill a gap in their portfolio of products?
3. Does the ODMs have something "close enough" already?
4. The patent landscape—what is the status?
   a. Application filed or already granted?
   b. The literature search—why you think your patent has value
   c. Freedom to practice.
5. What are the regulations (United States, European, Japan and the rest of the world) around this product/idea?
   a. You claim that the Big Idea will do certain things—how can you demonstrate that? In animal studies? Human clinical trials? Are there existing regulations that can be leveraged to bring this product to the market?
6. What is the cost? In your laboratory? For the manufacturing process, what will be different for an ODM company?
   a. To make this product, what will be required? Who will make it—the device manufacturer or the raw material manufacturer? For example, consider additive manufacturing—it is just a way to make what was being done via traditional coating technologies. If such is the case, is there a reason why companies will spend changing its entire manufacturing process to this new technology when this Big Idea does not solve a clinical need?
7. The ODM brings this device to the market but who pays for this device to the ODM?

In the following sections, the above are addressed in some detail.

12.3 THE RESEARCH TOPIC—THE BIG IDEA. IS IT REALLY THAT BIG?

It has been at least the author's experience and consequently his opinion that an original and unique idea is perhaps the hardest part of a journey to commercialization. In the field of biomaterials for orthopedic applications, this is getting even harder as the broad classes of biomaterials are well researched. These generally known biomaterials (e.g., calcium phosphates, titanium alloys, PMMA, and UHMWPE) are in common use and do the job well. The orthopedic industry has scores of calcium phosphate-based cements, so researching another one for the same application adds no value to ODM. However, researching these generally known biomaterials, especially for different and unique applications, has its own set of advantages as the industry is familiar with these biomaterials and has the infrastructure to commercialize this material. One way to start exploring for the Big Idea is to incorporate such known biomaterials and teach them new tricks. For example, though this is not a call for research initiation, could it be possible to process these biomaterials to make them selectively inhospitable to bacterial colonization, yet remain and retain their gross biomaterials functions? On the same theme, it is of value to research technology that can induce a specific surface texture on common hip or knee implants, where this specific surface texture is instrumental in inhibiting bacterial colonization and yet achieves necessary bone remodeling. Incorporation of such technologies in existing biomaterials and therefore in their existing manufacturing infrastructure would not be a seismic shift for ODMs. However, this new technology and the mundane biomaterial is worth another serious look only if this new claim is well substantiated.

12.4 THE BIG IDEA—SHORT-TERM AND NEAR-TERM RESEARCH

Research is expensive and a financial burden if it does not bear financial fruit. Plus the activity of successful research is almost always is followed by development, where the ODM tries to identify how to take this Big Idea and move it from the laboratory setting to manufacturing, while meeting all the necessary guidelines of regulatory, quality, and cost-effectiveness. The appetite of spending resources diminishes exponentially if there are no short-term deliverables that could be commercialized in short order. To illustrate this point, let us imagine that a research laboratory has come up with a unique approach to process titanium alloy that completely eliminates fatigue failure when subjected to clinically relevant mechanical loading. However, there is a catch with this technology—current data show that only small parts can be made and attempts at using these process parameters in making larger parts have been unsuccessful. Approaching larger and well-established ODMs, who have a diverse product portfolio, may still be valuable—such an ODM may consider acquiring this technology for its dental division. This could allow the ODM to start generating revenues and therefore justifying allocation of resources in this unique processing technology to make larger implants (hips, knees, etc.). The potential of near short-term revenue generation could prompt ODMs to seriously consider this research. As researchers evaluate their work, they must be considering applications—which of these could be brought to the market quickly and which application could take time? A strategy around this concept could help better position their research for acquisition.

So how to get these "short-term and near-term" research ideas? The answer is simple—talk to researchers at the ODMs. A few questions to consider for the overture—what are the projects they are working on? What kind of technical journal articles and trade newsletters are they reading? What kind of technical papers are they drafting to publish? What kind of patent applications are they filing? Where do they see the market headed? What kinds of questions are being asked by the regulatory bodies and what kind of standards are being drafted? Helping to answer these questions may not provide data that would be published in major scientific publications. However, helping answer these questions possibly gets the researcher a seat at the table of ODM research and development teams.

12.5 LONG-TERM RESEARCH

Finding a research topic that fits "long-term research" and that would be enticing to the ODM is much harder for two reasons—Based on what we know, how does one predict what we should start evaluating/researching now for a deliverable 8–10–15 years from now? Equally important, who will fund this long-term and long-shot research? And for this long shot to have a hope of being commercialized, what other unknowns must fall in place for this long-term really Big Idea to materialize. For example, additive manufacturing (3D printing) has been around for almost 30 years. But it saw an explosive growth only in the last few years when computers become fast and efficient ways were found to handle large amounts of data in the CAD files. Today, based on this success, many researchers are attempting to create printed tissue. And there has been some success in this endeavor too. But for this technology to be commercially successful and widespread, regulations would be needed. But other interesting hurdles must be crossed as well. For example, what is the source of this cell? How does the manufacturer ensure that the cell dispensing technology is accurate and does not destroy a portion of the cells? How do we demonstrate that these destroyed cells can be washed off or, at the least, would not affect the viability of the tissue formed? How long will these cells survive under manufacturing and storage conditions? Could these cells mutate? How do we detect such a change in the DNA—for every cell? Many such questions will need to be addressed before this technology can become mainstream. As a suggestion to academicians and researchers who undertake research on such long-term investigations—if they can mobilize committees related to standards for the generation of the needed standards and mobilize regulatory bodies for timely guidance documents—there is a strong possibility that their efforts could be commercialized in a shorter timeframe. If such documents are drafted only after many years of research, devices coming out of these technologies would be pushed many years out.

12.6 THE PATENT—A STEP TO MONETIZATION OF RESEARCH AND THE BIG IDEA

Patents are a legal mechanism to ensure that only the holder of the patent can practice what is taught in the patent. In simple terms, it is a legal authority to practice monopoly on the ideas described in the patent. In the business world, this implies that there would no competition in this space. And equally important, if the holder of the patent determines that another entity is practicing what is taught in the patent for financial gains, the patent holder can sue this entity for damages. Naturally, for a business, this is a very powerful tool and is always taken very seriously. The field of patent law is complicated and best addressed by professionals. The reader is director to the United States Patent and Trademark Office (USPTO), specifically the section on Learning and Resources. Fortunately, most universities have an office dedicated to help academicians file patents. Just as patents can be granted by USPTO, it is also possible that patents can be found to be invalid and not enforceable. For the uninitiated in patents—it is very important that they consult their university patent team or patent lawyers to properly file patents. Claims listed in patents define the scope of the patent—these describe what the patents teach. Anyone who is familiar with the art described in the patent should be able to read the claims and determine what the art teaches and how to practice this art. While it is important to describe the art in detail in the body of the patent, careful wording of claim language can and does add value to the patent. So how does the ODM evaluate the value of a patent? There are two important things to be mindful of here—Claims and Freedom to Practice.

12.7 CLAIMS—ARE THEY BROAD ENOUGH TO KEEP THE COMPETITION OUT OF THIS SPACE?

This is best explained with an example—suppose a patent claim reads "orthopedic device, composed of metal, when processed between room temperature to melt temperatures . . . ." If such a claim were to be awarded, the patent would encompass ALL metal in the periodic table, and alloys that could be designed or already in existence, and ALL orthopedic devices (spine, dental, large joints, etc.). The holder of such a patent can keep the competition away for a life of the patent. The owner of such a patent, being the single player, would capture this market. A patent could have two kinds of claim—independent and dependent claims. Independent claims define the self-standing aspects of the teaching. For example, a statement like "orthopedic implants comprising of magnesium with zinc," could be an independent claim but the additional language that qualify this claim to include better definition of composition, for example, "above claim with alloying elements in the ratio of 2:3" would be a dependent claim. As an advice to academicians and researchers, do pay special attention to language of the claims—have these drafted as broad as possible.

12.8 FREEDOM TO PRACTICE/OPERATE—CAN SOME OTHER PATENT STOP THIS TECHNOLOGY?

Again, an example to illustrate this point—suppose the claim language of your patent reads, "a hand-held tool, employing a gear reduction mechanism to make oblong holes, of suitable sizes to receive orthopedic implants, in the bone of a human patient." An ODM was developing an implant that needed this special instrument to better their surgical technique and the ODM is interested in the teachings of this patent so they can practice the art of designing and selling this instrument. However, during their investigation, it was discovered that there is another patent, in the hand-powered orthopedic space that claims and describes a device that will create openings in bone. It is possible that the opinion of the legal team could be that one cannot practice the teachings of your patent without violating the teachings of this newly discovered patent. Your patent lost its value because this discovered patent would need to be acquired or licensed to follow the teachings of your patents. Or worse, this newly discovered patent could do what you are describing and has already lived its enforceable life or is close to the end of its enforceable life. In that case, the teachings of this expired patent are now in the public domain—anyone is free to practice these teachings without the need to license this expired patent. Under this circumstance, the ODM will not acquire your patent.

So why are patents important—it indicates to the potential acquirer that the inventor believes in this market as they have put in both time and money to conduct the necessary research and believe in the market potential to have spent extra money to file for and obtain this patent. Though the validity or accuracy of the teachings of an issued patent by USPTO are not in any way the responsibility of the USPTO, it also provides the level of comfort that some other entity (other than the inventor) has reviewed the teachings of the patents and compared with the teachings of other patents in this space and has found this teaching to be different and well described to be awarded a patent. It has been the author's experience that the ODMs will conduct their own analysis of Freedom to Practice/Operate. However, if such a document is generated by the researching entity (possibly, conducted by a legal team), it provides a level of assurance to the ODM that they are acquiring a technology that likely does not infringe other patents.

The above is by no means an authoritative guide to patents. Nor is it a tutorial on possible ways to construct claim language. The important message here is that if researchers want to monetize their intellectual property, one step toward this goal is to consider the value of a patent. If the decision is made to file a patent, it is definitely advised to consult a patent lawyer to draft strong claim languages. Furthermore, though this may add to the cost, there may be value in conducting a Freedom of Practice search. These exercises have value as they indicate to a potential purchaser of the technology that while they may have to repeat some of this analysis, there is a good chance that findings would be similar. Therefore, the risk on the investment on behalf of the ODM is reduced.

12.9 WHAT ARE THE REGULATIONS AROUND THIS BIG IDEA PRODUCT?

Very early in the research phase, it is a good practice to start considering regulations that govern the product that may come out of this Big Idea. Though many things are unknown early in the ideation phase, a general understanding of what this product will do and, therefore, what aspects of the regulations would control commercialization could help shape the course of research. Imagine this—your research shows that if your recipe is followed, a material or process is created that does wonderful things. The Big Idea does solve a clinical problem and your research team has demonstrated that this technology solves this clinical problem. And very importantly, this has been proven over and over again. The good news is that you have crossed a very difficult barrier and now the entire industry is interested in your work. The bad news is that the next steps are related to navigating the world of regulations. On the onset, regulations and standards are necessary—while some think of these regulations as a burden to the industry and the cost is ultimately borne by the patient or taxpayers but the fact remains that regulations do serve a very important function. Regulations are designed to demonstrate that the product is safe and effective. There are two possibilities with regulations—either regulations exist and could cover the product that the ODM wants to introduce to the market or the field of research is so new that there are no regulations. In either case, the likelihood that a university-based research team would know about the regulations surrounding the area of research is quite low. This is in no way any criticism of the research team—it speaks more toward the complex and specialized world of regulations. Naturally, this aspect is generally managed by the ODMs.

So how does a research team get information on the possible regulations that govern the product that would come about due to the research activity at hand? There are many contract regulatory companies that could be consulted—but a simpler approach would be to call the R&D team of the target ODM. Conversations like "We would like to present none confidential (or already published) findings on a topic that could be of interest to you. It is about a device that can solve surgical failures due to avascular necrosis. In exchange, we would like your input of research direction and guidance on regulations surrounding this technology. We hope to understand the regulations and direct our research to address some possible questions from the regulatory agencies." This approach serves multiple purposes. At the least, your published research is now known to the ODM who may be a potential purchaser of this technology. But you can also get information on what kind of questions/hurdles would need addressing to commercialize this product. If regulations already exist, you are now aware of them. You now know how to expand the scope of your research to answer these regulatory questions. In all likelihood, the ODM that is interested in this technology may have to redo this work on their laboratories and manufacturing floor—but now with this extra work during the research phase, ODMs get a good sense of what the results would be during scale up and their risk related to investment of resources is reduced. From the ODM perspective, the bet is now more on a technology that is better understood.

The field of research where there are no regulations and the ODM does not have a clear pathway to take this technology to the market makes commercialization more difficult. It is not because regulations are designed to stifle innovation. The rationale for increased burden of proof is simply due to the fact that there is no experience with such a device. In today's world of high-volume production and rapid distribution of products, if there were a clinical issue with this new and unique product, many patients could be adversely affected. Therefore, to minimize large-scale patient risk, for devices for which there are no prior examples, there is higher burden of proof that the device is safe and effective. As before, the reader is advised to consult with regulatory bodies or consultants in the field. However, in spite of the lack of guidance documents dictating the course through regulatory bodies, a general course of research can be considered by asking the following questions:

1. What are the benefits of this unique and unprecedented technology? If the commercialization team intends to market this unique product and advertise to the general population (or practicing clinicians) these benefits, it is important that studies be conducted to demonstrate that the device does indeed deliver on these benefits. These studies could span from bench-top tests to controlled clinical trials where the regulatory bodies review the study protocols, end points, and outcomes to verify the validity of such claims.
2. What is the additional risk that a recipient patient will be subjected to when treated with this unique and new technology? Is this additional risk justified? Equally important is to determine exposure to additional risks in the administering of the unique treatment. For example, if there was a device under research that could treat a neurological disorder but the treatment required exposure to an electrical current pulse not employed by any medical device. In this particular instance, there is an additional risk that has not been addressed by any medical before. Exposing a patient to this additional risk would be justified only if the treatment provided a benefit at levels that are not achieved by current standard of care.

Regulation is a vast subject in itself. Additionally, regulations can also vary from country to country. It may not be possible to introduce a technology in one country but the regulations of another country may be favorable. There are consulting firms that specialize in this area. Moreover, for concepts where similar devices already exist (say a hip stem), there is generally good guidance at the websites of regulatory bodies. In the event that the research is cutting edge with no guidance available, it is best to consider risks that the patient will be exposed to and how can these risks be mitigated. For more information, the reader is advised to visit the websites of the Food and Drug Administration (FDA), American Standard for Testing and Materials (ASTM), and International Standards Organization (ISO) for device-specific guidance documents, regulations, and standards. Similarly, for the Japanese market, the Pharmaceuticals and Medical Devices Agency (PMDA) website would be useful.

12.10 WHAT IS THE COST OF MAKING THIS PRODUCT?

This is a good question to answer for multiple reasons. For the sake of discussion, let us assume that extensive research has unequivocally demonstrated that a particular kind of surface texturing at the nanoscale will always eliminate bacterial colonization. This is great news and possibly a way to eliminate infection at the implant. But what is the cost of making this coating in the laboratory? A simple way to determine the cost would be based on cost of ingredients, utilities, equipment, labor, etc. There are two points to discuss here:

1. The cost—if your laboratory cost was calculated to some astronomically high amount (compared to the cost of the traditional implant)—what are the chances that it can be brought to a reasonable amount so that an ODM would consider this technology? While it is very important to answer this question, this should never be a show-stopper. If industry is good at something, it is driving excess cost out of a process. And if the technology in question is so compelling clinically, the interested ODM would most likely find a way to adopt the technology.

2. ODM also must consider additional work (post research phase) that must be conducted before such a technology can be commercialized. To list a few:

a. Possibly, reproduce the results in the laboratory under various conditional to simulate what may happen during production and carve out a window of parameter ranges that produce the unique nanostructure;

b. Reproduce the results in a larger scale (pilot and/or full production);

3. Legal fees (license of technology, patent search and filling, conducting freedom of practice search, etc.);

4. Production equipment cost;

5. Equipment and process validations;

6. Quality control and equipment for quality control, possible destructive tests for quality control;

7. Cleaning, packaging, and sterilization and shelf-life studies;

8. Regulatory cost (including bench-top studies, animal studies, and clinical trials);

9. Marketing cost.

This is a list of possible action items that an interested ODM would most likely go through before the acquired technology and product would come to the store shelf.

12.11 CONCLUSION

Research with the intent of commercialization of the findings in the form of clinical applications is a daunting task. How do researchers or academicians determine what is it that the industry is looking for—what is that one clinical problem that could be solved? This chapter is designed to provide researchers and academicians a glimpse into the thought process at the manufacturer when they are evaluating research for acquisition. This chapter describes how to hone into industry-relevant questions and how to gather information on rules and regulations that may affect the products that may come out of the research. By no means is this chapter a compendium of every question that should be asked before research efforts are undertaken. Much less, neither does this chapter provides answers to every question raised here. But the point to remember is this—if questions considered here are addressed, before and during the course of the research, and if most are answered, the research team has made it so much easier for ODMs to better relate to the Big Idea and the research behind it. This approach would better the chances of this research and the Big Idea to be considered for acquisition.

CHAPTER 13

Current Challenges and Future Needs in Biomaterials and Devices for Bone Disorders

S. Bose and A. Bandyopadhyay
Washington State University, Pullman, WA, United States

Content

13.1 INTRODUCTION

The field of biomaterials is inherently complex and truly interdisciplinary. To use a biomaterial, a researcher needs to understand different properties of the material and its implications in a clinical setting. In terms of properties, it is not only the biological properties that matter, but also relevant physical, mechanical, and chemical properties are equally important. The need for such a multidisciplinary background forced scientists of different backgrounds to work on various aspects of biomaterials. Though biomaterials means both natural and synthetic materials, it is the design and the development of synthetic biomaterials with tailored properties that is mostly discussed in the context of this book. Natural materials are great to learn from, and we sometimes mimic them to achieve properties that are otherwise difficult to accomplish; however, those materials can be difficult to mass produce with reproducible properties for a variety of applications. As a final chapter of this book, it is our intent to write this chapter focusing on what are some of the unmet challenges that remain today, and how we feel the biomaterials field will grow in the future.

To start with, let us use a simple example—hip implants. Total hip prostheses have been practiced since the 1950s using solid metal implants that can alleviate pain for patients where cartilage between the two bony surfaces has worn out. Millions of patients have benefitted from this procedure worldwide, and millions more will feel the same way in the future. Every leading biomedical device manufacturer has multiple total hip implants in the market with some modifications in design or composition of the device. Yet, if we look at the success rate for these devices worldwide, we will see that there is very little variation in performance outcome. Most of those devices are performing at the same average level now compared to what it was even 30 years back. Most patients can expect an average of 15 years of implant life. However, if we look at those data carefully, we will see that about 7% of the patients require a revision surgery within about 7 years due to some form of complications. Since thousands of patients are using these implants, that 7% number itself is quite large, and improvements in device design or surgical procedure are still needed to bring that number close to 0%. Although not all of those 7% early failures are due to problems in implant materials or designs, innovation in biomaterials is needed to minimize premature device failure. It is important to note that the synthetic biomaterials act as foreign bodies inside the living system and hence are prone to microbial infections. Infections are often reasons for catastrophic failures of the implants and necessitate total removal or replacement of the implants that results in severe morbidity. Another aspect of load-bearing implants of concern is metal ion release. Though a significant amount of metal ion release is more of a concern for articulating surfaces that can even cause cancer, release of metal ions due to localized corrosion from any metallic implants in the neighboring bones is also possible. Researchers are looking into different surface treatments to minimize metal ion release from load-bearing implants. Even though this load-bearing implant example is focused on mature devices that are performing well, our purpose is to show that we still need further innovation to improve the quality of these implants to enhance the quality of life for the patients.

Let us look at another example in which good treatment options are still not available. It is infection control. In a planned surgery that is typically done in a hospital setting, infection is not a major concern, and typically below 1% of all cases are reported in most hospitals. However, for fracture management cases, where the fracture occurred outside, and patients are brought in the emergency room with injury, infection rates are much higher, and in some cases as high as 30%. The problem for patients with bone fracture is the late realization of infection, in some cases as late as 6–9 months after the accident. For example, if the infection is from meticillin-resistant *Staphylococcus aureus* (MRSA), physicians have very little option but to surgically remove the implant and then treat the patient for the infection. Once the infection is completely treated, then the physician can put an implant back into the same site. Such a scenario is not only cost-intensive, it is also very painful for the patients. Any new discoveries that can prevent biofilm formation on devices in vivo can significantly minimize infection-related concerns, a topic that is intensely researched at present and hopes to bring solutions in the future.

Long bone fracture is another example of a common bone-related disorder that has attracted a lot of attention from researchers as viable treatment options are still unavailable. Incompatible mechanical strength, mismatch in modulus of elasticity in the case of a metal implant, and inherent brittleness for ceramic implants remain key challenges to be solved. Besides the mechanical strength of the implant itself, proper mechanical load transfer, vascularized long bone tissue formation, and tissue integration or ingrowth from the host bone to the implant are also some of the critical issues that require consideration from researchers. Moreover, the clinical need of the implants varied by the loading conditions as well as location of implantation in the living system. Finally, short-term bone formation may not guarantee longer-term fixation of bone disorders.

With the above three simple yet very common examples, it is important to understand that the field of biomaterials is still young and has tremendous potential to make a significant contribution in the future to solve upcoming as well as long-standing challenges related to bone disorders. Innovations in materials and device designs will dominate the field of biomaterials for many years to come. From a materials perspective, metallic materials are the most mature, and only a few are used for most devices. Since metals offer excellent mechanical strength and fatigue resistance, metals are preferred for most load-bearing applications. A large variety of polymers are also currently being used to treat different bone disorders. The main challenges with polymeric materials are their low strength and low modulus. In recent years, some structural polymers, such as polyether ether ketone (PEEK), are used in spinal devices that are load-bearing. Otherwise, most of the applications for polymers are in nonload-bearing areas. Controlled degradation rates of various polymeric biomaterials are of significant interest. Though bone is mostly an inorganic material consisting of calcium phosphates with collagen polymers and water, ceramics are probably the least used biomaterials due to their inherent brittleness and processing difficulty. Ceramics are only used as coating, or in powder form in cements, and in void filling for dental, craniofacial, and orthopedic applications. It is anticipated that the use of ceramics will increase in the future in the pure form or as a filler in composites.

Apart from compositions, advances in manufacturing science are also making a significant impact toward devices for bone disorders. Though not in all cases, patient-matched implants are needed for some patients due to complex fractures, unique anatomy, or specific allergies toward certain elements. Using conventional manufacturing, such devices are not only difficult to process, they are cost-intensive. Use of 3D printing or additive manufacturing can alleviate those challenges, making it easy to customize implants for a specific patient. Application of an additive manufacturing approach also helps in design modifications and manufacturing parts with both compositional and structural gradation. Parts like acetabular cups, with both the dense and the porous areas, are now manufactured regularly in one 3D printing operation. The other advantage of additive manufacturing is on-demand manufacturing in which products can be made on an as-needed basis. Such flexibility in manufacturing is influencing the biomedical device industry and it is anticipated that more innovative products will be introduced in the future that can only be manufactured using 3D printing.

With this basic information, the following section looks at current challenges and future needs toward biomedical devices for bone disorders. Our goal is really to offer some global perspectives on some of these challenges to the reader in this chapter to make them aware of these issues related to bone disorders. Our comments are focused on materials and devices points of view, and not a clinical opinion. However, readers are suggested, if needed, to find more in-depth information on any of these challenges in various scientific literatures and patents.

13.2 CURRENT CHALLENGES AND FUTURE NEEDS

There are many critical issues about biomaterials and devices for bone disorders that are currently being researched by different groups worldwide. Instead of being very specific about those research challenges, in this section we plan to highlight our perspectives about some of those challenges and the future needs.

Resorbable biomaterials: Resorbable biomaterials are those materials that can dissolve in the body while helping to restore the body tissue to its normal function. Among different resorbable biomaterials, sutures for internal stitching are perhaps the most popular ones in which biopolymers such as poly(lactic acid)/poly(glycolic acid) (PLA/PGA) are used with controlled degradation rates. The use of resorbable materials avoids the need for another surgery for removal of the material, and that is the main advantage for these materials. Moreover, once the tissue heals and the resorbable material degrades, there is no residue or signature left about the synthetic material placed in the body at the defect site. Because of such advantages, naturally, resorbable materials can be viewed as a potential solution to many bone defects. For many years, only different biopolymers were used as resorbable biomaterials in vivo. However, in recent years, the use of controlled strength loss ceramics for bone tissue engineering has also become a reality. In these cases, mostly calcium phosphate-based ceramics or bioglasses are designed via compositional modification to tailor its degradation behavior in vivo. Those ceramic/glass compositions can then be used to treat different bone disorders in which the scaffold structures will support bone tissue migration, differentiation, and eventual healing. As the healing progresses, the scaffolds degrade, matching the in vivo tissue ingrowth kinetics, and are eventually removed completely from the defect site. The key challenge in this idea is not just to find the composition that can match the bone tissue healing rate, but that can also withstand the mechanical loading during healing. Moreover, the resorbable scaffold must encourage both osteogenesis and angiogenesis for functionally viable bone tissue repair. It has been shown that in the case of calcium phosphate ceramics with controlled resorption rates, trace elements can play a major role in modulating initial strength, strength degradation rates, as well as both osteogenesis and angiogenesis. Since tissue ingrowth and scaffold degradation are key factors toward the success of these structures, porosity plays an important role apart from compositional variations. Pore sizes between 300 and 600 μm proved to be more effective in these scaffolds, while a minimum pore size of 100 μm is needed for vascularization. However, key challenges remain to manufacture such porous scaffolds with interconnected porosity that has sufficient mechanical strength in vivo for tissue integration and maturation during healing. Also, tailoring compositional modification that can match patient needs is also a critical issue. Manufacturing some of these ceramic scaffolds using 3D printing has shown some promise in recent years. In terms of metals, most metals are bioinert and will not degrade in vivo. However, some active metals can degrade in the presence of water in vivo, and magnesium is one such metal, which is also commonly available in our body. Magnesium and magnesium alloys have been researched extensively in recent years for their applications in bone disorders after their successful applications in resorbable stents.

Though resorbable materials are exciting, with a lot of potential for treating bone disorders, there are many critical issues that require fundamental understanding before these materials can be used safely. Some of those critical issues include:

1. *Degradation product*—If the degradation product is harmful to body tissues or lowers the pH locally, then use of those materials in large structures will be challenging. A simple example is: hydrogen release from Mg may cause a detrimental effect toward bone tissue integration.
2. *Mechanical strength*—For bone disorders, it is important to maintain some minimum strength during healing. If biodegradation of the scaffold lowers the strength such that it cannot support the tissue ingrowth, then such structures may not be suitable for the repair of bone disorders.
3. *Processing ability*—Reliable and reproducible processing methods for these resorbable scaffold structures are very important, otherwise such materials cannot be used in different devices for bone disorders. Factors that influence processing ability include stability of the materials, phase purity, availability of raw materials, and sterilization ability.
4. *Tissue–materials interaction*—Perhaps the most important factors of all is biocompatibility of the material and its ability toward early-stage osseointegration. For successful osseointegration, materials should have a favorable surface for both osteogenesis and angiogenesis in vivo.

It is anticipated that further research and development will pave the way for resorbable materials use more frequently in various treatment options for bone disorders in the future.

Active devices: The concept of active devices to treat bone disorders is still in its infancy. Most devices that are used today are passive devices that will help the patient to enjoy a better quality of life. However, in an active device, like many new-generation cars, sensors can be placed to warn of malfunctions of the device or progress of healing that can be recorded remotely, and if needed fixed without the need for any surgical intervention. With the advancement of wireless technologies, such devices will become the hotbed of innovation in the future to treat bone disorders. The reader can extend her/his imagination to come up with any such device that can enhance the quality of life for patients. For example, in the case of bone fractures, frequent visits to the physician's office are needed to check healing of the fracture site using X-ray or magnetic resonance imaging techniques. If an active device could be designed and placed such that the patient can receive data about her/his healing, various postoperative procedures could be designed based on the specific needs of that patient. Similarly, we can imagine another set of devices that is loaded with specific drugs to treat site-specific bone cancer in which doses of the drugs can be altered based on patient healing in situ. A third set of devices that can be imagined would be able to generate electrical pulses at the fracture site in situ to enhance bone healing. Any such device will be patient-matched and tailored for that specific disorder—an approach that is generally classified as personalized medicine, which is becoming popular worldwide. It is anticipated that various innovative active device concepts will become a reality in the future to treat bone disorders.

Infection control: Infection control is still one of the most significant concerns related to treatment options for bone disorders. This can happen to simple and widely practiced procedures that generally have a good success rate, and cause significant trauma to patients. Infection is mostly common in fracture management devices due to outside exposure. Most treatment options call for extensive use of antibiotics, which is good for the first 1–2 weeks. However, in many cases, such an approach does not work. One such example is MRSA, which can stay dormant for many months, and yet form a biofilm at a later stage, even after 3 or 6 months. If biofilm is formed, unfortunately, nothing can be done but to remove the implant and treat the surface for infection before another implant can be placed there. As mentioned before, in some cases such as road traffic accidents, infection rates can be as high as even 30%.

Based on today's treatment options, there is no clear winner. The concept that is becoming popular is coated devices in which antimicrobial layers are placed at the outside surface of the device. If the antimicrobial layer is stable for many months, then such coatings can prevent the formation of any biofilm on the device. Among different coating options, silver is the most commonly studied coating material explored today. Silver has excellent antimicrobial properties. Silver can be placed at the outside surface using different coating methods, and controlled silver release to the vicinity of the bone disorder may prevent bacterial growth for many months. Among different critical issues, probably the most significant is the dose. The amount of silver should be such that it is effective in destroying the pathogens but is not detrimental to the tissue that is healing. The second issue is the time of silver release. If the loading is such that most of the silver will be released during the first few weeks, then the effectiveness of the coating may be limited. The need is for at least 1 year of silver release, if not longer, without any harmful effect to the local tissue and various organs.

Infection control will remain a challenge for many years to come. Based on specific cases, some local drug delivery options may become a common treatment option. However, better and more reliable treatment options are still elusive and need to be invented.

Patient-matched devices: With the advancement of treatment options for bone disorders, interest is growing toward devices that are patient-matched toward a particular defect. In some cases, this may be the only option left to a physician, such as in the case of complex craniofacial fractures. In other cases, such an approach may enhance healing time and patient comfort. Either way, technological advancements make it easy today to manufacture devices that are patient-matched. The most significant contribution toward patient-matched implants is coming from the rise of 3D printing technologies. Most biomedical device manufacturers have embraced 3D printing technologies and utilize them in various product lines. It is expected that such an approach will only grow with time. The main advantages of 3D printing technologies are: (1) on demand manufacturing over projection-based manufacturing; (2) easy to incorporate design modifications or multiple products can be manufactured from the same machine; and (3) ideal for low- to medium-volume part production. However, there are many challenges still remain, including product quality variation from machine to machine, variation in starting powders, and cost of machines. However, it is worth noting that patient-matched devices were there even before the widespread use 3D printing, though perhaps not as popular and easy to make.

Bone tissue engineering: Bone, having an almost 70% calcium phosphate-based inorganic component, is certainly a key material of choice for small-scale bone defects or low load-bearing applications. Bone tissue engineering is another important area that has perhaps the most significant prospects in the future. In an ideal scenario, autografts should be used toward bone tissue engineering. However, the trauma from the second surgery to harvest autografts, and in some cases lack of sufficient materials availability, force physicians to look at other options, such as allografts and xenografts. Unfortunately, both of these options suffer from other concerns. Synthetic bone grafts with tailored porosity and chemistry can be a good solution to replace autografts. Synthetic materials can be produced as needed, defect site-specific, and patient-matched. Significant research work has been done toward a variety of bone grafts to use in bone tissue engineering. Most of these are made of calcium phosphate-based ceramics with or without different growth factors, which can induce osteoinductivity. Though biological response is excellent in most cases, reliable mechanical strength is still a significant concern for most ceramic-based bone grafts. Also, tailorable strength loss is important to be used in different locations. Recent research results show that the addition of trace elements can tailor biocompatibility, mechanical strength, and strength loss kinetics. Overall, for small-scale bone defects, such as in bone cancers and segmental bone defects, bone tissue engineering still offers the best possible solution for thousands of patients worldwide, and more clinical success is expected in the future.

When polymeric biomaterial is used in bone tissue engineering, its lack of bioactivity, adverse effects on the surrounding tissue environment and the system due to its degradation products, along with poor mechanical properties, lead to suboptimum solutions for bone tissue engineering. Growth factor immobilized orthopedic implants have been reported to enhance osteogenesis and improve cellular functionalities, e.g., transforming growth factor beta (TGF-β) and bone morphogenic proteins (BMP), especially BMP-7 and BMP-2. These growth factors are either physically adsorbed or covalently attached to modify the surface of the implant to influence the bone remodeling process improving osseointegration. They can be used in tissue engineering scaffolds as well as in prosthetics. Optimized dosage, dual and sequential release, time of exposure, and rate of release of the growth factors are crucial to be harnessed to alleviate the detrimental effects of high burst release rate, short half-life, and ectopic bone formation.

Another approach includes cell-based therapy that has gained some interest in recent times to promote early bone regeneration. Implantation of purified human mesenchymal stem cells with unfractionated fresh bone marrow and differentiated osteoblasts is of interest to modulate bone formation. However, in all these cases, it is vital to understand the critical issues of keeping the biomolecules and cells viable without any adverse effects and the specific bone remodeling procedure that would involve the maturation and mineralization. Another aspect of developing a successful synthetic biomaterial is to understand the biological cues and related mechanisms. Signaling pathways involved in bone remodeling are still not well understood. The future of synthetic biomaterials lies in harnessing their osteoinductive properties and understanding the bone biology involved due to the incorporation of biologics and pharmacologics in a tissue engineering scaffold or a prosthetic device. Clinical applications of any biomaterial can be broadened using multimaterial and multifunctional devices having beneficial properties, while understanding the bone biology aspects for that specific clinical need.

Natural medicinal compounds for bone disorders: Understanding and utilization of natural materials toward improvement of current strategies to tackle bone disorders can be cost-effective, less prone to adverse effects of modern medicine and, most importantly, a healthy choice. For example, acemannan is a polysaccharide extracted from aloe vera which has been shown to augment the wound healing process in a variety of phases, such as fibroblast proliferation, extracellular matrix synthesis, and wound contraction. It has also been used in bone regeneration and reduction of inflammation in tooth extraction model by increasing alkaline phosphatase activity in rat. Another material that can be utilized in bone disorder treatment is curcumin. Curcumin is found in the natural turmeric plant. Although curcumin has not been used clinically due to its poor solubility in water, and thus reduced bioavailability, it has the potential to be used clinically as it has been shown to inhibit osteoclastogenesis, which can effect bone remodeling. Another important species that is used in cooking is garlic (*Allium sativum*). It has been demonstrated to have antimicrobial properties. Garlic plays an important role in the maintenance of skeletal health. Garlic intake in diets can increase calcium ion absorption in the small intestine, enhancing bone mass density.

In order to effectively combine the beneficial effects of natural medicinal compounds with modern technology such as 3D printed implants or prosthetics or bone tissue engineering scaffolds, one needs to keep in mind the rate of drug metabolism by proper fabrication of biomaterial–drug composition, and the need for continued release of drug or biomolecules from the implant or scaffolds to preserve therapeutic concentrations in the blood based on patients' needs. Although most research related to bone disorders and various treatment options is focused on synthetic biomaterials and devices, by combining advanced manufacturing techniques for devices along with the incorporation of natural materials, a whole new world of opportunities and solutions for clinical needs can be envisioned. It is also important to note that maintaining good bone health is critical with healthy food habits including calcium, vitamin D, whether from sunlight and/or food, and regular exercise from a young age.

Tooling for surgical planning: Among different treatment options being developed for bone disorders, one area that has been picked up by many device manufacturers in recent years is tooling. Even with the best-quality devices and treatment options, results can vary significantly based on physicians' skills and the complexity of the procedure. Advanced tooling options can minimize variations in surgical results from physician to physician. For example, in the case of robotic surgery, the depth to which drilling or other mechanical operations should be done can be performed accurately, reliably and repeatedly, measured precisely, and documented electronically. Such clarity helps physicians to focus on other aspects of surgery, and not to worry about those critical mechanical procedures. Also, for complex surgeries, presurgical tooling for planning is also becoming common and very useful. Three-dimensional printing or additive manufacturing is playing a role in some of these cases. One advantage for tooling is the relatively easy process to get regulatory approval for those class I devices. It is anticipated that in the future, more advanced tooling options will be available for most orthopedic and dental surgeries, and will be practiced regularly.

13.3 SUMMARY

The idea behind this perspective chapter is to identify some of the most significant challenges in bone disorders that need attention from the research community. Various FDA-approved bone replacement materials and devices have performed well over the years in many patients, improving their quality of life, which is encouraging. Although technological advancements have helped some of the clinical needs for biomedical implants, and made significant progress in a short time span, oftentimes the life time of the implants is challenged in the living system, demanding revision surgeries. Modification of the surface topography both physically and chemically, or by the incorporation of inorganic or organic molecules, will directly influence the cell material's interaction and tissue integration toward further understanding and development of clinically compatible systems. However, due to the inherent complexity of the field, some critical clinical challenges still remain, and there is certainly room for improvement for the current biomaterials and devices based on clinical needs which can try to mimic, as closely as possible, the physiological complexities at the micro- and macrolevels. We anticipate that solutions to many of these challenges will only come from collaborative interactions between scientists, engineers, and clinicians. With an aging population and increasing life expectancy worldwide, solutions to most of these problems will be needed to impact the quality of life for us, and future generations. Innovative, low-cost devices that can be used to address short- and long-term healthcare problems are changing healthcare practices around the world. As the editors of this book, we hope that this chapter and our book will help inspire the next generation to focus their attention to solve these and other types of bone disorders. A lifestyle including healthy food habits and regular exercise is still the best practice to maintain a good bone health, because it is difficult to mimic Mother Nature.

ACKNOWLEDGMENTS

The authors would like to acknowledge financial support from the National Institute of Arthritis and Musculoskeletal and Skin Diseases of the National Institutes of Health under Award Numbers R01 AR066361-01A1 and R01 AR067306-01A1. The content is solely the responsibility of the authors and does not necessarily represent the official views of the National Institutes of Health.

INDEX

Note: Page numbers followed by "*f*" and "*t*" refer to figures and tables, respectively.

C

N

O

P

Q

R

S

T

U

V

W

Kolibri 360 GmbH
Ferdinand-Jühlke-Straße 7
99095 Erfurt, Deutschland
produktsicherheit@kolibri360.de